Clinical Pharmacokinetics
Concepts and Applications

Boo

Clinical Pharmacokinetics
Concepts and Applications

third edition

MALCOLM ROWLAND, Ph.D.
Department of Pharmacy
University of Manchester
Manchester, England

THOMAS N. TOZER, Ph.D.
School of Pharmacy
University of California
San Francisco, California

A Lea & Febiger Book

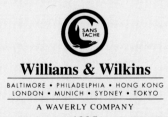

Williams & Wilkins
BALTIMORE • PHILADELPHIA • HONG KONG
LONDON • MUNICH • SYDNEY • TOKYO
A WAVERLY COMPANY
1995

Executive Editor: Donna Balado
Developmental Editors: Frances Klass, Lisa Stead
Production Manager: Laurie Forsyth
Project Editor: Robert D. Magee

Copyright © 1995
Williams & Wilkins
Rose Tree Corporate Center
1400 North Providence Road
Building II, Suite 5025
Media, PA 19063-2043 USA

Accurate indications, adverse reactions, and dosage schedules for drugs are provided in this book, but it is possible they may change. The reader is urged to review the package information data of the manufacturers of the medications mentioned.

Printed in the United States of America

First Edition 1980

Library of Congress Cataloging-in-Publication Data

Rowland, Malcolm.
    Clinical Pharmacokinetics : concepts and applications / Malcolm
Rowland, Thomas N. Tozer. — 3rd ed.
        p.   cm.
    "A Lea & Febiger Book."
    Includes bibliographical references and index.
    ISBN 0-683-07404-0
    1. Pharmacokinetics.   2. Chemotherapy.   I. Tozer, Thomas N.
II. Title.
    [DNLM: 1. Pharmacokinetics.   2. Drug Therapy.   QV 38 R883c 1994]
RM301.5.R68   1994
615.7—dc20
DNLM/DLC
for Library of Congress   94-26305
                                                                                            CIP

The Publishers have made every effort to trace the copyright holders for borrowed material. If they have inadvertently overlooked any, they will be pleased to make the necessary arrangements at the first opportunity.

95 96 97 98
1 2 3 4 5 6 7 8 9 10

Reprints of chapters may be purchased from Williams & Wilkins in quantities of 100 or more. Call Isabella Wise, Special Sales Department, (800) 358-3583.

To Margaret and Dawn

PREFACE

PURPOSE OF TEXT

The third edition, in keeping with the first two editions, is a primer in pharmacokinetics with an emphasis on clinical applications. The book should be useful to any student, practitioner, or researcher who is interested or engaged in the development, evaluation, or use of medicines. Such persons include pharmacists, physicians, veterinarians, pharmaceutical scientists, toxicologists, analytical chemists, biochemists, and clinical chemists. It is an introductory text and therefore presumes that the reader has little or no experience or knowledge in the area. Previous exposure to certain aspects of physiology and pharmacology would be helpful, but it is not essential. Some knowledge of calculus is also desirable.

Our intent is to help the reader learn to apply pharmacokinetics in therapeutics. To this end, we emphasize concepts through problem solving with only the essence of required mathematics. In this respect, the book is a programmed learning text. At the beginning of each chapter, objectives are given to identify the salient points to be learned. To further aid in learning the material, examples are worked out in detail in the text. At the end of each chapter, except the first, there are problems that allow the reader to grasp the concepts of the chapter and to build on material given in previous chapters. The order of the problems in each chapter reflects consideration of both difficulty and how well the problems apply to chapter principles. The questions start with the less difficult ones and those that emphasize the principles.

ORGANIZATION AND CONTENT

As in the second edition, the book is divided into five sections: Absorption and Disposition Kinetics, Therapeutic Regimens, Physiologic Concepts and Kinetics, Individualization, and Selected Topics. Those wishing to gain a general overview of the subject need only study Sections One and Two, together with Chapter 13, Variability, and Chapter 18, Monitoring. Section Three deals with the physiologic concepts relevant to an understanding of the processes of absorption, distribution, and elimination. This section forms the basis for an appreciation of the material in Section Four, which is concerned with the identification, description, and accounting of variability in patients' responses to drugs. Covered here are general aspects of variability, followed by considerations of genetics, age and weight, disease, interacting drugs, and monitoring of drug concentrations.

Section Five contains selected topics. These are intended for those readers who wish to gain a more detailed insight into various aspects of clinical pharmacokinetics. The topics are distribution kinetics, pharmacologic response, metabolite kinetics, dose and time dependencies, turnover concepts, and dialysis. Each topic is generally self-contained; they have not been arranged in any particular sequence.

CHANGES IN THIRD EDITION

The 6-year gap between this third edition and the second, published in 1989, is shorter than the 9 years between the second and first editions. This shortening of the time span between editions reflects the ever-gathering pace of progress and application of clinical pharmacokinetics. Despite this growth, which has required the inclusion of much new material, every effort has been made to contain the overall size of the book. This, in turn, has meant that some material has had to be condensed or deleted. It has also resulted in a much greater use of abbreviations, especially for units.

The number, topic, and sequence of chapters have been kept essentially the same as in the second edition. However, each chapter has been extensively revised and updated to ensure that the examples relate to currently prescribed drugs. A particular effort has been made to include stereochemistry, recognizing that isomers may have different kinetics and activity. There is also consideration of the increasing number of polypeptide and protein drugs emerging from advances in molecular biology and biotechnology. Although the kinetic concepts are the same, the physiologic handling of macromolecular compounds is quite distinct from that of typical small molecular weight drugs.

The presentation of the book has also been markedly improved through the use of color. The more important equations are now highlighted by means of color. Chapter number and section heading now appear at the top of each page layout to assist in cross-referencing. A table of frequently used symbols has been placed before Chapter 1 to facilitate redefining symbols, when necessary.

The range and number of problems at the end of each chapter and Appendix I (total of 87 new problems) have been substantially extended to assist in learning problem solving in pharmacokinetics. Most of the additional problems are taken from literature, rather than simulated, data.

The third edition contains 102 new figures and 20 new tables, reflecting, in large part, the advances made in recent years in our knowledge of the pharmacokinetics of drugs. The material on "Small Volume of Distribution" that comprised the last chapter of the second edition has been incorporated into Chapter 10, Distribution, and Appendix I–F.

We continue to adopt a uniform set of symbols and to use milligrams/liter (mg/L) as the standard measure of concentration. We do recognize, however, the increasing trend toward the adoption of molar units and have provided a factor for conversion between the two units of measurement in the pertinent figure captions. We shall only be convinced of the virtue of solely using the molar system of measurement when drugs are prescribed in such units.

ACKNOWLEDGMENTS

We wish to thank all the many students and readers who provided input that helped us shape this third edition. Their enthusiasm and encouragement have been a continual source of satisfaction. To the new reader, we hope that the book will succeed in helping you develop kinetic reasoning that will be of personal value in your professional practice.

We have been enormously gratified by the wide and diverse readership of the first two editions of the book. We would like to believe that the book has been instrumental in furthering rational management of drug therapy. We sincerely hope that the third edition will continue to do so.

Manchester, England   Malcolm Rowland
San Francisco, California   Thomas N. Tozer

CONTENTS

DEFINITIONS OF SYMBOLS*

A Amount of drug in body, mg or μmole.

Aa Amount of drug at absorption site remaining to be absorbed, mg or μmole.

Ae Cumulative amount of drug excreted unchanged in the urine, mg or μmole.

$Ael(m)$ Amount of metabolite eliminated, mg or μmole.

$Ae_{\tau,ss}$ Cumulative amount of drug excreted unchanged in the urine during a dosing interval at steady state, mg or μmole.

Ae_∞ Cumulative amount of drug excreted unchanged in the urine to time infinity after a single dose, mg or μmole.

$A(m)$ Amount of metabolite in body, mg or μmole.

A_{min} The minimum amount of drug in body required to obtain a predetermined level of response, mg or μmole.

$A_{N,max}$; $A_{N,min}$ Maximum and minimum amounts of drug in body after the Nth dose of fixed size and given at a fixed dosing interval, mg or μmole.

$A_{N,t}$ Amount of drug in body at time t after the Nth dose, mg or μmole.

ARE Amount of drug remaining to be excreted in urine after a single dose, mg or μmole.

A_{ss} Amount of drug in body at steady state during constant-rate intravenous infusion, mg or μmole.

$A_{ss,av}$ Average amount of drug in body during a dosing interval at steady state, mg or μmole.

$A_{ss,max}$; $A_{ss,min}$ Maximum and minimum amounts of drug in body during a dosing interval at steady state on administering a fixed dose at a fixed dosing interval, mg or μmole.

$A_{ss,t}$ Amount of drug in body at time t within a dosing interval at steady state on administering a fixed dose at a fixed dosing interval, mg or μmole.

AUC Area under the plasma drug concentration-time curve. Total area from time 0 to infinity is implied unless the local context indicates a specific time interval, e.g., dosing interval, mg-hr/L or μM-hr.

AUC_b Total area under the blood drug concentration time curve, mg-hr/L or μM-hr.

$AUC(m)$ Area under the plasma metabolite concentration time curve, mg-hr/L or μM-hr.

AUC_{ss} Area under the plasma drug concentration time curve within a dosing interval at steady state, mg-hr/L or μM-hr.

$AUMC$ Total area under the first moment-time curve, mg-hr^2/L or μM-hr^2.

C Concentration of drug in plasma, mg/L or μM.

*Usual units are given.

$C(0)$ Initial plasma concentration, usually obtained by extrapolation to time zero, mg/L or μM.

$C_1; C_2$ Coefficients with units of concentration, mg/L or μM.

Ca Concentration of drug in fluids at the absorption site, mg/L or μM.

C_A Concentration of drug in arterial blood, mg/L or μM.

C_b Concentration of drug in blood, mg/L or μM.

Cbd Concentration of bound drug in plasma, mg/L or μM.

C_D Drug concentration in dialysate leaving dialyzer, mg/L or μM.

C_l Concentration of inhibitor of metabolism, mg/L or μM.

CL Total clearance of drug from plasma, L/hr.

CL_b Total clearance of drug from blood, L/hr.

CL_{bD} Dialysis clearance based on drug concentration in blood, L/hr.

$CL_{b,H}$ Hepatic clearance of drug from blood, L/hr.

CL_{cr} Renal clearance of creatinine, mL/min or L/hr.

CL_D Dialysis clearance based on drug concentration in plasma, L/hr.

CL_f Clearance associated with formation of a metabolite from a drug, L/hr.

CL_H Hepatic clearance of drug from plasma, L/hr.

CL_{int} Intrinsic clearance of drug in organ of elimination, L/hr.

$CL(m)$ Total clearance of a metabolite, L/hr.

CL_{PD} Peritoneal dialysis clearance based on drug concentration in plasma, L/hr.

CL_R Renal clearance of drug, L/hr.

CLu Clearance of unbound drug, L/hr.

$C(m)$ Concentration of metabolite in plasma, mg/L or μM.

C_{max} Highest drug concentration observed in plasma following administration of an extravascular dose, mg/L or μM.

$C(m)_{ss}$ Concentration of a metabolite at steady state during a constant-rate intravenous infusion of drug, mg/L or μM.

C_{min} Minimum concentration required to obtain a predetermined intensity of response, mg/L or μM.

$C_{N,max}; C_{N,min}$ Maximum and minimum concentrations of drug in plasma after the Nth dose on administering a fixed dose at equal dosing intervals, mg/L or μM.

C_{PC} Concentration of drug in peritoneal cavity, mg/L or μM.

C_{ss} Concentration of drug in plasma at steady state during a constant-rate intravenous infusion, mg/L or μM.

$C_{ss,av}$ Average drug concentration in plasma during a dosing interval at steady state on administering a fixed dose at equal dosing intervals, mg/L or μM.

$C_{ss,max}; C_{ss,min}$ Maximum and minimum concentrations of drug in plasma at steady state on administering a fixed dose at equal dosing intervals, mg/L or μM.

C_T Average concentration of drug in fluids outside plasma, mg/L or μM.

C_{TW} Drug concentration unbound in total body water, mg/L or μM.

$C_{upper}; C_{lower}$ Maximum and minimum limits for plasma drug concentrations, mg/L or μM.

Cu Unbound drug concentration in plasma, mg/L or μM.

Cu_I Unbound plasma concentration of inhibitor, mg/L or μM.

C_V Concentration of drug in venous blood, mg/L or μM.

D_L — Loading dose, mg or μmole.

D_M — Maintenance dose of a fixed-dose regimen, mg or μmole.

$D_{M,max}$ — Maximum maintenance dose to ensure that the plasma drug concentration remains within C_{upper} and C_{lower} limits during a dosing interval at steady state, mg or μmole.

E — Extraction ratio, no units.

EC_{50} — Concentration giving one-half the maximum effect, mg/L or μM.

E_H — Hepatic extraction ratio, no units.

E_{max} — Maximum effect, units of response measurement.

F — Bioavailability of drug, no units.

f_{bd} — Ratio of bound to total drug concentrations in plasma, no units.

f_D — Dialysis clearance as a fraction of total clearance during a dialysis treatment, no units.

fe — Fraction of drug systemically available that is excreted unchanged in urine, no units.

FEV_1 — Forced expiratory volume in 1 second, L.

F_H — Fraction of drug entering the liver that escapes elimination on single passage through that organ, no units.

fm — Fraction of drug systemically available that is converted to a metabolite, no units.

Fm — Fraction of administered dose of drug that enters the general circulation as a metabolite, no units.

F_R — Fraction of filtered and secreted drug reabsorbed in the renal tubule, no units.

fu — Ratio of unbound and total drug concentrations in plasma, no units.

fu' — Ratio of unbound and total drug concentrations in plasma under conditions of altered binding, no units.

fu_b — Ratio of unbound concentration in plasma and total drug concentration in blood, no units.

fu_P — Ratio of unbound and total sites available for binding on a plasma protein, no units.

fu_R — Ratio of unbound and average total drug concentrations in intracellular fluids, no units.

fu_T — Ratio of unbound and total drug concentrations in tissues (outside plasma), no units.

γ — Shape factor in concentration-response relationship, no units.

GFR — Glomerular filtration rate, mL/min or L/hr.

k — Elimination rate constant, hr^{-1}.

K_A — Association constant for the binding of drug to protein, L/mole.

ka — Absorption rate constant, hr^{-1}.

k_D — Elimination rate constant while a patient is undergoing dialysis treatment, hr^{-1}.

ke — Urinary excretion rate constant, hr^{-1}.

k_f — Rate constant associated with the formation of a metabolite, hr^{-1}.

K_I — Inhibition equilibrium constant, mg/L or μM.

$k(m)$ — Rate constant for the elimination of a metabolite, hr^{-1}.

Km — Michaelis-Menten constant, mg/L or μM.

Km' — Michaelis-Menten constant, expressed in terms of total plasma concentration, mg/L or μM.

Kp — Equilibrium distribution ratio of drug between tissue and blood or plasma, no units.

k_T — Fractional rate at which drug leaves tissue, hr^{-1}.

k_t — Fractional turnover rate, hr^{-1}.

$\lambda_1; \lambda_2$ — Exponential coefficients, hr^{-1}.

m — Slope of the center of the intensity of response versus log concentration curve, units of response.

MRT — Mean time a molecule resides in body, hr.

n — A unitless number.

N — Number of doses, no units.

P — Permeability coefficient, cm/min or cm/hr.

Q — Blood flow, L/min or L/hr.

Q_D — Dialysate flow in hemodialysis system, mL/min or L/hr.

Q_f — Rate of filtrate flow from a hemofiltration system, mL/min or L/hr.

Q_H — Hepatic blood flow (portal vein plus hepatic artery), L/min or L/hr.

ρ — Ratio of concentration in blood cell to that unbound in plasma.

R_{ac} — Accumulation ratio (index), no units.

Rd — Ratio of unbound clearance of an individual patient to that of a typical patient, no units.

RF — Renal function in an individual patient as a fraction of renal function in a typical patient, no units.

R_o — Rate of constant intravenous infusion, mg/hr.

R_t — Turnover rate, mg/hr.

S — Salt form factor, no units.

SA — Surface area, m^2.

τ — Dosing interval, hr.

τ_{max} — Maximum dosing interval to remain within C_{upper} and C_{lower} limits, hr.

t_{max} — Time at which the highest drug concentration occurs following administration of an extravascular dose, min or hr.

t_d — Duration of effect, hr.

t_{inf} — Duration of a constant-rate infusion, hr.

Tm — Maximum rate of drug transport (secretion) into renal tubule, mg/hr.

$t_{1/2}$ — Half-life, hr.

t_t — Turnover time, hr.

V — Volume of distribution (apparent) based on drug concentration in plasma, L.

V_b — Volume of distribution (apparent) based on drug concentration in blood, L.

V_B — Blood volume, L.

V_D — Volume of dialysate solution collected during a hemodialysis treatment, L.

V_1 — Volume of initial dilution compartment, L.

Vm — Maximum rate of metabolism by an enzymatically mediated reaction, mg/hr or µmole/hr.

$V(m)$ — Volume of distribution (apparent) of a metabolite based on its plasma concentration, L.

V_P — Plasma volume, L.

V_{PC} — Volume of dialysate within the peritoneal cavity, L.

V_R — Aqueous volume of intracellular fluids, L.

V_T — Physiologic volume outside plasma into which drug distributes, L.

V_{ss} — Volume of distribution (apparent) under steady-state conditions based on drug concentration in plasma, L.

V_{TW} — Aqueous volume outside plasma into which drug distributes, L.

Vu — Volume of distribution (apparent) based on unbound drug concentration in plasma, L.

WHY CLINICAL PHARMACOKINETICS?

Those patients who suffer from chronic ailments such as diabetes and epilepsy may have to take drugs every day for the rest of their lives. At the other extreme are those who take a single dose of a drug to relieve an occasional headache. The duration of drug therapy is usually between these extremes. The manner in which a drug is taken is called a *dosage regimen*. Both the duration of drug therapy and the dosage regimen depend on the therapeutic objectives, which may be either the cure, the mitigation, or the prevention of disease. Because all drugs exhibit undesirable effects, such as drowsiness, dryness of the mouth, gastrointestinal irritation, nausea, and hypotension, successful drug therapy is achieved by optimally balancing the desirable and the undesirable effects. To achieve optimal therapy, the appropriate "drug of choice" must be selected. This decision implies an accurate diagnosis of the disease, a knowledge of the clinical state of the patient, and a sound understanding of the pharmacotherapeutic management of the disease. Then the questions How much? How often? and How long? must be answered. The question How much? recognizes that the magnitudes of the therapeutic and toxic responses are functions of the dose given. The question How often? recognizes the importance of time, in that the magnitude of the effect eventually declines with time following a single dose of drug. The question How long? recognizes that a cost (in terms of side effects, toxicity, economics) is incurred with continuous drug administration. In practice, these questions cannot be divorced from one another. For example, the convenience of giving a larger dose less frequently may be more than offset by an increased incidence of toxicity.

In the past, the answers to many important therapeutic questions were obtained by trial and error. The dose, interval between doses, and route of administration were selected, and the patient's progress followed. The desired effect and any signs of toxicity were carefully noted, and if necessary, the dosage regimen was adjusted empirically until an acceptable balance between the desired effect and toxicity was achieved. Eventually, after considerable experimentation on a large number of patients, reasonable dosage regimens were established (Table 1–1), but not without some regimens producing excessive toxicity or proving ineffective. Moreover, the above empirical approach left many questions unanswered. Why, for example, does tetracycline have to be given every 6 to 8 hours to be effective, while digoxin can be given once daily? Why must oxytocin be infused intravenously? Why is morphine more effective given intramuscularly than when given orally? Furthermore, this empirical approach contributes little, if anything, toward establishing a safe, effective dosage regimen of another drug. That is, our basic understanding of drugs has not been increased.

To overcome some of the limitations of the empirical approach and to answer some of the questions raised, it is necessary to delve further into the events that follow drug administration. *In vitro* and *in vivo* studies show that the magnitude of the response is a function of the concentration of drug in the fluid bathing the site(s) of action. From these observations the suggestion might be made that the therapeutic objective can be achieved by maintaining an adequate concentration of drug at the site(s) of action for the duration of therapy. However, rarely is a drug placed at its site of action. Indeed, most drugs are given orally, and yet they act in the brain, on the heart, at the neuromuscular junction, or elsewhere. A drug must therefore move from the site of administration to the site of action. Simultaneously, however, the drug distributes to all other tissues including those organs, notably the liver and the kidneys, that eliminate it from the body.

Figure 1–1 illustrates the events occurring after a dose of drug is administered orally. The rate at which drug initially enters the body exceeds its rate of elimination; the concentrations of drug in blood and other tissues rise, often sufficiently high to elicit the desired therapeutic effects and sometimes even to produce toxicity. Eventually, the rate of drug elimination exceeds the rate of its absorption, and thereafter, the concentration of drug in both blood and tissues declines and the effect(s) subsides. To administer drugs optimally, therefore, knowledge is needed not only of the mechanisms of drug absorption, distribution, and elimination but also of the kinetics of these processes, that is, *pharmacokinetics*. The application of pharmacokinetic principles to the therapeutic management of patients is *clinical pharmacokinetics*.

Table 1–1. Empirically Derived Usual Adult Dosage Regimens of Some Representative Drugs *Before* the Introduction of Clinical Pharmacokinetics[a]

DRUG	INDICATED USE	ROUTE	DOSAGE REGIMEN
Tetracycline	Treatment of Infections	Oral	250 mg every 6–8 hr
Digoxin	Amelioration of congestive cardiac failure	Oral	1.5–2 mg initially over 24 hr, thereafter 0.25–0.5 mg once a day
Oxytocin	Induction and maintenance of labor	Intravenous	0.2–4 milliunits/min by infusion
Morphine sulfate	Relief of severe pain	Intramuscular	10 mg when needed
		Oral	Not recommended because of reduced effectiveness

[a]Taken from American Medical Association: Drug Evaluations. 2nd Ed., Publishers Science Group, Acton, MA, 1973.

Fig. 1–1. Plasma concentration of theophylline in a subject following an oral dose of a 600-mg controlled-release formulation. Before the peak is reached, the rate of absorption exceeds that of elimination. At the peak, the two rates are equal; thereafter, the rate of elimination exceeds that of absorption. (Redrawn from Sauter, R., Steinijans, V.W., Diletti, E., Böhm, A., and Schulz, H.U.: Presentation of results in bioequivalence studies. Int. J. Clin. Pharmacol. Ther. Toxicol., *30*:S7–30, 1992.)

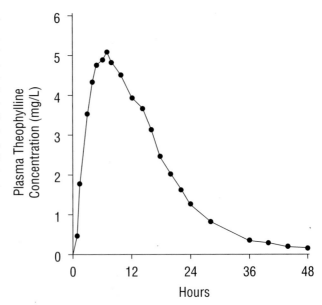

The events following drug administration can be divided into two phases, a *pharmaco-kinetic phase*, in which the adjustable elements of dose, dosage form, frequency, and route of administration are related to drug level–time relationships in the body, and a *pharma-codynamic phase*, in which the concentration of drug at the site(s) of action is related to the magnitude of the effect(s) produced (Fig. 1–2). Once both of these phases have been defined, a dosage regimen can be designed to achieve the therapeutic objective. Despite the greater amount of information required with this approach, it has several advantages over the empirical approach. First, and most obvious, distinction can be made between pharmacokinetic and pharmacodynamic causes of an unusual drug response. Second, the basic concepts of pharmacokinetics are common to all drugs; information gained about the pharmacokinetics of one drug can help in anticipating the pharmacokinetics of another. Third, understanding the pharmacokinetics of a drug often explains the manner of its use; occasionally such an understanding has saved a drug that otherwise may have been dis-carded or has suggested a more appropriate dosage regimen. Lastly, knowing the phar-macokinetics of a drug aids the clinician in anticipating the optimal dosage regimen for an individual patient and in predicting what may happen when a dosage regimen is changed.

A basic tenet of clinical pharmacokinetics is that the magnitudes of both the desired response and toxicity are functions of the drug concentration at the site(s) of action. Ac-cordingly, therapeutic failure results when either the concentration is too low, giving in-effective therapy, or is too high, producing unacceptable toxicity. Between these limits of concentration lies a region associated with therapeutic success; this region may be regarded as a "therapeutic window." Rarely can the concentration of the drug at the site of action be measured directly; instead the concentration is measured at an alternative and more accessible site, *the plasma*.

Based on the foregoing considerations, an optimal dosage regimen might be defined as one that maintains the plasma concentration of a drug within the therapeutic window. For many drugs, this therapeutic objective is met by giving an initial dose to achieve a plasma concentration within the therapeutic window and then maintaining this concentration by replacing the amount of drug lost with time. One popular and convenient means of main-tenance is to give a dose at discrete time intervals. Figure 1–3 illustrates the basic features associated with this approach by depicting the concentrations that follow the administration of two regimens, A and B. The dosing interval is the same but the dose given in regimen B is twice that given in regimen A. Because some drug always remains in the body from preceding doses, accumulation occurs until, within a dosing interval, the amount lost equals the dose given; a characteristic saw-toothed plateau is then achieved. With regimen A,

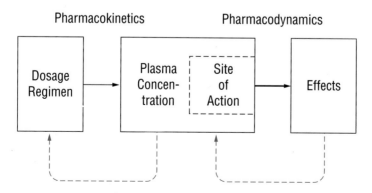

Fig. 1–2. An approach to the design of a dosage regimen. The pharmacokinetics and the pharmacodynamics of the drug are first defined. Then, either the plasma drug concentration-time data or the effects produced are used via pharmacokinetics as a feedback (dashed lines) to modify the dosage regimen to achieve optimal therapy.

several doses had to be given before drug accumulation was sufficient to produce a therapeutic concentration. Had therapy been stopped before then, the drug might have been thought ineffective and perhaps abandoned prematurely. Alternatively, larger doses might have been tried, e.g., regimen B. Although a therapeutic response would have been achieved fairly promptly, toxicity would have ensued with continued administration when the concentration exceeded the upper limit of the therapeutic window.

The synthetic antimalarial agent, quinacrine, developed during World War II to substitute for the relatively scarce quinine, is an example. Quinacrine was either ineffective acutely against malaria or eventually produced unacceptable toxicity when a dosing rate sufficiently high to be effective acutely was maintained. Only after its pharmacokinetics had been defined was this drug used successfully. Quinacrine is eliminated slowly and accumulates extensively with repeated daily administration. The answer was to give large doses over the first few days to rapidly achieve therapeutic success, followed by small daily doses to maintain the plasma concentration within the therapeutic window.

The plateau situation in Fig. 1–3 shows that both the width of the therapeutic window and the speed of drug elimination govern the size of the maintenance dose and the frequency of administration. When the window is narrow and the drug is eliminated rapidly, small doses must be given often to achieve therapeutic success. Both cyclosporine and digoxin have a narrow therapeutic window, but because cyclosporine is eliminated much more rapidly than digoxin, it has to be given more frequently. Oxytocin is an extreme example; it also has a narrow therapeutic window but is eliminated within minutes. The only means of adequately ensuring a therapeutic concentration of oxytocin therefore is to infuse it at a precise and constant rate directly into the blood. This degree of control is not possible with other modes of administration. Besides, had oxytocin been given orally, this polypeptide hormone would have been destroyed by the proteolytic enzymes in the gastrointestinal fluids. Morphine, given orally, is also destroyed substantially before entering the general circulation, but for a reason different from that of oxytocin. Morphine is extensively metabolized on passage through the liver, an organ lying between the gastrointestinal tract and the general circulation.

Awareness of the benefits of understanding pharmacokinetics and concentration–response relationships has led in recent years to the extensive application of such information by the pharmaceutical industry to drug design, selection, and development. For example, a potent compound found to be poorly and unreliably absorbed and intended for oral administration may be shelved in favor of a somewhat less potent but more extensively and reliably absorbed compound. Also, many of the basic processes controlling both pharmacokinetics and response are similar across mammalian species such that data can be extrapolated from animals to predict quantitatively the likely behavior in humans. This quan-

Fig. 1–3. When a drug is given in a fixed dose and at fixed time intervals (denoted by the arrows), it accumulates within the body until a plateau is reached. With regimen A, therapeutic success is achieved although not initially. With regimen B, the therapeutic objective is achieved more quickly, but the plasma drug concentration is ultimately too high.

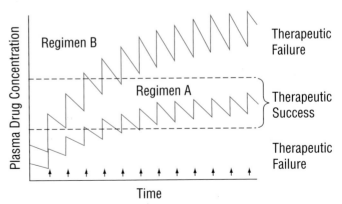

titative framework improves the chances of selecting not only the most promising compounds but also the correct range of safe doses to first test in humans. Incorporation of a pharmacokinetic element with these early Phase I studies, usually in healthy subjects, together with assessment of any side effects produced, helps to define candidate dosage forms and regimens for evaluation in Phase II studies conducted in a small number of patients. These Phase II studies are aimed at defining the most likely safe and efficacious dosage regimens for use in the subsequent larger Phase III clinical trials, often involving many thousands of patients. Ultimately, some compounds prove to be of sufficient benefit and safety to be approved for a particular clinical indication by drug regulatory authorities. Even then the drug undergoes virtually continuous postmarketing surveillance to further refine its pharmacotherapeutic profile. This sequence of events in drug development and evaluation is depicted schematically in Fig. 1–4.

Figure 1–5 illustrates an important problem identified during drug development and therapy, variability. There is a wide range of daily dose requirements of the oral antico-

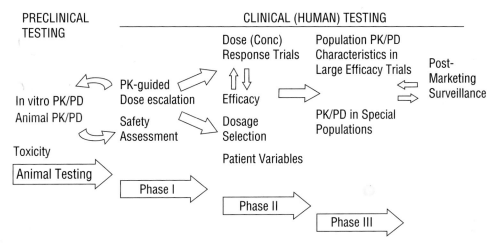

Fig. 1–4. The development and subsequent marketing of a drug. The prehuman data helps to identify promising compounds and to suggest useful doses for testing in humans. Phases I, II, and III of human assessment generally correspond to the first administration to humans, early evaluation in selected patients, and the larger trials, respectively. Pharmacokinetic (PK) and pharmacodynamic (PD) data gathered during all phases of drug development help to efficiently define safe and effective dosage regimens for optimal individual use. Postmarketing surveillance helps to refine the PK/PD information.

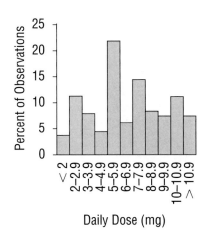

Fig. 1–5. The daily dose of warfarin required to produce similar prothrombin times in 200 adult patients varies widely. (1 mg/L = 3.3 μM). (Redrawn from Koch-Weser, J.: The serum level approach to individualization of drug dosage. Eur. J. Clin. Pharmacol. 9:1–8, 1975.)

agulant warfarin needed to produce a similar prothrombin time (an index of blood coagulability). Sources of variability in drug response include the patient's age, weight, degree of obesity, type and degree of severity of the disease, the patient's genetic makeup, other drugs concurrently administered, and environmental factors. The result is that a standard dosage regimen of a drug may prove therapeutic in some patients, ineffective in others, and toxic in still others. The need to adjust the dosage regimen of a drug for an individual patient is evident; this need is clearly greatest for drugs that have a narrow therapeutic window, that exhibit a steep concentration–response curve, and that are critical to drug therapy. Examples are digoxin, used to treat some cardiac disorders; phenytoin, used to prevent epileptic convulsions; theophylline, used to diminish chronic airway resistance in asthmatics; and cyclosporine, an immunosuppressant used in organ transplantation. With these drugs, and with many others, variability in pharmacokinetics is a major source of total variability in drug response.

It is becoming increasingly common to gain as much information on variability as possible during drug development by gathering, albeit limited, individual plasma concentration and response data in a large population of patients during Phase III clinical trials. Attempts are then made to account for this variability in terms of such patient characteristics as age and weight. These *population* pharmacokinetic/pharmacodynamic studies form a basis for dosage regimen recommendations in clinical practice.

Coadministration of several drugs to a patient, prevalent in clinical practice, can pose problems. Although the response produced by each drug alone may be predictable, that produced by the combination may be less certain and occasionally unpredictable. Ketoconazole, for example, devoid of immunosuppressant activity, potentiates the effect of cyclosporine. Possible causes of this kind of effect are many. In this instance, as in many others, the interaction involves a change in pharmacokinetics. Some drugs stimulate drug-

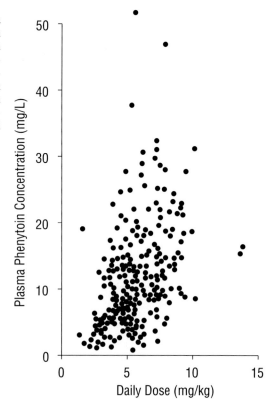

Fig. 1–6. Although the average plateau plasma concentration of phenytoin tends to increase with the dosing rate, there is considerable variation in the individual values. (One mg/L = 3.97 μM.) (Redrawn from Lund, L.: Effects of phenytoin in patients with epilepsy in relation to its concentration in plasma. *In* Biological Effects of Drugs in Relation to Their Plasma Concentration. Edited by D.S. Davies and B.N.C. Prichard, Macmillan, London and Basingstoke, 1973, pp. 227–238.)

metabolizing enzymes and hasten drug loss; others inhibit these enzymes and slow elimination. Still others interfere with drug absorption. Such interactions are graded; the change in the pharmacokinetics of a drug varies continuously with the plasma concentration of the interacting drug and hence with time. Indeed, given in sufficiently high doses, almost any drug can interact with another. It is always a question of degree. Understanding the quantitative elements of interactions ensures the more rational use of drugs that may need to be coadministered.

Figure 1–6 illustrates a situation in which monitoring of the drug concentration may be beneficial. Over the narrow range of the daily dose of the antiepileptic drug phenytoin, the plateau plasma drug concentration varies markedly within the patient population. Yet the therapeutic window of phenytoin is narrow, 7 to 20 mg/L; beyond 20 mg/L, the frequency and the degree of toxicity increase progressively with concentration. Here again, pharmacokinetics is the major source of variability. A pragmatic approach to this problem would be to adjust the dosage until the desired objective is achieved. Control on a dosage basis alone, however, has proved difficult. Control is achieved more readily and accurately when plasma drug concentration data and the pharmacokinetics of the drug are known.

Drug selection and therapy have traditionally been based solely on observations of the effects produced. In this chapter, the application of pharmacokinetic principles to decision making in drug therapy has been illustrated. Both approaches are needed to achieve optimal drug therapy. This book emphasizes the pharmacokinetic approach. It begins with a consideration of kinetic concepts basic to pharmacokinetics and ends with a section containing selected topics.

ABSORPTION AND
DISPOSITION KINETICS

BASIC CONSIDERATIONS

OBJECTIVES

The reader will be able to:

1. Define the following terms:
   Pharmacokinetics, intravascular and extravascular administration, absorption, disposition, distribution, metabolism, excretion, first-pass effect, enterohepatic cycling, compartment
2. Discuss the limitations to interpretation of pharmacokinetic data imposed by assays that fail to distinguish between compounds administered (e.g., R- and S-isomers) or between drug and metabolite.
3. Show the general contribution of mass balance concepts to drug absorption and drug and metabolite disposition.

Pharmacokinetics has many useful applications that stem from basic concepts. These concepts are developed in this section of the book. This chapter specifically defines terms and describes a basic model for drug absorption and disposition.

ANATOMIC AND PHYSIOLOGIC CONSIDERATIONS

Measurement of a drug in the body is limited usually to blood or plasma. Nonetheless, the information obtained has proved very useful. Such usefulness can be explained by anatomic and physiologic features that affect a drug following its administration.

Blood or plasma, in addition to being a practical and convenient site of measurement, is the most logical one for determining drug in the body. Blood receives drug from the site of administration as well as carries it to all the organs, including those in which the drug acts and those in which it is eliminated. This movement of drug is depicted schematically in Fig. 2–1. This scheme forms a basis for *physiologic modeling in pharmacokinetics*. Such modeling has applications not only in clinical pharmacokinetics but in drug development, veterinary medicine, and in assessing risk associated with exposures to environmental and occupational substances.

Sites of Administration

There are several sites at which drugs are commonly administered. These sites may be classified as either intravascular or extravascular. *Intravascular* administration refers to the placement of a drug directly into the blood, either intravenously or intra-arterially.

Extravascular modes of administration include the oral, sublingual, buccal, intramuscular, subcutaneous, dermal, pulmonary, and rectal routes. To enter the blood, drug administered extravascularly must be absorbed: No absorption step is required when a drug is administered intravascularly.

Drug may also be administered regionally, e.g., into the pleural or peritoneal cavities or into the cerebrospinal fluid. Regional administration includes intra-arterial injection into the vessel leading to a tissue to be treated, e.g., one containing a cancerous tumor. It is a potential means of gaining a selective therapeutic advantage. This advantage, in comparison with other routes of administration, comes about by increasing drug exposure locally, where it is needed, and decreasing or producing little or no change in exposure throughout the rest of the body, where it is not wanted.

Disposition

Once absorbed, a drug is distributed to the various organs of the body. Distribution is influenced by how well each organ is perfused with blood, organ size, binding of drug within blood and in tissues, and permeability of tissue membranes.

The two principal organs of elimination, the liver and the kidneys, are shown separately in Fig. 2–1. The kidneys are the primary site for excretion of the chemically unaltered, or unchanged, drug. The liver is the usual organ for drug metabolism; however, the kidneys and other organs can also play an important metabolic role for certain drugs. The metabolites so formed are either further metabolized or excreted unchanged. The liver may also secrete unchanged drug into the bile. The lungs are, or may be, an important route for

Fig. 2–1. Once absorbed from any of the many sites of administration, drug is conveyed by blood to all sites within the body including the eliminating organs. Sites of administration include: *a*, artery; *b*, peripheral vein; *c*, muscle and subcutaneous tissue; *d*, lung; and *e*, gastrointestinal tract. The dark- and light-colored lines with arrows refer to the mass movement of drug in blood and in bile, respectively. The movement of virtually any drug can be followed from site of administration to site of elimination.

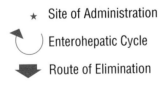

★   Site of Administration

)   Enterohepatic Cycle

➡   Route of Elimination

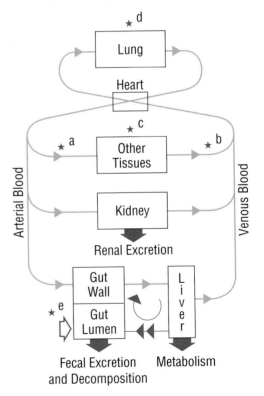

eliminating volatile substances, for example, gaseous anesthetics. Another potential route of elimination is via a mother's milk. Although an insignificant route of elimination in the mother, drug in the milk may be consumed in sufficient quantity to affect the suckling infant.

CHEMICAL PURITY AND ANALYTIC SPECIFICITY

A general statement needs to be made about the chemical purity of prescribed medicines and the specificity of chemical assays.

Over the years, a major thrust of the pharmaceutical industry has been to produce therapeutic agents that are not only as safe and effective as possible but also are well characterized to ensure reproducible qualities. The majority of administered drugs today are therefore essentially pure materials, and coupled with specific analytic techniques for their determination in biologic fluids, definitive information about their pharmacokinetics can be gained. However, a large number of drug substances are not single chemical entities but rather mixtures. This particularly applies to stereoisomers and proteins. The most common stereoisomers found together in medicines are optical isomers, or compounds for which their structures are mirror images; the drug substance is usually a racemate, a 50:50 mixture of the R- and S-isomers. Some drug substances contain geometric isomers, and still others, especially proteins of high molecular weight derived from natural products or through fermentation, may be a mixture of structurally related, but chemically distinct, compounds. Each chemical entity within the drug substance can have a different pharmacologic, toxicologic, and pharmacokinetic profile. Sometimes these differences are small and inconsequential, other times the differences can be therapeutically important. For example, dextroamphetamine (S-isomer) is a potent central nervous stimulant, whereas the R-enantiomer is almost devoid of such activity. Despite such differences, many commonly employed chemical assays do not distinguish between stereoisomers. Obviously, under these circumstances, attempting to quantify the various processes and to relate plasma concentration to response has many problems with no simple solutions. Notwithstanding these problems, specific information about each chemical entity should be sought whenever possible. Increasingly, stereoisomers are being produced as single chemical entities, such as S-naproxyn, which avoid these problems. In contrast, many new protein and polypeptide drugs are being introduced that may, in many instances, lack purity. Furthermore, these substances are often measured by assays that lack specificity.

An added problem exists following drug administration, namely, the formation of metabolites. To be of value, an analytic procedure must distinguish between drug and metabolite(s). Today, most assays have this desired specificity, except for some of those used to measure many proteins and polypeptides.

A potential problem exists when using radiolabeled drugs. Incorporation of one or more radionuclides, usually ^{14}C and ^{3}H, into the molecular structure allows for simple and ready detection within a complex biologic milieu, but not necessarily of the administered drug. Complete recovery of all of a radiolabeled dose in urine, following oral drug administration, is useful in identifying the ultimate location of drug-related material but may provide little to no information about the drug. For example, almost all of an orally administered drug may have been destroyed in the gastrointestinal tract, from which the degradation products enter the body and are eventually excreted in urine. A basic lesson is learned here. Distinguish carefully between drug and metabolite(s). Many metabolites are of interest, especially if they are active or toxic. Each chemical entity must be considered separately for kinetic data to be meaningful.

DEFINITIONS

Although the processes of absorption and elimination are descriptive and their meanings are apparent at first glance, it is only within the context of experimental observation that they can be quantified (Chaps. 3, 4, and 6). General definitions of the processes follow.

Absorption

Absorption is defined as the process by which unchanged drug proceeds from site of administration to site of measurement within the body. To illustrate why absorption is defined in this way, consider the events depicted in Fig. 2–2 as a drug, given orally, moves from the site of administration to the general circulation. There are several possible sites of loss. One site is the gastrointestinal lumen where decomposition may occur. Suppose, however, that a drug survives destruction in the lumen only to be completely metabolized by enzymes as it passes through the membranes of the gastrointestinal tract. One would ask, Is the drug absorbed? Even though the drug leaves the gastrointestinal tract, it would not be detected in the general circulation. Hence, the drug is not absorbed systemically. Taking this argument one step further, Is the drug absorbed if all of the orally administered drug were to pass through the membranes of the gastrointestinal tract into the portal vein only to be metabolized completely on passing through the liver? In an experiment performed *in vitro* in which the passage of a drug across the intestinal membranes is studied separately, the answer would be positive. If, however, as is common, blood or plasma in an arm vein is the site of measurement, then, because no drug would be detected, the answer would be negative. Indeed, loss at any site prior to the site of measurement contributes to a decrease in the systemic absorption. The gastrointestinal tissues and the liver, in particular, are often sites of elimination. The requirement for an orally administered drug to pass through these tissues, prior to reaching the site of measurement, makes the extent of

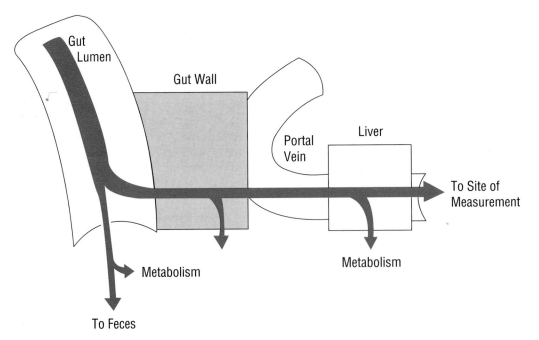

Fig. 2–2. A drug, given as a solid, encounters several barriers and sites of loss in its sequential movement during gastrointestinal absorption. Incomplete dissolution or metabolism in the gut lumen or by enzymes in the gut wall is a cause of poor absorption. Removal of drug as it first passes through the liver further reduces absorption.

absorption dependent on elimination. The loss as drug passes, for the first time, through sites of elimination, such as the gastrointestinal membranes and the liver, during absorption is known as the *first-pass effect.*

Absorption is not restricted to oral administration. It occurs as well following intramuscular, subcutaneous, and other extravascular routes of administration. Monitoring intact drug in blood or plasma offers a useful means of assessing the entry of drug into the systemic circulation.

Disposition

As absorption and elimination of drugs are interrelated for physiologic and anatomic reasons, so too are distribution and elimination. Once absorbed, a drug is delivered simultaneously by arterial blood to all tissues, including organs of elimination. Distinguishing between elimination and distribution as a cause for a decline in concentration in blood or plasma is often difficult. *Disposition* is the term used to embrace both processes. *Disposition* may be defined as all the processes that occur subsequent to the absorption of a drug. By definition, the components of disposition are distribution and elimination.

Distribution. Distribution is the process of reversible transfer of a drug to and from the site of measurement, usually the blood or plasma. An example is distribution between blood and muscle. The pathway for return of drug need not be the same as that leaving the circulation. For example, drug may be excreted in the bile, stored in and released from the gallbladder, transit into the small intestine, and be reabsorbed into the circulation. By doing so, the drug completes a cycle, the *enterohepatic cycle* (see Fig. 2–1). If all the drug is reabsorbed in this manner, biliary secretion is not a route of elimination; the cycling is then a component of distribution. The situation is analogous to one in which water is pumped from one reservoir into another, only to drain back into the original reservoir. Biliary secretion is truly a route of elimination only to the extent that the drug fails to be reabsorbed. This failure may result from decomposition in the intestine, poor absorption characteristics, or other complications. Unchanged drug in bile that is neither reabsorbed nor decomposed in the intestinal tract is eventually excreted in the feces.

Elimination. Elimination is the irreversible loss of drug from the site of measurement. Elimination occurs by two processes, excretion and metabolism. *Excretion* is the irreversible loss of chemically unchanged drug. *Metabolism* is the conversion of one chemical species to another. Occasionally, metabolites are converted back to the drug. As with enterohepatic cycling, this *metabolic interconversion* is a route of elimination only to the extent that the metabolite is excreted or otherwise irreversibly lost from the body.

BASIC MODEL FOR DRUG ABSORPTION AND DISPOSITION

The complexities of human anatomy and physiology would appear to make it difficult, if not impossible, to model how the body handles a drug. Perhaps surprisingly then, it is a simple pharmacokinetic model, depicted in Fig. 2–3 which has proved useful in many applications and is emphasized throughout much of this book. More complex models are necessary to describe the pharmacokinetics of some drugs. Examples of such models are described in Chaps. 10, 19, and 22.

The boxes in Fig. 2–3 represent *compartments* that logically fall into two classes, transfer and chemical. The site of administration, the body, and excreta are clearly different places. Each place may be referred to as a location or transfer compartment. In contrast, metabolism involves a chemical conversion; the metabolite in the body and in excreta are therefore in compartments that differ chemically from the drug.

The model is based on amounts of drug and metabolite. However, the amounts of drug and metabolite can only be measured in urine directly. The total amount of drug metabolized includes metabolites in, as well as eliminated from, the body. The amount in the body is usually determined from measurement of the blood or plasma concentration. Estimates of drug in the absorption compartment are also usually made indirectly from either blood or urine data. Drug at the absorption site includes that which is never absorbed, for example, drug that is ultimately decomposed in the gastrointestinal tract or lost in the feces after oral administration.

The model is readily visualized from mass balance considerations. The dose is accounted for at any one time by the molar amount of substance in each of the compartments:

$$\text{Dose} = \begin{array}{c}\text{Amount of}\\\text{drug at}\\\text{absorption site}\end{array} + \begin{array}{c}\text{Amount}\\\text{of drug}\\\text{in body}\end{array} + \begin{array}{c}\text{Amount}\\\text{of drug}\\\text{excreted}\end{array} + \begin{array}{c}\text{Amount of}\\\text{metabolite}\\\text{in body}\end{array} + \begin{array}{c}\text{Amount of}\\\text{metabolite}\\\text{eliminated}\end{array} \qquad 1$$

The mass balance of drug and related material with time is shown in Fig. 2–4. Since the sum of the molar amounts of drug in transfer and chemical compartments is equal to the dose, the sum of the rates of change of the drug in these compartments must be equal to zero so that:

$$\begin{array}{c}\text{Rate of change of}\\\text{drug in body}\end{array} = \begin{array}{c}\text{Rate of}\\\text{absorption}\end{array} - \begin{array}{c}\text{Rate of}\\\text{elimination}\end{array} \qquad 2$$

The relationships expressed in Eqs. 1 and 2 apply under all circumstances, regardless of the nature of the absorption and elimination processes. They are particularly useful in developing more complex models for quantifying drug absorption and disposition. *Pharmacokinetics* is the quantitation of the time course of a drug and its metabolites in the body

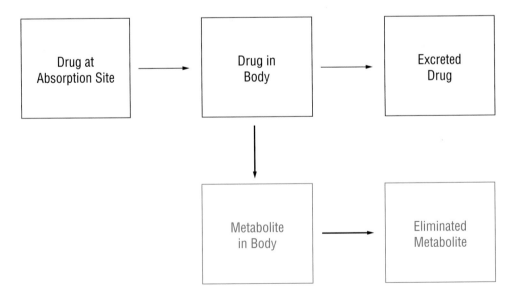

Fig. 2–3. A drug is simultaneously absorbed into the body and eliminated from it by excretion and metabolism. The processes of absorption, excretion, and metabolism are indicated with arrows and the compartments with boxes. The compartments represent different locations and different chemical species (color = metabolite). Metabolite elimination may occur by further metabolism (not shown) or excretion.

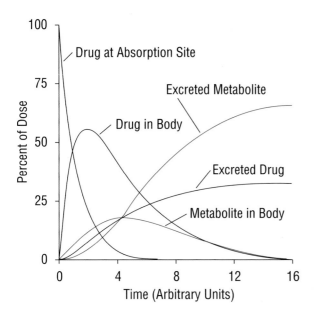

Fig. 2–4. Time course of drug and metabolite in each of the compartments shown in Fig. 2–3. The amount in each compartment is expressed as a percentage of the dose administered. In this example, all the dose is absorbed.

and the development of appropriate models to describe observations and predict outcomes in other situations.

STUDY PROBLEMS

(Answers to Study Problems are in Appendix II.)

1. Define the terms listed in the first objective at the beginning of this chapter.
2. Briefly state why an analytical method that does not distinguish between R- and S-isomers can lead to problems in the interpretation of plasma data following administration of a racemic mixture.
3. Using Figs. 2–3 and 2–4, speculate on how an assay that measures the sum of drug and inactive metabolite might influence a correlation between plasma concentration and therapeutic response.
4. Following oral administration of a drug labeled with a radioactive atom, all of the radioactivity is recovered in urine. Can one conclude that the drug is completely absorbed?
5. Answer each of the following questions, which relate to Fig. 2–4 and Eqs. 1 and 2.
   a. Does a 100% recovery of unchanged drug in urine following oral administration indicate that drug is completely absorbed and not metabolized?
   b. When does drug in body reach a peak following administration of an oral dose?
   c. Can the amount of drug absorbed up to a given time be determined?
   d. When is rate of change of drug in body equal to rate of drug elimination?
   e. When does rate of change of drug in body approach rate of absorption?

INTRAVENOUS DOSE

Administering a drug intravascularly ensures that all of the dose enters the general circulation. By rapid injection, elevated concentrations of drug in the blood can be promptly achieved; by infusion at a controlled rate, a constant concentration can be maintained. With no other route of administration can blood concentration be as promptly and efficiently controlled. Of the two intravascular routes, the intravenous (i.v.) one is the most frequently employed. Intra-arterial administration, which has greater inherent manipulative dangers, is reserved for situations in which drug localization in a specific organ or tissue is desired.

The disposition characteristics of a drug are defined by analyzing the temporal changes of drug and metabolites in blood, plasma, and occasionally urine following i.v. administration.

How this information is obtained following a rapid injection of the drug forms the basis of this chapter. The remaining chapter in this section deals with events following an extravascular dose. The pharmacokinetic information so derived forms a basis for making rational decisions in therapeutics, the subject of subsequent sections.

DISPOSITION VIEWED FROM PLASMA

Several methods are employed for graphically displaying plasma concentration-time data. One common method, shown with theophylline in Fig. 3–1A, is to plot concentration against time on regular (Cartesian) graph paper. Depicted in this manner, the plasma concentration is observed to fall rapidly immediately after a 500-mg bolus, in this case from approximately 29 to 18 mg/L within 30 min. Thereafter, the rate of decline becomes much slower, taking almost another 4 hrs before the concentration falls 50% to 9 mg/L. Another method of display is a plot of the same data on semilogarithmic paper (Fig. 3–1B). The time scale is the same as before, but now the ordinate (concentration) scale is logarithmic.

Notice the sharp break at about 1 hr when the plasma concentration is about 16 mg/L. Before this time, the fall is rapid. Thereafter, the decline is slower and, on this semilogarithmic plot, appears to continue linearly. The early phase is commonly called the *distribution phase* and the latter, the *elimination phase*. This distinction is sometimes not clear-cut, an aspect more completely discussed in Chap. 19, Distribution Kinetics.

Distribution Phase

The distribution phase is so called because distribution primarily determines the early rapid decline in plasma concentration. For theophylline, distribution is extremely rapid and occurs significantly even by the time of the first measurement, 5 min. This must be so because the amount of theophylline in plasma at the end of this period is only 99 mg. This value is calculated by multiplying the highest plasma concentration, 33 mg/L, by the plasma volume, 3 L. The majority, 401 mg or 80% of the total (500 mg) dose, must have already left the plasma and been distributed into other tissues. Among these tissues are the liver and the kidneys, which also clear drug from the body. However, although some drug is eliminated during the early moments, the fraction of the administered dose lost during the distribution phase is small for theophylline and many other drugs.

Elimination Phase

During the distribution phase, changes in the concentration of drug in plasma reflect primarily movement of drug within, rather than loss from, the body. However, with time, distribution equilibrium of drug in tissue with that in plasma is established in more and more tissues, and eventually, changes in plasma concentration reflect a proportional change in the concentrations of drug in all other tissues and, hence, in the amount of drug in the body. During this proportionality phase, the body acts kinetically as a single container or compartment. As decline of the plasma concentration is now due only to elimination of drug from the body, this phase is often called the elimination phase.

    Elimination Half-Life. The elimination phase is characterized by two parameters, the *elimination half-life* ($t_{1/2}$) and *the apparent volume of distribution* (V). The elimination half-

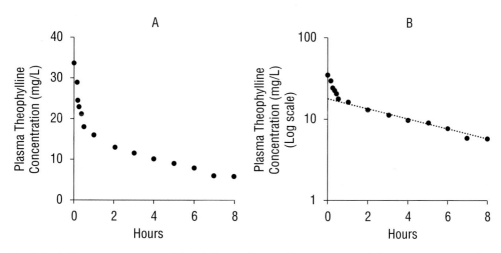

Fig. 3–1. *A*. Plasma concentration of theophylline with time after a 500-mg i.v. bolus injection into a 70-kg patient. *B*. The data in *A* are redisplayed as a semilogarithmic plot. Note the short distribution phase (1 mg/L = 5.5 μM). (Modified from the data of Mitenko, P.A., and Ogilvie, R.I.: Pharmacokinetics of intravenous theophylline. Clin. Pharmacol. Ther., *14*:509–513, 1973.)

life is the time taken for the plasma concentration, as well as the amount of the drug in the body, to fall by one-half. The half-life of theophylline, determined by the time taken to fall from 16 to 8 mg/L, is 5.0 hrs (Fig. 3–1B). This is the same time that it takes for the concentration to fall from 12 to 6 mg/L. In other words, for theophylline at the dose administered, the elimination half-life is independent of the amount of drug in the body. It follows, therefore, that less drug is eliminated in each succeeding half-life. Initially there are 500 mg in the body. After 1 half-life (5 hr), 250 mg remain. After 2 half-lives (10 hr), 125 mg remain, and after 3 half-lives (15 hr), 62.5 mg remain. In practice, all the drug (97%) may be regarded as having been eliminated by 5 half-lives (25 hr).

Volume of Distribution. The concentration in plasma achieved after distribution is complete is a function of dose and extent of distribution of drug into tissues. This extent of distribution can be determined by relating the concentration obtained with a known amount of drug in the body. This is analogous to the determination of the volume of a reservoir by dividing the amount of dye added to it by the resultant concentration, after thorough mixing. The volume measured is, in effect, a dilution space.

The apparent volume into which a drug distributes in the body at equilibrium is called the *(apparent) volume of distribution*. Plasma, rather than blood, is usually measured. Consequently, the volume of distribution, V, is the volume of plasma at the drug concentration, C, required to account for all the drug in the body, A.

$$V = A/C$$

$$\frac{\text{Volume of}}{\text{distribution}} = \frac{\text{Amount in body}}{\text{Plasma drug concentration}}$$

1

Volume of distribution is useful in estimating plasma concentration when a known amount of drug is in the body or, conversely, in estimating the dose required to achieve a given plasma concentration.

Calculation of volume of distribution requires that distribution equilibrium be achieved between drug in tissues and that in plasma. The amount of drug in the body is known immediately after an i.v. bolus; it is the dose administered. However, distribution equilibrium has not yet been achieved. An estimate is needed of the plasma concentration that would have resulted had all drug spontaneously distributed into its final volume of distribution. To do this, use is made of the linear decline during the elimination phase seen in the semilogarithmic plot (Fig. 3–1B).

Decline in plasma concentration during the elimination phase can be characterized by the linear equation

$$\ln C = \ln C(0) - kt$$

2

where k is the slope of the line in Fig. 3–1B and $C(0)$ is the concentration one would determine from this equation at zero time. The negative sign arises because concentration declines with time. The term $C(0)$ is an extrapolated value and is an estimate of the concentration which when multiplied by the volume term, V, accounts for the dose administered, i.e.,

$$\text{Dose} = V \cdot C(0)$$

3

In the example with theophylline, $C(0)$ is 18 mg/L. Since 500 mg was administered to the patient, the volume of distribution of theophylline is 28 L. Knowing the volume of distribution, the amount in the body can now be estimated at any time during the elimination phase. For example, when the concentration of theophylline in plasma is 5 mg/L, there are 140 mg in the body.

Volume of distribution is a direct measure of the extent of distribution. It rarely, however, corresponds to a real volume, such as plasma volume (3 L), extracellular water (16 L), or total body water (42 L). Drug distribution may be to any one or a combination of the tissues and fluids of the body. Furthermore, binding to tissue components may be so great that the volume of distribution is many times the total body size.

To appreciate the effect of tissue binding, consider the distribution of 100 mg of a drug in a 1-L system composed of water and 10 g of activated charcoal, and where 99% of drug is adsorbed onto the charcoal. When the charcoal has settled, the concentration of drug in the aqueous phase would be 1 mg/L; thus, 100 L of the aqueous phase would be required to account for all the drug in the system, a volume much greater than that of the total system. Volumes of distribution for selected drugs are shown in Fig. 3–2. The causes for this wide range of values are discussed in Chap. 10, Distribution.

First-Order Elimination. Why the elimination for theophylline (and for most other drugs) is linear when displayed semilogarithmically can be appreciated as follows. Taking the antilogarithm of both sides of Eq. 2 yields

$$C = C(0) \cdot e^{-kt} \qquad\qquad 4$$

And multiplying both sides by V, gives

$$A = \text{Dose} \cdot e^{-kt} \qquad\qquad 5$$

since $C \cdot V$ and $C(0) \cdot V$ are the amount in the body and the dose administered, respectively. Equations 4 and 5 enable the concentration and amount in the body at any time to be estimated. When decline in the plasma concentration or amount in the body can be described by a single exponential term as given by Eqs. 4 and 5, it is said to be (mono)exponential. Since the elimination half-life ($t_{1/2}$) is the time taken for the concentration and the amount in the body to fall by one-half, e.g., from $C(0)$ to 1/2 $C(0)$, it follows from Eq. 4 that:

$$0.5 = e^{-k \cdot t_{1/2}} \qquad\qquad 6$$

or, on inversion

$$e^{k \cdot t_{1/2}} = 2$$

Taking the natural logarithm of both sides,

$$k \cdot t_{1/2} = \ln 2 = 0.693$$

one obtains the important relationship,

$$t_{1/2} = \frac{0.693}{k} \qquad\qquad 7$$

Although the constant k is in the exponent in Eq. 4 and can be calculated from Eq. 7, its meaning may be better understood by examining the rate at which the amount in the body, A, is changing with time. This is obtained by differentiating Eq. 5,

$$\frac{dA}{dt} = -k \cdot \text{Dose} \cdot e^{-kt} \qquad\qquad 8$$

but since $A = \text{Dose} \cdot e^{-kt}$, it follows that

$$\frac{dA}{dt} = -k \cdot A \qquad\qquad 9$$

The term on the left-hand side of Eq. 9 is the rate of change of the amount in the body. This is also the rate of elimination of drug from the body. Processes such as this, in which

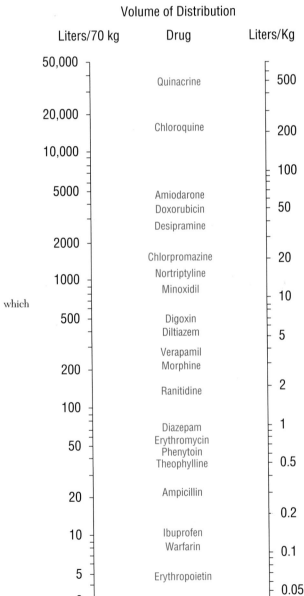

Fig. 3–2. The apparent volume into which drugs distribute varies widely.

the rate of reaction is proportional to the amount present, are known as *first-order processes*. The proportionality constant is known as the *first-order rate constant* with dimensions of time^{-1}. Because k characterizes the elimination process, it is known as the *elimination rate constant*. Since the rate constant can also be defined by rearranging Eq. 9 to yield

$$k = \frac{\text{Rate of elimination}}{\text{Amount in body}} \qquad\qquad 10$$

the elimination rate constant may simply be regarded as the *fractional rate of drug removal*. For example, since the half-life of theophylline is 5 hr, the value of its elimination rate constant is 0.14 hr^{-1}. Hence, the speed of the elimination process of theophylline can be characterized either by its half-life, 5 hr, or by saying that the fractional rate of elimination is 0.14 (or 14%) of the drug in the body per hour.

Fraction of Dose Remaining. Another view of the kinetics of drug elimination may be gained by examining how the fraction of the dose remaining in the body (A/Dose) varies with time. By reference to Eq. 5,

$$\text{Fraction of dose remaining in the body} = \frac{A}{\text{Dose}} = e^{-kt} \qquad\qquad 11$$

The fraction of the dose remaining is, therefore, given by e^{-kt}. Sometimes, it is useful to express time relative to the half-life. The value of doing so is seen by letting n be the number of half-lives elapsed after a bolus dose ($n = t/t_{1/2}$). Then, as $k = 0.693/t_{1/2}$,

$$\text{Fraction of dose remaining in the body} = e^{-kt} = e^{-0.693n} \qquad\qquad 12$$

Since $e^{-0.693} = \frac{1}{2}$, it follows that

$$\text{Fraction of dose remaining in the body} = (\frac{1}{2})^n \qquad\qquad 13$$

Thus, $\frac{1}{2}$ or 50% of the dose remains after 1 half-life, and $\frac{1}{4}$ ($\frac{1}{2} \times \frac{1}{2}$) or 25% remains after 2 half-lives, and so on.

Total Clearance. Just as the parameter volume of distribution is needed to relate concentration to amount in the body, so there is a need to have a parameter to relate concentration to rate of drug elimination. Clearance (total), denoted by CL, is that proportionality factor. Thus,

$$\text{Rate of elimination} = CL \cdot \text{Concentration} \qquad\qquad 14$$

The units of clearance, like those of flow, are volume per unit time. For example, if the clearance value is 1 L/hr, then at a concentration of 1 mg/L, the rate of drug elimination is 1 mg/hr. Ordinarily, as the concentration of a drug increases, so does its rate of elimination; clearance remains the same. From Eq. 9, rate of elimination = $k \cdot A$. Since $A = V \cdot C$; from Eq. 1, it follows that

$$\text{Rate of elimination} = k \cdot V \cdot C \qquad\qquad 15$$

Comparison of Eqs. 14 and 15 leads to the relationship

$$\text{Clearance} = k \cdot V \qquad\qquad 16$$

Using Eq. 16, the (total) clearance of theophylline is calculated to be 4 L/hr or 67 mL/min. So that at a plasma concentration of 1 mg/L, e.g., the rate of elimination of theophylline from the body is 4 mg/hr.

Clearance and Elimination Half-life. It is more common to refer to the half-life rather than to the elimination rate constant of a drug. Recall that $t_{1/2} = 0.693/k$, so that half-life is related to clearance by:

$$t_{1/2} = \frac{0.693 \cdot \text{Volume of distribution}}{\text{Clearance}} \qquad\qquad 17$$

Equation 17 is purposely arranged in the above manner to stress that half-life (and elimination rate constant) reflects rather than controls volume of distribution and clearance, two independent parameters. To show the application of Eq. 17, consider the use of creatinine, a product of muscle catabolism, as a marker of renal function. Creatinine has a clearance of 7.2 L/hr and is evenly distributed throughout the 42 L of total body water. As expected by calculation using Eq. 17, its half-life is 4 hr. Inulin, a polysaccharide also used to assess renal function, has the same clearance as creatinine. However, inulin has a half-life of only 1.5 hr because it is restricted to the 16 L of extracellular water.

Clearance, Area, and Volume of Distribution. Thus far, clearance has been estimated from half-life and volume of distribution. Clearance can be better estimated in another way. By rearranging Eq. 14, it can be seen that during a small interval of time, dt,

$$\text{Amount eliminated in interval } dt = \text{Clearance} \cdot C \cdot dt \qquad\qquad 18$$

where the product $C \cdot dt$ is the corresponding small area under the plasma concentration-time curve. For example, if the clearance of a drug is 1 L/min and the area under the curve between 60 and 61 min is 1 mg-min/L, then the amount of drug eliminated in that minute is 1 mg. The total amount of drug eventually eliminated, which for an i.v. bolus equals the dose administered, is assessed by adding up or integrating the amounts eliminated in each time interval, from time zero to infinite time, and therefore,

$$\text{Dose} = CL \cdot AUC \qquad\qquad 19$$

where AUC is the total area under the concentration-time curve. Thus, once AUC is known (Appendix I-A), clearance is readily calculated. Note that there is no need to know the half-life or volume of distribution to calculate clearance. Furthermore, this calculation of clearance is independent of the shape of the concentration-time profile.

The relationship between area and elimination can be applied at any time following drug administration, as illustrated in Fig. 3–3. Thus, multiplying the area up to a given time, $[AUC(o, t)]$ by clearance gives the amount of drug that has been eliminated up to that time. Alternatively, when the area is expressed as a fraction of the total AUC, one obtains the fraction of the dose eliminated. And the fraction of the total area beyond a given time is a measure of the fraction of dose remaining to be eliminated. For example, in the case of theophylline, by 3.6 hr the area is 40% of the total AUC, and hence 40% of the administered 500-mg dose, or 200 mg, has been eliminated from the body; 300 mg has yet to be eliminated.

Volume of distribution (V) is used to relate plasma concentration to amount of drug in the body during the elimination phase. Often the value obtained by extrapolation (Eq. 3) is a reasonable estimate of this volume term. Occasionally, when extensive elimination occurs in the distribution phase, it is not. The best method of calculating volume of distribution is to divide clearance by elimination rate constant

$$V = \frac{CL}{k} = \frac{Dose}{AUC \cdot k} \qquad\qquad 20$$

Unlike extrapolation, this method of estimating V is not restricted to the i.v. bolus situation but can be used under a variety of conditions, e.g., long-term i.v. infusions. Consequently, the value of V, estimated using Eq. 20, is applied throughout the remainder of this book, although other volume terms are examined in Chap. 19, Distribution Kinetics.

RENAL CLEARANCE

Elimination occurs by renal excretion and extrarenal pathways, usually hepatic metabolism. Not only is renal excretion an important route of elimination for many drugs, but useful pharmacokinetic information can be obtained from analysis of urinary data. Central to this analysis is the concept of *renal clearance*.

Analogous to total clearance, renal clearance (CL_R) is defined as the proportionality term between urinary excretion rate and plasma concentration:

$$Excretion\ rate = CL_R \cdot C \qquad\qquad 21$$

Renal clearance, like total clearance, has units of flow, usually milliliters/minute or liters/hour.

Practical problems arise, however, in estimating renal clearance. Urine is collected over a finite period, e.g., 4 hr, during which the plasma concentration is changing continuously. Shortening the collection period reduces the change in plasma concentration but increases the uncertainty in the estimate of excretion rate owing to incomplete bladder emptying. This is especially true for urine collection intervals of less than 15 min. Lengthening the

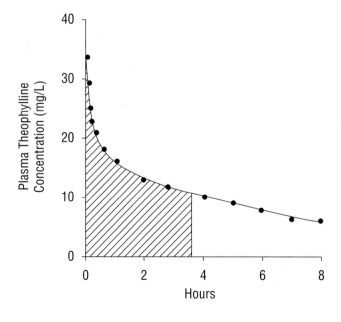

Fig. 3–3. A linear plot of the same plasma concentration-time data for theophylline as displayed in Fig. 3–1A. The area up to 3.6 hr is 40% of the total *AUC* indicating that 40% of the dose administered has been eliminated by then. The area beyond 3.6 hr represents the 60% of administered theophylline remaining to be eliminated.

collection interval, to avoid the problem of incomplete emptying, requires a modified approach for the estimation of renal clearance. This approach is analogous to that taken with total clearance. By rearranging Eq. 21, during a very small interval of time, dt,

$$\text{Amount excreted} = CL_R \cdot C \cdot dt \qquad\qquad 22$$

where $C \cdot dt$ is the corresponding small area under the plasma drug concentration-time curve. The urine collection interval (denoted by Δt) is composed of many such very small increments of time, and the amount of drug excreted in a collection interval is the sum of the amounts excreted in each of these small increments of time, that is,

$$\frac{\text{Amount excreted in}}{\text{collection interval}} = CL_R \cdot [AUC \text{ within interval}] \qquad\qquad 23$$

The problem in calculating renal clearance therefore rests with estimating the AUC within the time interval (see Appendix I–A). The average plasma drug concentration during the collection interval is given by $((AUC$ within interval)/$\Delta t)$. This average plasma concentration is neither the value at the beginning nor at the end of the collection time but at some intermediate point. By assuming that the plasma concentration changes linearly with time, the appropriate concentration is that at the midpoint of the collection interval. Because the plasma concentration of drug is in fact changing exponentially with time, this assumption of linear change is reasonable only when loss during the interval is small. In practice, the interval should be less than an elimination half-life.

Extending Eq. 23 over all time intervals, from zero to infinity, one obtains the useful relationship

$$\text{Renal clearance} = \frac{\text{Total amount excreted unchanged}}{AUC} \qquad\qquad 24$$

where AUC is the total area under the plasma drug concentration-time curve. To apply Eq. 24, care must be taken to ensure that all urine is collected and for a sufficient period of time to gain a good estimate of the total amount excreted unchanged. In practice, the period of time must be at least 5 to 6 elimination half-lives of the drug (see Appendix I–B). Thus, if the half-life of a drug is in the order of a few hours, no practical difficulties exist in ensuring urine collections taken over an adequate period of time. Severe difficulties with compliance in urine collection occur, however, for drugs such as phenobarbital with a half-life of about a week, since all urine formed over a period of at least 1 month must be collected.

DISPOSITION VIEWED FROM URINE ONLY

Lack of sufficiently sensitive analytic techniques can and previously has prevented measurement of the concentration of many drugs in plasma. In the absence of plasma measurements, neither volume of distribution nor clearance can be determined. Nonetheless, useful information can still be obtained from urine data alone, when such is necessary.

Elimination Half-Life

The elimination half-life of the reversible cholinesterase inhibitor, galanthamine, can be estimated from urine data. The approach is to plot the average excretion rate against the midpoint of the collection time semilogarithmically and, from the slope of the straight line, obtain an estimate of the half-life. Intuitively, the approach is easy to see. Assuming that renal clearance is constant, the urinary excretion rate is proportional to plasma concentration, and plotting urinary excretion rate against time is like plotting plasma concentration against time. The half-life is then taken as the time for the urinary excretion rate (or plasma concentration) to fall by one-half. For galanthamine this is approximately 6 hr in a healthy subject (Fig. 3–4). Conversely, when a straight line is obtained by plotting the urinary excretion rate against the midpoint time, constancy of renal clearance is inferred. The need for using midpoint time follows from the previous discussion; the measured urinary excretion rate reflects the average plasma concentration during the collection interval. Formal proof of the foregoing discussion is given in Appendix I–B.

Renal Excretion as a Fraction of Total Elimination

An important pharmacokinetic parameter is the fraction of the amount entering the general circulation that is excreted unchanged, fe. It is a quantitative measure of the contribution of renal excretion to overall drug elimination. Knowing fe aids in establishing appropriate modifications in the usual dosage regimen of a drug for patients with varying degrees of renal function. Among drugs, the value of fe ranges between 0 and 1.0. When the value is low, excretion is a minor pathway of drug elimination. Occasionally, renal excretion is the only route of elimination, in which case the value of fe is 1.0. By definition the difference, $1 - fe$, is the fraction of the amount entering the circulation that is eliminated by extrarenal mechanisms, usually metabolism.

An estimate of fe is most readily obtained from cumulative urinary excretion data following i.v. administration, since by definition.

$$fe = \frac{\text{Total drug excreted unchanged}}{\text{Dose}}$$ 25

In practice, care should always be taken to ensure complete urinary recovery (i.e., collect

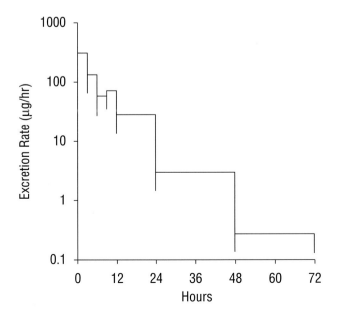

Fig. 3–4. Average urine excretion rate during each urine collection interval after an i.v. bolus dose of 10 mg of galanthamine to a healthy subject. (Redrawn from Bickel, U., Thomsen, T., Weber, W., Fischer, J.P., Bachus, R., Nitz, M., and Kewitz, H. Pharmacokinetics of galanthamine in humans and corresponding cholinesterase inhibition. Clin. Pharmacol. Ther., 50:420–428, 1991.)

urine for at least 5 elimination half-lives). In the case of galanthamine, *fe* is approximately 0.25 in subjects with normal renal function. At any instant, the fraction *fe* may be defined as the ratio of the rate of excretion to the rate of elimination,

$$fe = \frac{\text{Rate of excretion}}{\text{Rate of elimination}} \qquad\qquad 26$$

Appropriately substituting for numerator and denominator in Eq. 26, it is seen that

$$fe = \frac{CL_R \cdot C}{CL \cdot C} = \frac{CL_R}{CL} \qquad\qquad 27$$

Thus, *fe* may also be defined and estimated as the ratio of renal and total clearances. This is particularly useful in those situations in which total urine collection is not possible.

In practice, estimates of CL and CL_R are obtained directly, whereas extrarenal clearance is determined by difference. Thus, extrarenal clearance is $(1 - fe) \cdot CL$.

ESTIMATION OF PHARMACOKINETIC PARAMETERS

To appreciate how the pharmacokinetic parameters defining disposition are estimated, consider the plasma and urine data in Table 3–1 obtained following an i.v. bolus dose of 50 mg of a drug.

Table 3-1. Plasma and Urine Data Obtained Following an i.v. Bolus Dose

OBSERVATION					TREATMENT OF DATA		
PLASMA DATA		URINE DATA					
TIME (hr)	CONCEN- TRATION (mg/L)	TIME INTERVAL OF COLLEC- TION (hr)	VOLUME OF URINE (mL)	CONCENTRA- TION OF UNCHANGED DRUG IN URINE (mg/L)	*AUC* WITHIN TIME INTERVAL (mg-hr/L)	AMOUNT EXCRETED IN TIME INTERVAL (mg)	CUMULATIVE AMOUNT EXCRETED (mg)
1	2.0	0–2	120	133	4.00	16.0	16.0
3	1.13	2–4	180	50	2.26	9.0	25.0
5	0.70	4–6	89	63	1.40	5.6	30.6
7	0.43	6–8	340	10	0.86	3.4	34.0
10	0.20	8–12	178	18	0.80	3.2	37.2
18	0.025	12–24	950	2	0.43	1.9	39.1

Plasma Data Alone

A plot of plasma concentration versus time indicates that the values are dropping progressively, but only after the data are plotted semilogarithmically (Fig. 3–5) can the half-life and elimination rate constant be readily determined. The half-life, taken as the time for the concentration to fall in half (e.g., from 1.0 to 0.5 mg/L or 0.2 to 0.1 mg/L), is 2.8 hr, so that k is 0.25 hr^{-1}. Clearance is determined by dividing dose by AUC. The total AUC, estimated using the trapezoidal rule (Appendix I–A), is 10.2 mg-hr/L and when divided into the dose yields a value of 4.9 L/hr for clearance. Volume of distribution, estimated from CL/k (Eq. 20), is therefore 19.6 L. This value is virtually identical to that calculated by dividing dose by the intercept concentration at zero time, because no distinct distribution phase is apparent.

Plasma and Urine Data

Both plasma and urine data are required to estimate renal clearance. This parameter can be obtained from the slope of a plot of the amount excreted within a collection interval against *AUC* within the same time interval (Fig. 3–6). The straight line implies that renal clearance is constant and independent of plasma concentration. The slope of the line indicates that the renal clearance of this drug is 4 L/hr. Essentially the same value is obtained by multiplying total clearance (5.0 L/hr) by *fe* (0.78) (cf. Eq. 27). The cumulative amount excreted is 39.1 mg, so the fraction of the dose excreted unchanged, *fe*, is 39.1 mg/50 mg, or 0.78.

Urine Data Alone

The elimination half-life of the drug can be obtained from either excretion rate or cumulative excretion data. The appropriate methods are dealt with in Appendix I–B.

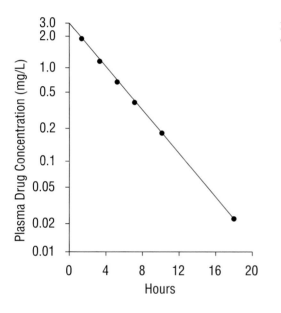

Fig. 3–5. Semilogarithmic plot of the plasma concentration-time data given in Table 3–1.

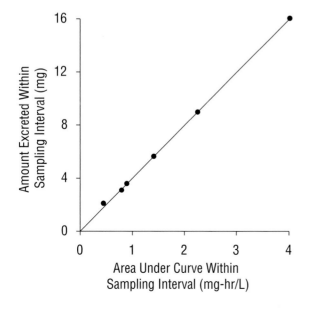

Fig. 3–6. The amount excreted is directly proportional to the *AUC* measured over the urine collection interval. Renal clearance is given by the slope of the line. Data from Table 3–1.

A Question of Precision

Had you, the reader, plotted the same data and calculated the pharmacokinetic parameters, you may have obtained answers that differ from those given. This is not unusual and will occur in many cases when you check your answers to the problems at the end of each chapter against those given in Appendix II. The reason lies in differences in the drawing of a line through data, after they have been plotted, and in rounding-off numbers. In addition, all measurements have errors associated with analytic methods, conditions of storage, and handling of samples prior to analysis.

Also, had the study just considered been repeated subsequently in the same individual, the estimated half-life may have been 3.1 hr instead of 2.8 hr. For almost all clinical situations, this degree of intraindividual variation is acceptable. To reflect the acceptable 5 to 10% variation, most answers here and throughout the remainder of the book are only given to two or three significant places.

In this chapter, many symbols are defined, as it is the first time that they are used. These symbols are reused repeatedly throughout the book. To avoid continually redefining them in every chapter and to facilitate reference to them, the Definitions of Symbols appear just before Chapter 1. Some infrequently used symbols that occur only in one chapter may not be included in the Definitions.

Measurement Fluid

So far, the pharmacokinetics of the drug within the body have been defined with reference to drug in plasma. Sometimes the reference is drug in serum or whole blood. The major difference between plasma and serum is the removal of fibrinogen in the latter case by clotting of blood, and as most drugs do not bind to fibrinogen, no difference between the concentrations of drug in plasma and serum is expected. Consequently, throughout the book the term *plasma* is taken to include serum.

Within blood, drug can bind to many constituents including plasma proteins and blood cells. Drug concentrations in whole blood and plasma can differ, thereby yielding different values for many pharmacokinetic parameters, an aspect discussed in some depth subsequently in the book (particularly Chap. 11, Elimination, and Chap. 12, Integration With Kinetics). Accordingly, unlike serum and plasma, blood and plasma cannot be considered to be equivalent, although for many applications in pharmacokinetics, the difference is relatively unimportant. Because of ease of clinical analysis, most measurements are made in plasma, rather than in blood.

Strictly speaking, one should use the terminology *concentration of drug in plasma (or blood, or plasma water)*. For expediency, in much of this chapter and throughout the rest of the book, this phrase is often shortened to *plasma (or blood) drug concentration*. Indeed, this is sometimes even further shortened to *plasma concentration (or blood concentration)* in many contexts in which concentration of a drug is understood. Similarly, the phrase *amount in body* refers to the amount of drug in the body.

Use of Computers

Today computers are used to analyze pharmacokinetic data and make predictions. Based upon statistical criteria, the pharmacokinetic parameter values are adjusted to give the best fit of the appropriate equation to the experimental data. This approach not only provides the best estimate of parameters but also increases one's confidence in them. Also, application of the same computer program results in the same answers independent of the operator. This consistency cannot be achieved by fitting graphical data by eye. Moreover, unlike an exponential equation, there are many situations in pharmacokinetics that require equations that cannot be linearized. Then, obtaining a best fit by eye becomes virtually impossible. This limitation does not arise using a computer; any equation can be fitted directly to the experimental data. Nonetheless, a great deal about data is learned by displaying them graphically. One gains a feeling for the quality of the data and the equation that is most likely to describe them appropriately. The parameter values obtained by eye also generally serve as suitable starting values in a computer program. Because of the great benefits to learning pharmacokinetics gained by plotting data, this element is incorporated into many problems throughout the book.

EFFECT OF DOSE

An adjustment in dose is often necessary to achieve optimal drug therapy. Adjustment is made more readily when the values of the pharmacokinetic parameters of a drug do not vary with dose or with concentration. The possibility for a change with dose exists, however, for many reasons, and these are dealt with in Chap. 22 under the title of Dose and Time Dependencies. Throughout the majority of the book, however, pharmacokinetic parameters are assumed not to change with either dose or time.

STUDY PROBLEMS

(Answers to Study Problems are in Appendix II.)

1. Given that the disposition kinetics of a drug is described by a one-compartment model, which one(s) of the following statements is correct?
   The half-life of a drug following therapeutic doses in humans is 4 hr, therefore,
   a. The elimination rate constant of this drug is 0.173 hr^{-1}.
   b. It takes 16 hr for 87.5% of an i.v. bolus dose to be eliminated.
   c. It takes twice as long to eliminate 0.375 g following a 0.5-g bolus dose as it does to eliminate 0.5 g following a 1-g dose.
   d. Complete urine collection up to 12 hr is needed to provide a good estimate of the ultimate amount of drug excreted unchanged.
   e. The fraction of the administered dose eliminated by a given time is independent of the size of the dose.
2. Calculate the following:
   a. The fraction of an i.v. dose remaining in the body at 3 hr, when the half-life is 6 hr.
   b. The half-life of a drug, when 18% of the dose remains in the body 4 hr after an i.v. bolus dose.
3. Prepare a semilogarithmic plot of the following plasma concentration–time relationship:

$$C = 0.9\, e^{-0.347t}$$

   where C is in mg/L and time is in hours.
4. A drug that displays one-compartment disposition kinetics is administered as a single bolus dose. Depicted in the left-hand graph of Fig. 3–7 are the plasma concentrations of drug observed initially (10 mg/L) and 60 min later (2.5 mg/L). Depicted in the right-hand graph of Fig. 3–7 is the total urinary excretion of unchanged drug [$Ae_\infty = 60$ mg]. Complete the figure by drawing continuous lines that depict the fall of drug concentration in plasma and the accumulation of drug in urine with time.
5. From 0 to 3 hr after a 50-mg i.v. bolus dose of drug, the AUC is 5.1 mg-hr/L. The total AUC is 22.4 mg-hr/L and the cumulative amount excreted unchanged, Ae_∞, is 11 mg.
   a. What percent of the administered dose remains in the body as drug at 3 hr?

    b. Calculate total clearance.

    c. Calculate the renal clearance of the drug.

    d. What's the fraction of the dose that is eliminated by renal excretion?

6. When 100 mg of a drug was given as an i.v. bolus, the following plasma concentration–time relationship (C in mg/L and t in hr) was observed,

$$C = 7.14\,e^{-0.173t}$$

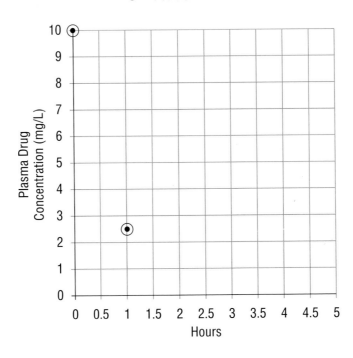

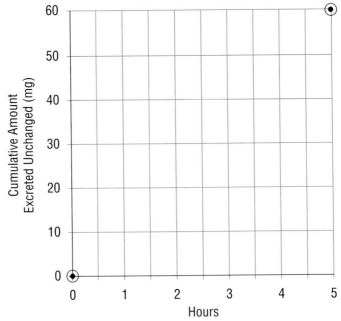

Fig. 3–7.

Calculate:

a. Volume of distribution

b. Elimination half-life

c. Total *AUC*

d. Total clearance

e. The plasma concentration 20 min after a 250-mg i.v. bolus dose.

7. Table 3–2 summarizes plasma data obtained after a bolus dose of ceftriaxone, a semi-synthetic cephalosporin antibiotic, in a newborn infant. (Adapted from Schaad, U.B., Hayton, W.L., and Stoeckel, K.: Single-dose ceftriaxone kinetics in the newborn. Clin. Pharmacol. Ther., 37:522–528, 1985.)

Table 3-2. Plasma Concentrations of Ceftriaxone After i.v. Administration of a 184 mg (50 mg/kg) Dose

Time (hr)	1	6	12	24	48	72	96	144
Concentration (mg/L)	137	120	103	76	42	23	12	3.7

a. Prepare a semilogarithmic plot of the plasma concentration of ceftriaxone versus time. Estimate the half-life of the drug.

b. Estimate the total *AUC* of ceftriaxone.

c. Calculate total clearance.

d. Calculate the volume of distribution.

8. The data given in Table 3–3 are the plasma concentrations of cocaine as a function of time after i.v. administration of 33 mg cocaine hydrochloride to a subject. (Molecular weight of cocaine hydrochloride = 340 g/mole; molecular weight of cocaine = 303 g/mole.) (Adapted from Chow, M.J., Ambre, J.J., Ruo, T.I., Atkinson, A.J., Bowsher, D.J., and Fischman, M.W.: Kinetics of cocaine distribution, elimination, and chronotropic effects. Clin. Pharmacol. Ther., 38:318–324, 1985.)

Table 3-3. Plasma Concentrations of Cocaine After a Single i.v. Dose of 33 mg

Time (hr)	0.16	0.5	1.0	1.5	2.0	2.5	3.0
Concentration (μg/L)	170	122	74	45	28	17	10

a. Prepare a semilogarithmic plot of plasma concentration versus time.

b. Estimate the half-life and total clearance of cocaine.

c. Given that the body weight of the subject is 75 kg, calculate the volume of distribution of cocaine in L/kg.

EXTRAVASCULAR DOSE

OBJECTIVES

The reader will be able to:

1. Describe the characteristics of, and the differences between, first-order and zero-order absorption processes.

2. Determine whether absorption or disposition rate limits drug elimination, given plasma concentration-time data following different dosage forms or routes of administration.

3. Anticipate the effect of altering rate of absorption, extent of absorption, clearance, or volume of distribution on the plasma concentration and amount of drug in the body following extravascular administration.

4. Estimate the bioavailability of a drug, given either plasma concentration or urinary excretion data following both extravascular and intravascular administration.

5. Estimate the relative bioavailability of a drug, given either plasma concentration or urinary excretion data following different dosage forms or routes of administration.

6. Estimate the renal clearance of a drug from plasma concentration and urinary excretion data following extravascular administration.

For systemically acting drugs, absorption is a prerequisite for therapeutic activity when they are administered extravascularly. The factors that influence drug absorption are considered in Chap. 9, Absorption. In this chapter the following aspects are examined: the impact of rate and extent of absorption on both plasma concentration and amount of drug in the body; the effect of alterations in absorption and disposition on body level-time relationships; and the methods used to assess pharmacokinetic parameters from plasma and urinary data following extravascular administration.

The term *bioavailability* is commonly applied to both rate and extent of drug input into the systemic circulation. Throughout this book the term will be limited to the extent of drug input and can be considered as the fraction, or percent, of the administered dose absorbed intact.

KINETICS OF ABSORPTION

The oral absorption of drugs often approximates first-order kinetics, especially when given in solution. The same holds true for the absorption of drugs from many other extravascular sites including subcutaneous tissue and muscle. Under these circumstances, absorption is characterized by an absorption rate constant, ka, and a corresponding half-life. The half-lives for the absorption of drugs administered orally in solution or in a rapidly disintegrating dosage form usually range from 15 min to 1 hr. Occasionally, they are longer.

Sometimes, a drug is absorbed at essentially a constant rate. The absorption kinetics are then called *zero order*. Differences between zero-order and first-order kinetics are illustrated in Fig. 4–1. For zero-order absorption, a plot of amount remaining to be absorbed against time yields a straight line, the slope of which is the rate of absorption (Fig. 4–1A). Recall from Chap. 3 that the fractional rate of decline is constant for a first-order process; the amount declines linearly with time when plotted semilogarithmically. In contrast, for a zero-order absorption process, the fractional rate increases with time, because the rate is constant but the amount remaining decreases. This is reflected in an ever-increasing gradient with time in a semilogarithmic plot of the amount remaining to be absorbed (Fig. 4–1B). A graphical method of examining the kinetics of absorption from plasma data following extravascular administration is given in Appendix I–C.

For the remainder of this chapter, and for much of the book, absorption is assumed to be first order. If absorption is zero order, then the equations developed in Chap. 6 (Constant-Rate Regimens) apply.

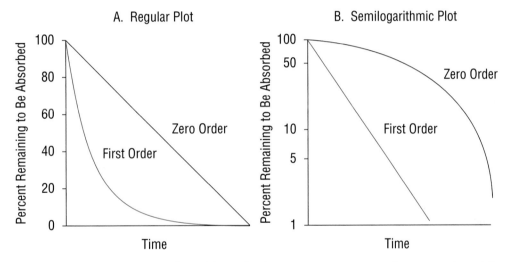

Fig. 4–1. A comparison of zero-order and first-order absorption processes. Depicted are: *A*, regular and *B*, semilogarithmic plots of the percent remaining to be absorbed against time.

BODY LEVEL-TIME RELATIONSHIPS

Comparison With an Intravenous Dose

Absorption delays and reduces the *magnitude of the peak* compared to that seen following an equal i.v. bolus dose. These effects are portrayed for aspirin in Fig. 4–2. The rise and fall of the drug concentration in plasma are best understood by remembering (Chap. 2, Eq. 2, p. 16) that at any time

$$\underset{\substack{\text{Rate of} \\ \text{change of} \\ \text{drug in} \\ \text{body}}}{\frac{dA}{dt}} = \underset{\substack{\text{Rate of} \\ \text{absorption}}}{\frac{dA_a}{dt}} - \underset{\substack{\text{Rate of} \\ \text{elimination}}}{k \cdot A} \qquad\qquad 1$$

where *Aa* is the amount of drug at the absorption site remaining to be absorbed. When absorption occurs by a first-order process, the rate of absorption is given by $ka \cdot Aa$.

Initially, with all drug at the absorption site and none in the body, rate of absorption is maximal and rate of elimination is zero. Thereafter, as drug is absorbed, its rate of absorption decreases, whereas its rate of elimination increases. Consequently, the difference between the two rates diminishes. However, as long as the rate of absorption exceeds that of elimination the plasma concentration continues to rise. Eventually, a time t_{max}, is reached when the rate of elimination matches the rate of absorption; the concentration is then at a maximum, C_{max}. Subsequently, the rate of elimination exceeds the rate of absorption and the plasma concentration declines.

The peak plasma concentration is always lower following extravascular administration than the initial value following an equal i.v. bolus dose. In the former case, at the peak time some drug remains at the absorption site and some has been eliminated, while the entire dose is in the body immediately following the i.v. dose. Beyond the peak time, the plasma concentration exceeds that following i.v. administration of the same dose because of the continual entry of drug into the body.

Frequently, the rising portion of the plasma concentration-time curve is called the *absorption phase* and the declining portion, the *elimination phase*. As will be seen, this description may be misleading. Also, if bioavailability is low, the drug concentration may remain lower than that observed after i.v. administration at all times.

Lag time, the delay between drug administration and the beginning of absorption, may be particularly important when a rapid onset of effect is desired. The lag time can be anywhere from a few minutes to many hours. Long lag times have been observed following ingestion of enteric-coated tablets. The coating is resistant to the gastric environment, thus protecting an acid-labile drug or preventing gastric irritation by a drug. Factors contributing to the lag time are the delay in emptying the product from the stomach and the time taken for the protective coating to dissolve or to swell and release the inner contents into the intestinal fluids. Once absorption begins, however, it may be as rapid as with uncoated tablets. Clearly, enteric-coated products should not be used when a prompt and predictable response is desired. A method for estimating lag time is discussed in Appendix I–C.

Bioavailability and *area* are also important factors. As discussed more fully in Chaps. 7 and 9, the completeness of absorption is of primary importance in therapeutic situations.

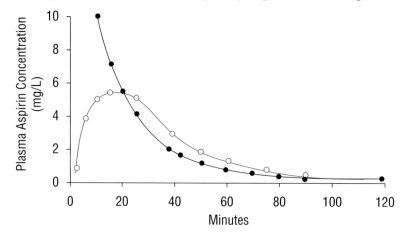

Fig. 4–2. Aspirin (650 mg) was administered as an intravenous bolus (●) and as an oral solution (○) on separate occasions to the same individual. Absorption causes a delay and a lowering of the peak concentration (1 mg/L = 5.5 µM). (Modified from the data of Rowland, M., Riegelman, S., Harris, P. A., and Sholkoff, S.D.: Absorption kinetics of aspirin in man following oral administration of an aqueous solution. J. Pharm. Sci., 67:379–385, 1972. Adapted with permission of the copyright owner.)

The bioavailability, F, is proportional to the total area under the plasma concentration-time curve (AUC) irrespective of its shape. This must be so. Recall from Chap. 3 that:

$$\text{Total amount eliminated} = \text{Clearance} \cdot AUC \qquad\qquad 2$$

but the total amount eliminated is the amount absorbed, $F \cdot \text{Dose}$, therefore:

$$F \cdot \text{Dose} = \text{Clearance} \cdot AUC \qquad\qquad 3$$

$$\begin{array}{cc}\text{Amount} & \text{Total amount} \\ \text{absorbed} & \text{eliminated}\end{array}$$

Thus, knowing dose, clearance, and area, bioavailability may be determined.

Changing Dose

Unless absorption half-life or bioavailability is altered, increasing the dose produces a proportional increase in plasma concentration at all times. The value of t_{max} remains unchanged, but C_{max} increases proportionally with dose.

Changing Absorption Kinetics

Alterations in either absorption or disposition produce changes in the time profiles of the amount in the body and the plasma concentration. This point is illustrated by the three situations depicted in the semilogarithmic plots of Fig. 4–3 involving only a change in the

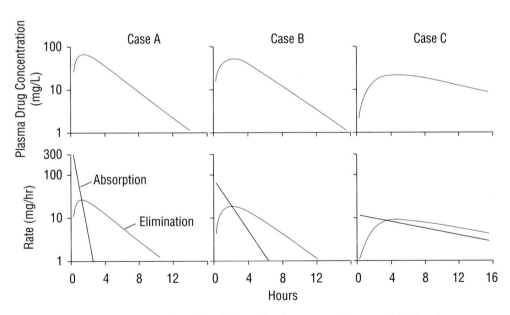

Fig. 4–3. A slowing (from left to right) of drug decline at the absorption site (lower graphs) delays the attainment and decreases the magnitude of the peak plasma drug concentration (top graphs). In Cases A and B (bottom two graphs), absorption (black line) is a faster process than elimination (colored line). In Case C (third graph on bottom), absorption (black line) rate limits elimination so that decline of drug in plasma reflects absorption rather than elimination; because there is a net elimination of drug during the decline phase, the rate of elimination is slightly greater than the rate of absorption. In all three cases, bioavailability is 1.0 and clearance is unchanged. Consequently, the areas under the plasma concentration-time curves (corresponding linear plots of the top three graphs) are identical. The $AUCs$ of the linear plots of the rate data are also equal because the integral of the rate of absorption, amount absorbed, equals the integral of the rate of elimination, amount eliminated.

absorption half-life. All other factors (bioavailability, clearance, and volume of distribution and hence elimination half-life) remain constant.

In Case A, the most common situation, absorption half-life is much shorter than elimination half-life. In this case, by the time the peak is reached, most of the drug has been absorbed and little has been eliminated. Thereafter, decline of drug in the body is determined primarily by the disposition of the drug, that is, *disposition is the rate-limiting step*. The half-life estimated from the decline phase is, therefore, the elimination half-life.

In Case B, absorption half-life is longer than in Case A but still shorter than elimination half-life. The peak occurs later because it takes longer for the amount in the body to reach the value at which rate of elimination matches rate of absorption; the C_{max} is lower because less drug has been absorbed by that time. Even so, absorption is still essentially complete before the majority of drug has been eliminated. Consequently, disposition remains the rate-limiting step, and the terminal half-life remains the elimination half-life.

Absorption Rate-Limited Elimination

Occasionally, absorption half-life is much longer than elimination half-life, and Case C prevails (Fig. 4–3). The peak occurs later and is lower than in the two previous cases. The half-life of decline of drug in the body now corresponds to the absorption half-life. During the rise to the peak, the rate of elimination increases and eventually, at the peak, equals the rate of absorption. However, in contrast to the previous situations, absorption is so slow that much of the drug remains to be absorbed well beyond the peak time. The drug is either at the absorption site or has been eliminated; little is in the body. In fact, during the decline phase, the drug is eliminated as fast as it is absorbed. *Absorption is now the rate-limiting step*. Under these circumstances, since the rate of elimination essentially matches the rate of absorption, the following approximation ($\approx$) can be written

$$\underset{\substack{\text{Rate of} \\ \text{elimination}}}{k \cdot A} \quad \approx \quad \underset{\substack{\text{Rate of} \\ \text{absorption}}}{ka \cdot Aa} \qquad\qquad 4$$

that is,

$$\underset{\substack{\text{Amount} \\ \text{in body}}}{\text{Amount}} \approx \left(\frac{ka}{k}\right) \cdot \underset{\substack{\text{Amount} \\ \text{remaining to} \\ \text{be absorbed}}}{} \qquad\qquad 5$$

Accordingly, amount in the body (and plasma concentration) during the decline phase is directly proportional to the amount remaining to be absorbed. For example, when amount remaining to be absorbed falls by one-half, so does amount in body. However, the time for this to occur is the absorption half-life.

Absorption influences the kinetics of drug in the body; but what of the *AUC*? Because bioavailability and clearance were held constant, it follows from Eq. 3 that the *AUC* must be the same for Cases A, B, and C.

Distinguishing Absorption From Disposition Rate-Limited Elimination

Although disposition generally is rate-limiting, the preceding discussion suggests that caution may need to be exercised in interpreting the meaning of half-life determined from the decline phase following extravascular administration. Confusion is avoided if the drug is also given intravenously. In practice, however, i.v. dosage forms of many drugs do not exist for clinical use. Distinguishing between absorption and disposition rate-limitations is achieved by altering the absorption kinetics of the drug. This is most readily accomplished by giving the drug either in different dosage forms or by different routes. To illustrate this point, consider data for theophylline and penicillin G.

Food and water influence the oral absorption kinetics of theophylline but not the half-life of the decline phase (Fig. 4–4). Here then, disposition rate-limits theophylline elimination. In contrast, for penicillin, with a very short elimination half-life, intramuscular (i.m.) absorption can become rate-limiting by formulation of a sparingly soluble salt (Fig. 4–5).

Changing Disposition Kinetics

What happens to the plasma concentration-time profile of a drug when the absorption kinetics remain constant, but modifications in disposition occur? When clearance is reduced, but bioavailability remains constant, the AUC must increase; so must both the time and magnitude of the peak concentration. These events are depicted in Fig. 4–6. With a

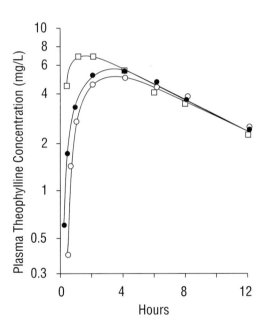

Fig. 4–4. Two tablets, each containing 130 mg theophylline, were taken by 6 healthy volunteers under various conditions. Absorption of theophylline was most rapid when the tablets were dissolved in 500 mL of water and taken on an empty stomach (□). Taking the tablets with 20 mL of water on an empty stomach (○) resulted in slower absorption than taking them with the same volume of water immediately following a standardized high carbohydrate meal (●). Despite differences in rates of absorption, however, the terminal half-life was the same (6.3 hours) and, therefore, it is the elimination half-life of theophylline (1 mg/L = 5.5 μM). (Modified from Welling, P.G., Lyons, L.L., Craig, W.A., and Trochta, G.A.: Influence of diet and fluid on bioavailability of theophylline. Clin. Pharmacol. Ther., 7:475–480, 1975.)

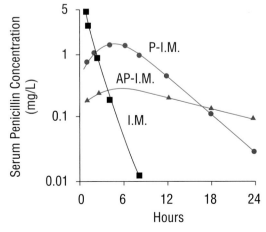

Fig. 4–5. Penicillin G (3 mg/kg) was administered intramuscularly to the same individual on different occasions as an aqueous solution (I.M.) and as procaine penicillin in oil (P-I.M.) and in oil with aluminum monostearate (AP-I.M.). The differing rates of decline of the plasma concentration of penicillin G point to an absorption rate-limitation when this antibiotic is given as the procaine salt in oil. Distinction between rate-limited absorption and rate-limited disposition following intramuscular administration of the aqueous solution can only be made by giving penicillin G intravenously. (1 mg/L = 3.0 μM). (Modified from Marsh. D.F.: Outline of Fundamental Pharmacology. Charles C. Thomas, Springfield, IL, 1951.)

reduction in clearance and, hence, elimination rate constant, a greater amount of drug must be absorbed, and the plasma concentration must be greater prior to the time when the rate of elimination equals the rate of absorption.

As shown in Fig. 4–7, the events are different when an increased volume of distribution is responsible for a longer elimination half-life. Under these circumstances the AUC is the same if bioavailability and clearance are unchanged. The peak occurs later and is lower, however. With a larger volume of distribution, more drug must be absorbed before the plasma concentration reaches a value at which the rate of elimination ($CL \cdot C$) equals the rate of absorption; the absorption rate is lower then and so is the plasma concentration.

Predicting Changes in Peak

Qualitative changes in C_{max} and t_{max} are difficult to predict when absorption or disposition is altered. To facilitate this prediction, a memory aid has been found to be useful. The basic principle of the method (Fig. 4–8) is simple; absorption increases and elimination decreases the amount of drug in the body. The faster the absorption process (measured by absorption rate constant), the greater is the slope of the absorption line, and the converse. The faster the elimination process (elimination rate constant), the steeper is the decline of the elimination line.

If absorption rate constant is increased, the new point of intersection indicates that peak amount is increased and that it occurs at an earlier time. If elimination rate constant is increased, the new point of intersection occurs at an earlier time, but at a lower amount.

The graph is designed for predicting changes in t_{max} and peak amount in the body. It applies as well to C_{max} with the exception of when volume of distribution is altered. An

Fig. 4–6. A twofold reduction in clearance increases the area under the plasma concentration-time (colored line, top graph) twofold compared to that of the control (black line) after a single extravascular dose. With no change in absorption kinetics (and hence absorption rate profile with time) (colored line, bottom graph), the rate of elimination (colored line, bottom graph) is observed to be lower at first but to become greater than that of the control (black line, bottom graph), as the area under the corresponding linear plots of these rate curves must be equal to the dose (see Fig. 4–3). The decrease in clearance causes the peak concentration to be greater and to occur at a later time (only slightly different here). The peak time occurs when the rate of elimination equals the rate of absorption (bottom graph). The terminal slope reflects the increased elimination half-life.

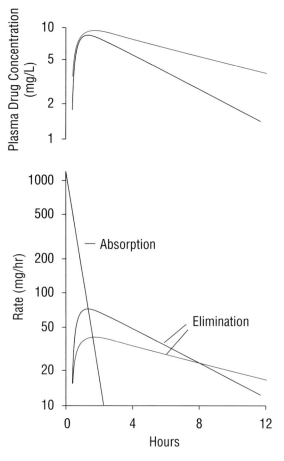

increase in volume of distribution causes a decrease in peak concentration, and the converse, as explained under Changing Disposition Kinetics. Specific relationships for estimating the values of C_{max} and t_{max} when absorption and disposition are first-order are given in Appendix I–C.

ASSESSMENT OF PHARMACOKINETIC PARAMETERS

How some parameter values are estimated following extravascular administration can be appreciated by considering both the plasma concentration-time curves in Fig. 4–9, obtained

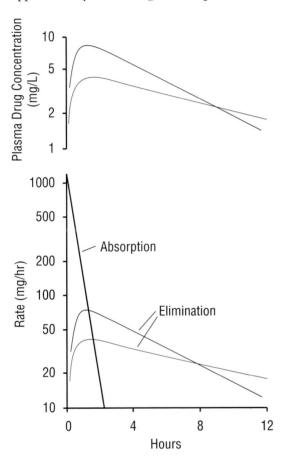

Fig. 4–7. A twofold increase in the volume of distribution causes a twofold increase in the elimination half-life and delays the time at which the peak plasma concentration occurs (colored line, top graph) compared to the control observation (black line) after a single extravascular dose. With no change in clearance, area (under linear concentration-time plot) is unchanged and peak concentration is thereby reduced. Because of a lower concentration, rate of elimination is initially slowed (colored line, bottom graph), but since the amount eliminated is the same (the dose), rate of elimination eventually is greater than that of the control (black line, bottom graph).

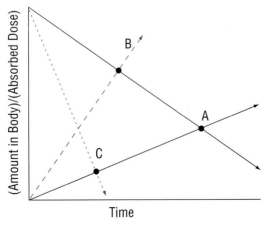

Fig. 4–8. Memory aid to assess changes in peak time and peak amount in the body after extravascular administration of a single dose when absorption or disposition is altered. The relative peak time and the relative peak amount are indicated by the intersection of the absorption and elimination lines (A) with slopes representing the absorption and elimination rate constants, respectively. The predictions for an increased absorption rate constant (colored line and point B) and an increased elimination rate constant (colored line and point C) are shown. (Modified from Øie, S. and Tozer, T.N.: A memory aid to assess changes in peak time and peak concentration with alteration in drug absorption or disposition. Am. J. Pharm. Ed., *46*:154–155, 1982.)

following i.m. and oral administrations of 500 mg of a drug, and the additional information in Table 4–1.

Plasma Data Alone

Bioavailability. Supplemental data from i.v. administration allow calculation of bioavailability, F. The total AUC following extravascular administration is divided by the area following an i.v. bolus, appropriately correcting for dose. The basis for this calculation, which assumes that *clearance remains constant*, is as follows:

Intravenous (i.v.) dose

$$\text{Dose}_{i.v.} = \text{Clearance} \cdot AUC_{i.v.} \qquad 6$$

Extravascular (e.v.) dose

$$F_{e.v.} \cdot \text{Dose}_{e.v.} = \text{Clearance} \cdot AUC_{e.v.} \qquad 7$$

which upon division yields

$$F_{e.v.} = \left(\frac{AUC_{e.v.}}{AUC_{i.v.}}\right)\left(\frac{\text{Dose}_{i.v.}}{\text{Dose}_{e.v.}}\right) \qquad 8$$

For example, appropriately substituting the area measurements in Table 4–1 into Eq. 8

Fig. 4–9. A 500-mg dose is given intramuscularly (●—●) and orally (○· · ·○) to the same subject on separate occasions. The drug is less bioavailable and is absorbed more slowly from the gastrointestinal tract. A parallel decline, however, implies that disposition is rate-limiting in both instances.

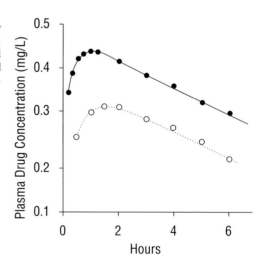

Table 4–1. Data Obtained Following Administration of 500 mg of a Drug in Solution by Different Routes

	PLASMA DATA		URINE DATA
ROUTE	AUC (mg·hr/L)	HALF-LIFE; DECAY PHASE (min)	CUMULATIVE AMOUNT EXCRETED UNCHANGED (mg)
Intravenous	7.6	190	152
Intramuscular	7.4	185	147
Oral	3.5	193	70

indicates that the bioavailability of the i.m. dose is 97%. Virtually all drug injected into muscle is absorbed systemically. In contrast, only 46% is bioavailable when drug is given orally in solution.

An alternative method of estimating bioavailability, which gives the same answer, is to substitute the value for clearance directly into Eq. 7. Clearance can be estimated from blood (or plasma) data following either an i.v. bolus dose or a constant-rate i.v. infusion (Chap. 6).

Relative bioavailability is determined when there are no i.v. data. Cost, stability, solubility limitations, and potential hazards are major reasons for the lack of an i.v. preparation. Relative bioavailability is determined by comparing different dosage forms, different routes of administration, or different conditions (e.g., diet, disease state). As with the calculation of bioavailability, clearance is assumed to be constant.

Thus, taking the general case:

Dosage form A

$$F_A \cdot Dose_A = Clearance \cdot AUC_A \qquad\qquad 9$$

Amount   Total amount
absorbed   eliminated

Dosage form B

$$F_B \cdot Dose_B = Clearance \cdot AUC_B \qquad\qquad 10$$

So that,

$$\text{Relative bioavailability} = \frac{F_A}{F_B} = \left(\frac{AUC_A}{AUC_B}\right)\left(\frac{Dose_B}{Dose_A}\right) \qquad\qquad 11$$

The reference dosage form chosen is usually the one with the highest bioavailability, that is, the one having the highest area-to-dose ratio. In the example considered, this is the i.m. dose; the relative bioavailability of the oral dose is then 46%. If only two oral doses had been compared, they may have been equally, albeit poorly, bioavailable. It should be noted that all the preceding relationships hold, irrespective of route of administration, rate of absorption, or shape of the curve. Constancy of clearance is the only requirement.

Fraction Eliminated. Based on the relationship between area and amount eliminated presented in Chap. 3, *AUC* up to a given time, for example, t_{max}, reflects the amount eliminated up to that time (see Fig. 4–10). The area beyond t_{max} reflects the amount remaining to be eliminated. The latter area represents drug in the body if absorption is fast compared to elimination, because absorption is essentially finished. Conversely, it approximates amount remaining to be absorbed if absorption is rate-limiting.

Other Pharmacokinetic Parameters. Given only extravascular data, it is sometimes difficult to estimate pharmacokinetic parameters. Indeed, no pharmacokinetic parameter can be determined confidently from observations following only a single oral dose. Consider: Area can be calculated without knowing bioavailability, but clearance cannot. Similarly, although a half-life can be ascribed to the decay phase, without knowing whether absorption or disposition is rate-limiting, the value cannot be assigned to either absorption or elimination. Without knowing any of the foregoing parameters, the volume of distribution clearly cannot be calculated.

Fortunately, there is a sufficient body of data to determine at least the elimination half-life of most drugs. Failure of food, dosage form, and, in the example in Fig. 4–7, route of administration to affect the terminal half-life indicate that this must be the elimination half-life. Also, a drug is often fully bioavailable ($F = 1$) from i.m. or subcutaneous sites. Hence, clearance can be calculated knowing area (Eq. 3), and the volume of distribution can be estimated once the elimination half-life is known. Consider, for example, just the i.m. data in Table 4–1. Clearance, obtained by dividing dose (500 mg) by AUC (7.4 mg-hr/L), is 1.1 L/min. Dividing clearance by the elimination rate constant (0.693/185 min) gives the volume of distribution, in this case 300 L.

Previously, a range of likely absorption half-lives was quoted. The values were estimated indirectly from plasma concentration-time data. Direct measurements of absorption kinetics are impossible because plasma is the site of measurement for both absorption and disposition. To calculate the kinetics of absorption, a method must therefore be devised to separate these two processes. Two relatively simple methods for achieving this separation are discussed in Appendix I-C.

Urine Data Alone

Given only urine data, neither clearance nor volume of distribution can be calculated. If renal clearance of drug is constant, rate of drug excretion is proportional to its plasma concentration, and under these circumstances, theoretically, excretion rate data can be treated in a manner similar to that for plasma data. In practice, during the first collection of urine, usually 1 or 2 hr after drug administration, absorption of many well-absorbed drugs is virtually finished. A shorter collection interval is needed to characterize absorption kinetics but is impractical because of incomplete emptying of the bladder and an inability of a subject to produce a urine sample on demand so frequently. Urinary excretion rate data are then often of little use in estimating absorption kinetics.

Cumulative urine data can be used to estimate bioavailability. The method requires that the value of fe remains constant. Recall from Chap. 3 that fe is the ratio of the total amount excreted unchanged (Ae_∞) to the total amount absorbed.

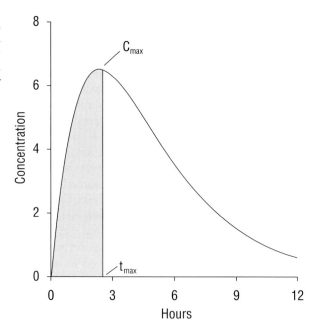

Fig. 4–10. The AUC up to t_{max}, the time of occurrence of the highest concentration, C_{max}, relative to the total AUC represents the amount eliminated at t_{max} relative to the total amount ultimately eliminated (see Fig. 3–3).

$$fe = \frac{Ae_\infty}{F \cdot Dose}$$ 12

Then, using the subscripts A and B to denote two treatments, it follows that

$$F_A \cdot Dose_A = Ae_{\infty,A}/fe$$ 13

$$F_B \cdot Dose_B = Ae_{\infty,B}/fe$$ 14

Amount   Total amount
absorbed   eliminated

which upon division gives:

$$\frac{F_A}{F_B} = \left(\frac{Ae_{\infty,A}}{Ae_{\infty,B}}\right) \cdot \left(\frac{Dose_B}{Dose_A}\right)$$ 15

The ratio of the dose-normalized cumulative amount excreted unchanged is therefore the ratio of the bioavailabilities. When Dose B is given intravenously, the ratio is the bioavailability of the drug. Otherwise the ratio gives the relative bioavailability. For example, from the cumulative urinary excretion data in Table 4–1, it is apparent that the i.m. dose is almost completely bioavailable; the corresponding value for the oral dose is only 46% [(70 mg/152 mg) $\times$ 100]. Notice that, as expected if fe is constant, this value is the same as that estimated from plasma data.

Urine data alone can be particularly useful for estimating bioavailability when the fraction excreted unchanged approaches 1. Under this condition, changes in renal clearance (and hence total clearance) affect AUC, but not the amount excreted, which is a direct measure of amount absorbed. The major problem here is in ensuring complete urine collection until virtually all the absorbed drug has been excreted.

Plasma and Urine Data

The renal clearance of a drug can be estimated when both plasma and urine data exist. The approach is identical to that taken for an i.v. dose (Chap. 3). Since no knowledge of bioavailability is required, the estimate of renal clearance from combined plasma and urine data following extravascular administration is as accurate as that obtained following i.v. drug administration.

BIOEQUIVALENCE

Laws mandate that new drug products be safe and effective. If a new product of a drug has the same molar dose and is of similar formulation to one already shown to be safe and effective, such laws allow marketing of the new product if it shows bioequivalence, i.e., similar efficacy and safety. The major concern is *switchability*, the ability of a patient to exchange one product for the other. Two products are considered to be bioequivalent if the concentration-time profiles are so similar that they are unlikely to produce clinically relevant differences in either therapeutic or adverse effects. The common measures used to assess differences in absorption are AUC, C_{max}, and t_{max}.

In practice, C_{max} and t_{max} are estimated from the highest concentration measured and the time of its occurrence. As the plasma concentration-time curve is quite flat near the peak and because of assay variability, the value of t_{max} chosen may not be a good representation of the actual value. Furthermore, the accuracy of the t_{max} estimate is limited by samples being obtained only at discrete times.

Bioequivalence testing usually arises when a patent on an innovator's drug expires. Other manufacturers may then wish to market the same formulation of the drug. Formulations that are bioequivalent with that of the innovator and bearing the generic name of the drug are called *generic* products. Bioequivalence testing is also performed during the course of development of new drugs, when a formulation is changed, or when the site or method of manufacture is altered.

STUDY PROBLEMS

(Answers to Study Problems are in Appendix II.)

1. Identify each of the statements below that are correct (see Fig. 4–8). For the one, or more, that is not correct, state why it is not or supply a qualification.
   a. All other parameters remaining unchanged, the slower the absorption process, the higher is the peak plasma concentration after a single oral dose.
   b. After a single oral dose, an increase in bioavailability causes the peak time to shorten.
   c. For a given drug in a subject, AUC is proportional to the amount of drug absorbed.
   d. If $ka \ll k$, then the terminal slope of the plasma concentration versus time curve reflects absorption, not elimination.
2. Graffner et al. (Graffner, C., Johnsson, G., and Sjögren, J.: Pharmacokinetics of procainamide intravenously and orally as conventional and slow-release tablets. Clin. Pharmacol. Ther., *17*:414–423, 1975), in evaluating different dosage forms of procainamide, obtained the following AUC and cumulative urine excretion data listed in Table 4–2.

Table 4-2.

ROUTE	DOSE (mg)	AUC (mg·hr/L)	AMOUNT EXCRETED (0–48 hr) (mg)
i.v.	500	13.1	332
Oral			
Formulation 1	1000	20.9	586
Formulation 2	1000	19.9	554

   a. Estimate both bioavailability and relative bioavailability of formulation 2 from both plasma and urine data. What are the assumptions made in your calculations?
   b. The half-life of procainamide found in this study was 2.7 hr. Was the urine collected over a long enough time interval to obtain a good estimate of the cumulative amount excreted at infinite time?
   c. Does renal clearance of procainamide vary much among the three treatments?
3. Depicted in Fig. 4–11 are curves of plasma concentration and amount in the body with time following the oral ingestion of a single dose of a drug. First draw five pairs of curves identical to those in Fig. 4–11. Then, draw another curve on each pair of these curves that shows the effect of each of the following alterations in pharmacokinetic parameters. In each case, the dose administered and all other parameters (among F, ka, V, and CL) remain unchanged.

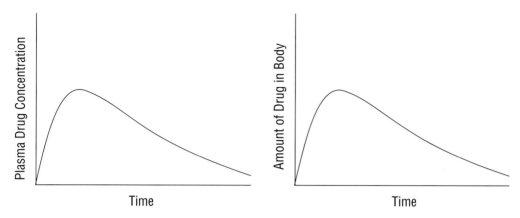

Fig. 4–11.

    a. *F* decreased

    b. *ka* increased

    c. *CL* increased, *k* increased by same factor

    d. *CL* decreased, *k* decreased by same factor

    e. *V* increased, *k* decreased by same factor

4. Kampf et al. studied the pharmacokinetics of recombinant human erythropoietin, a glycosylated protein (M.W. = 34,000 g/mole) used to increase red blood cell formation, in patients with end-stage renal disease after single i.v. and subcutaneous (s.c.) administrations of 40 units/kg on separate occasions. Table 4–3 lists the salient findings of these studies. The mean weight of the patients was 60 kg.

Table 4–3. Mean AUC, Maximum Plasma Concentration, and Terminal Half-life of Erythropoietin in End-Stage Renal Disease Patients Following i.v. and s.c.[A] Administration

ADMINISTRATION	AUC (Units·hr/L)	MAXIMUM CONCENTRATION (Units/L)	TIME OF MAXIMUM CONCENTRATION	TERMINAL HALF-LIFE (hr)
Intravenous	3010	417	5 min[b]	6.7
Subcutaneous	1372	40.5	12 hr	16.1

[A]Abstracted from Kampf, D., Eckardt, K.U., Fischer, H.C., Schmalisch, C., Ehmer, B., and Schostak, M.: Pharmacokinetics of recombinant human erythropoietin in dialysis patients after single and multiple subcutaneous administration. Nephron, 61:393–398, 1992.
[b]Time when first blood sample was taken.

    a. Determine the clearance and volume of distribution of this drug.

    b. Calculate the bioavailability of erythropoietin after s.c. administration in these patients. How might you explain your answer?

    c. The maximum concentration observed was much lower after the s.c. dose. How do you explain this observation?

5. Channer and Roberts (1985) studied the effect of delayed esophageal transit on the absorption of acetaminophen. Each of 20 patients awaiting cardiac catheterization swallowed a single tablet containing acetaminophen (500-mg) and barium sulfate. The first 11 subjects swallowed the tablet while lying down; in 10 of these subjects, transit of the tablet was delayed, as visualized by fluoroscopy. In the other 9 subjects who swallowed the tablet while standing, it entered the stomach immediately. In both groups the tablet was taken with a sufficient volume of water to ease swallowing. Table 4–4 lists the average plasma acetaminophen data obtained over 6 hr after swallowing the tablet.

Table 4–4.[a]

TIME (min)	PLASMA ACETAMINOPHEN CONCENTRATION (mg/L)[b]	
	SUBJECTS STANDING	SUBJECTS LYING DOWN
0	0	0
10	2.1	0.1
20	5.6	0.3
30	5.8	1.1
40	6.3	1.9
50	4.7	2.8
60	4.1	3.2
90	3.5	3.9
120	2.8	3.1
150	2.2	2.9
180	1.7	1.8
210	1.8	1.7
240	1.5	1.5
360	0.75	0.7

[a]Abstracted from Channer, K.S. and Roberts, C.J.C.: Effect of delayed esophageal transit on acetaminophen absorption. Clin. Pharmacol. Ther., *37*:72–76, 1985.
[b]One mg/L = 6.6 µM.

  a. What effect does delayed esophageal transit have on the speed and extent of absorption of acetaminophen?
  b. What process, absorption or disposition, rate-limits the decline in plasma drug concentration?
  c. Acetaminophen is used for the relief of pain. Do the findings of this study affect the recommendation for the use of this drug?
6. Beshyah et al. (Beshyah, S.A., Anyaoku, V., Niththyananthan, R., Sharp, P., and Johnston, D.G.: The effect of subcutaneous injection site on absorption of human growth hormone: Abdomen versus thigh. Clin. Endocrinol., 35:409–412, 1991) examined the effect of s.c. injection site on the absorption of human growth hormone. Table 4–5 lists the mean serum concentrations in 11 subjects observed during the first 12 hr after the administration of 4 IU (international units) of biosynthetic human growth hormone. The drug was injected, on separate occasions, into a lifted fold of skin on the anterior thigh and a lower quadrant of the abdomen.

Table 4–5. Mean Serum Concentrations of Growth Hormone for 12 hr following s.c. Injection of 4 IU in the Abdomen and Thigh

TIME (hr) INJECTION SITE	0	1	2	3	4	5	6	7	8	9	10	11	12
					SERUM CONCENTRATION (milliunits/L)								
Abdomen	<2	34	55	92	84	75	74	51	31	24	20	12	8
Thigh	<2	16	27	27	37	28	28	23	20	19	14	12	10

  a. Is there information in these data, gleaned from graphical analysis, to suggest whether absorption or disposition of growth hormone rate-limits the terminal decline? Briefly discuss.
  b. Many proteins given subcutaneously or intramuscularly are partially degraded within the lymphatic system before reaching the systemic circulation. Calculate the relative bioavailability of the drug after s.c. injection into the thigh (relative to abdomen).
  c. The clearance of growth hormone has been reported in the literature to average about 5 L/hr. Roughly estimate the bioavailability of the drug following abdominal s.c. injection.

7. Phenylethylmalonide (PEMA) is one of the major metabolites of the antiepileptic drug primidone. As part of a program to assess the potential use of PEMA as an antiepileptic drug itself, its pharmacokinetics were studied following i.v. and oral administration of 500 mg. Table 4–6 below lists the resultant plasma concentrations in one subject. Also, 81% of the i.v. dose was recovered in urine unchanged.

Table 4–6. Plasma Concentrations following i.v. and Oral Administration of 500 mg of PEMA to a Subject[a]

TIME (hr)		0.33	0.5	0.67	1	1.5	2	4	6	10	16	24	32	48
Plasma concentration	i.v.	14.7	12.6	11.0	—	9.0	8.2	7.9	6.6	6.2	4.6	3.2	2.3	1.2
(mg/L)	oral	—	2.4	—	3.8	4.2	4.6	8.1	5.8	5.1	4.1	3.0	2.3	1.3

[a]Abstracted from Pisani, F., and Richens, A.: Pharmacokinetics of phenylethylmalonamide (PEMA) after oral and intravenous administration. Clin. Pharmacokinet., 8:272–276, 1983.

a. From a semilogarithmic plot of the plasma concentrations, estimate the elimination half-life of PEMA in the subject.
b. Calculate the total *AUC* following i.v. and oral administration.
c. From the i.v. data, estimate the clearance and volume of distribution of PEMA.
d. Calculate the oral bioavailability of the drug.
e. Calculate the renal clearance.

8. Rowland *et al.* (Rowland, M., Epstein, W., and Riegelman, S.: Absorption kinetics of griseofulvin in man. J. Pharm. Sci., 57:984–989, 1968) gave griseofulvin orally, 0.5 g of a micronized drug formulation and, on another occasion intravenously, 100 mg, to volunteers. The plasma concentration-time data obtained in one subject are given in Table 4–7 below.

Table 4–7.

	ROUTE	TIME (hr)	0	1	2	3	4	5	7	8	12	24	28	32	35	48
Plasma Griseofulvin Concentration	i.v.		0	1.4	1.1	0.98	0.90	0.80	—	0.68	0.55	0.37	—	0.24	—	0.14
(mg/L)[A]	Oral		0	0.4	0.95	1.15	1.15	1.05	1.2	1.2	0.90	1.05	0.90	0.85	0.80	0.50

[A]One mg/L = 2.8 μM.

From appropriate plots and calculations, what can be concluded from these data with respect to:
a. Rate of absorption of griseofulvin with time on oral administration in this individual?
b. Completeness of absorption?

9. Kostenbauder et al. (1975) measured plasma phenytoin concentrations after the administration of sodium phenytoin intramuscularly (500 mg) and intravenously (250 mg). The average data obtained in 12 subjects, each of whom received both treatments, are listed in Table 4–8.

Table 4–8.[a]

TIME (hr)	ROUTE	0	1	2	4	6	8	12	24	48	72	96	120
Plasma Phenytoin Concentration	Intramuscular	0	3.0	3.2	3.5	3.2	3.6	3.8	4.1	3.2	1.6	0.8	0.4
(mg/L)[b]	Intravenous	5.6	5.4	5.2	4.9	—	3.9	3.2	2.2	0.88	0.42	—	—

[a]Abstracted from Kostenbauder, H.B., Rapp, R.P., McGovren, J.P., Foster, T.S., Perrier, D.G., Blacker, H.M., Hulon, W.C., and Kinkel, A.W.: Bioavailability and single-dose pharmacokinetics of intramuscular phenytoin. Clin. Pharmacol. Ther., 18:449–456, 1975.
[b]One mg/L = 4.0 μM.

a. Estimate the bioavailability of phenytoin from the i.m. site based on area comparisons.
b. From an appropriate plot of the data, comment on the process limiting the decline of the plasma phenytoin concentration following i.m. administration.
c. The authors analyzed the plasma concentration-time data and found that, following i.m. administration, 23% of the dose was absorbed within the first hour, and thereafter absorption was much slower. The cumulative absorption data are shown in Table 4–9. After the rapid absorption in the first hour, is the subsequent absorption better characterized by a zero-order or a first-order process?

Table 4-9.

TIME (hr)	1	6	19	40	65
Percent of bioavailable drug absorbed from i.m. site	23	40	60	80	90

THERAPEUTIC REGIMENS

THERAPEUTIC RESPONSE AND TOXICITY

OBJECTIVES

The reader will be able to:

1. Explain why effect (desired or toxic) of a drug is often better correlated with plasma concentration than with dose.

2. Define the terms: graded response, all-or-none response, therapeutic concentration range, utility curve, and tolerance.

3. List the range of plasma concentrations associated with therapy for any of the drugs given in Table 5–2.

4. Discuss briefly situations in which poor plasma drug concentration–response relationships are likely to occur.

5. Explain briefly why modality of administration of a given daily dose can affect therapeutic outcome.

The rational design of safe and efficacious dosage regimens is now examined. In this section, fundamental aspects of dosage regimens are covered primarily from the point of view of treating a patient population with a given disease. It is realized, of course, that individuals vary in their responses to drugs, and subsequently, in Section Four, focus is turned toward the establishment of dosage regimens in individual patients.

A therapeutic dosage regimen is basically derived from the kinds of information shown in Table 5–1. One consideration includes those factors that relate to both efficacy and safety of the drug, that is, its pharmacodynamics and toxicology. Another consideration is how the body acts on the drug and its dosage form, the essence of pharmacokinetics. A third consideration is that of the clinical state of the patient and his or her total therapeutic regimen. A fourth category includes all other factors such as genetic differences, tolerance, and drug interactions. All of these determinants are, of course, interrelated and interdependent.

Dosage regimens are designed to produce a therapeutic objective. This objective may be achieved by various modalities of drug administration, extending from a single occasional dose to continuous and constant input. An example of the former is the use of aspirin to treat an occasional headache; the continuous i.v. infusion of heparin to maintain a desired degree of anticoagulation is an example of the latter. More commonly, drugs are administered repeatedly in discrete doses. The frequency and duration vary with the condition being treated. Some drugs are administered relatively infrequently, producing large fluctuations in the plasma concentration. Reasons for this approach include the development of tolerance to the drug and the need to produce high concentrations for short periods of time, as occurs in some antibiotic and anticancer chemotherapies. In other situations, maintenance of a relatively constant concentration of drug is needed. In all cases, attempts are made to minimize undesirable and toxic effects and prevent ineffective therapy.

Evidence exists that response is often better correlated with plasma concentration than with dose administered. Accordingly, it would seem to be most appropriate to apply pharmacokinetic principles to the design of dosage regimens. Thus, given pharmacokinetic data following a single dose, the plasma concentration or amount of drug in the body following any dosing scheme can be estimated. Ultimately, however, the value of a dosage regimen must be assessed by the therapeutic and toxic responses produced. Pharmacokinetics facilitates the achievement of an appropriate dosage regimen and serves as a useful means of evaluating existing dosage regimens.

In this chapter, various elements of the concentration–response relationship are explored. Principles for attaining and maintaining a therapeutic level of drug in the body are discussed in the subsequent two chapters of this section.

RESPONSE AND CONCENTRATION

Response may be as vague as a general feeling of improvement or as precise as a lowering of the diastolic blood pressure by 30 mm Hg.

Information relating concentration to response is obtained at three levels: *in vitro* experiments, animal studies, and investigations in human volunteers and patients. The last level is the most relevant to human drug therapy but, unfortunately, only limited information is often obtainable here about the nature of the drug–receptor interaction. *In vitro* experiments, which include studies of the action of drugs on enzymes, receptors, microorganisms, and isolated tissues and organs, serve this purpose best. However, in isolating the variables, many of the complex interrelationships that exist *in vivo* are destroyed. Animal studies bridge much of the gap between *in vitro* experimentation and human investigation. Studies in animals introduce both the variable time, with all that it connotes, and

Table 5-1. Determinants of a Dosage Regimen

ACTIVITY-TOXICITY	PHARMACOKINETICS
Therapeutic window	Absorption
Side effects	Distribution
Toxicity	Metabolism
Concentration–response relationships	Excretion

Dosage Regimen

CLINICAL FACTORS

STATE OF PATIENT	MANAGEMENT OF THERAPY	OTHER FACTORS
Age, weight	Multiple drug therapy	Route of administration
Condition being treated	Convenience of regimen	Dosage form
Existence of other disease states	Compliance of patient	Tolerance-dependence
		Pharmacogenetics-idiosyncrasy
		Drug interactions
		Cost

the elements of absorption and disposition as well as the feedback control systems that operate to maintain homeostasis. Animal studies are often most useful for evaluating the pharmacologic spectrum of activity of a potential therapeutic agent and for determining aspects of its toxicity profile. Irrespective of the level of information, however, the conclusion is the same: A relationship, although sometimes complex, exists between the concentration of active agent at the site of measurement and the response.

The majority of drugs used clinically act reversibly in that the effect is reversed upon reducing concentration at the site of action. Many responses produced are *graded*, so called because the magnitude of the response can be scaled or graded. An example of a graded response, shown in Fig. 5–1, is the improvement of pulmonary function produced by the bronchodilator terbutaline, after its s.c. administration. The intensity of the response varies with the drug concentration in plasma. Many other pharmacologic and toxic responses do not occur on a continuous basis; these are known as *quantal* or *all-or-none* responses. An obvious but extreme example is death. Another is the suppression of an arrhythmia. The arrhythmia either is or is not suppressed. Sometimes, a limit is set on a graded response below which an effect is said not to occur clinically. For example, a potentially toxic effect of antihypertensive therapy is an excessive lowering of blood pressure. The lowering of blood pressure produced by the antihypertensive agents is a graded response, but hypotensive toxicity is said to occur only if the blood pressure falls to too low a value. Here the clinical endpoint is all-or-none, but the pharmacologic response is graded.

Returning to terbutaline, Fig. 5–1 is a plot of the forced expiratory volume in 1 second, a measure of pulmonary function, against plasma concentration. The plot is characteristic of most graded response curves. A nearly linear relationship between the intensity of response and the concentration at low concentrations and a tendency to reach a maximal response at high concentrations are apparent.

Unlike a graded response, the correlation between a quantal response and concentration is explored by examining the *frequency* of the event with concentration. This is illustrated in Fig. 5–2 by a plot of frequency of the suppression of ventricular arrhythmias as a function of the plasma concentration of the antiarrhythmic agent procainamide. In most patients

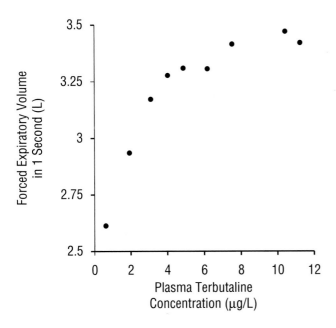

Fig. 5–1. The mean forced expiratory volume in 1 second (FEV_1) increases with the mean plasma concentration at preselected times in 10 patients given 0.75 mg of terbutaline subcutaneously. The improvement in pulmonary function increases with plasma concentration but appears to approach a limiting value. (Redrawn from Oosterhuis, B., Braat, P., Roos, C.M.J., and Van Boxtel, C.J.: Pharmacokinetic-pharmacodynamic modeling of terbutaline bronchodilation in asthma. Clin. Pharmacol. Ther., *40*:469–475, 1986.)

the arrhythmias are suppressed at concentrations of 2 to 8 mg/L. However, this belies the entire picture.

THERAPEUTIC PLASMA CONCENTRATION RANGE

Figure 5–3 shows the percent of those patients who did not respond to procainamide, those who responded, those who exhibited minor side effects, and those who exhibited serious toxicity. Side effects were considered minor when cessation of the drug was unnecessary and serious when disturbances of cardiovascular function or other adverse effects necessitated discontinuation of the drug. It should be noted in particular that serious toxicity begins to appear above 8 mg/L and occurs with increasing frequency at higher concentrations. Above 16 mg/L, the toxic effects may prove fatal. From these data, it can be concluded that the range of plasma concentrations of procainamide associated with effective therapy and without undue toxicity is 4 to 8 mg/L. This range is commonly known as the *therapeutic concentration range* of the drug.

Clearly, not all patients receiving procainamide for the treatment of ventricular arrhythmias need plasma concentrations between 4 and 8 mg/L. In a few, the arrhythmias are suppressed at concentrations below 4 mg/L; in others, toxicity occurs before efficacy, and for them procainamide is certainly not the drug of choice. Thus, a therapeutic concentration is most appropriately defined in terms of an individual patient's requirement. Usually, this information is unknown, and on initiating therapy, the therapeutic concentration must be estimated from consideration of the probability of therapeutic success within the typical patient population.

Also shown in Fig. 5–3 is a curve that represents the frequency of therapeutic effectiveness, i.e., the frequency of effective therapy minus the frequency of all toxic effects. This may be an inappropriate means of estimating the concentration at which therapeutic success is most probable. Perhaps the minor toxic effects should not be weighted equally against the desired response. Obviously, the major toxic effects should be given more weight. These are considerations requiring judgment.

Fig. 5–2. The concentration of procainamide was determined in over 3000 plasma samples obtained from 291 patients receiving this drug for the treatment of cardiac arrhythmias. The frequency, expressed as a percent of the number of plasma samples with which a serum concentration correlates with effective therapy, increases with each interval of increasing concentration. The value above each bar refers to the number of samples within the respective concentration range (1 mg (base)/L = 4.3 μM). (From Koch-Weser, J.: *In* Pharmacology and the Future: Problems in Therapy. Edited by G.T. Okita and G.H. Archeson. Karger, Basel, 1973, Vol. 3, pp. 69–85.)

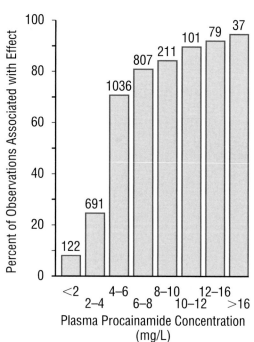

Therapeutic Window

Let us expand philosophically on this concept of weighting developed for procainamide using the information in Fig. 5–3, adding hypersensitivity and assigning values to the responses according to our best judgment. Figure 5–4 shows the probabilities of the responses, plus that of hypersensitivity, each weighted by a judgmental factor versus the logarithm of the plasma concentration. The factor is negative for undesirable effects and positive for desirable effects. On algebraically adding the weighted probabilities, a *utility curve* is obtained that simply shows the chance of therapeutic success as a function of the plasma concentration. Both low and high concentrations have a negative utility; i.e., at these concentrations, the drug is potentially more harmful than helpful. There is an optimal concentration (8 mg/L) at which therapeutic success is most likely, and there is a range of concentrations (about 4 to 10 mg/L) within which the chances of successful therapy are high. This is the *therapeutic window* or *therapeutic concentration range*. Precise limits, of course, are not definable, particularly considering the subjective nature of the utility curve. Each drug produces its own peculiar responses, and the weighting assigned to these responses differ, but both the incidence of the drug effects and the relative importance of each effect must be evaluated to determine the therapeutic concentration range.

There are problems associated with the acquisition of the incidence of the various responses. For example, the procainamide data were obtained in patients who were sometimes titrated with the drug. That is, the dosage was adjusted when the patient had not adequately responded or when toxicity was present. However, patients even on the usual

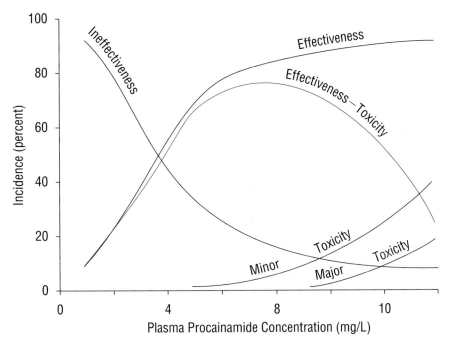

Fig. 5–3. Schematic representation of the frequency of ineffective therapy, effective therapy, minor side effects, serious toxicity, and "therapeutic effectiveness" with plasma concentration of procainamide in patients receiving this drug for the treatment of arrhythmias. Therapeutic effectiveness is defined arbitrarily as the difference in the frequency between effective therapy and toxic effects; the therapeutic effectiveness (colored line) of procainamide reaches a peak of 8 mg/L (1 mg/L = 4.3 µM). (Adapted from the data of Koch-Weser, J.: *In* Pharmacology and the Future: Problems in Therapy. Edited by G.T. Okita and G.H. Archeson. Karger, Basel, 1973, Vol. 3, pp. 69–85.)

dosage show a wide range of concentrations, leading one to question if selection of patients showing toxicity might have occurred. To avoid this bias, each of the patients should be titrated through all the responses. This is, of course, ethically unacceptable. Our information on toxicity must come from the patient who, for one reason or another, exhibits toxicity because the drug concentration is excessive or who has an unusual response at a low concentration.

For the majority of patients, knowledge of a drug's therapeutic plasma concentration range and pharmacokinetics should lead to a more rapid establishment of a safe and efficacious dosage regimen. However, the narrower this range, the more difficult is the maintenance of values within it. The plasma concentration ranges associated with successful therapy of specific conditions are shown in Table 5–2 for a number of representative drugs.

Several points are worth noting about the data in Table 5–2. First, for most of these drugs, the therapeutic concentration range is narrow; the upper and lower limits differ by a factor of only 2 or 3. Of course, for many other drugs, this concentration range is much wider. Second, some drugs are used to treat several diseases, and the therapeutic plasma concentration range may differ with the disease. For example, a lower concentration of theophylline is needed to abolish episodes of recurring apnea in premature infants than is needed to substantially improve pulmonary function in patients with chronic airway diseases. Next, the upper limit of the plasma concentration may be either, like nortriptyline, a result of diminishing effectiveness at higher concentrations without noticeable signs of increasing toxicity or, like cyclosporine, a result of the possibility of nephrotoxicity. The upper limit may also be due to limiting effectiveness of the drug, as with the use of salicylic acid to relieve pain. Finally, toxicity may be either an extension of the pharmacologic property of the drug or totally dissociated from its therapeutic effect. The hemorrhagic tendency associated with an excessive plasma concentration of the oral anticoagulant, war-

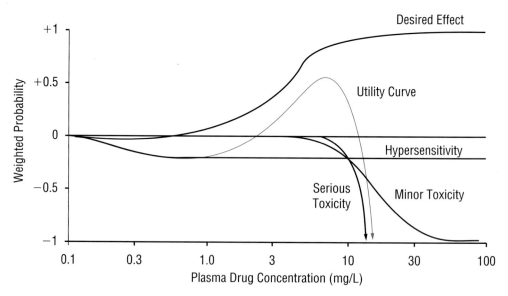

Fig. 5–4. Schematic diagram of the weighted probabilities of responses versus the plasma concentration of a drug. The probabilities from Fig. 5–3 (plus a hypothetical hypersensitivity reaction) are weighted by the following factors: desired effect, 1; hypersensitivity, −5; minor toxicity, −1; serious toxicity, −5. The algebraic sum of the weighted probabilities is the utility curve. According to this scheme, the highest weighted probability of therapeutic success occurs at 8 mg/L, and concentrations below 2 mg/L and above 12 mg/L are potentially more harmful than beneficial.

farin, is an example of the former; the ototoxicity caused by the antibiotic gentamicin is an example of the latter.

Distinction also needs to be made between the steepness of a concentration–response curve and the width of a therapeutic window. This point is illustrated schematically in Fig. 5–5. Figure 5–5A shows a drug with a wide therapeutic window. The wide window occurs despite steep concentration–response curves for both efficacy and toxicity. Here toxicity occurs at concentrations well above those needed to achieve maximum desired effect. The normal strategy would be to ensure that all patients receive a dosage regimen that produces plasma concentrations that achieve maximal efficiency without toxicity. Figure 5–5B shows a drug with a narrow therapeutic window. The narrow window occurs despite shallow concentration–response curves for both efficacy and toxicity. This narrowness arises because the response curves overlap well below maximal efficacy, so that it is difficult to find plasma concentrations that produce efficacy without some degree of limiting toxicity.

It is to be stressed that significant interindividual variability may occur in both the efficacy and toxicity response curves, leading to differences among individuals in the location and width of the therapeutic window. This should be kept in mind when considering the therapeutic windows listed in Table 5–2. The values are derived from patient populations requiring the drugs and apply to the average patient within those populations. Also, keep in mind that the ultimate objective is to treat each individual patient as efficaciously and safely as possible and not to keep his or her plasma concentrations within the rec-

Table 5–2. Representative Drugs and Their Plasma Concentrations Usually Associated With Successful Therapy

DRUG	DISEASE/CONDITION	THERAPEUTIC WINDOW (mg/L)	(µM)
Acetazolamide	Glaucoma	10–30	50–150
Amikacin	Gram-negative infection	12–25[a]	—
Amitriptyline	Depression	0.12–0.25[b]	0.43–0.90
Carbamazepine	Epilepsy	4–12	17–51
Cyclosporine	Organ transplantation	0.15–0.4[c]	0.13–0.34
Desipramine	Depression	0.12[d]	0.45
Digitoxin	Cardiac dysfunction	0.01–0.02	0.013–0.026
Digoxin	Cardiac dysfunction	0.0006–0.002	0.0008–0.003
Ethosuximide	Epilepsy	25–75	180–540
Gentamicin	Gram-negative infection	4–12[a]	7–21
Lidocaine	Ventricular arrhythmias	2–6	4–25
Lithium	Manic and recurrent depression	—	0.4–1.4[e]
Nortriptyline	Endogenous depression	0.05–0.15	0.2–0.6
Phenobarbital	Epilepsy	10–30	40–120
Phenytoin	Epilepsy	10–20	30–60
	Ventricular arrhythmias	10–20	30–60
Procainamide	Ventricular arrhythmias	4–8	17–34
Propranolol	Angina	0.02–0.2	0.08–0.8
Salicylic Acid	Aches and pains	20–100	150–750
	Rheumatoid arthritis	100–300	750–2200
	Rheumatic fever	250–400	1800–3000
Theophylline	Asthma and chronic obstructive airway diseases	6–20	33–100
	Apnea	5–10	28–55
Tobramycin	Gram-negative infection	4–12[a]	35–120
Warfarin	Thromboembolic diseases	1–4	3–13
Valproic Acid	Epilepsy	40–100	280–690
Vancomycin	Penicillin-resistant infection	5–15[f]	3.3–10

[a] Thirty minutes after a 30-min infusion.
[b] Parent drug plus N-desmethyl metabolite.
[c] Whole blood, trough concentration.
[d] Suggested threshold concentration.
[e] Milliequivalents/liter.
[f] Sample obtained just before next dose.

ommended therapeutic window. This window does serve as a useful guide, however, particularly in the absence of additional information about the individual.

Therapeutic Correlates

So far, plasma concentration has been assumed to be a better correlate of a drug's therapeutic response and toxicity, in a population of patients needing a drug, than any other measure. However, since doses are administered, why not use dose as a therapeutic correlate? Certainly, in most cases, response, plasma concentration, and amount of drug in the body all increase with dose. Still, plasma concentration is expected to be a better

Fig. 5–5. The width of a therapeutic window depends on the degree of overlap of the efficacy (black lines) and toxicity (colored lines) concentration-response curves. *A*, The therapeutic window (shaded) is wide despite steep concentration-response curves for both efficacy and toxicity, as there is virtually no overlap between the two response curves. *B*, The therapeutic window (shaded) is narrow because of a high degree of overlap between efficacy and toxicity even though both the response curves are shallow.

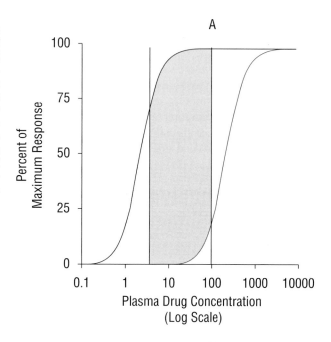

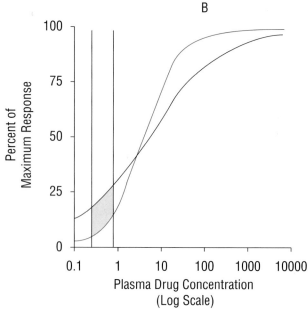

correlate than dosage. This must be true following a single dose of drug, since with dose alone no account is taken of time. It may also be true for continuous drug administration but for a different reason.

The objective of most drug therapy is to maintain a stable therapeutic response, usually by maintaining an effective plasma concentration. Figure 1–6 (Chap. 1, p. 6) shows the relationship between the steady-state plasma concentration and the rate of administration of phenytoin, expressed as the daily dose per kilogram of body weight. There are large interindividual deviations in the plasma concentration at any dosing rate; in the patient cohort studied, the plasma concentration ranged from nearly 0 to 50 mg/L when the dosing rate is 6 mg/day/kg of body weight. Had no correction been made for body weight, the deviations would have been even greater. In contrast, plasma concentration correlates reasonably well with effect. Thus, seizures are usually effectively controlled at concentrations between 10 and 20 mg/L; side effects occur with increasing frequency and severity as the plasma concentration exceeds 20 mg/L, as shown in Fig. 5–6. The first sign of toxicity is usually nystagmus, which appears above a concentration of approximately 20 mg/L; gait ataxia usually appears with a concentration approaching 30 mg/L, and prolonged drowsiness and lethargy may be seen at concentrations in excess of 40 mg/L.

For phenytoin, plasma concentration is a better correlate than dose during chronic administration because pharmacokinetics is the major source of variability between dose and response. For other drugs, such as ampicillin, pharmacokinetic variability within the patient population is relatively small, and variability in the concentration–response curve is large. In such cases, plasma concentration is no better a correlate with response than dose and indeed may be worse if, for example, metabolites contribute to activity and toxicity (see below, Additional Considerations).

ADDITIONAL CONSIDERATIONS

Despite the appeal, measurement of plasma concentration is relatively uncommon in clinical practice (See Concentration Monitoring, Chap. 18). The major reason is the wide margin of safety of many drugs with direct and simple means of assessing the therapeutic and toxic responses. Another is that plasma concentration often correlates poorly with measured response. Some examples of poor correlations with explanations, where known, follow. This subject is considered further in Chap. 20, Pharmacologic Response.

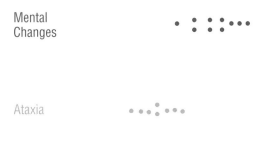

Mental Changes

Ataxia

Fig. 5–6. The severity of the untoward effects of phenytoin increases in proportion to its concentration in plasma (1 mg/L = 4.0 μM). (Modified from Kutt, H., Winters, W., Kokenge, R., and McDowell, F.: Diphenylhydantoin metabolism, blood levels, and toxicity. Arch. Neurol., 11:642–648, 1964. Copyright 1964, American Medical Association.)

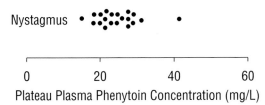

Nystagmus

0   20   40   60
Plateau Plasma Phenytoin Concentration (mg/L)

Active Metabolites

Unless active metabolites are also measured, poor correlations may exist. For example, based on its plasma concentration, alprenolol is more active as a β-blocker when given as a single oral dose than when administered intravenously. This drug is highly cleared by the liver, and so in terms of the parent drug, the oral dose is poorly bioavailable. However, large amounts of metabolites, including an active species, 4-hydroxyalprenolol, are formed during the absorption process, which explains the apparent discrepancy. The tricyclic antidepressant amitriptyline offers a second example. Its antidepressant activity correlates poorly with the plasma concentration of parent drug. Only when the contribution of its active desmethyl metabolite is also considered can useful correlations be established. Other examples of active metabolites and the implications with respect to their pharmacologic response are discussed in Chap. 21, Metabolite Kinetics.

Chirality

About 40% of drugs contain one or more asymmetric (chiral) centers in the molecule. For each center, there are two possible mirror images or enantiomers, the R- and S-forms, which often differ in their pharmacokinetic and pharmacodynamic properties. Because of difficulty and cost of separation, the majority of synthetic chiral drugs are marketed as racemic mixtures. Failure to use a stereospecific chemical assay to measure the individual enantiomers can therefore lead to problems when attempting to correlate plasma concentration with response following administration of the racemate. Even when a stereospecific assay is employed, it is not always easy to know how to combine the enantiomer concentrations to relate to response when both enantiomers contribute to activity. For example, although R-warfarin is less potent than S-warfarin, it can still produce full anticoagulation. Thus, response cannot be related simply to the sum of the concentrations of warfarin enantiomers.

Tolerance and Acquired Resistance

The effectiveness of a drug can diminish with continual use. Acquired resistance denotes the diminished sensitivity of a population of cells (microorganisms, neoplasms) to a chemotherapeutic agent; tolerance denotes a diminished pharmacologic responsiveness to a drug. The degree of acquired resistance varies; it may be complete, thereby rendering the agent, e.g., an antibiotic, ineffective against a microorganism. The degree of tolerance also varies but is never complete. For example, within days or weeks of its repeated use, subjects can develop a profound tolerance but not total unresponsiveness to the pharmacologic effects (euphoria, sedation, respiratory depression) of morphine. Tolerance can develop slowly; e.g., tolerance to the central nervous system effects of ethanol takes weeks. Tolerance can also occur acutely (tachyphylaxis). Thus, tolerance, expressed by a diminished cardiovascular responsiveness, develops within minutes following repetitive administration of many β-phenethylamine-type sympathomimetics, such as isoproterenol. At any moment, a correlation might be found between the intensity of response and the plasma concentration of the drug, but the relationship varies with time.

Single-Dose Therapy

One dose of aspirin can often relieve a headache, which does not return even when all the drug has been eliminated. Other examples of effective single-dose therapy include the use of isoproterenol to relieve an acute asthmatic attack, colchicine to treat an acute gouty attack, nitroglycerin to relieve acute episodes of angina, and morphine to relieve acute pain. Although the specific mechanism of action is often poorly understood, the overall effect is known; the drug returns an out-of-balance physiologic system to within normal bounds. Thereafter, feedback control systems within the body maintain homeostasis. The need for drug has now ended. In these instances of single-dose therapy, a correlation between effect and peak plasma concentration may exist, but beyond the peak, any such correlation is unlikely.

Duration Versus Intensity of Exposure

Some chemotherapeutic agents, e.g., methotrexate, exhibit peculiar relationships between response and dose. The response observed relates more closely to the duration of dosing than to the actual dose used or concentrations produced. This behavior for methotrexate can be explained by its activity as an antimetabolite. It inhibits dihydrofolate reductase, thereby preventing many methylation reactions in the body. These reactions can be inhibited for short periods of time, a few days, without causing irreversible damage. When the exposure is sufficiently prolonged, however, the damage is irreversible and potentially lethal.

Time Delays

It often takes some time for a measured response to fully reflect a given plasma concentration of drug. Until then, the continuously changing response makes any correlation between response and plasma concentration extremely difficult to establish. One source of the delay is the time required for equilibration to occur between drug in plasma and that at the site of action, usually in a tissue. This delay may be short if the drug enters the tissue rapidly; when effective, lidocaine suppresses ventricular arrhythmias within a few minutes of giving a bolus dose; thiopental induces anesthesia even more quickly. When the target organ resides in a slowly equilibrating tissue, the delay may be many hours. For example, the maximum cardiac effects of digoxin are not seen for an hour or more after administering an i.v. bolus of the drug.

Another source of delay can arise when the response monitored is an indirect measure of drug effect. A change in blood pressure is an indirect measure of either a change in peripheral resistance, in cardiac output, or in both. Plasma uric acid is another example; here, the direct effect is an alteration in uric acid synthesis or elimination. Yet another example of an indirect response is the change in the serum prothrombin complex activity produced by coumarin oral anticoagulants. The more direct effect of these anticoagulants is to inhibit synthesis of the prothrombin complex.

The delay between attainment of a plasma concentration and maximal indirect effect varies. Full response in blood pressure to a change in peripheral resistance or in cardiac output occurs within minutes, whereas maximal response of the prothrombin complex activity to warfarin is not seen for 1 to 2 days after an oral dose of this anticoagulant (Fig. 5–7).

Uric acid and the prothrombin complex are examples of endogenous materials. Such materials are continuously being renewed, with the pool size reflecting the balance between input and loss. The impact of changes in input and loss on the kinetics of endogenous compounds and the appropriate interpretation of such data are covered in greater detail in Chap. 23, Turnover Concepts.

MODALITY OF ADMINISTRATION AND THERAPEUTIC OUTCOME

As mentioned at the beginning of this chapter, maintenance of a plasma concentration is not always a desirable therapeutic objective. Sometimes, a fluctuating concentration is more desirable. Much depends on the pharmacodynamic features of efficacy and toxicity. This point is well illustrated with the antimicrobial agents. The purpose of antimicrobial therapy is the eradication of an infection with minimal toxicity. Figure 5–8 shows major differences in the effect of dosing frequency on the daily dose of ceftazidime and gentamicin required to produce 50% of maximal efficacy in pneumonia that is due to *Klebsiella pneumoniae* in neutropenic mice. Whereas decreasing the frequency of administration, and hence increasing the degree of fluctuation in plasma concentration, drastically diminished the efficacy of ceftazidime, it had minimal effect on gentamicin. The explanation lies in the different pharmacodynamic profiles of these two drugs.

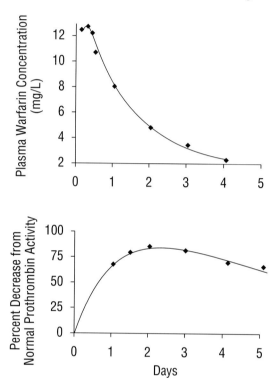

Fig. 5–7. The sluggish response in the plasma prothrombin complex activity to inhibition of its synthesis by warfarin reflects the indirect nature of the measurement and the slow elimination of this complex. For the first 2 days after giving a dose of warfarin, the complex activity steadily decreases. During the first day, the concentration of warfarin is sufficient to almost completely block complex synthesis. As warfarin concentration falls, the synthesis rate of the complex increases and by 48 hr equals the rate of degradation of the complex. Thereafter, with the synthesis rate exceeding the rate of degradation, the complex activity rises and eventually, when all the warfarin has been eliminated, returns to the normal prewarfarin steady-state level. The data points are the averages following the oral administration of 1.5 mg warfarin sodium per kg body weight in 5 male volunteers (1 mg/L = 3.3 μM). (From Nagashima, R., O'Reilly, R.A., and Levy, G.: Kinetics of pharmacologic effects in man: The anticoagulant action of warfarin. Clin. Pharmacol. Ther., *10*:22–35, 1969.)

Fig. 5–8. The influence of lengthening the dosing interval on the daily dose needed to produce 50% of maximal efficacy in treating pneumonia due to *Klebsiella pneumoniae* in neutropenic mice varies with the antimicrobial agent. Whereas no change in daily dose is needed with gentamicin (black curve), much larger doses of ceftazidime (colored curve) are needed when administered less frequently. (From Leggett, J.E., Fantin, B., Ebert, S.C., Totsuka, K., Vogelman, R., and Craig, W.F.: Comparative antibiotic dose-effect relationships of several dosing intervals in murine pneumonitis and thigh-infection models. J. Infect. Dis., *159*:281–292, 1989.)

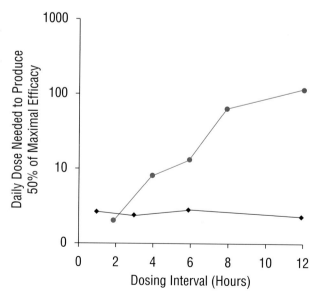

Ceftazidime, like other β-lactam antibiotics, exhibits only minimal concentration-dependent bactericidal activity, so that bacterial killing is more dependent on time above the minimal bactericidal concentration than on the magnitude of the drug concentration. Greater benefit is therefore achieved with more frequent administration that minimizes the possibility of the plasma concentration falling too low. An additional reason for frequent administration is that the duration of the postantibiotic effect—whereby bacterial growth is suppressed for some time after intermittent exposure of bacteria to the antimicrobial agent—is very short with the β-lactam antibiotics.

In contrast to ceftazidime, gentamicin and other aminoglycosides produce a prolonged postantibiotic effect. They also exhibit marked concentration-dependent killing over a wide range of concentrations with higher values having a more pronounced effect on the rate and extent of bactericidal activity. Accordingly, large infrequent doses of gentamicin are as effective and potentially more so than smaller more frequent ones.

Although data in patients with infections, of necessity, are more variable than those obtained in the experimental mouse model, they do tend to bear out the findings in Fig. 5–8. Moreover, studies indicate that the nephrotoxicity of the aminoglycosides can be reduced by a once-daily regimen compared to more frequent administration. This may explain the tendency, in some quarters, to move from a thrice-daily to a once-daily administration of gentamicin.

ACHIEVING THERAPEUTIC GOALS

Chapters 6 and 7 present the basic principles for establishing and evaluating dosage regimens for those drugs that show reasonably valid correlations of response with dose and concentration. Chapter 6 examines features of constant-rate input, while Chap. 7 examines the principles underlying the administration of drug in discrete doses to attain and maintain therapeutic concentrations. Some additional complexities of the concentration–response relationship are addressed in Chap. 20, Pharmacologic Response.

STUDY PROBLEMS

(Answers to Study Problems are in Appendix II.)

1. Define the terms:
   a. All-or-none response.
   b. Graded response.
   c. Therapeutic window.
   d. Utility curve.
   e. Tolerance.
2. Explain why effect (desired or toxic) is often better correlated with plasma concentration than with dose.
3. List and briefly discuss four situations in which poor plasma drug concentration–response relationships are likely to occur.
4. List the plasma concentration ranges commonly associated with therapeutic responses of cyclosporine, digoxin, gentamicin, lithium, phenobarbital, phenytoin, and theophylline.
5. Briefly discuss, with examples, two situations for which frequency of administration of the same daily dose affects the therapeutic outcome.

CONSTANT-RATE REGIMENS

OBJECTIVES

The reader will be able to:

1. Define plateau and describe the factors controlling it.
2. Describe the relationship between half-life of a drug and time required to approach the plateau following a constant-rate input with or without a bolus dose.
3. Estimate the values of half-life, volume of distribution, and clearance of a drug from plasma concentration data obtained during and following constant-rate input.
4. Estimate the values of half-life, elimination rate constant, and fraction excreted unchanged from urine data obtained during and following constant-rate input.
5. Estimate the value of renal clearance from combined plasma and urine data.
6. Use pharmacokinetic parameters to predict the plasma drug concentration and the amount of drug in the body with time during and following constant-rate input with or without a bolus dose.

A single dose may rapidly produce a desired therapeutic concentration, but this mode of administration is unsuitable when maintenance of plasma or tissue concentrations and effect is desired. To maintain a constant plasma concentration, drug must be administered at a constant rate. This is most reliably accomplished by infusing drug intravenously via either drip or a pump, when greater precision is desired. No other mode of administration provides such precise and readily controlled drug administration. It is, however, restricted primarily to hospital settings.

A wider application of constant-rate therapy has become possible with the development and use of constant-rate release devices, which can be ingested or placed at a variety of body sites and which deliver drug for a period of time extending from hours to years. Some examples of these devices and their applications are given in Table 6–1. Such devices are administered extravascularly. When given to produce a systemic effect, absorption is a prerequisite to attain effective plasma concentrations. However, for the purpose of understanding the principles in this chapter, drug delivery from these systems is assumed to be equivalent to a constant-rate i.v. infusion.

The salient features of the events following a constant-rate infusion are shown in Fig. 6–1 for tissue-type plasminogen activator (t-PA), a substance used to treat myocardial infarctions. The plasma concentration rises toward a constant value and drops off immediately after the infusion of 1.4 mg/min is stopped at 80 min. The half-life of the compound in this patient is 5.2 min, so the drug is infused for about 15 half-lives.

DRUG LEVEL–TIME RELATIONSHIPS

A drug is said to be given as a constant (rate) infusion when the intent is to maintain a stable plasma concentration or amount in the body. In contrast to the short duration of infusion of a bolus dose, the duration of constant infusion is usually much longer than the half-life of the drug. The essential features of the events following a constant infusion can be appreciated by considering the events depicted in Fig. 6–2.

The Plateau Value

At any time during an infusion, the rate of change in the amount of drug in the body (dA/dt) is the difference between the rates of drug infusion and elimination;

$$\frac{dA}{dt} = \underset{\substack{\text{Constant rate} \\ \text{of infusion}}}{R_0} - \underset{\substack{\text{Rate of} \\ \text{elimination}}}{k \cdot A} \qquad\qquad 1$$

or expressing the equation in terms of the concentration of drug in plasma,

Table 6–1.   Representative Constant-Rate Devices and Their Applications

TYPE OF THERAPEUTIC SYSTEM	DRUG	RATE SPECIFICATION	APPLICATION/COMMENTS
Intravenous	Many drugs	Rate controlled by device	Used for i.v. infusion Some devices are portable, others are implantable
Oral	Nifedipine	30, 60, or 90 mg/day administered daily	Calcium channel blocker Nondisintegrating system is designed to provide a constant rate of release for 24 hr
	Phenylpropanolamine	25 mg immediate release and 3.4 mg/hr for 16 hr	Appetite suppressant System aims to provide a constant and effective plasma concentration of phenylpropanolamine for 16 hr
Transdermal	17β-Estradiol	0.05 or 0.1 mg/day	Treatment of menopausal symptoms and prevention of osteoporosis Applied to trunk of body, including buttocks and abdomen, twice weekly
	Nicotine	7, 14, and 21 mg/day (40 μg/cm²/hr) changed daily	Aid to stop smoking Provides a reasonably constant plasma concentration of nicotine Patch placed on front or back above waist or on upper outer part of arm
	Nitroglycerin	2.5, 10, and 15 mg over 24 hr	Prophylaxis against attack of angina pectoris System aims to provide a constant plasma concentration of nitroglycerin Recommended application site is lateral chest wall
	Scopolamine	0.5 mg over 3 days	Used for prevention of motion sickness Applied to hairless area behind ear at least 4 hr before the antiemetic effect is desired

Fig. 6–1. The plasma concentration of recombinant tissue-type plasminogen activator (t-PA) rapidly approaches a limiting value in a patient who receives 0.93 Megaunits/min (1.4 mg/min) by constant-rate infusion for 80 min. At the end of the infusion, the plasma t-PA concentration drops rapidly toward zero with a 5.2-min half-life. The line is the function $C = 1320 \cdot (1 - e^{-0.133t})$ during the infusion and $C = 1320 \cdot e^{-0.133t_{post}}$ thereafter. The value of 0.133 min^{-1} corresponds to a half-life of 5.2 min. (Adapted from Koster, R.W., Cohen, A.F., Kluft, C., Kasper, F.J., van der Wouw, P.A., and Weatherly, B.C.: The pharmacokinetics of double-chain t-PA (duteplase): Effects of bolus injection, infusions, and administration by weight in patients with myocardial infarction. Clin. Pharmacol. Ther., 50:267–277, 1991.)

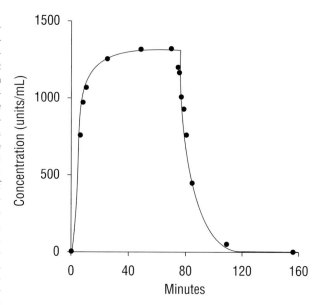

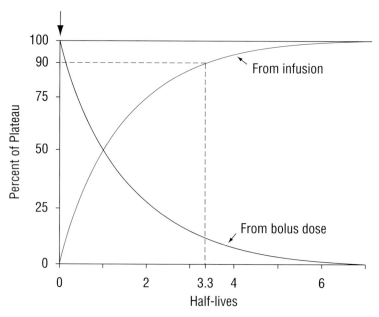

Fig. 6–2. The approach to plateau is controlled only by the half-life of the drug. Depicted is a situation in which a bolus dose (↓) immediately attains and a constant infusion thereafter maintains a constant amount in the body. As the amount of the bolus dose remaining in the body falls, there is a complementary rise resulting from the infusion. By 3.3 half-lives, the amount in the body associated with the infusion has reached 90% of the plateau value.

$$V \cdot \frac{dC}{dt} = R_0 - CL \cdot C \qquad\qquad 2$$

On starting a constant infusion, the amount in the body is zero, and hence there is no elimination; therefore, amount in the body rises. The rise continues until the rate of elimination matches the rate of infusion. Amount in the body and plasma concentration are then said to have reached a *steady state* or *plateau*, which continues as long as the same infusion rate is maintained. Since the rate of change of amount in the body at plateau is zero, it follows that Eqs. 1 and 2 simplify to:

$$
\begin{array}{ccc}
A_{ss} & = & R_0/k \\
\text{Amount at} & & \text{Infusion rate} \\
\text{steady state} & & \overline{\text{Elimination rate constant}}
\end{array}
\qquad 3
$$

$$
\begin{array}{ccc}
C_{ss} & = & R_0/CL \\
\text{Concentration} & & \text{Infusion rate} \\
\text{at steady state} & & \overline{\text{Clearance}}
\end{array}
\qquad 4
$$

Clearly, the only factors governing amount at plateau are the rate of infusion and the elimination rate constant. Similarly, only infusion rate and clearance control the steady-state plasma concentration. Suppose, for illustrative purposes, that a steady-state plasma theophylline concentration of 15 mg/L is desired in the patient whose i.v. bolus data are shown in Fig. 6–1. Since the clearance of this drug is 4 L/hr (Chap. 3), the required infusion rate is 60 mg/hr. As the elimination rate constant of theophylline is $0.14 \ hr^{-1}$, the corresponding amount of drug in the body at steady state is 428 mg. Alternatively, the amount can be calculated by multiplying the plateau concentration (15 mg/L) by the volume of distribution of theophylline (29 L).

To emphasize the factors that control the plateau, consider the following statement: All drugs infused at the same rate and having the same clearance reach the same plateau concentration. This statement is true. The liver and kidneys can clear only what is presented to them; they are insensitive to differences in tissue distribution. The rate of elimination depends only on clearance and plasma concentration. At plateau, rate of elimination is equal to rate of infusion. The plasma concentration must therefore be the same for all drugs with the same clearance if administered at the same rate. However, amount in the body varies with volume of distribution. Only with drugs for which clearance and volume of distribution are the same are both plasma concentration and amount in the body at plateau the same when infused at the same rate. Now consider the next statement: When infused at the same rate, the amount of drug in the body at plateau is the same for all drugs with the same half-life. This statement is also true. Drugs with the same half-life have the same elimination rate constant. The elimination rate constant is the fractional rate of drug elimination, that is, the rate of elimination divided by the amount of drug in the body. At plateau, rate of elimination equals rate of infusion. Hence amount in the body at plateau must be the same for all drugs with the same half-life. Although the amount in the body is the same, the corresponding plateau concentration varies inversely with the drug's volume of distribution.

Knowledge of the plateau value at one particular infusion rate allows prediction of the infusion rate needed to achieve other plateau values. Thus, provided that clearance is constant, a change in infusion rate produces a proportional change in plateau concentration. Returning to the theophylline example, one expects that a rate of 40 mg/hr is needed to produce a plateau concentration of 10 mg/L, since an infusion rate of 60 mg/hr results in a plateau concentration of 15 mg/L.

Mean Residence Time

Conceptually, a useful parameter to describe the sojourn of drug in the body is *mean residence time (MRT)*. To appreciate its relationship to other pharmacokinetic parameters, consider the infusion situation. For a given constant rate of infusion, the amount of drug in the body at steady state (rate of elimination = rate of infusion) depends on the time an average molecule resides in the body. For example, if 2×10^{20} molecules are eliminated per hour and they reside in the body for 10 hr, then only one-tenth of the molecules in the body are removed per hour. There must therefore be 20×10^{20} molecules in the body. Thus, *MRT* is related to the infusion rate and the amount in the body by the relationship:

$$MRT = \frac{A_{ss}}{R_0} \qquad\qquad 5$$

From Eq. 3, it is evident that

$$MRT = \frac{1}{k} \qquad\qquad 6$$

or, as $k = 0.693/t_{1/2}$

$$MRT = 1.44 \times t_{1/2} \qquad\qquad 7$$

Furthermore, as $k = CL/V$, it follows from Eq. 6 that

$$MRT = V/CL \qquad\qquad 8$$

For theophylline ($V = 29$ L, $CL = 4$ L/hr in the patient example), the *MRT* is 7.25 hr, a value corresponding (Eq. 7) to a half-life of 5.0 hr. The mean residence time concept is further discussed in Appendix I–D.

Time to Reach Plateau

A delay always exists between the start of an infusion and the establishment of plateau. The sole factor controlling the approach to plateau is the half-life of the drug. To appreciate this point, consider a situation in which a bolus dose is given at the start of a constant infusion to immediately attain the amount achieved at plateau; clearly, the size of the bolus dose must be A_{ss}. Thereafter, the amount in the body is maintained at the plateau value by constant infusion. Imagine that a way exists to monitor separately drug remaining in the body from the bolus and that accumulating due to the infusion. The events are depicted in Fig. 6–1. Drug in the body associated with each mode of administration is eliminated as though the other were not present. The amount associated with the bolus dose declines exponentially and at any time,

$$\text{Amount remaining in the body from bolus dose} = A_{ss} \cdot e^{-kt} \qquad\qquad 9$$

However, as long as the infusion is maintained, this decline is always exactly matched by the gain resulting from the infusion. This must be so since the sum always equals the amount at plateau, A_{ss}. It therefore follows that the amount in the body associated with a constant infusion (A_{inf}) is always the difference between the amount at plateau (A_{ss}) and the amount remaining from the bolus dose, namely,

$$A_{inf} = A_{ss} - A_{ss} \cdot e^{-kt} \qquad\qquad 10$$

Or, by dividing through by the volume of distribution,

$$C_{inf} = C_{ss}[1 - e^{-kt}] \qquad\qquad 11$$

Thus, both the amount in the body and the plasma concentration (C_{inf}) rise asymptotically toward respective plateau values following constant-rate drug infusion without a bolus dose.

The amount of drug in the body, or plasma concentration, expressed as a percent of the plateau value at different times after initiation of an infusion, is shown in Table 6–2. In 1 half-life, the value in the body is 50% of the plateau value. In 2 half-lives, it is 75% of the plateau value. Theoretically, a plateau is only reached when the drug has been infused for an infinite number of half-lives. For practical purposes, however, the plateau may be considered to be reached in 3.3 half-lives (90% of the plateau). Thus, the shorter the half-life, the sooner is the plateau reached. For example, t-PA (half-life of 5 min) reaches a plateau within minutes (3.3 half-lives is 17 min), whereas it takes 2 to 3 weeks of constant phenobarbital administration (half-life of 100 hr) before the plateau is reached (3.3 half-lives is 14 days). The important point to remember is that the approach to plateau depends *solely* on the half-life of the drug. For example, because the half-life of theophylline in the example patient is 5 hr, it must be infused for 17 hr before plateau is reached. This is so whether 60 mg/hr is infused to maintain a plateau concentration of 15 mg/L or the infusion rate is halved (30 mg/hr) to maintain a plateau concentration of 7.5 mg/L. In the former case, the theophylline plasma concentration at one half-life is one-half the corresponding plateau value of 15 mg/L. So, if one wanted to achieve a plateau concentration of 7.5 mg/L in 2.5 hr, one would infuse at a rate of 60 mg/hr for 1 half-life and then maintain this concentration by halving the infusion rate to 30 mg/hr.

Postinfusion

After stopping an infusion, the amount falls by one-half each half-life. Indeed, given only the declining values of a drug, one cannot clearly deduce whether a bolus or an infusion has been given. In the example of theophylline, 428 mg are in the body at plateau following an infusion rate of 60 mg/hr. Approximately 17 hr (3.3 half-lives) after stopping the infusion,

Table 6–2. Percent of the Plateau Level Reached at Various times Following a Constant Infusion of Drug

TIME (in half-lives)	PERCENT OF PLATEAU
0.5	29
1	50
2	75
3	88
3.3	90
4	94
5	97
6	98
7	99

only one-tenth of the plateau value, or 43 mg, remains in the body. The same amount of drug would be found in the body 17 hr after an i.v. bolus dose of 428 mg of theophylline.

After removing some transdermal constant-rate release devices, drug continues to be released from binding sites in skin for appreciable periods of time. In these instances, the plasma drug concentration falls more slowly than after stopping an i.v. infusion.

Changing Infusion Rates

The rate of infusion of a drug is sometimes changed during therapy because of excessive toxicity or an inadequate therapeutic response. If the object of the change is to effect a new plateau, then the time to go from one plateau to another, whether higher or lower, depends *solely* on the half-life of the drug.

Consider, for illustrative purposes, a patient stabilized on a 30-mg/hr infusion rate of theophylline, which according to Fig. 6–3 should produce a plateau concentration of 7.5 mg/L. Suppose the situation now demands a plateau concentration of 15 mg/L. This new plateau value is achieved by doubling the infusion rate to 60 mg/hr. Imagine that instead

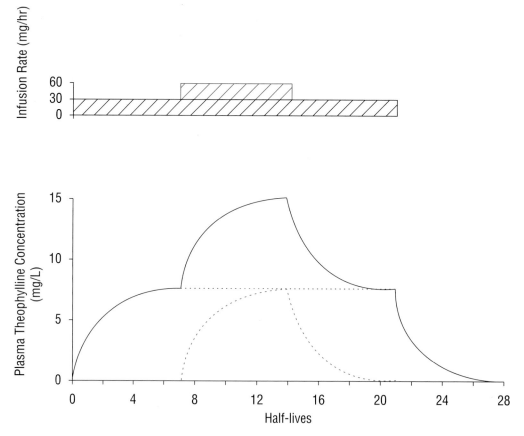

Fig. 6–3. Situation illustrating that the time to reach a new plateau, whether higher or lower than the previous value, depends only on the half-life of a drug. A plateau concentration of 7.5 mg/L is reached in approximately 3.3 half-lives after starting a constant infusion of 30 mg/hr of theophylline. Doubling the infusion rate is like maintaining 30 mg/hr and starting another constant infusion of 30 mg/hr (colored line). In approximately 3.3 half-lives, the theophylline concentration rises from 7.5 mg/L to 15 mg/L. Halving an infusion rate of 60 mg/hr is analogous to stopping the supplementary 30 mg/hr infusion. The plasma concentration of theophylline approaches a plateau of 7.5 mg/L in approximately 3.3 half-lives.

of increasing the infusion rate, the additional 30 mg/hr was administered at a different site and that a way existed of separately monitoring theophylline in the body from the two infusions. The events illustrated in Fig. 6–3 show that the theophylline concentration associated with the new infusion will rise to 7.5 mg/L in exactly the same time as in the first infusion; half the plateau concentration (3.75 mg/L) in one elimination half-life (5 hr) and so on. Addition of this rising concentration to the pre-existing plateau concentration shows that the half-life is the *sole* determinant of the time required to go from 7.5 to 15 mg/L. Needless to say, any readjustment in the infusion rate in less than 3.3 half-lives means that a new plateau concentration will not be established.

The decline from a high plateau to a low one is likewise related to the half-life. Consider, for example, the events after stopping the supplementary 30-mg/hr infusion rate discussed previously. The theophylline concentration associated with this supplementary infusion will fall to half the existing value in 1 half-life. In 3.3 half-lives, the total concentration will have almost returned to the pre-existing 7.5 mg/L concentration. Also, it will take another 3.3 half-lives for most of the theophylline to be removed from the body once the original 30-mg/hr infusion is stopped.

An example of the change in plasma concentration on changing from one infusion rate to another is again demonstrated by data on t-PA in Fig. 6–4. The half-life is the determinant of the speed of attaining the new steady state. Clearance determines the steady-state concentration.

Bolus and Infusion

It takes approximately 17 hr of constant infusion of theophylline before the plateau concentration is reached. An even longer time is required for drugs with half-lives greater than that of theophylline. Situations sometimes demand that the plateau be reached more rapidly. Figure 6–2 suggests a solution. That is, at the start of an infusion, give a bolus dose equal to the amount desired in the body at plateau. Usually the bolus dose is a therapeutic dose, and the infusion rate is adjusted to maintain the therapeutic level. When the bolus dose and infusion rate are exactly matched, as in Fig. 6–2, the amounts of drug in the body

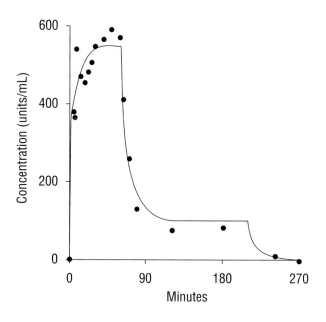

Fig. 6–4. The plasma concentration of plasminogen activator (t-PA) starts at about 350 IU/mL (1.2 µg/mL) and approaches plateau of 550 IU/mL (1.8 µg/mL) following an i.v. bolus of 10 mg and a constant-rate infusion of 1.6 mg/min for 60 min to an individual subject. Subsequently, the plasma concentration drops as the drug infusion is decreased to 0.3 mg/min. The time from the first steady state to the second depends on the half-life of the drug, 6.6 min in this subject. (Adapted from Koster, R.W., Cohen, A.F., Kluft, C., Kasper, F.J., van der Wouw, P.A., and Weatherly, B.C.: The pharmacokinetics of double-chain t-PA (duteplase): Effects of bolus injection, infusions, and administration by weight in patients with myocardial infarction. Clin. Pharmacol. Ther. *50*:267–277, 1991.)

associated with the two modes of administration are complementary; the gain of one offsets the loss of the other.

Now consider two situations. The first, shown in Fig. 6–5, is one in which different bolus doses are given at the start of a constant-rate infusion. In Case A, drug is infused alone and the amount rises, reaching a plateau of 200 mg in approximately 4 half-lives. In Case B, the bolus dose of 200 mg immediately attains, and the infusion rate thereafter maintains the plateau amount. In Case C, the bolus dose of 400 mg is excessive; because the rate of loss is initially greater than the rate of infusion, amount in the body falls. This fall continues until the same plateau as in Case B is reached. It should be noticed that the time to reach the plateau depends solely on the half-life of the drug. Thus, in Case C at 1 half-life, 300 mg, composed of 200 mg remaining from the bolus and 100 mg from the infusion, lies midway between the bolus dose and the plateau value. By 2 half-lives, the 250 mg in the body lies 75% of the way toward the plateau. By approximately 4 half-lives, little of the bolus dose remains and the plateau is reached. In Case D, the bolus dose of 100 mg is below the plateau amount. Because the rate of infusion now exceeds the rate of drug elimination, the amount in the body continuously rises until the same plateau as in the

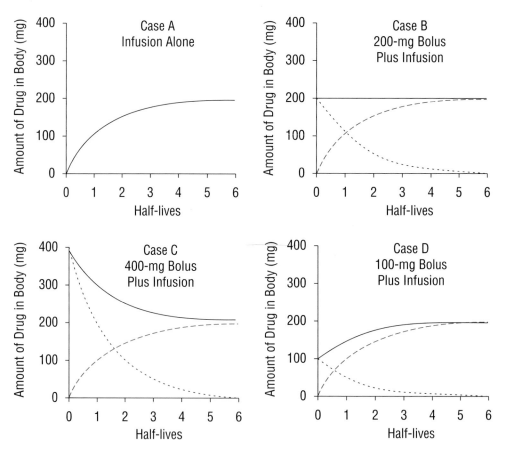

Fig. 6–5. Situations illustrating that the plateau depends upon the infusion rate and not upon the initial bolus dose. Whether a bolus dose is given (Cases B, C, D) or not (Case A) at the start of the infusion, the amount of drug in the body at the plateau is the same. The amount of the bolus dose remaining in the body declines exponentially (. . .) while the amount associated with infusion in all cases rises asymptotically toward plateau (– – –), as portrayed by Case A. In Cases B, C, and D, the observed concentration (———) is the sum of the two. When not initially achieved, it takes approximately 3.3 half-lives to reach plateau (Cases A, C, D). Note also in Cases A, C, and D that at 1 half-life amount in the body lies midway between initial and plateau values.

previous cases is reached. Once again the time to approach the plateau is controlled solely by the half-life of the drug.

Case D is demonstrated by t-PA in Fig. 6–4. The bolus dose of 10 mg was insufficient to attain the steady state achieved on infusing 1.6 mg/min. This result is expected from the 6.6 min half-life in this patient, as the amount in the body at plateau (R_o/k) is 15 mg.

In the second and more common situation, depicted in Fig. 6–6, the same bolus dose and infusion rate are administered to three patients, A, B, and C, with different clearance and associated half-life values. The half-lives in these patients are 3, 6, and 9 hr, respectively. All patients start with the same amount of drug in the body. In patient B, this amount is maintained because rate of infusion is exactly matched by rate of elimination. Since elimination is slower, the amount in patient C rises until rate of elimination equals infusion rate. The time to reach this higher plateau value is governed solely by the half-life of the drug in this patient. Thus, by 1 half-life (9 hr), the amount of drug in patient C is midway between the bolus dose and that at plateau. By the time the plateau is reached, all the bolus dose has been eliminated. Also, it follows from Eq. 3 that for a given infusion rate, amount at plateau is proportional to the half-life. This is seen in Fig. 6–6, where amount in patient C at plateau is 50% higher than that in patient B. Patient A eliminates the drug more rapidly than does patient B. Accordingly, the amount of drug in patient A falls until a new plateau value, one-half that of patient B, is reached. As always, the approach to plateau is governed solely by the half-life, which in patient A is only 3 hr. Thus, by 3 hr (1 half-life), the value has fallen 50% of the way toward the plateau, and by 10 hr plateau is reached.

The approach to plateau during an infusion has been presented so far in terms of the time required to go from the initial concentration (amount) to the plateau. The time to reach any value on approach to plateau can be determined by combining the principles already learned. Recall that plasma concentration after an i.v. bolus dose is $C = C(0)e^{-kt}$. The concentration resulting from a constant-rate infusion is given in Eq. 11. As each event is independent of the other, by summing these quantities, one obtains concentration at any time during an infusion. That is,

$$C = C(0)e^{-kt} + C_{ss}(1 - e^{-kt}) \qquad 12$$

For example, if the initial value is 500 µg/L, the plateau value is 100 µg/L, and the concentration to be reached is 110 µg/L, then the time to reach this concentration can be calculated as follows. Rearranging Eq. 12 and taking into account that $(1/2)^n = e^{-kt}$ (Chap. 3, p. 23),

$$e^{-kt} = \left(\frac{1}{2}\right)^n = \frac{C_{ss} - C}{C_{ss} - C(0)} \qquad 13$$

Substituting for C(0), C_{ss} and C into Eq. 13 yields $(1/2)^n = 0.025$. Solving for n, a concentration of 110 µg/L is reached in 5.3 half-lives.

Practical Issues

So far, the approach to plateau has been considered in absolute terms. Practically, it is helpful to establish a tolerance, such as $\pm 10\%$, for the final value. The time required to be within this tolerance varies with the starting and final values. This may be seen by application of Eq. 13. For example, if one begins at 80% of the final plateau, the time to reach the lower limit of tolerance (90%) is only 1 half-life. In contrast, if the starting concentration is 500% of the final value, it takes 5.3 half-lives to reach the upper limit of

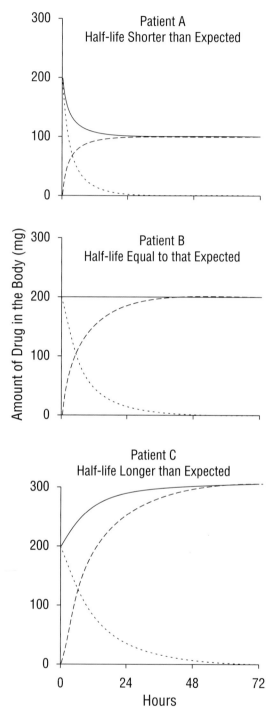

Fig. 6–6. Situations illustrating that the amount at plateau depends on half-life. The same bolus dose and, constant infusion are given to patients A, B, and C, with half-lives of 3, 6, and 9 hr, respectively. Although amount of drug in the initial bolus is the same (200 mg) in all three patients, amount in the body at the plateau differs in direct proportion to their respective half-lives. Amount of the bolus dose remaining (. . .) with time depends on the individual's half-life, as does the rise in amount in the body associated with the constant infusion (– – –). Only when rate of loss is immediately matched by rate of infusion is the plateau immediately attained and maintained (patient B). Otherwise amount in the body (———) changes, until after approximately 3.3 half-lives, a plateau is reached (patients A and C).

tolerance, 110% of the final value. Accepting a tolerance clearly modifies the statement: The time taken to reach plateau is determined solely by the half-life of the drug. Now both the initial and final values must also be considered.

The constant-rate release systems marketed may contain a loading dose to facilitate the more rapid achievement of therapeutic concentrations. Administered extravascularly, however, with the additional absorption step, the attainment of both therapeutic concentrations and plateau will therefore be longer, although perhaps inconsequentially, than that following an equivalent i.v. regimen.

ASSESSMENT OF PHARMACOKINETIC PARAMETERS

Pharmacokinetic parameters are generally determined just as readily from constant-rate data as from i.v. bolus data. Certainly, this is so for an i.v. infusion. Following the use of constant-rate release devices administered extravascularly, uncertainty exists about bioavailability, which therefore requires reference to i.v. data. Nonetheless, how estimates of pharmacokinetic parameters are made is seen by considering the plasma concentration data in Table 6–3, obtained during and after an i.v. infusion of a drug.

Plasma Data Alone

Consider, for the moment, that measurements only during the infusion are available. What can be estimated?

First, dividing the infusion rate of 40 mg/hr by the plateau concentration of 9.5 mg/L gives clearance, in this case 4.2 L/hr. Indeed, this is the preferred method for estimating clearance since the plateau concentration can be determined with great precision by averaging those concentrations that clearly lie at plateau.

Second, the half-life is easily ascertained, being the time taken to reach half the plateau concentration. However, in this example and in most cases, no sample was taken at this time, and so one must interpolate between the observed data. The half-life, estimated in this manner. (Fig. 6–7), is approximately 1.5 hr. A more accurate method of estimating the half-life uses all the data obtained during the infusion. On rearranging Eq. 11, one obtains

Table 6–3. Plasma Concentration of a Drug During and After a Constant Infusion (40 mg/hr) for 12 hr

OBSERVATION		TREATMENT OF DATA
TIME (hr)	PLASMA CONCENTRATION (C, mg/L)	$C_{ss}^{a} - C$ (mg/L)
During infusion		
1	3.3	6.2
2	5.4	4.1
4	7.6	1.9
6	8.7	0.8
8	9.3	0.2
10	9.6	−0.1
12	9.5	0.0
Postinfusion		
2	4.1	
4	1.8	
6	0.76	
8	0.33	
10	0.14	

^{a}The concentration at the 12th hr of infusion.

$$C_{ss} - C_{inf} = C_{ss} \cdot e^{-kt}$$ 14

which upon taking natural logarithms yields

$$\ln (C_{ss} - C_{inf}) = \ln C_{ss} - k \cdot t$$ 15

Thus, the decline obtained by plotting semilogarithmically the difference between the plateau concentration and that at earlier times against the corresponding time should be a straight line. The intercept at time zero is the plateau concentration (C_{ss}) and the slope is $-k$. These differences in concentration shown by vertical lines in Fig. 6–7, are presented in Table 6–3 and have been plotted in Fig. 6–8. The data indicate a half-life of 1.7 hr. It should be noted that the longer the infusion, the closer the concentration is to the plateau value and the greater is the error in the difference measurement. Generally, difference values calculated from concentrations beyond 90% of the plateau have excessive error.

Last, the volume of distribution is calculated knowing clearance and half-life; in this case it is 10 L.

Consider now the concentration data at and after the end of the infusion. Plotting these data on semilogarithmic paper also gives a straight line, from which half-life can be determined, since after stopping the infusion

Fig. 6–7. Estimation of pharmacokinetic parameters from plasma data during and after a constant infusion. The vertical arrows represent the differences between concentrations at plateau and observed during the infusion.

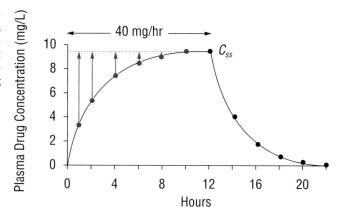

Fig. 6–8. Semilogarithmic plot of the difference (●) between plateau drug concentration and that observed during the infusion against time. Also plotted are the declining values of plasma drug concentration (○) against time after stopping the infusion.

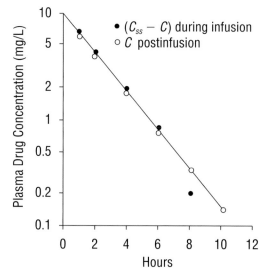

$$C = C_{ss} \cdot e^{-kt} \qquad\qquad 16$$

When these data are so plotted, they are observed to superimpose on the previous difference data (Fig. 6–8). In the particular example studied, the half-lives determined from the rising and declining curves are equal. Occasionally they differ, thereby indicating that drug disposition has changed over the period of study.

Urine Data Alone

If renal clearance is constant, the rate of excretion is proportional to the plasma concentration. Then excretion rate data can be treated in a manner analogous to that of plasma data, and estimates can be made of elimination half-life and fraction excreted unchanged (fe). An estimate of fe is obtained at plateau from

$$fe = \frac{\text{Rate of excretion at plateau}}{\text{Rate of infusion}} \qquad\qquad 17$$

because the rate of infusion is equal to the rate of elimination. For example, when the infusion rate is 40 mg/hr, the observed excretion rate at plateau for the drug is 12 mg/hr, so fe is 0.3.

Plasma and Urine Data

Without plasma data, values for volume of distribution and clearance cannot be estimated. When both plasma and urine data are obtained, renal clearance can be estimated in addition to all other pharmacokinetic parameters. Moreover, a steady-state experiment achieved with constant infusion is the preferred method for estimating renal clearance. At plateau, accurate measurements can be made of both plasma concentration and urine excretion rate. In the preceding example renal clearance, obtained by dividing excretion rate at plateau by C_{ss}, is 1.26 L/hr.

STUDY PROBLEMS

(Answers to Study Problems are in Appendix II.)

1. Which one or more of the following statements pertaining to constant rate infusion is correct?
   a. The time to reach a plateau concentration depends upon the rate of infusion.
   b. All drugs having the same clearance reach the same plateau concentration when given at the same i.v. infusion rate.
   c. Drugs with the same clearance generally reach the plateau concentration at the same time.
   d. The amount of drug in the body at plateau cannot be the same when drugs with different clearance values are infused at the same rate.
   e. All of the above.
   f. None of the above.
2. For prolonged surgical procedures, succinylcholine chloride is given by i.v. infusion for sustained muscle relaxation. A typical initial dose is 20 mg followed by continuous infusion of 4 mg/min. The infusion must be individualized because of variation in the kinetics of metabolism of succinylcholine. Estimate the elimination half-lives of succinylcholine in patients requiring 0.4 mg/min and 4 mg/min, respectively, to maintain 20 mg in the body.

3. In the graphs on the left below (Fig. 6–9) are two multiple infusion-rate scenarios. Sketch the anticipated plasma concentration-time profiles on the graphs on the right using concepts presented in this chapter. The total clearance of the drug is 200 mL/min. Note that the time scale is expressed in half-life units.

4. During an investigational program, the calcium channel blocking agent nifedipine was infused at a constant rate (1.5 mg/hr) via a rectal osmotic pump device for 24 hr. Table 6–4 lists the plasma nifedipine concentration during and after the infusion. These data indicate that an average plateau concentration of 21 µg/L was attained. Given that all the infused drug was absorbed and that nifedipine disposition can be characterized by a one-compartmental model:

Table 6–4. Nifedipine Kinetics During Rectal Infusion to Steady State With an Osmotic System[a]

TIME (hr)	PLASMA NIFEDIPINE CONCENTRATION (µg/L)
0	0
1	4.2
2	14.5
4	21.0
6	23.0
7.5	19.8
10.5	22.0
14	20.0
18	18.0
24	21.0
25	18.0
26	11.6
27	7.1
28	4.2

[a]Abstracted from Kleinbloessem, C.H., van Harten, J., de Leede, L.G.J., van Brummelen, P., and Briemer, D.D.: Nifedipine kinetics and dynamics during rectal infusion to steady state with an osmotic system. Clin. Pharmacol. Ther., 36:396–401, 1984.

  a. Calculate the clearance, half-life, volume of distribution, and *MRT* of the drug.
  b. Is the approach of the concentration to plateau in agreement with the half-life of nifedipine observed on removing the infusion pump?
  c. If the infusion rate were 3.0 mg/hr instead of 1.5 mg/hr, what would be the expected concentrations at 1 hr, 2 hr, and at plateau?
  d. If the desire is to achieve the plateau concentration associated with the 3.0 mg/hr infusion rate instantly, what is the loading dose required?

5. Droperidol, a butyrophenone derivative, has been used for the prevention and treatment of nausea and vomiting in postoperative patients and in patients undergoing chemotherapy. Droperidol is currently administered intravenously and intramuscularly, both invasive procedures. The oral route creates a problem for patients who are nauseous or vomiting. Gupta et al. (1992) evaluated a continuous-release rectal drug-delivery system as a means of achieving therapy for an extended period. Table 6–5 lists the mean plasma concentration of droperidol obtained following use of this device, designed to deliver drug at a constant rate for 15 hr, in comparison with a 24-hr constant rate i.v. infusion, rate 0.125 mg/hr. The rectal device contained a total of 3 mg droperidol. No drug was found in the recovered device.

Table 6-5. Mean Plasma Droperidol Concentrations Following an i.v. Infusion and the Use of a Rectal Device in Eight Subjects[a]

TIME (hr)		0	0.5	2	4	6	8	10	14	18	24	26	28	30
Plasma Concentration (mg/L)	i.v. infusion	0	0.90	1.80	2.60	2.50	2.50	2.70	2.70	2.90	3.10	1.40	0.67	0.36
	rectal device	0	0		0.49	0.99	1.83	1.84	1.93	1.52	1.43	1.63	0.65	0.29	0.10

[a]Abstracted from Gupta, S.K., Southam, M., and Hwang, S.: Pharmacokinetics of droperidol in healthy volunteers following intravenous infusion and rectal administration from an osmotic drug delivery module. Pharm. Res., 9:694–696, 1992.

      a. From the plasma concentration data after stopping the i.v. infusion, estimate the elimination half-life of droperidol.
      b. Calculate the expected *MRT* following an i.v. bolus.
      c. Estimate the systemic bioavailability of the drug.
      d. Calculate clearance.
      e. What is the volume of distribution of droperidol?

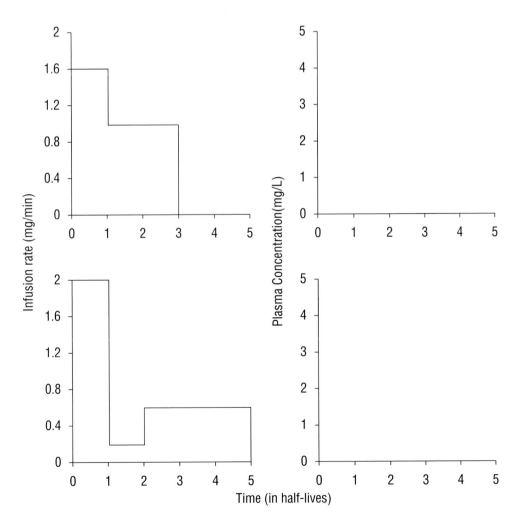

Fig. 6–9.

6. Hadgraft et al. explored the feasibility of transdermal delivery of a new antidepressant drug, rolipram. Table 6–6 lists the mean plasma rolipram concentrations in six subjects during and after a 24-hr application of a 25-cm² patch made of silicone adhesive, drug, and 5% isopropyl myristate on a polymer backing. The patches (5 cm × 5 cm), applied to forearm skin areas, were covered for 24 hr. At this time, the patches were removed and the skin area cleaned with alcohol swabs. The average clearance and half-life of rolipram are 8.4 L/hr and 3 hr, respectively.

Table 6–6. Mean Rolipram Concentrations During and After 24-hr Dermal Application in Six Male Subjects[a]

Time (hr)	0	1	2	4	6	8	10	12	14	24	25	26	28	30
Plasma Concentration (μg/L)	0	0	0.05	0.8	1.1	1.5	1.6	1.5	1.6	1.55	1.45	1.3	0.9	0.55

[a]Adapted from Hadgraft, J., Hill, S., Hümpel, M., Johnston, L.R., Lever, L.R., Marks, R., Murphy, T.M., and Rapier, C.: Investigations on the percutaneous absorption of the antidepressant rolipram in vitro and in vivo. Pharm. Res., 7:1307–1312, 1990.

a. Calculate the average rate that rolipram is being absorbed from the patch between 12 and 24 hr.
b. Determine the total amount of rolipram absorbed during the 24-hr application of the patch.
c. Does the approach to steady state follow the expectation of 50% in 1 half-life, 75% in 2 half-lives, and so on? If not, briefly discuss how the absorption-time profile differs from that expected following constant-rate input.

7. Estimate the volume of distribution, elimination rate constant, half-life, and clearance from the data in Table 6–7 obtained on infusing a drug at the rate of 50 mg/hr for 7.5 hr.

Table 6–7.

Time (hr)	0	2	4	6	7.5	9	12	15
Plasma drug concentration (mg/L)	0	3.4	5.4	6.5	7.0	4.6	2.0	0.9

8. A drug that displays one-compartment characteristics was administered as an i.v. bolus of 250 mg followed immediately by a constant infusion of 10 mg/hr for the duration of a study. Estimate the values of volume of distribution, half-life, and clearance from the data in Table 6–8.

Table 6–8.

Time (hr)	0.3	5.0	20	50
Plasma drug concentration (mg/L)	9.8	7.6	4.8	4.0

9. In the text on page 75, the practical view of the approach to plateau was presented. If the tolerance at plateau had been 15%, instead of 10%, what would be the time, in half-lives, needed to reach this tolerance when the initial concentration is:
a. 80% of the final (plateau) value.
b. 500% of the final (plateau) value.

MULTIPLE-DOSE REGIMENS

OBJECTIVES

The reader will be able to:

1. Predict the rate and extent of drug accumulation for a given regimen of fixed dose and fixed interval.

2. Develop a dosage regimen from knowledge of the pharmacokinetics and therapeutic window of a drug.

3. Evaluate the kinetics of a drug given in a multiple-dose regimen.

4. Evaluate the kinetics of a drug following a multiple-dose regimen of a controlled-release formulation.

5. Derive pharmacokinetic parameters for a drug from plasma concentration (or urine) data following a multiple-dose regimen.

The previous chapter dealt with constant-rate regimens. Although these regimens possess many desirable features, they are not the most common ones. The more common approach to the maintenance of continuous therapy is to give multiple discrete doses. This chapter covers the pharmacokinetic principles associated with such multiple-dose regimens.

DRUG ACCUMULATION

Drugs are most commonly prescribed to be taken on a fixed dose, fixed time interval basis; e.g., 100 mg three times a day. In association with this kind of administration, the plasma concentration and amount in the body fluctuate and, similar to an infusion, rise toward a plateau.

Consider the simplest situation of a dosage regimen composed of equal bolus doses administered intravenously at fixed and equal time intervals. Curve A of Fig. 7–1 shows how amount in the body varies with time when each dose is given successively twice every half-life. Under these conditions drug accumulates substantially. Accumulation occurs because drug from previous doses has not been completely removed.

Maxima and Minima on Accumulation to the Plateau

To appreciate the phenomenon of accumulation, consider what happens when a 100-mg bolus dose is given intravenously every elimination half-life. The amounts in the body just after each dose and just before the next dose can readily be calculated; these values correspond to the maximum (A_{max}) and minimum (A_{min}) amounts obtained within each dosing interval. The corresponding values during the first dosing interval are 100 mg ($A_{1,max}$) and 50 mg ($A_{1,min}$), respectively. The maximum amount of drug in the second dosing interval ($A_{2,max}$), 150 mg, is the dose (100 mg) plus the amount remaining from the previous dose

(50 mg). The amount remaining at the end of the second dosing interval ($A_{2,min}$), 75 mg, is that remaining from the first dose, 25 mg (100 mg $\times$ $^1/_2$ $\times$ $^1/_2$, because two half-lives have elapsed since its administration) plus that remaining from the second dose, 50 mg. Alternatively, the value, 75 mg, may simply be calculated by recognizing that one-half of the amount just after the second dose, 150 mg, remains at the end of that dosing interval. Upon repeating this procedure, it is readily seen (curve B, Fig. 7–1) that drug accumulation, viewed in terms of either maximum or minimum amount in the body, continues until a limit is reached. At the limit, the amount lost in each interval equals the amount gained, the dose. In this example, the maximum and the minimum amounts in the body at steady state are 200 mg and 100 mg, respectively. This must be so since the difference between the maximum and minimum amounts is the dose, 100 mg, and since at the end of the interval, one half-life, the amount must be half that at the beginning.

Following a constant rate input, the *plateau* is reached when rate of elimination matches rate of input. Then the level of drug in the body is constant. With discrete dosing, the level is not constant within a dosing interval, but the values at a given time within the interval are the same from one dosing interval to another, that is, when the amount lost equals the amount gained within the interval. The term *plateau* is also applied to this interdosing steady-state condition.

The foregoing considerations can be expanded for the more general situation in which a drug is given at a dosing interval, τ, which may differ from the half-life. The general equations derived in Appendix I–E for the maximum and minimum amounts in the body after the Nth dose ($A_{N,max}$; $A_{N,min}$) and at plateau ($A_{ss,max}$; $A_{ss,min}$) are

$$\text{Maximum amount in body after Nth dose, } A_{N,max} = \text{Dose} \cdot \left[\frac{1 - e^{-NK\tau}}{1 - e^{-k\tau}} \right] \qquad 1$$

$$\text{Minimum amount in body after Nth dose, } A_{N,min} = A_{N,max} \cdot e^{-k\tau} \qquad 2$$

$$\text{Maximum amount in body at plateau, } A_{ss,max} = \frac{\text{Dose}}{1 - e^{-k\tau}} \qquad 3$$

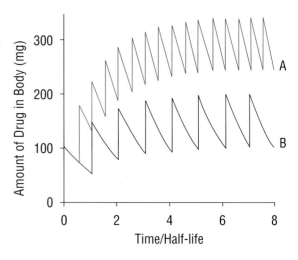

Fig. 7–1. Dosing frequency controls the degree of drug accumulation. Curve A, i.v. bolus dose (100 mg) administered twice every half-life; curve B, same bolus dose administered once every half-life. Note that time is expressed in half-life units.

$$\text{Minimum amount in body at plateau, } A_{ss,min} = A_{ss,max} \, e^{-k\tau} = A_{ss,max} - \text{Dose} \qquad 4$$

Recall from Chap. 3 that the function e^{-kt} is the fraction of the initial amount remaining in the body at time t. Similarly, the amount in the body at the end of a dosing interval τ of a multiple-dose regimen, $(A_{N,min})$, is obtained by multiplying the corresponding maximum amount by $e^{-k\tau}$, that is, $A_{N,min} = A_{N,max} \, e^{-k\tau}$ or $A_{ss,min} = A_{ss,max} \, e^{-k\tau}$.

To further appreciate the phenomenon of accumulation, consider an oral dosage regimen of 0.1 mg daily of digitoxin, used in the treatment of certain cardiac dysfunctions. Although not as widely used as the more popular drug, digoxin, digitoxin nicely illustrates many of the aspects of accumulation and design of dosage regimens. Given that absorption is complete and virtually instantaneous, oral administration can be simulated using i.v. bolus doses.

The average half-life of digitoxin is 6 days; therefore, from Eq. 3 the maximum amount at plateau is 0.92 mg, and from Eq. 4 the minimum amount at plateau is 0.82 mg. Digitoxin clearly undergoes considerable accumulation when given daily.

These calculations of the maximum and minimum values at plateau strictly apply only to intravascular bolus administration. They are reasonable approximations following extravascular administration, when absorption is complete and virtually instantaneous. The following discussion deals with a less restrictive view of accumulation, which applies to all routes of administration.

Average Amount and Concentration at Plateau

In many respects the accumulation of drugs, administered in multiple doses is the same as that observed following a constant-rate i.v. infusion. The average amount in the body at steady state, plateau, is readily calculated using the steady-state concept: Average *rate in* must equal average *rate out*. The average rate in is $F \cdot \text{Dose}/\tau$. The average rate out is $k \cdot A_{ss,av}$, where $A_{ss,av}$ is the average amount of drug in the body over the dosing interval at plateau. Therefore,

$$\frac{F \cdot \text{Dose}}{\tau} = k \cdot A_{ss,av} \qquad 5$$

or

$$\frac{F \cdot \text{Dose}}{\tau} = CL \cdot C_{ss,av} \qquad 6$$

where $C_{ss,av}$ is the average plasma concentration at the plateau. Since $k = 0.693/t_{1/2}$, it also follows that

$$A_{ss,av} = 1.44 \cdot F \cdot \text{Dose} \cdot t_{1/2}/\tau \qquad 7$$

and

$$C_{ss,av} = \frac{F}{CL} \cdot \frac{\text{Dose}}{\tau} \qquad 8$$

These are fundamental relationships; they show how the average amount in the body at steady state depends on rate of administration (Dose/τ), bioavailability, and half-life, and how the corresponding average concentration depends on the first two factors and clearance.

Drug accumulation is not a phenomenon that depends on the property of a drug, nor are there drugs that are cumulative and others that are not. Accumulation, in particular the extent of it, is a result of the frequency of administration relative to half-life ($t_{1/2}/\tau$ or $1/k\tau$) as shown in Figs. 7–1 and 7–2.

Notice that the average amount of digitoxin (0.87 mg), calculated from Eq. 7, lies midway between the maximum 0.92 mg and the minimum 0.82 mg. Since calculating the average value is the much simpler procedure, under these circumstances the maximum and minimum values can easily be calculated by adding and subtracting one-half the maintenance dose absorbed, respectively, to the average value. With digitoxin, for example, $A_{ss,max}$ is 0.87 + 0.05 = 0.92 mg; $A_{ss,min}$ is 0.87 − 0.05 = 0.82 mg. This simple method is a reasonable approximation as long as the dosing interval does not exceed the half-life.

Comparison of Maximum, Average, and Minimum Amounts at Plateau

Fluctuation in the amount of drug in the body, like accumulation, depends on both frequency of drug administration and half-life. Fluctuation also depends on rate of absorption; it is greatest for i.v. bolus administration. Figure 7–2A illustrates how maximum, minimum, and average amounts in the body at plateau depend on the frequency of i.v. bolus administration. Several observations are pertinent: (1) The average amount increases in direct proportion to frequency of administration (inverse of the dosing interval). (2) The maximum amount is not much greater than dose if drug is administered less frequently than once every 3 half-lives, $t_{1/2}/\tau$ = 0.33 or less. Then most of the drug from all previous doses has

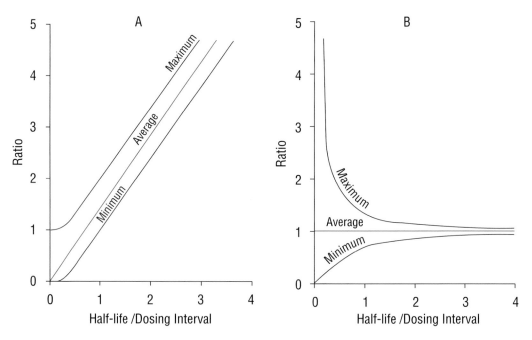

Fig. 7–2. More frequent administration results in a greater degree of drug accumulation and hence smaller relative differences among the maximum ($A_{ss,max}$), average ($A_{ss,av}$) and minimum ($A_{ss,min}$) amounts of drug in the body at plateau. Note that frequency is the reciprocal of the dosing interval expressed here in half-life units. *A,* Ratios of the maximum, average (colored line), and minimum amounts of drug at plateau to the maintenance dose following chronic i.v. bolus administration, as a function of the dosing frequency. *B,* Ratios of maximum to average (colored line), and minimum to average amounts of drug in the body as a function of the dosing frequency.

been eliminated before the next dose is administered. (3) Defining fluctuation as the ratio, $A_{ss,max}/A_{ss,min}$, given by $e^{k\tau}$ (Eq. 4), the greater the relative frequency of administration (1/$k\tau$) the smaller is the fluctuation. Figure 7–2B demonstrates how fluctuation at plateau depends on frequency of administration. The maximum and minimum amounts are each compared with the average amount in the body. Note that the average is arithmetically closer to the minimum than to the maximum value. This is particularly evident for low frequencies of administration.

Rate of Accumulation to Plateau

The amount in the body rises on multiple dosing just as it does following a constant-rate i.v. infusion (Chap. 6). That is, the approach to the plateau depends solely on the drug's half-life. The data for digitoxin, in Table 7–1 which show the ratio of the minimum amount during various dosing intervals to the maximum amount at plateau, illustrate this point. Observe that it takes 1 half-life (6 days), or 6 doses, to be at 50% of the value at plateau, 2 half-lives (12 days), or 12 doses, to be at 75% of the plateau value, and so on.

  Accumulation of digitoxin takes a long time because of its long half-life. The degree of accumulation is extensive, because of relatively frequent administration. The frequency of administration also determines the small fluctuation in the amount of drug in the body at plateau; 0.1 mg is lost every dosing interval, when there is about 0.9 mg in the body.

  The approach to steady state, observed for the minimum amounts of digitoxin in the body, also holds true for the maximum (proof in Appendix I–D), and average amounts, that is,

$$\frac{A_{N,max}}{A_{ss,max}} = \frac{A_{N,av}}{A_{ss,av}} = \frac{A_{N,min}}{A_{ss,min}} = 1 - e^{-Nk\tau} \qquad\qquad 9$$

where $A_{N,av}$ is the average amount in the body in the dosing interval after the Nth dose.

Accumulation Index

If the amounts at steady state are compared to the corresponding values at time τ after the first dose, then

$$\frac{A_{ss,max}}{A_{max,1}} = \frac{A_{ss,av}}{A_{av,1}} = \frac{A_{ss,min}}{A_{min,1}} = \frac{1}{(1 - e^{-k\tau})} \qquad\qquad 10$$

The quantity, $1/(1 - e^{-k\tau})$, is an index of the extent of accumulation. For digitoxin ($k = 0.116$ day^{-1}, $\tau = 1$ day), the *accumulation index* (R_{ac}) is 9.2. Thus, the maximum, average, and minimum amounts (and for that matter the amount at any time within the dosing interval at plateau) are 9.2 times the values at the corresponding times after a single dose.

Table 7-1. Approach to Plateau on Daily Administration of Digitoxin

Time (days)[a]	0	1	2	3	6	12	18	24	30	∞
Number of doses (N)		1	2	3	6	12	18	24	30	∞
$\left[\dfrac{\text{Minimum amount}}{\begin{array}{c}\text{Minimum amount}\\\text{at plateau}\end{array}}\right]^{b}$	0	0.11	0.21	0.29	0.5	0.75	0.875	0.94	0.97	1.00

[a] Time after first dose
[b] $A_{N,min}/A_{ss,min} = 1 - e^{-0.116N}$

Change in Regimen

Suppose that the decision is made to halve the amount of digitoxin in the body at plateau. The need for a twofold reduction in the rate of administration, to 0.05 mg/day, follows from Eq. 7.

As with i.v. infusion, it takes 1 half-life to go one-half the way from 0.90 to 0.45 mg, 2 half-lives to go three-quarters of the way, and so on. For digitoxin it would take about 12 days to go 75% of the way to the new plateau. (The same principle applies to an increase in the rate of digitoxin administration.) The fastest way to achieve 0.45 mg would be to discontinue drug for 1 week (approximately 1 half-life) before initiating the reduced rate of administration.

RELATIONSHIP BETWEEN INITIAL AND MAINTENANCE DOSES

It might be therapeutically desirable to establish the required amount of digitoxin in the body on the first day. When the first or initial dose is intended to be therapeutic it is referred to as the *priming* or *loading dose*. In this case, the patient would require 0.9 mg initially, followed by 0.1 mg daily. For digitoxin the initial dose is often administered in divided doses. Several procedures are followed, but the divided dose is commonly given every 6 hours until the desired therapeutic response is obtained. In this way each patient is titrated to the initial therapeutic dose required.

Instead of determining the loading dose when the maintenance dose is given, it is more common to determine the maintenance dose required to sustain a therapeutic amount in the body. The initial dose rapidly achieves the therapeutic response; subsequent doses maintain the response by replacing drug lost during the dosing interval. The maintenance dose, D_M, therefore, is the difference between the loading dose, D_L, and the amount remaining at the end of the dosing interval, $D_L \cdot e^{-k\tau}$. That is,

$$\text{Maintenance dose} = \left[\begin{array}{c} \text{Loading} \\ \text{dose} \end{array} \right] \cdot (1 - e^{-k\tau}) \qquad\qquad 11$$

Likewise, if the maintenance dose is known, the initial dose can be estimated:

$$\text{Loading dose} = \frac{\text{Maintenance dose}}{(1 - e^{-k\tau})} \qquad\qquad 12$$

Thus, for digitoxin, a daily maintenance dose of 0.1 mg requires a loading dose of 0.9 mg.

The similarity between Eqs. 3 and 11 should be noted. From the view point of accumulation, Eq. 3 relates to the maximum amount at plateau on administering a given dose repetitively. If the maximum amount were put into the body initially, then Eq. 11 indicates the dose needed to maintain that amount. The relationships are the same, although they were derived using different logic. These equations form the heart of multiple-dose drug administration and might well be called the "dosage regimen equations."

The ratio of loading to maintenance doses depends on the dosing interval and the half-life and is equal to the accumulation index, R_{ac}. For example, tetracycline has approximately an 8-hour half-life in man, and a dose in the range of 250 to 500 mg is considered to provide effective antimicrobial drug concentrations. Therefore, a reasonable schedule is 500 mg (two 250-mg capsules) initially, followed by 250 mg every half-life, as shown in Fig. 7–3. A dosage regimen consisting of a priming dose equal to twice the maintenance dose and a dosing interval of one half-life are convenient for drugs with half-lives between 8 and 24 hr. The frequency of administration for such drugs varies from 3 times a day to once daily, respectively. For drugs with very short to short half-lives, less than 3 hr, or with very long half-lives, greater than 24 hr, this regimen is often impractical.

Although a loading or initial dose greater than the maintenance dose seems appropriate for drugs with half-lives longer than 24 hr, such is often not the case. There are a variety of reasons why this is so. For piroxicam, an analgesic/antipyretic with a half-life of 48-hr, the most common adverse effects are gastrointestinal reactions. Such reactions may be increased if the loading dose is three to four times the maintenance dose ($D_L = D_M/(1 - e^{-k\tau})$, $\tau = 1$ day). Another example is that of warfarin (half-life $= 37$ hr), for which the anticoagulant effect develops slowly with time. A third example is that of protriptyline (an antidepressant with a half-life of 78 hr), for which larger doses slow gastric emptying and gastrointestinal activity (anticholinergic effect), resulting in slower and more erratic absorption of this and other drugs. Furthermore, for protriptyline, the development of therapeutic effects is also delayed, usually for 2 to 3 weeks.

MAINTENANCE OF DRUG IN THE THERAPEUTIC RANGE

Dosage regimens that achieve therapeutic concentrations are listed in Table 7–2 for drugs with both medium to high and low therapeutic indices and with various half-lives.

Half-Lives Less Than 30 Min

Great difficulty is encountered in trying to maintain therapeutic concentrations of such drugs. This is particularly true for a drug with a low therapeutic index, e.g., heparin, which has a half-life of approximately 30 min. Such a drug must be either infused or discarded unless intermittent concentrations are permissible. Drugs with a high therapeutic index may be given less frequently, but the greater the dosing interval, the greater is the maintenance dose required to ensure that drug in the body stays above a minimum effective value. Penicillin is a notable example of a drug for which the dosing interval (4 to 6 hr) is many times longer than its half-life (approximately 30 min). The dose given greatly exceeds that required to yield plasma concentrations of antibiotic equivalent to the minimum inhibitory concentration for most microorganisms.

Half-Lives Between 30 Min and 8 Hr

For such drugs, the major considerations are therapeutic index and convenience of dosing. A drug with a high therapeutic index need only be administered once every 1 to 3 half-lives, or even less frequently. A drug with a low therapeutic index must be given approximately every half-life, or more frequently, or be given by infusion. Lidocaine, for example,

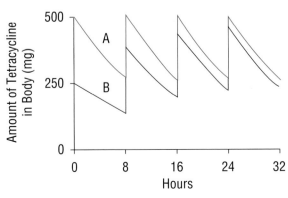

Fig. 7–3. Sketch of the amount of tetracycline in the body with time; simulation of the i.v. administration of 500 mg initially and 250 mg every 8 hr thereafter, curve A. When the initial and maintenance doses are the same, curve B, it takes approximately 30 hr (3 to 4 half-lives) before the plateau is practically reached. Thereafter, curves A and B are essentially the same.

has a half-life of 90 min, and the range of plasma concentrations associated with the treatment of cardiac arrhythmias is only about threefold. This drug must be given by infusion to ensure prolonged suppression of arrhythmias and minimal toxicity.

Half-Lives Between 8 and 24 Hr

Here, the most convenient and desirable regimen is one in which a dose is given every half-life. If immediate achievement of steady state is desired, then, as previously mentioned, the initial dose must be twice the maintenance dose; the minimum and maximum amounts in the body are equivalent to one and two maintenance doses, respectively.

Half-Lives Greater Than 24 Hr

For drugs with half-lives greater than 1 day, administration once daily is convenient and promotes patient compliance. If an immediate therapeutic effect is desired, a therapeutic dose needs to be given initially. Otherwise the initial and maintenance doses are the same, in which case several doses may be necessary before the drug accumulates to therapeutic levels. The decision whether or not to give larger initial doses is often a practical matter. Side effects to large oral doses (gastrointestinal side effects) or to acutely high concentrations of drug in the body may necessitate a slow accumulation.

Table 7-2.   Dosage Regimens for Continuous Maintenance of Therapeutic Concentrations

THERAPEUTIC INDEX[a]	HALF-LIFE	RATIO OF INITIAL DOSE TO MAINTENANCE DOSE	RATIO OF DOSING INTERVAL TO HALF-LIFE	GENERAL COMMENTS	DRUG EXAMPLES
Medium to High	<30 min	—	—	Candidate for constant-rate administration and/or short-term therapy.	Nitroglycerin
	30 min to 3 hr	1	3–6	To be given any less often than every 3 half-lives, drug must have very high therapeutic index.	Cephalosporins
	3–8 hr	1–2	1–3		Tetracycline
	8–24 hr	2	1	Very common and desirable regimen.	Sulfamethoxazole
	>24 hr	>2	<1	Once daily is practical. Occasionally given once weekly, or less frequently. Initial dose may need to be much greater than maintenance dose.	Chloroquine (suppression of malaria)
Low	<30 min	—	—	Not a candidate except under very closely controlled infusion.	Nitroprusside
	30 min to 3 hr	—	—	Only by infusion.	Lidocaine
	3–8 hr	1–2	~1	Requires 3–6 doses per day, but less frequently with controlled-release formulation.	Theophylline
	8–24 hr	2–4	0.5–1		Clonidine[b]
	>24 hr	>2	<1	Requires careful control; once toxicity is produced drug concentration and toxicity decline slowly.	Digitoxin

[a]Usually toxic maintenance dose/usual therapeutic maintenance dose.
[b]As with many other drugs in this category, rather than administering a loading dose, dosage is progressively elevated until the desired response is achieved.

To summarize the foregoing discussion, consider the antibiotic drug tetracycline, the nasal congestant phenylpropanolamine, and the antiepileptic agent phenobarbital, and their dosage regimens given in Table 7–3. Listed in Table 7–4 are the corresponding fractions of the initial amount remaining at the end of a dosing interval, the average amounts at steady state, and the maximum and minimum values. Instantaneous and complete absorption is assumed.

Dosing intervals for all three drugs are identical. The doses of phenylpropanolamine and phenobarbital are also the same, but the amounts of them in the body with time are certainly not. The explanation is readily visualized with a sketch.

As with any graph, consideration should first be given to scaling the axes. The amount of drug in the body should be scaled to the maximum amount at steady state. The time axis should be scaled to 4 to 5 half-lives, by which time plateau is achieved.

For tetracycline the amount in the body immediately after the first dose is 500 mg. At the end of the dosing interval, the fraction remaining is 0.5, and the amount therefore is 250 mg. A maintenance dose of 250 mg returns the level to 500 mg and so on. Figure 7–3, curve A, is thus readily drawn. Now consider the sketch had no loading dose been given. The initial amount, 250 mg, would then decline to 125 mg at the end of the first interval. The amount in the body immediately after the next dose would be 375 mg. At the end of the second interval, 187 mg would remain, and so on (curve B of Fig. 7–3).

For phenylpropanolamine the maximum and minimum amounts in the body at plateau are 40 mg and 10 mg, respectively, and a period of 4 half-lives is 16 hr. The fraction remaining at the end of each dosing interval is 0.25; therefore, the values of $A_{ss,max}$ and $A_{ss,min}$ are:

Dose	Time (hr)	$A_{ss,max}$ (mg)	$A_{ss,min}$ (mg)
1	0	30	
	8		7.5
2	8+	37.5	
	16		9.4
3	16+	39.4	

By the third dose (24 hr), the plateau is virtually achieved. Being given every two half-lives, the accumulation of phenylpropanolamine is minimal. Figure 7–4 is a sketch of the amounts of phenylpropanolamine in the body with time.

Table 7–3. Dosage Regimens and Half-lives of Three Drugs

DRUG	LOADING DOSE (mg)	MAINTENANCE DOSE (mg)	DOSING INTERVAL (hr)	HALF-LIFE (hr)
Tetracycline	500	250	8	8
Phenylpropanolamine	30	30	8	4
Phenobarbital	30	30	8	100

Table 7–4. Amount of Drug in Body (mg) on Regimens Given in Table 7–3

DRUG	FRACTION REMAINING AT END OF INTERVAL[a]	AVERAGE AT STEADY STATE[b]	MAXIMUM AT STEADY STATE[c]	MINIMUM AT STEADY STATE[d]
Tetracycline	0.5	360	500	250
Phenylpropanolamine	0.25	22	40	10
Phenobarbital	0.946	540	556	526

[a]Given by $e^{-k\tau}$
[b]$1.44 \cdot t_{1/2} \cdot D_M / \tau$.
[c]$F \cdot D_M (1 - e^{-k\tau})$
[d]$A_{ss,max} - F \cdot D_M$.

The same dosage regimen for phenobarbital produces a dramatically different result. At the end of each dosing interval, the fraction remaining is 0.946. Accumulation then occurs until the 5.4% lost in each interval is equal to the dose, and the amount in the body at steady state is therefore about 19 times the dose. From the calculated value of the maximum amount at plateau (556 mg) and the half-life, it is apparent that a sketch must be scaled to 600 mg and to about 15 days (Fig. 7–5). The curve is similar to that obtained with constant-rate infusion. The amounts in the body at 100 hr is one-half of the steady-state amount, and at 200 hr the level is 75% of the plateau amount, and so on. Practically, there is little need to consider the minor fluctuations.

The clinical implications of these regimens are manifold. The tetracycline regimen is designed to attain and maintain therapeutic levels. The phenylpropanolamine regimen gives rise to large fluctuations that may be desirable. Tolerance to the drug develops readily; the maintenance of high, effective, decongesting concentrations is questionable. With pheno-

Fig. 7–4. Sketch of the amount of phenyl-propanolamine in the body with time; simulation of 30 mg given i.v. every 8 hr. Because the half-life, 4 hr, is short relative to the dosing interval, the degree of accumulation is small and the fluctuation is large.

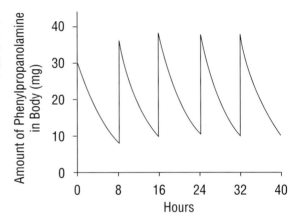

Fig. 7–5. Sketch of the amount of phenobarbital in the body with time; simulation of 30 mg given i.v. every 8 hr. Because the half-life, 4 days, is extremely long relative to the dosing interval, the degree of accumulation is large, and the fluctuation is low. The maximum and minimum values at steady state, 556 and 526 mg, are shown on the right.

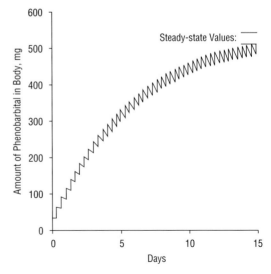

barbital the appropriate regimen depends on whether the drug is used for sedation or as an antiepileptic. For sedation, the omission of a loading dose is desirable, in that tolerance to the sedative effect develops with time and a large priming dose, 600 mg, causes too great a central depressive effect. As an antiepileptic, however, a loading dose may be appropriate. Although previously prescribed as such, chronic administration of phenobarbital three times daily is unnecessary; once daily administration may lead to better chances of compliance.

Lack of compliance is a major problem in pharmacotherapy. The most frequent pattern of noncompliance is the occasional omitted dose or failure to take several consecutive doses. Regimens of multiple daily doses tend to produce greater frequencies of missed doses than those in which a drug is taken once or twice daily. However, decreasing the frequency of dosing (with corresponding increase in each dose) may not improve the maintenance of concentrations within the effective range. The impact of a missed dose is shown in Fig. 7–6 for regimens of 300-mg once daily and 100-mg every 8 hr. In both regimens the total daily dose is the same. Omission of a single daily 300-mg dose produces a much lower minimum concentration than omission of a 100-mg dose for two reasons. First, the amount lost during the longer interval of the former regimen is greater. Second, the average minimum concentration at steady state is lower for the once daily regimen. Thus, omitting a single dose during a once daily regimen may have a much greater impact on therapeutic response than omitting an 8 hourly dose.

Note that even omitting three consecutive doses of the 8 hourly regimen (the equivalent of a once-daily dose) does not produce as low a concentration as the omission of a single daily dose.

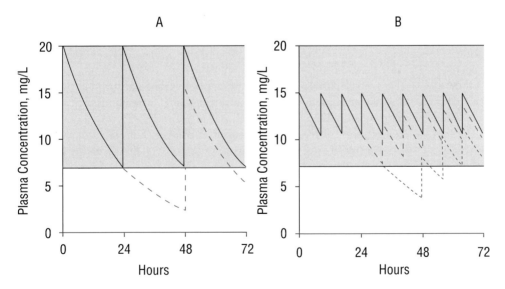

Fig. 7–6. From a kinetic perspective, the impact of a missed dose is greater the larger the dose and the less frequent the administration. Consider steady-state multi-dose conditions for a drug with a therapeutic window of 7 to 20 mg/L (color screened), a volume of distribution of 23.1 L, and a half-life of 15.9 hr. **Panel A:** When a 300-mg dose is given once daily to maintain therapeutic concentrations, a missed dose results in a trough concentration of 2.5 mg/L, a value well below the lower limit of the therapeutic window. **Panel B:** When a 100-mg dose is given every 8 hr (colored long dashed line), the lowest concentration achieved after a single missed dose is 7.3 mg/L, a value within the therapeutic concentration range. If 3 consecutive doses are missed (colored short-dashed line) the minimum concentration (3.7 mg/L) is still above that observed when a single daily dose of 300-mg is missed. The figure was adapted from concepts presented by Levy G., A pharmacokinetic perspective on medicament noncompliance. Clin. Pharmacol. Ther. 54:242-244, 1993.

The increased probability of compliance by once daily dosing is countered by kinetic arguments in favor of more frequent dosing. Where the optimum regimen lies depends on many factors. For example, for phenobarbital, with a half-life of 4 days, the omission of a single daily dose of 90 mg or an 8 hourly dose of 30 mg is of minor importance because the average amount in the body at steady state is 556 mg (see Fig. 7–5). Thus, the smaller the ratio of the dosing interval to half-life, the less the kinetic impact of a missed dose. Other determinants of the optimal regimen include factors such as those affecting the likelihood of compliance (severity and nature of disease, occupation of patient, personality of patient) and those relating to the pharmacodynamic characteristics of the drug (steepness of concentration-response curves, width of therapeutic window).

PRACTICAL ASPECTS OF MULTIPLE-DOSE ADMINISTRATION

So far, consideration has been given primarily to the amount of drug in the body following multiple i.v. bolus injections, or their equivalent, at equally spaced intervals. In practice, chronic administration is usually by the oral route. Furthermore, only drug concentration in plasma or in blood can be measured and not amount of drug in the body. These aspects are now considered. Problems related to unequal doses and dosing intervals and to missed doses are covered in Chap. 18, Concentration Monitoring.

Extravascular Administration

The oral (also intramuscular [i.m.], buccal, subcutaneous [s.c.], and rectal) administration of drugs requires an added step, absorption. Eqs. 1 to 4 apply to extravascular administration, provided that absorption has essentially ended within a small fraction of a dosing interval, a condition similar to i.v. bolus administration. Even so, a correction must be made if bioavailability is less than 1. When absorption continues throughout a dosing interval, or longer, then the relationships of Eqs. 7 and 8 still apply. These relationships allow estimation of the average plateau amount in the body and the average plateau concentration, respectively. The slowness of drug, absorption affects the degree of fluctuation around, but not the value of, the average concentration. The exception is when absorption becomes so slow that there is insufficient time for complete absorption, e.g., when limited by the transit time within the gastrointestinal tract.

The therapeutic impact of differences in absorption kinetics, but not in bioavailability, of extravascularly administered drug products given continuously depends on the frequency of their administration. As illustrated in Fig. 7–7, major differences seen following a single dose only persist and are of potential therapeutic concern at plateau when the drug products are given infrequently, relative to the half-life of the drug. Differences between them almost disappear at plateau when the products are given frequently. In the latter case, as stated previously, with extensive accumulation of drug, the concentration at plateau is relatively insensitive to variations in absorption rate.

Plasma Concentration Versus Amount in Body

During multiple dosing, the plasma concentration can be calculated at any time by dividing the corresponding equations defining amount by volume of distribution. Distribution equilibrium between drug in the tissues and that in plasma takes time. Thus, observed maximum concentrations may be appreciably greater than those calculated by dividing Eqs. 1 and 3 by V (see Chap. 19).

The average plateau concentration may be calculated using Eq. 8. This equation is applicable to any route, method of administration, or dosage form, as long as bioavailability and clearance remain constant with both time and dose.

DESIGN OF DOSAGE REGIMENS FROM PLASMA CONCENTRATIONS

Dosage regimens can be designed to maintain concentrations within a therapeutic window. The window is defined by a lower limit (C_{lower}) and an upper limit (C_{upper}). The maximum dosing interval, τ_{max}, and maximum maintenance dose, $D_{M,max}$, can be readily computed from these limits as follows:

$$C_{lower} = C_{upper} \cdot e^{-k\tau_{max}} \qquad\qquad 13$$

where τ_{max} is the maximum time interval over which these upper and lower concentrations can occur. By rearrangement of Eq. 13, the value of τ_{max} is

$$\tau_{max} = \frac{\ln\left(C_{upper}/C_{lower}\right)}{k} \qquad\qquad 14$$

and, from the relationship, $k = 0.693/t_{1/2}$,

$$\tau_{max} = 1.44 \cdot t_{1/2} \cdot \ln\left(C_{upper}/C_{lower}\right) \qquad\qquad 15$$

The corresponding maximum maintenance dose, $D_{M,max}$, that can be given every τ_{max} is

$$D_{M,max} = \frac{V}{F}\left(C_{upper} - C_{lower}\right) \qquad\qquad 16$$

When $D_{M,max}$ is administered every τ_{max}, there is an average concentration produced within the dosing interval, defined by

$$\frac{D_{M,max}}{\tau_{max}} = \frac{CL}{F} \cdot C_{ss,av} \qquad\qquad 17$$

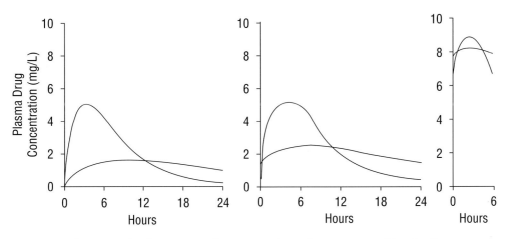

Fig. 7–7. Differences in the absorption rates between two dosage forms, exaggerated here for illustrative purposes, following a single extravascular dose (left panel) can have a major therapeutic impact at plateau during multiple dosing. The relative fluctuation of the plasma concentration when the drug products are given infrequently (middle panel) is much greater than when given frequently (right panel).

By dividing Eq. 16 by Eq. 14 and comparing this ratio to Eq. 17, it is apparent that the value of $C_{ss,av}$ is given by

$$C_{ss,av} = \frac{(C_{upper} - C_{lower})}{\ln(C_{upper}/C_{lower})} \qquad 18$$

A dosage regimen may be designed by setting the dosing rate either to achieve the average concentration, $C_{ss,av}$, or to maintain a peak concentration. In both approaches, concentrations are maintained within the therapeutic window throughout the dosing interval.

Maintenance of an Average Concentration

Choosing the average concentration within the dosing interval at plateau to be $C_{ss,av}$ allows the greatest possible dosing interval. This dosing interval (Eq. 15) and the corresponding maintenance dose (Eq. 16) may not be practical, however. Both values may need to be adjusted to make the frequency of administration convenient for patient compliance and to accommodate the dose strengths of the drug products available. The guiding principle is to maintain the same rate of administration and therefore the same chosen average steady-state concentration.

Having chosen a convenient dosing interval, τ smaller than τ_{max}, the maintenance dose is

$$D_M = (D_{M,max}/\tau_{max}) \cdot \tau \qquad 19$$

and the loading dose, appropriate to attain the steady-state concentration, initially, is

$$D_L = D_M/(1 - e^{-k\tau}) \qquad 20$$

If more (or less) vigorous therapy is desired, resulting in the setting of the average targeted concentration to be higher (or lower) than $C_{ss,av}$, the dosing rate can be increased (or decreased) proportionately. However, one may wish to adjust the dosing interval to ensure that concentrations remain within the therapeutic window.

Maintenance of a Peak Concentration

The second approach to the design of dosage regimens is based on the desire to maintain a given peak concentration. The peak concentration chosen, C_{peak}, depends on how aggressively one wishes to pursue therapy but usually lies in the upper half of the therapeutic window. The maximum dosing interval is:

$$\text{Maximum dosing interval} = \frac{\ln(C_{peak}/C_{lower})}{k} \qquad 21$$

On choosing a convenient interval, τ, less than the maximum defined in Eq. 21, the maintenance dose then becomes

$$D_M = V \cdot C_{peak}(1 - e^{-k\tau}) \qquad 22$$

and the loading dose, if necessary, is $V \cdot C_{peak}$. Note that C_{peak} is the same as $C_{ss,max}$. This method of regimen design tends to be simpler than the previous one.

For example, consider a drug with a therapeutic window of 2–10 mg/L, a volume of distribution of 25 L and a 16-hr half-life ($k = 0.043 \text{ hr}^{-1}$). The maximum dosing interval is then 37 hr (ln $(10/2)/0.043 \text{ hr}^{-1}$). If an interval of 12 hr is chosen, the maintenance dose needed is then about 100 mg ($V \cdot C_{peak}(1 - e^{-k\tau})$). The loading dose ($V \cdot C_{peak}$) is 250 mg. If the regimen is designed on the basis of attaining and maintaining the average concentration, the maintenance dose (Eqs. 17 and 19) is then 65 mg and the loading dose (Eq. 20) is 160 mg. Figure 7–8 illustrates the differences in these two approaches.

Following extravascular administration, fluctuations in the plasma concentration of drug are less than those after intravascular administration. Depending on the slowness of the absorption process, it may be possible to administer the drug less frequently than indicated in the regimens designed by either of the last two methods.

When Bioavailability and Volume Are Unknown

Oral dosage regimens can also be designed without determining bioavailability. This is accomplished using the area under the plasma concentration-time curve (AUC) following a single dose. From the relationship $F \cdot \text{Dose} = CL \cdot AUC$ after a single dose (Eq. 7, Chap. 4) and the relationship $F \cdot \text{Dose}/\tau = CL \cdot C_{ss,av}$ during steady state after multiple doses (Eq. 6), it follows that

$$C_{ss,av} = AUC \text{ (single dose)}/\tau \qquad\qquad 23$$

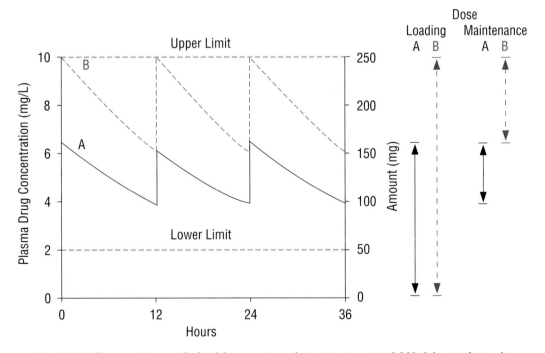

Fig. 7–8. Differences in two methods of dosage regimen design. Regimen A (solid black line) is designed to maintain the same average concentration as that obtained when the concentration fluctuates between the upper (10 mg/L) and lower (2 mg/L) limits. Regimen B (colored stippled line) is designed to ensure that the peak concentration does not exceed the upper limit. Of course, a lower peak value may have been chosen. The loading doses required to achieve the steady-state concentrations immediately and the maintenance doses for both regimens are indicated on the right side of the graph.

Consequently, either the dosing interval necessary to achieve a desired average steady-state concentration or the average concentration resulting from administering the dose every dosing interval can be calculated.

By definition of $C_{ss,av}$, the value of $\tau \cdot C_{ss,av}$ is the AUC within a dosing interval at steady state. Thus, this area is equal to that following a single dose. This principle is shown in Fig. 7–9, and a practical illustration is shown in Fig. 7–10.

Given the plasma concentrations with time after a single oral dose, the concentration at any time during repeated administration of the same dose can be readily calculated by adding the concentrations remaining from each of the previous doses. For example, if doses are given at 0, 12, and 24 hr, then the concentration at 30 hr is equal to the sum of the values at 30, 18, and 6 hr after a single dose.

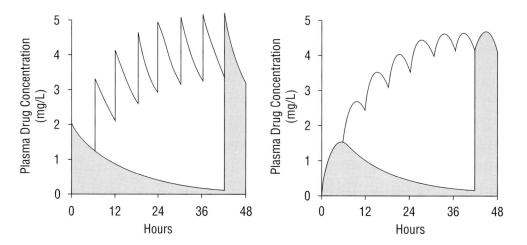

Fig. 7–9. Plasma concentrations of a drug given intravenously (left) and orally (right) on a fixed dose of 50 mg and fixed dosing interval of 6 hr. The half-life is 12 hr. Note that the AUC during a dosing interval at steady state is equal to the total area under the curve following a single dose. The fluctuation of the concentration is diminished when given orally (absorption half-life is 1.4 hr), but the average steady-state concentration is the same as that after i.v. administration, when, as in this example, $F = 1$. The equations used for the simulations are given in Appendix I-D.

Fig. 7–10. Twenty-four subjects each received a single 20-mg oral dose of the benzodiazepine, clobazam, followed 1 month later by an oral regimen of 10 mg of clobazam daily for 22 consecutive days. The observed average plateau clobazam concentration was well predicted by the value calculated from the single dose data, obtained by dividing the AUC by the dosing interval and correcting for dose. The solid line is the perfect prediction (1 mg/L = 33 µM) (Redrawn from Greenblatt, D.J., Divoll, M., Puri, S.K., Ho, I., Zinny, M.A., and Shader, R.I.: Reduced single-dose clearance of clobazam in elderly men predicts increased multiple-dose accumulation. Clin. Pharmacokinet., 8:83–94, 1983. Reproduced with permission of ADIS Press Australasia Pty Limited.)

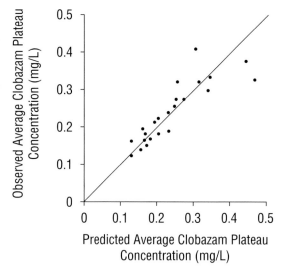

Useful relationships have been derived for designing and evaluating a dosage regimen in which the dose and the dosing interval are fixed. Table 7–5 summarizes some of the more important relationships and their limitations.

CONTROLLED RELEASE

The maintenance of a constant plasma concentration, and usually a relatively constant response, is achieved by constant-rate administration. While some constant-rate release systems have been developed (Chap. 6), other dosage forms exist from which drug release is much slower than from conventional dosage forms and for which the release kinetics are closer to first-order, than to zero-order. Such controlled-release products do not completely obliterate but do reduce considerably the fluctuation in the plasma concentration at plateau, when compared with conventional therapy, and are particularly useful when maintenance of therapeutic concentrations is difficult or inconvenient.

To illustrate the potential value of controlled-release products, consider the events at plateau simulated in Fig. 7–11 following oral administration in a child of theophylline, a therapeutic window of 6–20 mg/L, with a half-life of 4 hr. With the usual dosage forms, absorption is rapid and, to maintain the plasma concentration within the therapeutic window, the drug must be administered every 6 hr, an inconvenience. Administering the controlled-release dosage form at the same frequency as the conventional formulation leads to a marked reduction in the fluctuation at plateau. Indeed, the controlled-release formulation can be given at a more convenient dosing interval, 12 hr, and still maintain the plasma concentration within the therapeutic window. To maintain the same average concentration at plateau for the 12-hr interval, the dose of the less frequently administered controlled-release product must be twice that of the conventional product. Obviously, controlled-release products must perform reliably. If all the drug were released immediately, an unacceptable fluctuation in the plasma concentration would result.

For oral administration, once or twice daily is desirable. Accordingly, for drugs with half-lives greater than 12 hr, oral controlled-release products may be of little value, not only

Table 7–5. Relationships for Evaluating Dosage Regimens[a]

	RELATIONSHIP	I.V. BOLUS	RAPID ABSORPTION $(k_s \gg k)$	SLOW ABSORPTION $(k_s > k)$	$(k > k_s)$
Maintenance dose	$D_M = D_L \cdot (1 - e^{-k\tau})$	$\star\star\star$[b]	$\star\star\star$	$\star\star$	N[d]
Accumulation index	$R_{AC} = \dfrac{1}{(1 - e^{-k\tau})}$	$\star\star\star$	$\star\star\star$	$\star\star$	N
PLATEAU Average amount	$A_{ss,av} = 1.44 \cdot F \cdot D \cdot \left(\dfrac{t_{1/2}}{\tau}\right)$	$\star\star\star$	$\star\star\star$	$\star\star\star$	$\star\star\star$
Average concentration	$C_{av} = \dfrac{F \cdot D_M}{Cl \cdot \tau}$	$\star\star\star$	$\star\star\star$	$\star\star\star$	$\star\star\star$
	$C_{ss,av} = \dfrac{AUC \text{ (single dose)}}{\tau}$	$\star\star\star$	$\star\star\star$	$\star\star\star$	$\star\star\star$
Maximum concentration	$C_{ss,max} = \dfrac{F \cdot D_M}{V(1 - e^{-k\tau})}$	c	$\star\star$	$\star$	N
Minimum concentration	$C_{ss,min} = \dfrac{F \cdot D_M \cdot e^{-k\tau}}{V(1 - e^{-k\tau})}$	$\star\star\star$	$\star\star\star$	$\star\star$	N

[a]For regimens of equal doses and dosing intervals.
[b]$\star\star\star$Generally useful.
$\star\star$A reasonable approximation.
$\star$Limited usefulness.
[c]Should not be encouraged because distribution is not instantaneous.
[d]N Not Valid.

because the usual regimen is convenient but because protracted release may put drug into the lower intestine or perhaps out of the body before the release is complete. Decreased bioavailability then becomes a major concern, especially in patients with diseases in which gastrointestinal transit is shortened.

For a drug that is usually given i.m. or s.c., multiple injections are inconvenient and a controlled-release injectable dosage form may be advantageous. Depending on the total dose required and on the local effects of the injection mixture, it may only be necessary to administer the injection weekly, monthly, or perhaps as a single dose.

Evaluation of a Multiple-Dose Regimen and Assessment of Pharmacokinetic Parameters

The development of dosage regimens proceeds in two stages. The first involves establishing whether the events on multiple dosing are predicted from single-dose data. Often there is good accord between observation and prediction, indicating that the pharmacokinetic parameters have not changed upon multiple dosing. Occasionally, prediction is poor, signifying that one or more pharmacokinetic parameters has changed, evidence of some dose or time dependency (see Chap. 22). If prediction is good, the second stage is relatively straightforward. It involves varying the regimen to achieve particular plasma concentration-time profiles, which can be evaluated against therapeutic response and toxicity. The task is much more difficult when dose and time dependencies prevail.

This section deals with how to both evaluate a multiple-dose regimen, with or without single-dose data, and estimate pharmacokinetic parameters. It builds on what has been covered in the preceding parts of the chapter.

Clearance/Bioavailability. Stability in this ratio (CL/F) on multiple dosing is given by the equation

$$AUC_{ss} = AUC \text{ (single)} \qquad\qquad 24$$

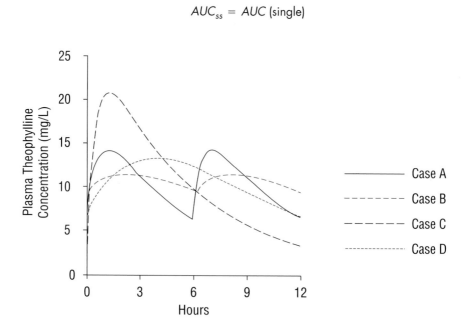

Fig. 7–11. Administering a drug, like theophylline, in a controlled-release dosage form (colored lines) may not only decrease the fluctuation in plasma concentration at plateau (Case A) compared to that seen with the usual regimen (Case B), but may also permit the drug to be given less frequently (Case C). Case D shows the concentration-time profile after the usual dosage form (360 mg) every 12 hr. In this example, $t_{1/2}$ = 4 hr, V = 35 L, F = 1, the half-life of release from the controlled-release product is 3 hr, and the therapeutic window is 3 to 10 mg/L. The dosage regimens are 180 mg every 6 hr (Cases A and B) and 360 mg every 12 hr (Cases C and D).

where AUC_{ss} is the AUC within a dosing interval at plateau. Equation 24 is a recasting of Eq. 23, where $AUC_{ss} = F \cdot \text{Dose}/CL$. A plateau is taken to be reached when several consecutive trough concentrations, determined from blood samples taken just before the next dose, show no trend with time. The accuracy of the estimates of AUC_{ss} and AUC (single) are heavily dependent on the number and timing of blood samples. If needed, the estimate of AUC_{ss} can be improved using several dosing intervals, which in turn improves the estimate of CL/F at plateau. As shown in Fig. 7–9 for clobazam, CL/F does not change on multiple dosing.

Half-Life. This parameter may be difficult to estimate during multiple dosing. Certainly, half-life cannot be estimated within a dosing interval with any confidence when the dosing interval is shorter than the half-life, as the decline in plasma concentration is too small over this time interval. The problem is made impossible if absorption continues throughout the dosing interval as often occurs with controlled-release products. Theoretically, half-life could be estimated from trough values taken on the approach to plateau, in much the same way as done with plasma data obtained on the rise to plateau following a constant-rate input regimen (pp. 70–71). In practice, however, this method is generally not very precise, especially when the dosing interval approaches the half-life, resulting in only a few trough values before plateau is reached.

The best way to estimate half-life is after stopping drug administration. At plateau, plasma concentrations are often much higher than those achieved after a single dose and so can be measured over much longer periods of time after stopping dosing, thereby facilitating an accurate estimate of half-life.

Degree of Accumulation. Accumulation always occurs. The major question is whether the degree of accumulation differs from that anticipated. One predictor of the degree of accumulation, given in Eq. 10, is the quantity $1/(1 - e^{-k\tau})$, the accumulation index (R_{ac}). This quantity predicts the ratio of the amount in the body at some time within the dosing interval at plateau to that at the same time after the first dose. However, plasma concentrations and not amounts are measured, and the ratio of amount to concentrations is only constant when the body acts as a single compartment. In practice, because distribution equilibrium between drug in tissues and that in plasma takes time, discrepancies arise between observed concentration and calculated values, assuming complete distribution. The discrepancy is greatest at early times. For this reason and because the value is difficult to estimate in practice, C_{max} is a poor choice to estimate the degree of accumulation. A trough value is a better choice, as distribution equilibrium is more likely to have been achieved at the end of the dosing interval. The observed degree of accumulation is $C_{ss,min}/C_{1,min}$, where $C_{1,min}$ is the trough concentration at the end of the first dosing interval. However, this last method relies on values obtained at only one time. This limitation is avoided using a commonly employed method based on AUC considerations, namely,

$$\begin{matrix} \text{Observed} \\ \text{accumulation} \\ \text{index} \end{matrix} = \frac{AUC_{ss}}{AUC(1, \tau)} \qquad \qquad 25$$

where $AUC (1,\tau)$ is the area under the plasma concentration-time profile during the first dosing interval to time τ. The procedure, analogous to the use of A_{av} values (Eq. 10), is illustrated in Fig. 7–12. Obviously, a prediction based on the ratio $AUC(\text{single})/AUC(1,\tau)$ will match the observed ratio if $AUC_{ss} = AUC(\text{single dose})$. The last term is the total AUC after a single dose. The value determined by Eq. 25 is approximately equal to $1/(1 - e^{-k\tau})$ if absorption is virtually complete at time τ after a single dose.

Degree of Fluctuation at Plateau. Fluctuation is an important consideration of any dosing regimen. It is usually evaluated at plateau. One common measure of the degree of fluctuation is the ratio $(C_{ss,max} - C_{ss,min})/C_{ss,min}$. An advantage of this measure is that it deals with direct observations, $C_{ss,max}$, $C_{ss,min}$, which are thought to have relevance with respect to correlates of safety and minimum efficacy. A disadvantage of this measure, however, is that it relies on only two observations, one of which $(C_{ss,max})$ is often difficult to estimate accurately, unless many blood samples are taken within the dosing interval, a relatively uncommon clinical practice. Another more stable measure of fluctuation, which is less dependent on single observations, is given by

$$\text{Fluctuation} = \frac{AUC\ (\text{above } C_{ss,av}) + AUC\ (\text{below } C_{ss,av})}{AUC_{ss}} \qquad 26$$

where AUC (above $C_{ss,av}$) and AUC (below $C_{ss,av}$) are the areas above and below the average concentration at plateau (AUC_{ss}/τ), respectively. Estimation of these values is shown in the inset to Fig. 7–12.

Other Parameters. Equation 27 forms a useful basis for determining relative bio-availability of a drug administered extravascularly (e.g., orally), between two treatments (e.g., dosage forms A and B). If clearance remains unchanged, then

$$\text{Relative bioavailability} = \frac{(AUC_{ss})_B}{(AUC_{ss})_A} \cdot \frac{(\text{Dose})_A}{(\text{Dose})_B} \qquad 27$$

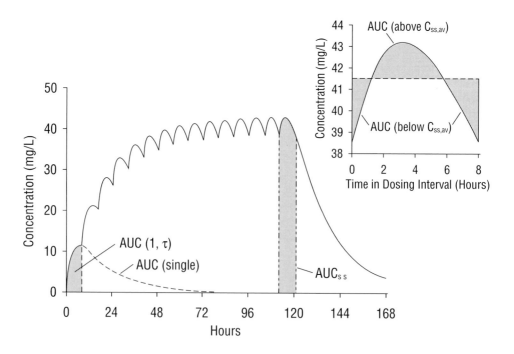

Fig. 7–12. Evaluation of a multiple-dose regimen. The stability of the CL/F ratio with dosing can be assessed by comparing the area during a dosing interval at plateau (AUC_{ss}) to that of the total area after a single dose $(AUC(\text{single}))$. The degree of accumulation is taken as the ratio of AUC_{ss} to the area during the first dosing interval to time τ $(AUC(1, \tau))$. The half-life is best determined after stopping drug administration. The inset shows the method for estimating the degree of fluctuation based on AUC (Eq. 26) above and below the average concentration, $C_{ss,av}$, within the dosing interval at plateau. Alternatively, it can be calculated from the observed maximum and minimum concentrations at plateau, $C_{ss,max}$, $C_{ss,min}$; degree of fluctuation $= (C_{ss,max} - C_{ss,min})/C_{ss,min}$.

Renal clearance can be estimated from the amount of drug excreted unchanged in a dosing interval at steady state, $Ae_{ss,\tau}$ and the value of AUC_{ss}

$$\text{Renal clearance} = \frac{Ae_{ss,\tau}}{AUC_{ss}} \qquad\qquad 28$$

The relative bioavailability of an extravascular dose may be determined from urine, as well as plasma, data as follows.

$$\text{Relative bioavailability} = \frac{(Ae_{ss,\tau})_B}{(Ae_{ss,\tau})_A} \cdot \frac{(Dose)_A}{(Dose)_B} \qquad\qquad 29$$

STUDY PROBLEMS

(Answers to Study Problems are in Appendix II.)

1. Comment on the accuracy of the following statements with regard to drugs given as an oral multiple-dose regimen.
   a. Accumulation always occurs.
   b. The extent of accumulation increases when drug is given less frequently.
   c. The time to reach plateau following a multiple-dose regimen depends on the frequency of drug administration.
   d. At plateau, the amount of drug lost within a dosing interval equals the oral maintenance dose.
   e. The larger the volume of distribution, the lower is the average plateau concentration.
   f. The average plateau concentration depends on the absorption kinetics of the drug following administration of a regimen of a fixed daily dose.
2. Gaffner et al. (Gaffner, C., Johnsson, G., and Sjögren, J.: Pharmacokinetics of procainamide intravenously and orally as conventional and slow-release tablets. Clin. Pharmacol. Ther., 17:414–423, 1975) compared a rapid-release with a controlled-release formulation of procainamide at steady state. To ensure comparability, the data (presented in Table 7–6) were collected over an 8-hr interval at steady state after administration of 0.5 g every 4 hr as the rapid-release tablet and 1 g every 8 hr as the controlled-release formulation.

Table 7–6.

	AUC (0,8) (mg·hr/L)	Ae_{ss}(0–8) (mg)
Rapid-release formulation	22.6	664
Controlled-release formulation	21.1	667

   a. Calculate the relative bioavailability of the controlled-release formulation compared with the rapid-release product.
   b. Calculate the renal clearance of procainamide.
3. The population pharmacokinetics of the oral diuretic agent, chlorthalidone, for a 70-kg person are

$$F = 0.64$$

$$V = 280 \text{ L}$$

$$CL = 4.5 \text{ L/hr}$$

    a. Given that absorption is instantaneous relative to elimination, calculate the following when a 50-mg dose of chlorthalidone is taken daily at breakfast.
      1. The maximum and minimum amounts of drug in the body at plateau
      2. The accumulation ratio
      3. The minimum plasma concentration at plateau
      4. The time required to achieve 50% of plateau
    b. Complete the table below for the dosage regimen of chlorthalidone given in (a).

	Amount of Chlorthalidone in Body (mg)							
Dose	1	2	3	4	5	6	7	∞
$A_{N,max}$								
$A_{N,min}$								

    c. Prepare a sketch on regular graph paper of the amount of chlorthalidone in the body with time. Show the salient features of accumulation of this drug during therapy.
    d. If required, what is the loading dose of chlorthalidone needed to immediately attain the condition at plateau?

4. Mr. J.M., a nonsmoking 60-kg patient with chronic obstructive pulmonary disease, is to be started on an oral regimen of aminophylline (85% of which is theophylline). The pharmacokinetics parameter values for a typical patient population with this disease are:

$$F = 1.0 \text{ (for theophylline)}$$

$$V = 0.5 \text{ L/kg}$$

$$CL = 40 \text{ mL/hr/kg}$$

Design an oral dosage regimen of *aminophylline* (100- and 200-mg tablets are marketed) for this patient to *attain* and *maintain* a plasma concentration within the therapeutic window, 10 to 20 mg/L. The absorption of theophylline is complete and rapid.

5. Table 7–7 lists a typical plasma concentration-time profile obtained following an oral 500-mg dose of a drug. The AUC is 80.6 mg-hr/L, and the terminal half-life is 5 hr.

Table 7-7.

Time (hr)	0	1	2	4	8	12	24	36	48
Plasma drug concentration (mg/L)	0	2.3	4.7	5.2	4.0	2.8	0.6	0.14	0.03

    a. What oral dosing rate of drug is needed to maintain an average plateau concentration of 10 mg/L?
    b. The decision has been made to give the drug once every 12 hr. What is:
      1. The unit dose strength of product needed?
      2. The plateau trough concentration expected?

6. The therapeutic dose of a rapidly (compared to elimination) and completely absorbed drug is 50 mg. A controlled-release dosage form to be given every 8 hr is designed to release its contents *evenly* and *completely* (no loading dose) over this dosing interval. Given that the half life of the drug is 4 hr:
    a. How much drug should the controlled-release dosage form contain?

b. To achieve a prompt effect, a rapidly absorbed dosage form is administered initially. When should the first controlled-release dosage form be given?

c. Following the dosage regimen in (b) what is the total dose (i) for day 1? (ii) for day 2?

d. In tabular form or on the same graph, provide the relative amounts of drug in the body versus time curves expected when the controlled-release preparation only is given (i) every 4 hr (ii) every 8 hr (iii) every 12 hr.

7. Adinazolam is a drug under investigation for the treatment of depression and panic disorders. Table 7–8 summarizes some of the salient pharmacokinetic information following single and multiple doses of immediate-release and controlled-release products.

Table 7-8. Mean Adinazolam Pharmacokinetic Information Following Single and Multiple Doses of Immediate-Release and Controlled-Release Preparations to a Group of 16 Subjects[a]

	IMMEDIATE RELEASE		CONTROLLED RELEASE	
	SINGLE DOSE 40 mg	MULTIPLE DOSES 40 mg every 8 hr	SINGLE DOSE 60 mg	MULTIPLE DOSES 60 mg every 12 hr
AUC (mg·hr/L)	0.57[b]	1.72[c]	0.88[b]	1.57[c]
C_{max} (mg/L)	0.15	0.20	0.07	0.11
T_{max} (hr)	1.00	—	2.50	—
Terminal $t_{1/2}$ (hr)	2.20	—	5.50	—

[a]Abstracted from Fleishaker, J.C. and Wright, C.E. Pharmacokinetic and pharmacodynamic comparison of immediate-release and sustained-release adinazolam mesylate tablets after singe-dose and multiple-dose administration. Pharm. Res. 9: 457–462, 1992.
[b]AUC (0–∞)
[c]AUC (0–24) after 7 days of dosing.

a. What rate-limits the decline of plasma adinazolam concentration following the administration of the controlled-release product?

b. On multiple dosing, have the immediate-release and controlled-release products been given long enough to ensure that a plateau should have been reached? In your answer, indicate whether any difference is expected in the time to reach plateau between the two products.

c. For both products, are the plasma concentration data observed on multiple dosing (Table 7–8) those predicted from single-dose data?

d. What is the relative bioavailability of adinazolam of the controlled-release product compared to the immediate-release product?

e. Are the pharmacokinetics of adinazolam after administration of the immediate-release and the controlled-release products such that the terminal half-life can be determined within the respective dosing intervals at plateau?

f. What are the degrees of accumulation associated with the immediate-release and the controlled-release regimens given that the AUC (0 to 8 hr) and AUC (0 to 12 hr) following the single 40-mg immediate-release product and the 60-mg controlled-release products are 0.45 and 0.44 mg-hr/L, respectively? Base your calculations on AUC considerations.

PHYSIOLOGIC CONCEPTS
AND KINETICS

MOVEMENT THROUGH MEMBRANES

So far in the book, emphasis has been placed on kinetic events following drug administration and application of pharmacokinetic principles to the design and evaluation of dosage regimens. Little has been said about how underlying physiologic processes control pharmacokinetic parameters, yet such information provides an insight into the interrelationships between drug and body. It also lays a foundation for individualization of drug therapy, the subject of the next section.

This section explores the physiologic concepts basic to pharmacokinetics. It begins with a chapter dealing with the passage of drugs through membranes, proceeds through the processes of absorption, distribution and elimination, and ends with a chapter on the integration of kinetics and physiologic concepts. Such information helps not only to interpret pharmacokinetic data, obtained under a variety of circumstances, but also to predict the likely outcome when pharmacokinetic parameters change.

Absorption, distribution, and elimination are all processes that require movement through membranes. This movement is known as drug transport. The anatomic and physiologic factors that determine the rapidity of drug transport are the substance of this chapter.

TRANSPORT PROCESSES

Cellular membranes appear to be composed of an inner, predominantly lipoidal, matrix covered on each surface by either a continuous layer or a lattice work of protein (Fig. 8–1, upper section of drawing). The hydrophobic portions of the lipid molecules are oriented toward the center of the membrane and the outer hydrophilic regions face the surrounding aqueous environment. Narrow aqueous-filled channels exist between some cells as in capillary membranes and intestinal epithelia.

The transport of drugs is often viewed as movement across a series of membranes and spaces which, in aggregate, serve as a "functional" macroscopic membrane. The cells and interstitial spaces that lie between the gastric lumen and the capillary blood and the structures between the sinusoidal space and the bile canaliculi in the liver, as well as the skin (Fig. 8–1), are examples. Each of the interposing cellular membranes and spaces impede drug transport to varying degrees, and any one of them can rate-limit the overall process. In the skin, the stratum corneum is the major site of impedance. It is this complexity of structure that makes quantitative extrapolation of drug transport from one membrane to another difficult. A description of the qualitative features of the processes of drug transport across these "functional" membranes follows.

Diffusion and Convection

Most drugs pass through membranes by *diffusion*, the natural tendency for molecules to move down a concentration gradient. Movement results from the kinetic energy of the molecules, and since no work is expended by the system, the process is known as *passive diffusion*.

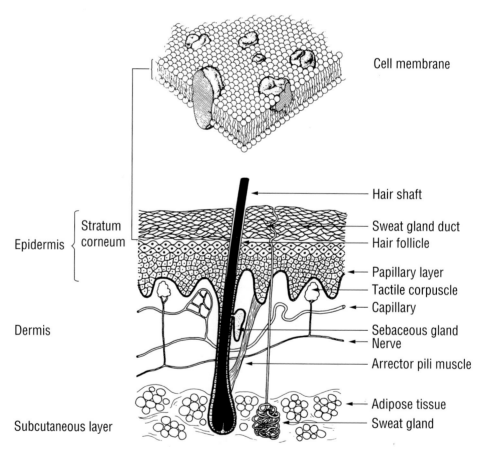

Fig. 8–1. Functional membranes vary enormously in structure and thickness. They can be as thin as a single-cell membrane, of approximately 1×10^{-6} cm thickness (top), to as thick as the multicellular barrier of the skin. This multicellular barrier extends from the stratum corneum to the upper part of the papillary layer of the dermis, adjacent to the capillaries of the microcirculation; a distance of approximately 2×10^{-2} cm (bottom). The cell membrane comprises a bimolecular leaflet, with a lipid interior and a polar exterior, dispersed through which are globular proteins, depicted as large solid irregular shaped bodies (Cell membrane—reproduced from Singer, S.J. and Nicolson, G.L.: The fluid mosaic model of the structure of cell membranes. *SCIENCE, 175*:720, 1972, copyright 1982 by the AAAS; skin was kindly drawn by Mandy North.)

To appreciate the properties of passive diffusion consider a simple system in which a membrane separates two well-stirred aqueous compartments. The driving force for drug transfer is the concentration of the diffusing species in each of the compartments on either side of the membrane. The net rate of penetration is

$$\text{Net rate of penetration} = \underset{\substack{\text{Permeability}}}{P} \cdot \underset{\substack{\text{Surface} \\ \text{area}}}{SA} \cdot \underset{\substack{\text{Concentration} \\ \text{difference}}}{(C_{side1} - C_{side2})} \qquad 1$$

The importance of the surface area of the membrane is readily apparent. For example, doubling the surface area doubles the probability of collision with the membrane and thereby increases the penetration rate twofold. Some drugs readily pass through a membrane, others do not. This difference in ease of penetration is quantitatively expressed in terms of the *permeability*. Note that the product $P \cdot SA$ has the units typical of flow, volume/time. Permeability therefore has units of velocity, distance/time.

The three major sources of variation in permeability of a given membrane to a drug are molecular size, lipophilicity, and charge. Molecular size has little impact on diffusion of substances in water but has a major effect on movement through membranes. This is presumably related to the structure of membranes. For some membranes, water-soluble materials move paracellularly through narrow channels between cells. Here again, molecular size is important, as are shape and charge of the molecule. For example, oxytocin, a cyclic monopeptide, paracellularly crosses the relatively loosely knit nasal membranes quite rapidly but is almost totally unable to cross the more tightly knit gastrointestinal membranes. Movement of water through the paracellular channels (a convective process) aids in the transport of substances by this route. The second source of variation, lipophilicity, is often characterized by partition between oil and water. Small lipid-soluble un-ionized drugs tend to penetrate lipid membranes with ease. This tendency and the effect of molecular size are shown in Fig. 8–2 for transdermal passage of a variety of uncharged molecules. Charge is the third major constraint to transmembrane passage. Again, there is considerable variation in the impedance of different membranes to charged molecules, but the effect of the charge is, with few exceptions (e.g. capillary membranes), always large.

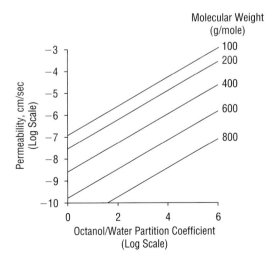

Fig. 8–2. Permeability across skin as a function of molecular size and lipophilicity. Lipophilicity is expressed as the octanol/water partition coefficient. Each line represents substances of the same molecular weight but different lipophilicity. (Modified from Potts, R.O. and Guy, R.H.: Predicting skin permeability. Pharm. Res., 9:663–669, 1992. Reproduced with permission of Plenum Publishing Corporation.)

Thus, the larger and more polar a molecule, the slower is its movement across membranes. Movement is slowed even more if the molecule is charged.

Another determinant of permeability is membrane thickness, the distance a molecule has to traverse from the site of interest (e.g., an absorption surface) to a blood capillary. The shorter the distance, the higher is the permeability. This distance can vary from about 0.005 to 0.01 μm (for cell membranes) to several millimeters (at some skin sites, Fig. 8–1, lower figure).

Drug transport continues toward equilibrium, a condition in which the concentrations of the diffusing species are the same in the aqueous phases on both sides of the membrane. Movement of drug between regions still continues at equilibrium, but the net flux is zero. Equilibrium is achieved more rapidly with highly permeable drugs, when there is a large surface area of contact with the membrane, and when the volumes of the compartments, to and from which the drug is transported, are small.

Initially, when all the drug is placed on one side of the membrane, it follows from Eq. 1 that rate of drug transport is directly proportional to concentration (Fig. 8–3). For example, rate of transport is increased twofold when concentration of drug is doubled. Stated differently, each molecule diffuses independently of the other, and the system cannot be saturated. Unless a drug alters the nature of the membrane, the last statement also applies when the other molecule is a different drug. Both absence of competition between molecules and lack of saturation are characteristics of passive diffusion.

Carrier-Mediated Transport

Membranes are not inert barriers; they have a specialized function. Membranes maintain the internal cellular environment by excluding or removing some materials and sequestering or selectively retaining vital substances. Many of these compounds are polar, with low lipid solubility. Yet they penetrate membranes much faster than anticipated for passive diffusion through an inert lipoidal barrier. Specialized carrier-mediated transport systems appear to be responsible. The substrates are often endogenous compounds, or close analogs.

The concept of a carrier stems from the observation of a limited rate of transport at increased substrate concentrations (Fig. 8–3). Two types of specialized transport processes have been proposed, passive facilitated diffusion and active transport.

Passive facilitated diffusion is exemplified by the movement of glucose into erythrocytes. It is a passive process; glucose moves down a concentration gradient without expenditure of energy, and at equilibrium, the concentrations in and surrounding the red blood cells are equal. At high plasma glucose concentrations, however, the rate of transport of glucose

Fig. 8–3. Initial rate of drug transport is plotted against the concentration of drug placed on one side of a membrane. With passive diffusion, the rate of transport increases linearly with concentration. With carrier-mediated transport, the rate of transport approaches a limiting value at high concentrations.

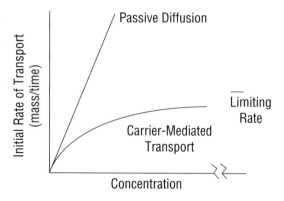

into the erythrocyte reaches a limiting value or *transport maximum*. Furthermore, in common with other carrier-mediated systems, glucose transport is reasonably specific and is inhibited by other substrates. Few drugs undergo passive facilitated diffusion. An example is the transport of vitamin B_{12} across the gastrointestinal epithelium.

Examples of *active transport* abound and include renal and biliary secretion of many acids and bases, secretion of certain acids out of the central nervous system, and intestinal absorption of some amino-β-lactam antibiotics and angiotensin-converting enzyme inhibitors via the dipeptide transport system. Characteristics in common with passive facilitated diffusion are saturability, specificity, and competitive inhibition. Active transport is distinguished from passive facilitated diffusion by the net movement of substance against a concentration gradient, which can be large. The maintenance of this gradient requires metabolic energy. Active transport can therefore be impeded by metabolic inhibitors.

BLOOD FLOW

Blood, perfusing tissues, delivers and removes substances. Accordingly, viewing any tissue as a whole, the movement of drug through membranes cannot be divorced from perfusion considerations. Perfusion is usually expressed in units of mL/min per volume (or mass) of tissue.

When membranes offer virtually no barrier, the slowest or rate-limiting step is perfusion, not permeability, as shown in Fig. 8–4. This perfusion limitation is exemplified in Fig. 8–5 for the passage of certain substances across the jejunal membranes of a rat, from lumen to blood. Tritiated water moves freely through the membrane, and its rate of passage increases with increasing perfusion. The passage of ethanol and many small drugs across the small intestine is similarly perfusion rate-limited.

As membrane resistance to drug increases, the rate limitation moves away from one of perfusion to one of permeability. The problem now lies in penetrating the membrane, not in delivering drug to, or removing it from, the tissue (Fig. 8–4B). This increase in resistance may arise for the same drug crossing membranes of increasing thickness; e.g., the multiple cell layers of the epidermis are less permeable to a drug than is the single cell layer of the capillary epithelium. For the same membrane, resistance increases with increasing size and polarity of the molecule. Thus, transport across the jejunum is slower for ribitol and many

A. Perfusion-Rate Limitation

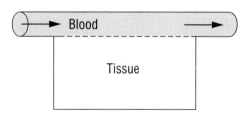

B. Permeability-Rate Limitation

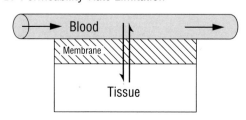

Fig. 8–4.   The limiting step controlling rate of movement of drug across a membrane, from blood to tissue or the converse, varies. *A,* If the membrane offers no resistance, drug in the blood leaving the tissue is in virtual equilibrium with that within tissue; blood and tissue may be viewed as one. Here movement of drug is limited by blood flow. *B,* A permeability-rate limitation exists if membrane resistance to drug movement becomes high; movement here is both slow and insensitive to changes in perfusion. Also, equilibrium is not achieved by the time the blood leaves the tissue; blood and tissue must now be viewed as separate compartments.

other larger polar compounds than for ethanol or water, which results in insensitivity to changes in perfusion (Fig. 8–5).

Some compounds, like urea, have intermediate permeability characteristics across the jejunum. At low blood flow rates, the compound has sufficient time to traverse the membrane so that perfusion becomes rate-limiting. At higher blood flow rates, however, membrane permeability becomes the rate-limiting step, and absorption becomes relatively insensitive to blood flow (Fig. 8–5).

IONIZATION

Most drugs are weak acids or weak bases and exist in solution as an equilibrium between un-ionized and ionized forms. Increased accumulation of drug on the side of a membrane where pH favors greater ionization of drug has led to the *pH partition hypothesis*. According to this hypothesis, only un-ionized nonpolar drug penetrates the membrane, and at equilibrium, the concentrations of the un-ionized species are equal on both sides.

The majority of evidence supporting the pH partition hypothesis stems from studies of gastrointestinal absorption, renal excretion, and gastric secretion of drugs. The pH of gastric fluid varies between 1.5 and 7.0; urine pH fluctuates between 4.5 and 7.5. Elsewhere in the body, changes in pH tend to be much smaller and to show less deviation from the pH of blood, 7.4.

The un-ionized form is assumed to be sufficiently lipophilic to traverse membranes. If it is not, theory predicts that there is no transfer, irrespective of pH. The fraction un-ionized is controlled by both the pH and the *pKa* of the drug according to the Henderson-Hasselbalch equation. Thus, for acids,

$$pH = pKa + \log_{10}\left(\frac{\text{Ionized concentration}}{\text{Un-ionized concentration}}\right) \qquad 2a$$

and for bases

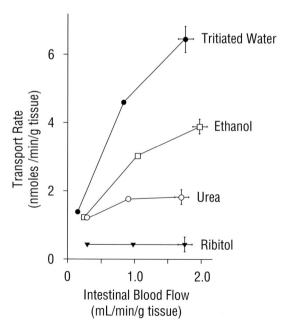

Fig. 8–5. The rate of passage of a substance across the jejunum of a rat was determined by measuring its rate of appearance in intestinal venous blood. The passage is blood flow limited when, like tritiated water, the molecule freely permeates the membrane. With poorly permeable substances, like the polar molecule ribitol, the passage is limited by transmembrane penetration, not by blood flow. (Redrawn from Winne, D., and Remischovsky, J.: Intestinal blood flow and absorption of non-dissociable substances. J. Pharm. Pharmacol., 22:640–641, 1970.)

$$pH = pKa + \log_{10}\left(\frac{\text{Un-ionized concentration}}{\text{Ionized concentration}}\right) \qquad 2b$$

As $\log_{10}(1) = 0$, the pKa of a compound is the pH at which the un-ionized and ionized concentrations are equal. The pKa is a characteristic of the drug (Fig. 8–6). Consider, for example, the anticoagulant warfarin. Warfarin is an acid with pKa 4.8, i.e., equimolar concentrations of un-ionized and ionized drug exist in solution at pH 4.8. Stated differently, 50% of the drug is un-ionized at this pH. At one pH unit higher, 5.8, the ratio is 10 to 1 in favor of the ionized drug; i.e., 10 out of 11 total parts or 91% of the drug now exists in the ionized form, and only 9% is un-ionized. At one pH unit lower than the pKa, 3.8, the percentages in the ionized and un-ionized forms are 9 and 91, the converse of those at pH 5.8.

Figure 8–7 shows changes in the percent of un-ionized drug with pH for acids of different pKa values. The pH range 1.0 to 8.0 encompasses values seen in the gastrointestinal tract and the renal tubule. Several considerations are in order and are exemplified by transport across the gastrointestinal barrier. First, very weak acids, such as phenytoin and many barbiturates, whose pKa values are greater than 7.5 are essentially un-ionized at all pH values. For these acids drug transport should be rapid and independent of pH, provided the un-ionized form is permeable. Second, the fraction un-ionized only changes dramatically for acids with pKa values between 3.0 and 7.5, and for these compounds a change in rate of transport with pH is expected and has been observed. Third, although transport of still stronger acids, those with pKa values less than 2.5, should theoretically also depend upon pH, in practice the fraction un-ionized is so low that transport across the gut membranes may be slow even under the most acidic conditions.

A similar analysis indicates that a base must be very weak, pKa less than 5, for transport to be independent of pH. Caffeine (pKa 0.8) is an example of a base that is rapidly trans-

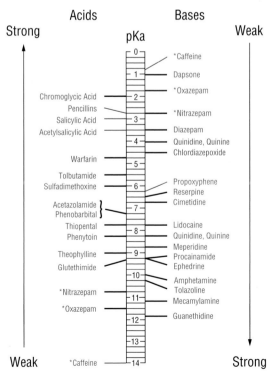

Fig. 8–6. The pKa values of acidic and basic drugs vary widely. Some drugs are amphoteric (*), i.e., they have both acidic and basic functional groups.

ported and shows no pH-dependent absorption. Only with stronger bases, those with *pKa* values between 5 and 11, is pH-dependent transport expected. At the usually low pH of the gastric fluid, these bases exist almost exclusively in the ionized form, and for these, gastric transport should be slow. Passage of these bases should be more rapid from a less acidic environment. All evidence supports these expectations.

As originally proposed, the pH partition hypothesis relates to events at equilibrium, yet it has been applied most widely to predict the influence of pH on the rates of absorption and distribution. The likely influence of pH on a rate process depends, however, on where the rate limitation lies. Only if the limitation is in permeability is an effect of pH on rate expected. If the limitation is in perfusion, the problem is not one of movement of drug through membranes and, therefore, any variation in pH is unlikely to have much effect on the rate process. Where the equilibrium lies, however, is independent of what process rate-limits the approach toward equilibrium. Accordingly, pH is predicted to affect the distribution of an ionizable drug across a membrane at equilibrium in all cases in which the membrane is permeable only to un-ionized drug.

Despite its general appeal, the pH partition hypothesis fails to explain certain observations. A variety of quaternary ammonium compounds (e.g., propantheline bromide) which are always ionized elicit systemic effects when given orally. Movement of these compounds through the gastrointestinal membranes occurs, although at a slow and erratic rate. Animal studies also indicate penetration of the ionized form of many acids and bases through membranes, though at a slower rate than the un-ionized form. These observations suggest that quantitative prediction of the influence of pH on the movement of drugs across a membrane is unlikely to be accurate.

PROTEIN BINDING

Many drugs bind to plasma proteins and tissue components (discussed in Chap. 10). Such binding is reversible and usually so rapid that an equilibrium is established within milliseconds. Consequently, the associated (bound) and dissociated (unbound) forms of the drug can be assumed to be at equilibrium at all times and under virtually all circumstances.

Only unbound drug is thought to be generally capable of passing through membranes, the protein-bound form being too large to do so. The influence of protein binding on the rate of movement through a membrane can be viewed in much the same way as that of the influence of pH on the movement of weak acids and bases. Both binding and ionization are virtually instantaneous reactions, with only one species (unbound, un-ionized form) capable of traversing membranes. If there is a perfusion limitation, dissociation of the

Fig. 8–7. Very weak acids, *pKa* values greater than 8.0, are predominantly (above dashed line) un-ionized at all pH values between 1.0 and 8.0. Profound changes in the fraction un-ionized occur with pH for an acid whose *pKa* value lies within the range of 2.0 to 8.0. Although the fraction un-ionized of even stronger acids increases with hydrogen ion concentration, the absolute value remains low at most pH values shown.

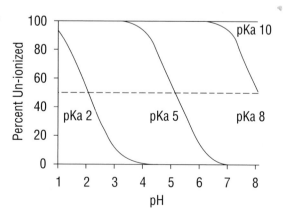

bound drug and diffusion of the unbound drug through the membrane must occur so rapidly that rates of delivery and transport are equal. Thus, an alteration in protein content is not expected to affect rate at a given concentration. If permeability is rate-limiting, little of the drug presented moves into the tissue. For a given rate of delivery, altered protein binding, by affecting the unbound concentration, now influences the rate of transport.

REVERSIBLE NATURE OF TRANSPORT

It is important to remember that drug transport is generally bidirectional. One tends, for example, to think of drug absorption in the gastrointestinal tract as being unidirectional. Normally, with very high concentrations of drug placed into the gastrointestinal tract, following oral administration, the net rate of transport is toward blood in mesenteric capillaries. However, important applications can be made of transport in the opposite direction. For example, repeated oral administration of charcoal can hasten removal from the body of drugs such as digoxin, phenylbutazone, phenobarbital, and digitoxin in cases of drug overdose. Because of extensive adsorption of drug to charcoal, the lumen of the gastrointestinal tract acts as a sink for removal of drug from blood. In this case, the site of transfer may be restricted to only a small region of the gastrointestinal tract or may apply to a much larger area. The restriction depends on the distribution of charcoal along the gastrointestinal tract. Even with complete distribution of charcoal, whether the overall transfer from blood to gut lumen is perfusion rate-limited or not depends on the permeability of the various functional membranes along the length of the gut as well as on blood flow to these various sites.

As previously stated, the concepts of this chapter on passage of drugs across membranes are important to an understanding of movement of drugs into, within, and out of the body. In the next three chapters, these concepts are incorporated with other principles dealing with drug absorption, distribution, and elimination.

STUDY PROBLEMS

(Answers to Study Problems are in Appendix II.)

1. Define the terms: passive diffusion, passive facilitated diffusion, active transport, and permeability.
2. How accurate are each of the following statements?
   a. When distribution is perfusion-rate limited, the ratio of concentrations across the capillary membrane of the tissue is virtually one at all times.
   b. When the surface area of a membrane is doubled, so is its permeability.
   c. Passive diffusion across a membrane stops when the concentrations on both sides are the same.
   d. Carrier-mediated transport is one in which energy is needed to transfer drug across a membrane.
   e. Protein binding in the aqueous phases diminishes the permeability of membranes.
3. Molecular size is an important determinant of permeability. Figure 8–2 summarizes the results of skin penetration for a variety of un-ionized compounds. Using the figure, describe the effect of doubling molecular weight on the permeability for a series of compounds of equal lipophilicity (octanol/water partition coefficients on log scale are all equal to 2).
4. Briefly discuss the role of ionization in the movement of weak acids and weak bases across membranes.
5. Table 8–1 shows the effect of oral administration of activated charcoal on removal of phenobarbital from the body.

Table 8–1. Effect of Repeated Doses of Activated Charcoal on the Half-life (Hours) of Phenobarbital[a]

DURING COADMINISTRATION OF ACTIVATED CHARCOAL[b]	ABSENCE OF CHARCOAL ADMINISTRATION
36 ± 13	93 ± 7

[a]Pond, S.M., Olson, K.R., Osterloh, J.D., and Tong, T.G.: Randomized study of the treatment of phenobarbital overdose with repeated doses of activated charcoal. JAMA, 251:3104–3108, 1984.
[b]17 g of charcoal in 70 mL of 70% sorbitol every 4 hr administered through a nasogastric tube.

a. Knowing that the volume of distribution of phenobarbital is 0.55 L/kg, calculate the clearance of phenobarbital into the alimentary canal during treatment with charcoal. Hint: CL (during treatment) = CL (no treatment) + CL (by charcoal).

b. The clearance value determined in "a" should apply as well to movement of drug from the lumen of the gastrointestinal tract into the bloodstream. If the majority of drug removal and absorption occurs in the small intestine, estimate the half-life associated with absorption when 0.4 L of fluid is in the small intestine. For this problem, conceive the small intestine as a single compartment.

ABSORPTION

OBJECTIVES

The reader will be able to:

1. Describe the steps involved in the oral absorption of a drug.
2. Distinguish between dissolution and permeability rate-limitations in absorption.
3. Anticipate the influence of physicochemical properties of a drug on its absorption from different sites of administration.
4. Anticipate the role of gastric emptying and intestinal transit in the gastrointestinal absorption of a drug, with particular reference to the physicochemical properties of the drug and its dosage form.
5. List the factors influencing dissolution rate of a drug.
6. Describe the influence of decreased permeability and surface area along the intestinal tract on the performance of oral constant-rate release systems *in vivo*.

Drugs are most frequently administered extravascularly. The majority are intended to act systemically, and for these, absorption is a prerequisite for activity. Delays or losses of drug during absorption may contribute to variability in drug response and, occasionally, may result in failure of drug therapy. It is primarily in this context, as a source of variability in systemic response and as a means of controlling the concentration-time profile of drug in the body, that absorption is considered here and throughout the remainder of the book. It should be kept in mind, however, that even for those drugs intended to act locally (e.g., mydriatics, local anesthetics, nasal decongestants, topical agents, and aerosol bronchodilators), movement of drug from the site of application to the systemic circulation influences time of onset, intensity, and duration of effect.

This chapter deals with the general principles governing rate and extent of drug absorption. Although absorption from other sites is discussed, emphasis is placed on absorption following oral administration. This is not only because the oral mode of administration is the most prevalent for systemically acting drugs, but also because it illustrates many sources of variability encountered in drug absorption.

Figure 9–1 depicts the numerous steps involved in the absorption of a drug given orally. Being a complex structure, many anatomic and physiologic factors affect the overall rate and extent of drug absorption from the gastrointestinal tract, making a precise quantitative prediction difficult. Nonetheless, much can be understood and appreciated of the events occurring at this and other sites of absorption.

Absorption is favored because the body acts as a large sink. A concentration gradient is present until virtually no drug remains to be absorbed. The gradient is maintained longer, the larger the volume of distribution of the drug.

Passage of drug through the membranes dividing the absorption site from the blood is a prerequisite for absorption to occur. To do so, the drug must be in solution. Most drugs are administered as solid preparations. Common examples are tablets and capsules. Because solid particles cannot pass through membranes, a drug must dissolve to be absorbed. Many factors influence the release of drug from a solid pharmaceutical formulation. *Biopharmaceutics* is a comprehensive term denoting the study of the influence of pharmaceutical formulation variables on the performance of a drug *in vivo*.

ABSORPTION FROM SOLUTION

Several physiologic and physical factors that determine movement of drug through membranes have been discussed generally in Chap. 8. Included among them are the physicochemical properties of the molecule, the nature of the membrane, perfusion, and pH. These factors and others are now considered with respect to drug absorption.

Gastrointestinal Absorption

In accordance with the prediction of the pH partition hypothesis, weak acids are absorbed more rapidly from the stomach at pH 1.0 than at pH 8.0, and the converse holds for weak bases. Absorption of acids, however, is always much faster from the less acidic small intestine (pH 6.6 to 7.5) than from the stomach (Fig. 9–2). These apparently conflicting observations can be reconciled. Surface area, permeability, and for perfusion rate-limited absorption, blood flow are important determinants of the rapidity of absorption. The intestine, especially the small intestine, is favored on all accounts. The total absorptive area of the small intestine, composed largely of microvilli, has been calculated to be about 200 M^2, and an estimated 1 L of blood passes through the intestinal capillaries each minute. The corresponding estimates for the stomach are only 1 M^2 and 150 mL/min. The permeability

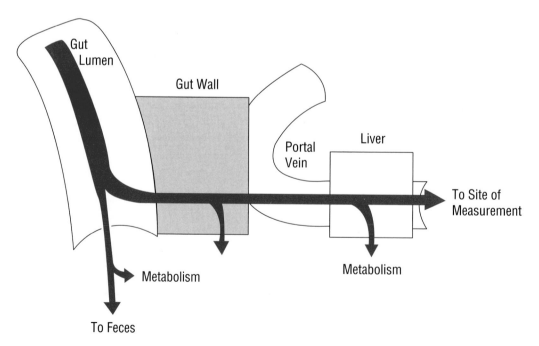

Fig. 9–1. A drug, given as a solid, encounters several barriers and sites of loss in its sequential movement during gastrointestinal absorption. Dissolution, a prerequisite to movement across the gut wall, is the first step. Incomplete dissolution or metabolism in the gut lumen or by enzymes in the gut wall is a cause of poor bioavailability. Removal of drug as it first passes through the liver further reduces bioavailability.

of the intestinal membranes to drugs may also be greater than that of the stomach. These increases in surface area, permeability, and blood flow more than compensate for the decreased fraction of un-ionized acid in the intestine. Indeed, the absorption of *all* compounds, be they acids, bases, or neutral compounds, is faster from the (small) intestine than from the stomach. Because absorption is greater in the small intestine, the rate of gastric emptying is a controlling step in the speed of drug absorption.

Gastric Emptying. Gastric emptying of liquids is approximately zero-order. Food, especially fat, slows gastric emptying, which explains why drugs are frequently recommended to be taken on an empty stomach when a rapid onset of action is desired. Drugs that influence gastric emptying also affect the rate of absorption of other drugs (Fig. 9–3).

Retention of drug in the stomach increases the percentage of a dose absorbed through the gastric mucosa, but usually the majority of drug is still absorbed through the intestinal epithelium. In this regard, the stomach may be viewed as a repository organ from which pulses of drug are ejected by peristalsis onto the absorption sites in the small intestine.

Intestinal Absorption. Throughout its length, the intestine varies in its multifaceted properties and luminal composition. The intestine may be broadly divided into the small

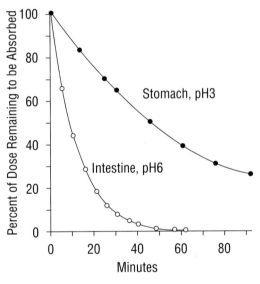

Fig. 9–2. Despite an environment favoring a greater percentage of un-ionized drug, absorption of salicylic acid (*pKa* 3) is slower from the rat stomach at pH 3 (●) than from the rat intestine at pH 6 (○). (Modified from Doluisio, J.T., Billups, N.F., Dittert, L.W., Sugita, E.G., and Swintosky, J.V.: Drug absorption I. An *in situ* rat gut technique yielding realistic absorption rates. J. Pharm. Sci., 58:1196–1199, 1969. Adapted with permission of the copyright owner.)

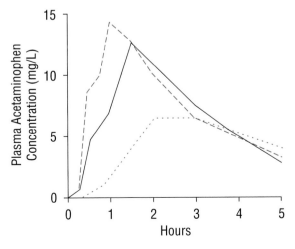

Fig. 9–3. Slowing gastric emptying by propantheline (30 mg i.v.) slows the rate of absorption of acetaminophen (1500 mg), administered orally in a 22-year-old male, as seen by a decrease in the maximum plasma concentration and a longer time to reach this concentration (· · · · ·) compared to values when acetaminophen is given alone (———). Metoclopramide (10 mg i.v.), which hastens gastric emptying, hastens the absorption of acetaminophen (– – –) (1 mg/L = 6.6 μM). (Redrawn from Nimmo, J., Heading, R.C., Tothill, P., and Prescott, L.F.: Pharmacological modification of gastric emptying: Effects of propantheline and metoclopramide on paracetamol (acetaminophen) absorption. Br. Med. J., *1*:587–588, 1973.)

and large intestine separated by the ileocecal junction. Surface area per unit length decreases from the duodenum to the rectum. Electrical resistance, a measure of the degree of tightness of the junctions between the epithelial cells, is much higher in the colon than in the small intestine. Proteolytic and metabolic enzymes, as well as active and facilitated transport systems are distributed along the intestine, often in restrictive regions. The colon abounds with anaerobic microflora. The mean pH, 6.6 in the proximal small intestine rising to 7.5 in the terminal ileum, falls sharply to 6.4 at the start of the cecum before finally rising to 7.0 in the descending colon. Transit time of materials is around 3 to 4 hr in the small intestine and from 10 to 24 hr or even longer in the large bowel. Although these and other complexities make precise quantitative prediction of intestinal drug absorption difficult, several general features emerge.

The permeability-surface area product $(P \cdot SA)$ tends to decrease progressively from duodenum to colon. This applies to all drug molecules traversing the intestine epithelium by non carrier-mediated processes, whether via the transcellular or paracellular route. The decrease in $P \cdot SA$ is seen as a decrease in the kinetics of absorption when drugs are placed in different parts of the intestine, as illustrated in Fig. 9–4 for ranitidine.

Permeability in the small intestine can be sufficiently high so that absorption from the lumen is perfusion rate-limited (Fig. 8–5, p. 114). Under these conditions, overall gastric emptying would rate-limit absorption from an oral solution. As shown in Fig. 8–5, at any one site along the intestine, in this case the jejunum, small molecules permeate more freely than larger ones. The issue of molecular size is particularly important for polar drugs. These substances move paracellularly via the tight functions between epithelial cells. Permeability appears to drop off sharply with molecular weights above 350 g/mole. Molecular size has

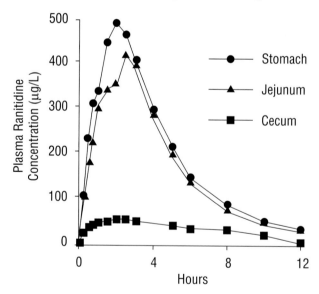

Fig. 9–4. The gastrointestinal absorption of ranitidine varies with site of application. Shown are the mean plasma concentration-time profiles of ranitidine observed after placing an aqueous solution (6 mL) containing 150 mg of ranitidine hydrochloride into the stomach (●), jejunum (▲), and colon (■) of eight volunteers, via a nasoenteric tube. The much less extensive absorption of this small (M.W. = 313 g/mole) polar molecule from the colon is consistent with the idea that the permeability-surface area $(P \cdot SA)$ product is much lower in the colon than in the small intestine. Notice that absorption of ranitidine effectively ceases (in terminal decline phase) by 3 hr when placed in the stomach or jejunum, even though the drug is incompletely bioavailable ($F \sim 0.6$, data not shown) suggesting that the small intestine is the major site of absorption when rantidine is taken orally. (Adapted from Williams, M.F., Dukes, G.E., Heizer, W., Han, Y-H., Hermann, D.J., Lampkin, T., and Hak, L.J.: Influence of gastrointestinal site of drug delivery on the absorption characteristics of ranitidine. Pharm. Res., 9:1190–1194, 1992.)

less of an effect on permeability for lipophilic drugs, which trasverse transcellularly. The ultimate limit to permeability is size, however. Thus, large polypeptides, proteins, and other macromolecular drugs are virtually unable to pass through the intestine wall even if they are metabolically stable, unless they can be processed by one of the specialized systems that traffic vital materials, such as vitamin B_{12}, from the apical to the basolateral surface of the epithelial cell.

Causes of Low Oral Bioavailability. When a drug is given in solution and passes readily across membranes, absorption from most sites of administration is complete. This is not always so, especially when drugs are placed into the gastrointestinal tract.

A drug must pass sequentially from the gastrointestinal lumen, through the gut wall, and through the liver, before entering the general circulation (Fig. 9–1). This sequence is an anatomic requirement because blood perfusing virtually all gastrointestinal tissues drains into the liver via the hepatic portal vein. If the only cause of loss is incomplete time for absorption, then the bioavailability is less than one and the complement, the fraction appearing in feces unchanged, is a measure of luminal retention. Drug may also be lost by decomposition in the lumen; the fraction entering the tissues, F_F, is then the fraction neither lost in the feces nor decomposed in the lumen. Of this permeating drug, only a fraction may escape destruction within the walls of the gastrointestinal tract, F_G, thereby reducing the fraction of dose reaching the portal vein to $F_F \cdot F_G$. If drug is also eliminated in the liver, an additional fraction, F_H, of that reaching the liver escapes extraction there. The measured overall systemic bioavailability, F, clearly is then

$$F = F_F \cdot F_G \cdot F_H \qquad 1$$

For example, if 50% of the drug is lost at each step, the bioavailability of the drug, measured systematically, would be $0.5 \times 0.5 \times 0.5$ or 12.5%. Note that the drug can be rendered totally unavailable at any one of these steps.

The lungs are excluded from the foregoing considerations of bioavailability even though they may occasionally be an important site of elimination. As discussed in Chap. 4, drug given intravenously is used as a standard to measure bioavailability, with calculation based on measurement of drug at a peripheral venous site. Both intravenously and orally administered drugs must first pass through the lungs to reach this site of measurement. Consequently, the effect of the lungs on the measurement of bioavailability need not be considered.

Insufficient Time for Absorption. The $P \cdot SA$ term for drugs appears to drop sharply with movement from the small intestine to colon. How much of this drop is due to a decrease in permeability and how much to a decrease in surface area between small and large intestine is not known for certain. For permeable drugs, absorption is rapid and probably complete within the small intestine. Even if some drug were to enter the large intestine, the permeability there would still be sufficiently high to ensure that all that entered was absorbed. Absorption of less permeable, generally polar, drugs still primarily occurs within the small intestine but is unlikely to be complete within the limited 2- to 4-hr transit period. Evidence supporting this notion is provided with the H_2-antagonist ranitidine. This relatively polar stable compound is almost totally excreted unchanged when given intravenously. When given orally, 60% is absorbed but all within the first 3 to 4 hr after administration (Fig. 9–4); the rest is recovered unchanged in feces. Evidently, very little ranitidine is absorbed from the large intestine even though drug can be there for up to 24 hr.

Table 9–1 lists representative drugs for which oral bioavailability is very low (0.1 to 14%), most likely due to poor intestinal permeability with most of that absorbed having occurred within the small intestine. The drugs share the common properties of being polar and, with the exception of pyridostigmine, relatively large (molecular weight greater than 400 g/mole). Pyridostigmine is a quaternary ammonium compound, which may explain its low bioavailability despite its small molecular weight (181 g/mole). Most of the compounds listed in Table 9–1 cannot be given orally for effective systemic activity; they must be given parenterally.

Finally, there are small molecular weight, 200 to 350 g/mole, polar drugs for which absorption, although incomplete (50 to 80%), is sufficiently high to render them useful given orally. These include cimetidine, ranitidine, hydrochorothiazide, and atenolol. As with ranitidine, though, the small intestine is likely to be the predominant site of absorption.

The rectum has a small surface area, and a drug given rectally is not always retained for a sufficient length of time to ensure complete absorption. No time limitation exists for a drug injected into muscle, subcutaneous tissue, and most other sites within the body; complete absorption is anticipated unless destruction occurs between site of administration and systemic circulation.

Competing Reactions. Any reaction that competes with absorption may reduce the oral bioavailability of a drug. Table 9–2 lists various reactions that can occur within the gastrointestinal tract. Reactions can be both enzymatic and nonenzymatic. Acid hydrolysis is a common nonenzymatic reaction. Enzymes in the intestinal epithelium and within the intestinal microflora, which normally reside in the large bowel, metabolize some drugs. The reaction products are often inactive or less potent than the parent molecule. Interactions with constituents of the gastrointestinal fluids also occur; the result may be low drug bioavailability. For example, one reason why tetracycline is incompletely absorbed when coadministered with milk and with certain antacids is that this antibiotic forms spar-

Table 9-1. Representative Drugs Showing Low Oral Bioavailability That Is Due to Poor Intestinal Permeability[a]

Amikacin	Gentamicin
Carbenicillin	Neomycin
Cefamandole	Pyridostigmine
Cefazolin	Streptomycin
Cefotaxime	Teicoplanin
Ceftazidime	Vancomycin

[a]Less than 20% bioavailable. Administered either in solution or as an immediate-release dosage form.

Table 9-2. Representative Reactions within the Gastrointestinal Tract That Compete for Drug Absorption From Solution

REACTION	DRUG	COMMENT
Complexation	Tetracycline	Unabsorbed insoluble complexes with polyvalent metal ions, e.g., Ca^{2+}, Al^{3+}, Fe^{3+}
Conjugation		
Sulfoconjugation	Isoproterenol	Loss of activity: product inactive
Glucuronidation	Salicylamide	Loss of activity: product inactive
Decarboxylation	Levodopa	Loss of activity: given with a peripheral dopa decarboxylase inhibitor to reduce gastrointestinal metabolism
Hydrolysis		
Acid	Penicillin G	Loss of activity: product inactive
	Erythromycin	Loss of activity: product inactive
	Digoxin	Products (digitoxides) have variable activity
Enzymatic	Aspirin	Salicylic acid formed, active anti-inflammatory compound
	Pivampicillin	Active ampicillin formed: pivampicillin (ester) is inactive
	Insulin	Loss of activity: product inactive
Oxidation	Cyclosporine	Loss of activity: product less active
Reduction (microflora)	Sulfasalazine	Intended for local (intestinal) anti-inflammatory action; parent drug may have some activity; product, 5-aminosalicylic acid, active
Adsorption	Digitoxin	Adsorption to cholestyramine: adsorbed material not absorbed

ingly soluble complexes with the polyvalent cation (e.g., Ca^{2+}, Fe^{3+} and Al^{3+}) contained in these preparations.

The complexities that occur *in vivo* preclude accurate prediction of the contribution of a competing reaction to decreased bioavailability. Sometimes the problem of incomplete absorption can be circumvented by physically protecting the drug from destruction in the stomach (see enteric coating discussion, p. 36) or by synthesizing a more stable derivative, which is converted to the active molecule within the body. Similarly, to enhance absorption, more permeable derivatives are made, which are rapidly converted to the active molecule, often during passage through the intestinal wall. For example, absorption of the polar antibiotic ampicillin is incomplete. Its systemic delivery is improved substantially by administering a more lipophilic and permeable inactive ester prodrug, pivampicillin. The hydrolysis of this ester within the intestinal wall is so rapid that only ampicillin is detected in the circulation. Derivatives, such as pivampicillin, are generally referred to as *prodrugs*, as they are pharmacologically inactive.

Hepatic Extraction. Aspirin (acetylsalicylic acid) is one of the first synthetic prodrugs. It was marketed at the turn of the century to overcome the unpleasant taste and the gastrointestinal irritation associated with the parent drug, salicylic acid. Aspirin was originally thought to be inactive, being designed to be rapidly hydrolyzed within the body to salicylic acid. Only subsequently was aspirin shown to be pharmacologically active. Yet the original design worked; upon ingestion, aspirin, a labile ester, is rapidly hydrolyzed, particularly by esterases in the liver. Indeed, hepatic hydrolysis is so rapid that a sizeable fraction of aspirin is converted to salicylic acid in a single passage through the liver, resulting in a substantial "first-pass effect."

Drugs that show a substantial first-pass effect due to hepatic elimination are listed in Table 9–3. Apart from this feature, they have little in common. They are of diverse chemical structure, possess different pharmacologic activities, and are metabolized via a number of pathways. When the metabolite(s) formed during the first pass through the liver is less potent than the parent drug, the oral dose is larger than the i.v. or i.m. dose required to achieve the same therapeutic effect. This occurs for many of the drugs listed in Table 9–3. In some instances, e.g., isoproterenol, hepatic extraction is so high as to essentially preclude the oral route. Here, no amount of pharmaceutical formulation helps. Either the drug must be given by a parenteral route, or it must be discarded in favor of another drug candidate. A method of estimating the maximum likely decrease in oral bioavailability due to this first-pass effect is discussed in Chap. 11, Elimination.

Table 9–3.   Representative Drugs Showing Low Oral Bioavailability That Is Due to Extensive[a] First-Pass Hepatic Elimination[b]

Alprenolol	Hydralazine	Naltrexone
Amitriptyline	Imipramine	Neostigmine
Chlormethiazole	Isoproterenol	Nicardipine
Chlorpromazine	Isosorbide dinitrate	Nicotine
Cytarabine	Ketamine	Nifedipine
Desipramine	Labetolol	Nitroglycerin
Dextropropoxyphene	Lidocaine	Papaverine
Dihydroergotamine	Lorcainide	Phenacetin
Diltiazem	Mercaptopurine	Pentazocine
Doxepin	Methylphenidate	Pentoxifylline
Doxorubicin	Metoprolol	Propranolol
Encainide	Morphine	Scopolamine
Estradiol	Nalbuphine	Testosterone
5-Fluorouracil	Naloxone	Verapamil

[a]$F = 0.5$ or less, on average.
[b]Adapted and expanded from Pond, S.M., and Tozer, T.N.: First-pass elimination: Basis concepts and clinical consequences. Clin. Pharmacokinet., 9:1–25, 1984.

Avoiding first pass through the liver probably explains most of the activity of nitroglycerin administered sublingually for an acute anginal attack. Blood perfusing the buccal cavity bypasses the liver and enters directly into the superior vena cava. This antianginal drug is almost completely metabolized as it passes through the liver, and any drug swallowed is not systematically available. The metabolites seen in blood are only weakly active but under certain circumstances may reach concentrations high enough to contribute to overall activity.

The rectal route has a definite advantage over the oral route for drugs destroyed by gastric acidity or by enzymes in the intestinal wall and microflora. Potentially, the rectal route may also partially reduce first-pass hepatic loss. Part of the rectal blood supply, particularly the inferior and middle hemorrhoidal veins, bypasses the hepatic portal circulation and dumps directly into the inferior vena cava. Achieving a reproducible bioavailability, which is important in drug therapy, may be difficult, however, since bioavailability strongly depends on the site of absorption within the rectum.

Absorption From Intramuscular and Subcutaneous Sites

The General Case. In contrast to the small intestine, and indeed to the entire gastrointestinal tract, absorption of most drugs in solution from muscle and subcutaneous tissue is perfusion rate-limited; increases in blood flow hasten absorption. For example, consider the data in Table 9–4 for the local anesthetic lidocaine. Shown are the peak plasma concentrations observed when the same dose of lidocaine is administered at different sites in the body. Recall, for a given dose, the higher the peak concentration, the faster is drug absorption. Large differences in speed of absorption are clearly evident, the speed decreasing from intercostal muscle to s.c. tissue, in line with a decreasing tissue perfusion.

This dependence of absorption on perfusion may be explained by the nature of the barrier (the capillary wall) between the site of injection (interstitial fluid) and blood. This capillary wall, a much more loosely knit structure than the epithelial lining of the gastrointestinal tract, offers little impedance to the movement of drugs into blood, even for polar ionized drugs. For example, gentamicin, a water-soluble, ionized, polar base of molecular weight 477 g/mole, has great difficulty penetrating the gastrointestinal mucosa but is rapidly and completely absorbed from an intramuscular site. This low impedance by the capillary wall in muscle and s.c. tissue applies to drugs, independent of pKa, degree of ionization, and molecular size up to approximately 5000 g/mole.

Macromolecular and Lymphatic Transport. In contrast to small molecules, size, polarity, and charge pose a particular problem for administration of protein, and large polypeptide drugs; their transport across many membranes is hindered. Furthermore, be-

Table 9–4. Influence of Site of Injection on the Peak Venous Lidocaine Concentration Following Injection of a 100-mg Dose[a]

INJECTION SITE	PEAK PLASMA LIDOCAINE CONCENTRATION (mg/L)[b]
Intercostal	1.46
Paracervical	1.20
Caudal	1.18
Lumbar epidural	0.97
Brachial plexus	0.53
Subarachnoid	0.44
Subcutaneous	0.35

[a]Taken from Covino, B.G.: Pharmacokinetics of local anaesthetic drugs. In: Pharmacokinetics of Anaesthesia. Edited by C. Prys-Roberts and C.C. Hug. Blackwell Scientific Publications, Oxford, 1984, pp. 270–292.
[b]One mg/L = 4.3 µM.

cause of decomposition by proteolytic enzymes in the gastrointestinal tract, their oral absorption is extremely low and erratic. Most of the information on these kinds of drugs has been obtained following nonvascular parenteral administration. For the s.c., i.m., and intraperitoneal routes, drug reaches the systemic circulation by two mechanisms: diffusion through the interstitial fluids and fenestrations in the linings of the vascular capillaries and by convective flow of the interstitial fluids through lymphatic channels. Molecular size is of primary importance for passage across the capillary endothelium. Polypeptides of less than approximately 5000 g/mole primarily pass through the capillary pathway. Those of greater than about 20,000 g/mole are less able to traverse the capillary wall; they primarily enter the blood via the lymphatic pathway.

Lymph flow is slow and causes absorption from nonvascular parenteral sites to continue for many hours, as shown in Fig. 9–5 for glycosylated recombinant human granulocyte-macrophage colony-stimulating factor (molecular weight = 15,000 to 34,000 g/mole). The drug has a half-life of 68 min after i.v. administration, but following s.c. administration, the plasma concentration is prolonged for at least 42 hr, with a rate of decline indicating continuing input.

The nonvascular parenteral routes offer the advantage of providing prolonged input for short half-life proteins. Thus, nonvascular parenteral administration allows for less frequent administration than the i.v. route. A main concern here relates to the reproducibility of the release into the systemic circulation from the site of administration. Absorption kinetics from both i.m. and s.c. administration has been shown to be highly dependent on the site of injection, temperature, and degree of rubbing at the injection site.

Because of the short half-life often observed and decomposition in the gastrointestinal tract, there is clearly a need for the development of novel delivery systems for protein drugs. Smaller polypeptides have been tested in controlled-release (microencapsulated) injectable systems. They have also been shown to be absorbed across nasal membranes. Higher molecular weight polypeptides and proteins may require more creative methods to

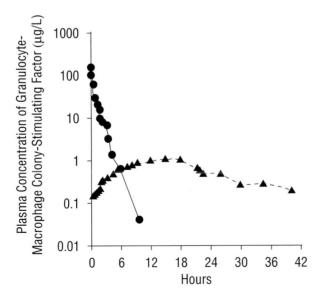

Fig. 9–5. Plasma concentrations of glycosylated recombinant human granulocyte-macrophage colony-stimulating factor following i.v. (●, solid line) and s.c. (▲, dashed line) bolus injection of 8 µg/kg. The results, obtained in two different individuals, typify the kinetics of the drug following these two modes of parenteral administration. (Adapted from Hovgaard D., Mortensen, B.T., Schifter, S., and Nissen, N.I.: Clinical pharmacokinetic studies of a human haemopoietic growth factor, GM-CSF. Euro. J. Clin. Invest., 22:45–49, 1992.)

ensure consistent and more complete bioavailability or may require the development of more specific methods for delivering these drugs to the site of action.

Absorption From Other Sites

Drugs may be administered to virtually any site of the body. This is certainly true of local anesthetics. In recent years there has been considerable interest in exploiting some of the less conventional sites, such as the lung, nasal cavity, and buccal cavity as a means of delivering drugs systemically. The new polypeptide and protein drugs that are poorly and erratically absorbed when given orally have received particular attention. Transdermal application has become popular for systemic delivery of small, generally lipophilic, potent molecules that require low input rates to achieve effective therapy. In all cases, consideration has to be given to the particular properties of the site and the drug. Nonetheless, the factors influencing absorption from these sites are likely to be the same as those influencing absorption from the oral, i.m., and s.c. sites.

ABSORPTION FROM SOLID DOSAGE FORMS

Formulation

Equality of drug content does not guarantee equality of efficacy. The presence of different excipients (ingredients in addition to drug) and manufacturing processes may result in dosage forms containing the same dose of drug behaving differently *in vivo*. Hence the reason for testing for bioequivalence of preparations of a drug intended to be switchable (p. 45). Generally, the primary concern is with the extent of absorption. Occasionally, variations in absorption rate may be important. Much often depends on the degree of accumulation that occurs on multiple dosing (Fig. 7–6, p. 87).

The major cause of differences in absorption of a drug from various products is dissolution. Standards exist for content and purity of the numerous inactive ingredients used to stabilize the drug; to facilitate manufacture and maintain integrity of the dosage form during handling and storage; and to facilitate, or sometimes control, release of drug following administration of the dosage form. Intended, or otherwise, each ingredient can influence the rate of dissolution of the drug, as can the manufacturing process. The result is a large potential for differences in drug absorption among products. Indeed, a large variety of dosage forms of drugs are marketed in which release may be immediate, delayed, prolonged, or sustained, regardless of the physicochemical properties of the drug itself. Sometimes, differences in absorption can be correlated with differences in dissolution measured in an *in vitro* apparatus. There are dissolution requirements for an increasing number of important drug products. On occasion, however, *in vitro* dissolution tests fail to correlate with absorption. At present, assessment in humans continues to be the primary means of evaluating drug products and discriminating between satisfactory and unsatisfactory formulations.

Dissolution

The reason why dissolution is so important may be gained by realizing that absorption following administration of a solid is a two-step process:

$$\text{Drug in product} \xrightarrow{\text{Dissolution}} \text{Drug in solution} \xrightarrow{\text{Entry into the body}} \text{Absorbed drug}$$

Two situations are now considered. The first, depicted in Fig. 9–6A, is one in which dissolution is a much faster process than is entry of drug into the body. Consequently, most of the drug is dissolved before an appreciable amount is absorbed. Here, permeability rather than dissolution rate-limits absorption. An example is the gastrointestinal absorption of neomycin given as a tablet. This polar antibiotic dissolves rapidly but has difficulty penetrating the gastrointestinal epithelium. So, little is absorbed. Differences in rates of dissolution of neomycin from different tablets have little or no effect on the speed of absorption of this drug.

In the second and much more common situation, shown in Fig. 9–6B, dissolution proceeds relatively slowly, and any dissolved drug readily traverses the gastrointestinal epithelium. Absorption cannot proceed any faster, however, than the rate at which the drug dissolves. That is, absorption is dissolution rate-limited. In this case, changes in dissolution profoundly affect the rate, and sometimes the extent, of drug absorption. Evidence supporting dissolution rate-limited absorption comes from the noticeably slower absorption of most drugs from solid dosage forms than from a simple aqueous solution.

Factors Controlling Dissolution

Many factors influence the dissolution of a drug. Among these are surface area, solubility, pH, and stirring.

Expanding the surface exposed to body fluids hastens dissolution. Reducing the size of the solid particles is the most common means of achieving this goal. To this effect, for example, materials (disintegrants) are incorporated into tablets that cause them to swell upon contact with water and then to disintegrate into granules that finally deaggregate into the original fine drug particles.

In dissolution rate-limited absorption, the concentration of drug in solution at the absorption site is kept low because dissolved drug rapidly enters the body. The driving force for dissolution is directly related to the solubility of the drug at the surface of the dissolving

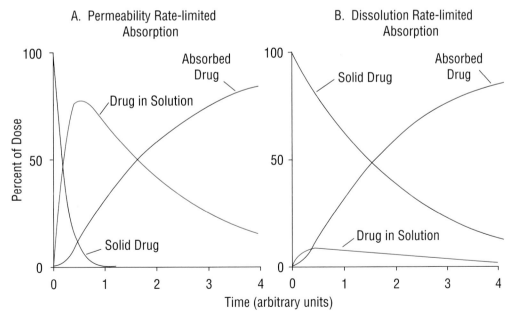

Fig. 9–6. When absorption is permeability rate-limited (Case A), most of the drug has dissolved (colored line) before an appreciable fraction has been absorbed. In contrast, when dissolution rate-limits absorption (Case B), very little drug is in solution (colored line) at the absorption site at any time; drug is absorbed as soon as it dissolves. Notice that the majority of drug not absorbed is always found at the rate-limiting step: in solution in Case A and as a solid in Case B.

solid. This explains why tablets, capsules, and even suspensions of sparingly soluble drugs are prone to absorption problems. Even if dissolution were not the rate-limiting step and a saturated solution at the absorption site could be maintained, the rate of absorption of these drugs would still be low, owing to the low aqueous solubility.

For weak acids and bases, the rate of dissolution can be markedly increased by using a salt form. The explanation lies in the different concentrations at the surface of the dissolving solid. This concentration is much higher for the much more soluble salt than for the free acid or base. Adjusting pH of the medium also increases dissolution of weak acids and bases, by helping to maintain such conditions around the dissolving material. This is generally, however, not as effective as using a salt form.

Peristaltic movements in the stomach are generally feeble and variable. Mixing in the antrum can be quite vigorous. The disintegration rate, deaggregation rate, location of the dosage form in the stomach, food, and the state of the patient each influences the stirring rate around the dissolving particle. Stirring is generally sufficient to ensure complete and rapid drug absorption from solid dosage forms containing soluble drugs.

As mentioned previously, little drug is generally absorbed from the stomach. Nonetheless, dissolution in the gastric fluid is a prerequisite to the absorption of some drugs. This point is well illustrated by tetracycline hydrochloride. Only that which dissolves in the stomach is apparently absorbed. This amphoteric antibiotic, freely soluble in both strongly acidic and alkaline solutions, is minimally soluble at pH 5.8, a pH typical of the intestinal fluid. Perhaps the sparingly soluble tetracycline precipitates onto undissolved particles entering the intestine, thereby limiting further dissolution.

Gastric Emptying and Intestinal Transit

Before discussing the role of gastric emptying on absorption of drugs given as solids, consider the information provided in Fig. 9–7. Shown are the mean transit times in the stomach and small intestine of small nondisintegrating pellets (diameters between 0.3 and 1.8 mm) and of large single nondisintegrating units (either capsules, 25 mm by 9 mm or tablets, 8 to 12 mm in diameter).

During fasting, gastric emptying of both small and large solids is seen, on average, to be rapid, with a mean transit time of around 1 hr, although there is considerable individual variability. In this state, the stomach displays a complex temporal pattern of motor activity with alternating periods of quiescence and moderate contraction of varying frequency, culminating in an intense contraction, the "housekeeping wave," that propels all gastric contents, including solids almost irrespective of size, into the small intestine. The exact ejection time of a solid particle therefore depends on when the solid is taken during the motor activity cycle, an unpredictable period varying from 20 min to a few hours.

The situation is very different after eating. As shown in Fig. 9–7, when taken on a fed stomach, the gastric transit time of solids is increased. This increase is greater after a heavy meal than after a light one and is much greater for a large single unit than for small pellets. For example, the mean gastric transit time for large single unit systems is now almost 7 hr, with some of them still in the stomach 11 hr after ingestion. These observations are explained by the sieving action of a fed stomach. The irregular "housekeeping waves" are now replaced by regular and more gentle contractions, which continuously mix and triturate the gastric contents. Furthermore, only solids with diameters less than 7 to 10 mm are allowed to pass into the small intestine with gastric fluid. Larger food particles are retained until reduced to the requisite size by trituration and partial digestion. With conventional tablets, disintegration and subsequent deaggregation into fine particles achieves the same objective. As long as the stomach remains in a fed state, the conditions above prevail. For those persons who eat three good meals a day, this is most of the waking hours of the day.

In contrast to events in the stomach, the transit time of solids within the small intestine varies little among subjects, appears to be independent of either the size of a solid or the presence of food in the stomach, and is remarkably short, approximately 3 hr (Fig. 9–7), a time similar to that found for the transit of liquids. Both solids and liquids appear to move down the small intestine as a plug with relatively little mixing. As the mouth-to-anus transit time is typically 1 to 2 days, these data on gastric and small intestinal transit times indicate that, for the majority of this time, unabsorbed materials are in either the large bowel or rectum. Provided with the physiologic information above, the possible role of gastric emptying and intestinal transit on the absorption of drugs given in solid dosage forms can be understood. Consider the following situations.

Rapid Dissolution in Stomach. This is the common situation seen with many conventional tablets and capsules. Drug dissolves so rapidly that most is in solution before much has entered the intestine. Here, gastric emptying clearly influences the rate of drug absorption. Hastening gastric emptying, for example, quickens drug absorption from solution.

Rapid Dissolution in Intestine. In this situation, drug does not dissolve in the stomach, whereas in the intestine it rapidly both dissolves and passes across the intestinal wall. Gastric emptying then dramatically affects the time and perhaps the rate of drug absorption. An enteric-coated product is an extreme example of this situation. Erythromycin and pen-

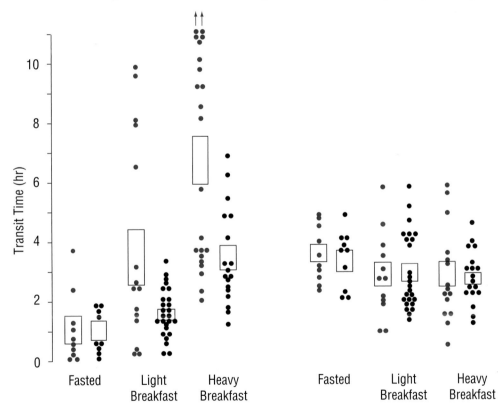

Fig. 9–7. Food, particularly a heavy meal, increases the gastric transit time of small pellets (black circles) and, even more markedly, of large single units (colored circles). In contrast, neither food nor the physical size of the solid affects the small intestine transit time. The data (individual points, black or colored circles, and their mean ± S.E., indicated by the rectangles) were obtained in healthy young adults using drug-free nondisintegrating materials. The points with an arrow indicate the solid was still in the stomach at the time of the last observation, the time indicated. (Adapted from Davis, S.S., Hardy, J.G., and Fara, J.: Transit of pharmaceutical dosage forms through the small intestine, Gut, 27:886–892, 1986.)

icillin G are rapidly hydrolyzed to inactive products in the acidic environment of the stomach. Salicylic acid is a gastric irritant. A solution to both types of problems has been to coat these drugs with a material resistant to acid but not to the intestinal fluids. Many such enteric-coated products are large single tablets, and the time taken for an intact tablet to pass from the stomach into the intestine varies unpredictably from 20 min to several hours when taken on an empty stomach and up to 12 hr or even more when taken on a fed stomach. Accordingly, such enteric-coated products are not to be used when a rapid and reliable rate of absorption is required. A product composed of enteric-coated granules is an improvement because the rate of delivery of the granules to the intestine is expected to be more reliable, being less dependent on a single event and on food.

Poor Dissolution. Some drugs, such as the oral antifungal agent griseofulvin, are sparingly soluble in both gastric and intestinal fluids. When these drugs are administered as a solid, there may already be insufficient time for complete dissolution and absorption. With a fixed short time within the small intestine, retention in the stomach increases the time for drug to dissolve before entering the intestine, thereby favoring increased bioavailability. As mentioned, food, and fat in particular, delays gastric emptying. This delay may be one of the explanations for the observed increase in the bioavailability of griseofulvin when taken with a fatty meal or with fats. Subsequently, as the intestinal fluid and contents move into the large intestine and water is reabsorbed, the resulting compaction of the solid contents may severely limit further dissolution and hence absorption of drug.

Controlled-Release Products. The conclusions drawn for sparingly soluble drugs may also apply to certain controlled-release dosage forms. Some of these are coated with, or contained within, a nondisintegrating material through which the release rate of drug is independent of both pH and agitation. In such cases, gastric emptying has little effect on the rate of drug absorption. Even though the solid dosage form may be retained in the stomach, the released drug is continuously emptied with the gastric fluid into the duodenum and is available for absorption. Any delay in the gastric emptying of such products prolongs the total period for drug release and absorption. For reasons discussed above, this delay is most likely to be seen with large single units taken on a fed stomach. It would be unwise, however, to depend too much on this delay to achieve a prolonged absorption profile given the well-known unpredictability of patients' eating habits and their general lack of compliance in taking medications. Furthermore, some concern must exist that compaction in the large intestine may preclude reliable input of drug beyond 12 to 16 hr. This would severely limit the design of controlled-release dosage forms of drugs with short half-lives intended for once-a-day administration. That said, data for some drug-delivery systems indicate that reliable and sustained absorption for up to 22 hr can be achieved. Future work in this area is needed to understand the scope and limitations of the approach. One limitation can be the properties of the drug itself, as now discussed.

Changing Rate Control

The rate of absorption is controlled by a delivery device as long as release from the device is the rate-limiting step in the absorption process. With the $P \cdot SA$ term for drugs decreasing along the length of the intestinal tract, the rate limitation could change from the device to the intestinal membrane as the device moves down the intestine (Fig. 9–8). Much depends on the relative impedances for drug movement in the device and in the intestinal wall. In the small intestine, $P \cdot SA$ is at its highest and control may then well lie with the delivery device. However, on movement into the colon, $P \cdot SA$ may drop enough so that the rate-limiting step becomes passage across the wall, in which case, control of drug input is lost. This situation is more likely to occur with relatively polar molecules, for which permeability may be a problem. Even with rapid-release dosage forms, absorption of these compounds is essentially restricted to the small intestine (e.g., Fig. 9–4). Currently, however, it is difficult to make any quantitative prediction of those drugs for which controlled drug delivery can be achieved beyond the small intestine. But clearly, whenever release of drug beyond the stomach continues for 4 hr or more, some of the drug is likely to be released in the large intestine (Fig. 9–7). More needs to be known about the relationship between the physicochemical properties of a molecule and intestinal permeability. Currently, the only recourse is to evaluate the drug delivery system *in vivo*.

Precipitation and Redissolution

Absorption is normally complete within 1 or 2 hr of i.m. or s.c. administration of an aqueous solution of a drug. There are exceptions, as seen with protein drugs (Fig. 9–5) and when injecting a solution of a salt of either a sparingly soluble acid or base. For example, although, chlordiazepoxide hydrochloride, in solution, is eventually completely absorbed, absorption is slow from the i.m. site. However, large doses sometimes appear to be poorly effective or ineffective. Indeed, absorption is even slower than from the gastrointestinal tract, when capsules of chlordiazepoxide hydrochloride are administered (Fig. 9–8). The explanation involves consideration of pH, solubility, perfusion, and stirring.

In the study referenced in Fig. 9–8, the same dose, 50 mg of chlordiazepoxide hydrochloride, was administered by both routes. The i.m. dose was dissolved in 1 mL of an aqueous vehicle. Chlordiazepoxide is sparingly soluble; its aqueous solubility is approximately 2 mg/mL. To achieve this high concentration of 50 mg of chlordiazepoxide hydrochloride/mL, the vehicle contains 20% propylene glycol and 4% polysorbate 80, both water-miscible materials that permit a greater solubility of the drug. Being the salt of a strong acid and a weak base (*pKa* 4.5), the final pH is low, approximately 3.0. Upon injection, the buffer capacity of both the tissue and the blood perfusing it gradually restores the pH at the injection site to 7.4. This rise in pH and the absorption of the injected water and water-miscible materials cause chlordiazepoxide base to precipitate out of solution. As movement and hence spreading is minimal, a large mass of drug is deposited around the injection site. The rate of absorption now becomes limited by dissolution of the precipitated drug. However, the small surface area, low solubility, limited perfusion, and minimal stirring tend to keep the rate of dissolution down. The result is protracted absorption over many hours or

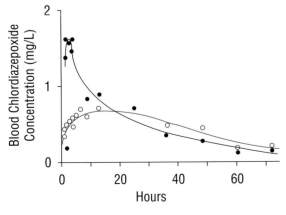

Fig. 9–8. A delayed and lower peak blood concentration of chlordiazepoxide, when given intramuscularly (○—○), as compared to when given orally (●—●), indicates slower absorption from the intramuscular site than from the oral site. On both occasions 50 mg of chlordiazepoxide hydrochloride were administered (1 mg/L = 3.3 μM). (Redrawn from Greenblatt, D.J., Shader, R.I., and Koch-Weser, J.: Slow absorption of intramuscular chlordiazepoxide. N. Engl. J. Med., *291*:1116–1118, 1974. Reprinted by permission.)

even days. In contrast, absorption following oral administration is relatively rapid. For reasons already discussed, a greater degree of agitation, a larger volume of fluid at the site, and a higher rate of blood flow to the gastrointestinal tract promote more rapid dissolution and absorption following ingestion of chlordiazepoxide hydrochloride. Another example is diazepam, a drug that is sparingly soluble and slowly absorbed when injected intramuscularly. This essentially neutral drug is kept in solution with the aid of propylene glycol. Precipitation at the injection site occurs with dilution and absorption of this water-miscible solvent.

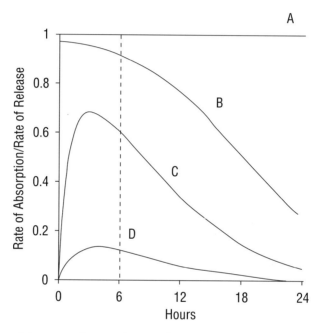

Fig. 9–9. The rate of absorption relative to the rate of constant release from an oral 24-hr sustained-release delivery device varies with time when movement across the membranes of the gastrointestinal tract, rather than release, becomes rate limiting. The change in rate control from release to membrane occurs for a drug with low membrane permeability. The rate control imposed by permeability is more apparent in the colon (6 hr is shown as the time for the device to leave the stomach and transit the small intestine, dashed vertical line), where permeability is much lower than that in the small intestine. The simulations are conducted with the model

$$
\underset{\substack{\text{Net rate of change of} \\ \text{released drug} \\ \text{in lumen}}}{dA_R/dt} \quad = \quad \underset{\substack{\text{Rate of} \\ \text{release}}}{R} \quad - \quad \underset{\substack{\text{Rate of} \\ \text{absorption}}}{\dfrac{P \cdot SA}{Va} \cdot e^{-bt} \cdot A_R}
$$

where A_R is amount of released drug residing in the gastrointestinal tract, Va is the volume of luminal fluid into which the released drug is distributed, and b is the rate constant for the decrease in $P \cdot SA/Va$ with time. As the actual changes in P, SA, and Va with time are unknown, an exponential (half-life of 3 hr) decline in the composite is used. The following conditions are simulated: **A**, $P \cdot SA/Va$ is sufficiently high (approaches ∞) to ensure that the rate-controlling step is always in the device with rate of absorption matching rate of release. **B**, $P \cdot SA/Va$ is $10 \ hr^{-1}$, a value for which drug is absorbed virtually as quickly as it is released while in the proximal small intestine but not so further down the gastrointestinal tract where rate control by the device is lost. **C**, $P \cdot SA/Va$ is $1 \ hr^{-1}$. The rate of absorption never matches the rate of release. The product fails to control absorption. **D**, $P \cdot SA/Va$ = $0.1 \ hr^{-1}$. Rate control lies almost entirely with the membranes of the gastrointestinal tract at all times. In cases *B to D*, drug accumulates in the lumen of the intestines. The area under each curve relative to the area under the release curve (curve A) is the fraction of released drug that is absorbed.

STUDY PROBLEMS

(Answers to Study Problems are in Appendix II.)

1. List at least three reasons for reduced oral bioavailability of a drug.
2. Indicate the accuracy of the following statements:
   a. When administered orally in solution, gastric emptying rate-limits the absorption of small lipophilic drugs.
   b. For rapidly dissolving products of a drug, differences in rates of dissolution markedly affect the plasma concentration-time profile, when intestinal permeability is the rate-limiting step.
   c. Polar drugs are primarily absorbed from the small intestine via the transcellular route.
   d. A substantial fraction of bioavailable drug enters the systemic circulation via the lymphatic route for large (M.W. greater than 100,000 g/mole) protein drugs administered intramuscularly.
   e. Large nondisintegrating controlled-release dosage forms commonly remain in the stomach for 6 hr when taken just after a heavy meal.
3. List six drugs for which oral bioavailability is low due to a substantial first-pass hepatic loss.
4. List four factors that can influence the rate of dissolution of a drug from a solid dosage form.
5. Comment on the statement: Drugs administered in solution are more slowly absorbed from muscle (i.m. administration) than from the small intestine (oral administration).
6. Listed in Table 9–5 are four drugs together with some of their physical properties.

Table 9–5.

PROPERTY OR CHARACTERISTIC	DRUG A	DRUG B	DRUG C	DRUG D
Molecular weight (g/mole)	327	273	315	378
pKa	8.4 (Acid)	7.8 (Amine)	Neutral	Quaternary ammonium compound
Polarity of un-ionized form	Nonpolar	Nonpolar	Polar	—
Solubility of un-ionized form (mg/L)	1.3	150	—	—

Given that the conventional single dose of both Drug A and Drug B is 100 mg and that both drugs are stable in the gastrointestinal fluids, circle the most appropriate drug, word, or phrase (in italics) that completes the following statements.

a. The sodium salt of Drug A dissolves *much faster, much slower, at essentially the same rate*, in a solution of pH 3.0 than (as) does the free acid in a solution of pH 8.0. (Other factors, such as surface area and stirring, are the same.)
b. The hydrochloride salt of Drug B should dissolve *much faster, much slower, at essentially the same rate*, in the stomach of a patient with achlorhydria (no gastric acid secretion) than (as) in a patient with normal gastric function.
c. Drug A is poorly absorbed when taken orally as the free acid with 100 mL of water. The bioavailability of this drug should be significantly increased by taking the drug *with 200 mL of water, in divided doses during the day, on an empty stomach*.
d. Absorption problems are likely to be greater with Drug *A, B*, when administered intramuscularly as an aqueous solution of the *sodium, hydrochloride* salt.

7. In Table 9–6 below are listed the *AUC* values of ciprofloxacin, a drug with a broad antimicrobial activity, following its delivery (180 mg) in solution to various regions of

the gastrointestinal tract. Ciprofloxacin appears to be stable in all parts of the gastro-intestinal tract.

Table 9–6. *AUC* Values of Ciprofloxacin after Delivery of 180 mg to Various Regions of the Gastrointestinal Tract[a]

REGION:	STOMACH	JEJUNUM	ILEUM	ASCENDING COLON	DESCENDING COLON
AUC (mg-L/hr)	1.48	0.38	0.24	0.08	0.05

[a]Abstracted from Harder, S., Fuhr, U., Beermann, D., and Staib, A.H.: Ciprofloxacin absorption in different regions of the human gastrointestinal tract. Investigation with the hf-capsule. Br. J. Clin. Pharmacol., *30*:35–39, 1990.

a. From which site of the gastrointestinal tract, stomach, small intestine, or large intestine is the majority of ciprofloxacin likely to be absorbed following oral administration of the drug?

b. Based on the difference in *AUC* values following delivery into the stomach and jejunum, suggest a possible primary site of absorption of ciprofloxacin.

c. For drugs that exhibit absorption patterns similar to that of ciprofloxacin, comment on the chances of success fully achieving a constant systemic input for up to 12 hr following administration of an oral drug-delivery system.

DISTRIBUTION

OBJECTIVES

The reader will be able to:

1. Define the following terms:
   a. Perfusion limitation in distribution
   b. Permeability limitation in distribution
   c. Tissue-to-blood equilibrium distribution ratio
   d. Fraction unbound
   e. Plasma protein binding

2. Determine the plasma concentration, the amount of drug in the body, and the apparent volume of distribution when any two of these values are known.

3. Describe the effects of perfusion limitation, permeability limitation, and the tissue-to-blood equilibrium distribution ratio on the time required for drug distribution to the tissues.

4. Ascertain whether, for a given amount of drug in the body, the unbound plasma concentration is likely to be sensitive to variation in plasma protein binding when the volume of distribution is known.

5. Calculate the fraction of drug in the body that is:
   a. unbound
   b. in the extracellular fluids
   c. outside the extracellular fluids
   d. bound to plasma proteins
   e. bound to plasma proteins in the extracellular fluids
   f. bound intracellularly (in or on tissue cells)

   from knowledge of the volume of distribution and the fraction unbound in plasma.

6. Anticipate the effect of altered plasma protein binding on the half-life of a drug, bound to albumin and with a volume of distribution less than 0.2 L/kg.

Distribution refers to the reversible transfer of drug from one location to another within the body. Definitive information on the distribution of a drug requires its measurement in various tissues. Such data have been obtained in animals, but are essentially lacking in humans. Much useful information on rate and extent of distribution in humans can be derived, however, from observations in blood or plasma. This chapter explores distribution and its applications in clinical pharmacokinetics. It begins with kinetic considerations and ends with equilibrium concepts.

RATE OF DISTRIBUTION

Distribution of drugs to and from blood and other tissues occurs at various rates and to various extents. Several factors determine the distribution pattern of a drug with time.

Included are delivery of drug to tissues by blood, ability to cross tissue membranes, binding within blood and tissues, and partitioning into fat. Tissue uptake, commonly called *extravasation*, continues toward equilibrium of the diffusible form between tissue and blood perfusing it.

Perfusion Limitation

Distribution, like absorption (see Chap. 9), can be rate-limited by either perfusion or permeability. A *perfusion-rate limitation* prevails when the tissue membranes present essentially no barrier to distribution. As expected, this condition is likely to be met by small lipophilic drugs diffusing across most membranes of the body and, by almost all drugs, except macromolecules diffusing across loosely knit membranes, such as capillary walls of muscle and subcutaneous tissue (see Chap. 8).

Perfusion is usually expressed in units of milliliters of blood per minute per volume of tissue. As seen in Table 10–1, the perfusion rate of tissues varies from approximately 10 mL/min/mL for lungs down to values of only 0.025 mL/min/mL for resting muscle or fat. All other factors remaining equal, well-perfused tissues take up a drug much more rapidly than do poorly perfused tissues. Moreover, as the subsequent analysis shows, there is a direct correlation between tissue perfusion rate and the time required to distribute a drug to a tissue.

Table 10–1. Blood Flow, Perfusion Rate, and Relative Size of Different Organs and Tissues Under Basal Conditions in a Standard 70-kg Human[a]

ORGAN[b]	PERCENT OF BODY VOLUME	BLOOD FLOW (mL/min)	PERCENT OF CARDIAC OUTPUT	PERFUSION RATE (mL/min/mL of tissue)
1. Adrenal glands	0.03	25	0.2	1.2
2. Blood	7	(5000)[b]	(100)	—
3. Bone	16	250	5	0.02
4. Brain	2.0	700	14	0.5
5. Fat	20[c]	200	4	0.03
6. Heart	0.4	200	4	0.6
7. Kidneys	0.5	1100	22	4
8. Liver	2.3	1350	27	0.8
Portal	1.7 (Gut)	(1050)	(21)	—
Arterial	—	(300)	(6)	—
9. Lungs	1.6	(5000)	(100)	10
10. Muscle (inactive)	43	750	15	0.025
11. Skin (cool weather)	11	300	6	0.04
12. Spleen	0.3	77	1.5	0.4
13. Thyroid gland	0.03	50	1	2.4
Total Body	100	5000	100	0.071

[a]Compiled and adapted from data in Guyton, A.C.: Textbook of Medical Physiology. 7th Ed. Philadelphia, W.B. Saunders, 1986, p. 230; Lentner, C. (ed.): Geigy Scientific Tables. Vol. 1. Edison, NJ, Ciba-Geigy, 1981; and Davies, B., and Morris, T.: Physiological parameters in laboratory animals and humans. Pharm. Res., 10:1093–1095, 1993.
[b]Some organs, e.g., stomach, intestines, spleen and pancreas are not included.
[c]Includes fat within organs.

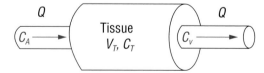

Fig. 10–1. Drug is presented to a tissue at an arterial blood concentration of C_A and at a rate equal to the product of blood flow, Q, and C_A. The drug leaves the tissue at a venous concentration of C_V and at a rate equal to $Q \cdot C_V$. The tissue concentration, C_T, increases when rate of presentation exceeds rate of leaving in the venous blood, and the converse. The amount in the tissue is the product of V_T, the volume of the tissue, and the tissue drug concentration.

Figure 10–1 shows blood perfusing a tissue in which distribution is perfusion rate-limited and no elimination occurs. The rate of presentation to the tissue is the product of blood flow, Q, and arterial blood concentration, C_A, i.e.,

$$\text{Rate of presentation} = Q \cdot C_A \qquad\qquad 1$$

The net rate of extravasation is the difference between rates of presentation and leaving, $Q \cdot C_V$, where C_V is the emergent venous concentration. Therefore,

$$\text{Net rate of uptake} = Q \cdot (C_A - C_V) \qquad\qquad 2$$

The maximum initial rate of uptake is the rate of presentation, $Q \cdot C_A$. Further, with no effective impedance to movement into the tissue, blood and tissue can be viewed kinetically as one compartment, with the concentration in emergent venous blood (C_V) in equilibrium with that in the tissue, C_T.

At any time, therefore,

$$\text{Amount of drug in tissue} = V_T \cdot K_P \cdot C_V \qquad\qquad 3$$

where V_T is the tissue volume and K_P is the equilibrium distribution ratio (C_T/C_V). Furthermore, the fractional rate of exit, k_T, is given by

$$k_T = \frac{\text{Rate of exit}}{\text{Amount in tissue}} = \frac{Q \cdot C_V}{V_T \cdot K_P \cdot C_V}$$

or   4

$$k_T = \frac{(Q/V_T)}{K_P}$$

where Q/V_T is the perfusion rate of the tissue. The parameter k_T, a distribution rate constant with units of reciprocal time, may be regarded as a measure of how rapidly drug would leave the tissue if the arterial concentration were suddenly to drop to zero. It is analogous to the elimination rate constant for loss of drug from the whole body and, like elimination, the kinetics of tissue distribution can be characterized by a tissue distribution half-life for which

$$\text{Half-life} = \frac{0.693}{k_T} = \frac{0.693\, K_P}{(Q/V_T)} \qquad\qquad 5$$

Thus, drug leaves slowly from tissues that have a high affinity (K_P) for it and that are poorly perfused.

Suppose now, that the arterial concentration is maintained constant with time. Then tissue uptake continues, but at a decreasing rate as tissue concentration rises, until equilibrium is achieved, when the net rate of uptake is zero, $C_V = C_A$ and $C_T = K_P \cdot C_A$. This situation is analogous to events occurring during a constant-rate infusion of drug into the body (Chap. 6, p. 71), with the equation defining the rise of tissue concentration to its plateau being given by

$$\text{Tissue concentration} = K_P \cdot C_A [1 - e^{-k_T \cdot t}] \qquad\qquad 6$$

Thus, the approach to plateau is determined solely by the tissue distribution half-life. In one half-life, the tissue concentration is 50% of its plateau value; in two half-lives, it is 75%; and so on.

To appreciate the foregoing, consider the events depicted in Fig. 10–2. Shown are plots of concentration in various tissues with time during the maintenance of a constant arterial concentration of 1 mg/L. First consider panel A in which the K_p values of a drug in kidneys, brain, and fat are the same and equal to one. Given that the perfusion rates to these tissues are 4, 0.5, and 0.03 mL/min/mL of tissue, respectively (Table 10–1), it follows that the corresponding half-lives for distribution are 0.17, 1.4, and 23 min. Thus, by 1 min (more than 4 half-lives), drug in the kidneys has reached equilibrium with that in blood, while it takes closer to 5 and 75 min for 90% of equilibrium to be reached in brain and fat, tissues of lower perfusion. Next consider panel B, in which events in fat are shown for drugs with different K_p values, namely 1, 2, and 5. Here the corresponding half-lives are 23, 46, and 115 min. Now, not only is the time taken for drug in tissue to reach equilibrium different, but so are the equilibrium tissue concentrations.

These simple examples illustrate two basic principles. Namely, both the approach toward equilibrium and the loss of drug from a tissue take longer the poorer the perfusion and the greater the partitioning of drug into a tissue. The latter is contrary to what one might intuitively anticipate. However, the greater the tendency to concentrate in a tissue, the longer it takes to deliver to that tissue the amount needed to reach distribution equilibrium and the longer it takes to redistribute drug out of that tissue. Stated differently, an increased affinity for a tissue accentuates an existing limitation imposed by perfusion.

Permeability Limitation

A permeability-rate limitation arises particularly for polar drugs diffusing across tightly knit lipoidal membranes, as demonstrated in Fig. 10–3 for the passage of compounds into the cerebrospinal fluid. In this study, the concentration of each drug was measured in cerebrospinal fluid, relative to that in plasma water (unbound), with time following attainment and maintenance of a constant plasma concentration. Differences in ease of entry are a

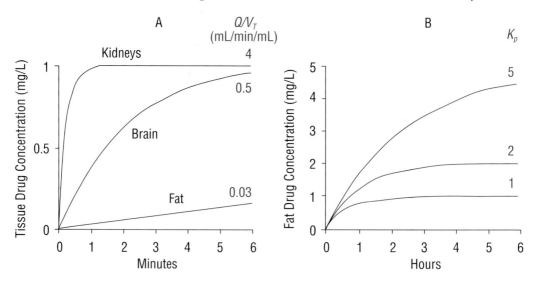

Fig. 10–2. If distribution is perfusion rate-limited, the time to reach equilibrium in tissue, when the arterial concentration is constant (1 mg/L), depends on perfusion and equilibrium distribution ratio. *A*, Concentrations with time in kidneys, brain, and fat tissues with different perfusion rates for a drug with a $K_p = 1$ in all three tissues. *B*, Concentrations with time in fat of three drugs with different K_p values of 1, 2, and 5, respectively. Note the difference in time scales of A (min) and B (hr).

function of both lipid-to-water partition coefficient and degree of ionization (Table 10–2), suggesting that only the un-ionized drug penetrates brain. For example, the partition coefficients of salicylic acid and pentobarbital are similar, yet the time required to reach distribution equilibrium is far shorter for pentobarbital than for salicyclic acid because, being the weaker acid, a greater fraction of pentobarbital is un-ionized in plasma, pH 7.4.

With large differences in perfusion and permeability of various tissues, it would appear to be impossible to predict tissue distribution of a drug. However, either of these two factors may limit the rate of extravasation, thereby simplifying the situation and allowing some conclusion to be drawn. Consider, for example, the following question: "Why, on measuring total tissue concentration, does the general anesthetic thiopental enter the brain much more rapidly than it does muscle tissue; yet, for penicillin the opposite is true?" The explanation lies in the properties of these drugs and of tissue membranes.

Thiopental is nonpolar, lipophilic and, being a weak acid (pKa 7.6), only partially ionized at plasma pH. As such, its entry into both brain and muscle occurs readily and is perfusion rate-limited. Since perfusion of the brain, particularly gray matter, is one or two orders of

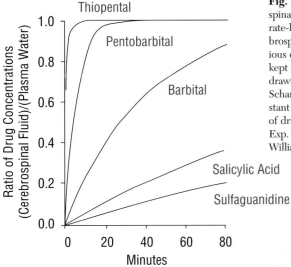

Fig. 10–3. Equilibration of drug in the cerebrospinal fluid with that in plasma is often permeability rate-limited. The ratio of drug concentrations (cerebrospinal fluid/unbound in plasma) is shown for various drugs in a dog. The plasma concentration was kept relatively constant throughout the study. (Redrawn from the data of Brodie, B.B., Kurz, H., and Schanker, L.S.: The importance of dissociation constant and lipid solubility in influencing the passage of drugs into the cerebrospinal fluid. J. Pharmacol. Exp. Ther., *130*:20–25, 1960. Copyright 1960, The Williams & Wilkins Co., Baltimore.)

Table 10–2. Physicochemical Properties and Time for Cerebrospinal Fluid Concentration to Reach 50% of Equilibrium Value for Selected Acidic Compounds[a] of Fig. 10–3[b]

DRUG	pKa	FRACTION UN-IONIZED AT pH 7.4	PARTITION COEFFICIENT OF UN-IONIZED FORM (n-HEPTANE/WATER)	EFFECTIVE PARTITION COEFFICIENT AT pH 7.4[c]	TIME TO REACH 50% OF EQUILIBRIUM VALUE (MIN)
Thiopental	7.6	0.6	3.3	2.0	1.4[d]
Pentobarbital	8.1	0.8	0.05	0.042	4
Barbital	7.5	0.6	0.002	0.0012	27
Salicylic acid	3.0	0.004	0.12	0.0005	115
Sulfaguanidine	>10	1.0	0.001	<0.001	231

[a]Similar correlation is observed for basic compounds.
[b]Data from reference in Fig. 10–3 and Hogben, C.A.M., Tocco, D.J., Brodie, B.B., and Schanker, L.S.: On the mechanism of intestinal absorption of drugs. J. Pharmacol. Exp. Ther., *125*:275–286, 1959.
[c]Fraction un-ionized at pH 7.4 times partition coefficient of un-ionized form.
[d]Probably perfusion rate-limited.

magnitude greater than that of muscle (Table 10–1), entry of thiopental into the brain is the more rapid process.

Penicillin, a relatively large polar compound, does not readily pass through membranes. The faster rate of entry of penicillin into muscle than into brain arises from the greater porosity of muscle capillaries. Recall from Chap. 9 (p. 126) for many tissues, e.g., muscle, capillary membranes appear to be very porous and have little influence on the entry of drugs of usual molecular weight (100 to 400 g/mole) into the interstitial fluids, regardless of the drug's physicochemical properties. There may be a permeability limitation at the tissue cell membrane, but in terms of measurement of drug in the *whole* tissue, there would appear to be only a partial impedance to the entry of either ionized or polar compounds, or both. Other tissues, for example, much of the central nervous system, anatomically have a permeability limitation at the capillary level that impedes movement of drug into the tissue as a whole, as observed with penicillin. This observation, especially with a number of polar organic dyes, led to the concept of *blood-to-brain* and *blood-to-cerebrospinal fluid* barriers.

The effect of a high equilibrium distribution ratio (K_p) on the time to achieve distribution equilibrium, discussed previously for a perfusion-rate limitation, applies equally well to a permeability-rate limitation. A permeability-rate limitation simply decreases the rate of entry and hence increases the time to reach distribution equilibrium over that of perfusion. Where the equilibrium lies is independent, however, of which process is rate-limiting.

If the arterial concentration is maintained long enough, the unbound concentration in tissue becomes the same as that in plasma. Sometimes, however, this equality is not observed. Reasons for lack of equality include maintenance of sink conditions by metabolism, active transport, bulk flow of interstitial fluids through both lymphatic channels and ducts, and pH gradients across cell membranes. Inequality in unbound concentration is frequently observed in the cerebrospinal fluid relative to plasma for large polar molecules, e.g., many antibiotics. The most likely explanation here is that the rate of fluid formation is sufficiently fast and the rate of diffusion sufficiently slow so that the resulting concentration, even at steady state, remains below that of the diffusible unbound drug in plasma. Another example is that of the distribution of albumin in the body (Table 10–3). Albumin slowly diffuses across the endothelial linings of the capillaries. The bulk flow of water in the interstitial fluids and lymphatic vessels provides a means of removing albumin from the tissues. The resulting tissue concentration is much below that of plasma. Albumin also diffuses into the cerebrospinal fluid, but the rate is so slow compared to the rate of production of the fluid that the concentration is virtually immeasurable. When there is a breakdown in the blood–cerebrospinal fluid barrier, as occurs for example in meningitis, albumin is found in the fluid as a result of an increased rate of entry.

Table 10–3. Distribution of Albumin in the Body[a]

ORGAN	AMOUNT (g/70-kg subject)	CONCENTRATION (g/kg organ)
Intravascular		
Plasma	140	43
Extravascular		
Muscle	50	2.3
Skin	40	7.7
Liver	2	1.4
Gut	8	5
Other tissues	110	3
Total:	210	
Total body	350	

[a]Adapted from compilation of data of Peters, T.: Serum albumin. *In* The Plasma Proteins. 2nd Ed., Vol. 1. Edited by F.W. Putnam. New York, Academic Press, 1975, p. 162.

EXTENT OF DISTRIBUTION

Multiple equilibria occur within plasma where drug can bind to various proteins, examples of which are listed in Table 10–4. Acidic drugs commonly bind to albumin, the most abundant plasma protein. Basic drugs often bind to α_1-acid glycoprotein and to lipoproteins. Proteins, such as γ-globulin, transcortin, fibrinogen, and thyroid-binding globulin, bind specific compounds. Distribution within each tissue also involves multiple equilibria. Tissue distribution can involve both binding to a wide variety of substances and partitioning into fat.

Apparent Volume of Distribution

The concentration in plasma achieved after distribution is complete is a result of the dose administered and the extent of tissue distribution. Recall from Chap. 3 that, at equilibrium, the extent of distribution is defined by an apparent volume of distribution (V):

$$V = \frac{\text{Amount in body at equilibrium}}{\text{Plasma drug concentration}} = \frac{A}{C} \qquad 7$$

This parameter is useful in relating amount in body to plasma concentration, and the converse. Recall, also, that volumes of distribution vary widely, with illustrative values ranging from 3 L/70 kg body weight to 40,000 L/70 kg body weight, a value far in excess of total body size.

Knowing plasma volume, V_P, and volume of distribution, V, the fraction of drug in body in and outside plasma can be estimated. The amount in plasma is $V_P \cdot C$; the amount in the body is $V \cdot C$. Therefore,

$$\text{Fraction of drug in body in plasma} = \frac{V_P}{V} \qquad 8$$

It is evident that the larger the volume of distribution, the smaller is the fraction in plasma. For example, for a drug with a volume of distribution of 100 L, only 3% resides in plasma.

The remaining fraction, given by

$$\text{Fraction of drug in body outside plasma} = \frac{(V - V_P)}{V} \qquad 9$$

includes drug in the blood cells. For the example considered above, 97% is outside plasma. Although this fraction can be readily determined, the actual distribution of drug outside plasma cannot.

The reason why the volume of distribution is an apparent volume and why its value differs among drugs may be appreciated by considering the simple model shown in Fig. 10–4.

Table 10–4. Representative Proteins to Which Drugs Bind in Plasma

PROTEIN	MOLECULAR WEIGHT (g/mole)	NORMAL CONCENTRATIONS	
		g/L	µM
Albumin	67,000	35–50	500–700
α_1-Acid glycoprotein	42,000	0.4–1.0	9–23
Lipoproteins	200,000–2,400,000	Variable	
Cortisol binding globulin (transcortin)	53,000	0.03–0.07	0.6–1.4

In this model, drug in the body is entirely accounted for in plasma, of volume V_P, and one tissue compartment, of volume V_T. At distribution equilibrium, the amount of drug in each location can be expressed in terms of plasma concentration, C, volumes of plasma and tissue and distribution ratio, as follows:

$$A = \underset{\substack{\text{Amount} \\ \text{in plasma}}}{V_P \cdot C} + \underset{\substack{\text{Amount} \\ \text{in tissue}}}{V_T \cdot K_P \cdot C} \qquad 10$$

And since $A = V \cdot C$ (Eq. 7), it follows, on dividing the equation above by C, that

$$V = V_P + V_T \cdot K_P \qquad 11$$

The product $V_T \cdot K_P$ is the apparent volume of a tissue viewed from measurement of drug in plasma. Thus, by expanding the model to embrace all tissues of the body, it is seen that the volume of distribution of a drug is the volume of plasma plus the sum of the apparent volumes of distribution of each tissue. For some tissues the value of K_P is large, which explains why the volume of distribution of some drugs can be much greater than total body size. Fat, for example, occupies approximately 20% of body volume. If the K_P value in fat is 5, then this tissue alone has an apparent volume of distribution equal to that of body volume. Remember, however, even when a perfusion rate limitation applies, it takes approximately 7 hrs for distribution equilibrium to occur in fat (Fig. 10–2B).

The volume of distribution of a specific drug can vary widely among patients. The reasons for such differences are now explored. Before doing so, however, a general point is considered.

Binding Within Blood. Within blood, drug can bind to many components including blood cells and plasma proteins. As a consequence of binding, the concentration of drug in whole blood (C_b), in plasma (C) and unbound in plasma water (Cu) can differ greatly. For ease of chemical analysis, plasma is the most common fluid analyzed. In many respects this choice is unfortunate. One of the primary goals of measuring concentration is to relate the measurement to pharmacologic response and toxicity. However, only unbound drug can pass through most cell membranes, the protein-bound form being too large. Accordingly, the unbound drug concentration is undoubtedly more closely related to the activity of the drug than is the total plasma concentration. Yet unbound concentration is only occasionally measured, primarily because the methods for doing so are often tedious, lack

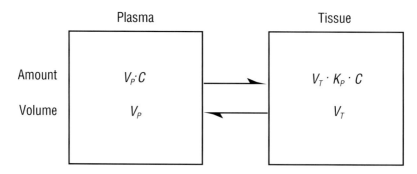

Fig. 10–4. The effect of tissue binding on drug distribution is illustrated by a drug that distributes between plasma and a tissue. The physiologic volumes are V_P and V_T, respectively. At equilibrium the amount of drug in each location depends on the equilibrium distribution (partition) ratio, K_P, the plasma and the tissue volumes, and the plasma concentration.

accuracy and precision, and are costly. Nonetheless, it is helpful to define an unbound volume of distribution, Vu,

$$Vu = \frac{\text{Amount in body at equilibrium}}{\text{Unbound plasma concentration}} = \frac{A}{Cu} \qquad 12$$

which permits the amount of drug in the body to be related to the unbound drug concentration.

Sometimes whole blood concentration is measured. Once again an appropriate volume term, V_b, can be defined. Namely,

$$V_b = \frac{\text{Amount in body at equilibrium}}{\text{Concentration in whole blood}} = \frac{A}{C_b} \qquad 13$$

As the amount of drug in body is independent of the site of measurement, it follows from Eqs. 7, 12, and 13 that

$$V \cdot C = Vu \cdot Cu = V_b \cdot C_b \qquad 14$$

The values of these volume terms can differ markedly for a given drug. The term most often quoted in the literature is based on measurement of drug in plasma (i.e., V). Examples of drugs with differing values of V are given in Fig. 3–2 (p. 22).

Plasma Protein Binding. The principal concern with plasma protein binding is related to its variability within and among patients in various therapeutic settings. The degree of binding is frequently expressed as the bound-to-total concentration ratio. This ratio has limiting values of 0 and 1.0. Drugs with values greater than 0.9 are said to be highly bound.

As stated previously, unbound, rather than bound, concentration is frequently more important in therapeutics. Therefore, the fraction of drug in plasma unbound, fu,

$$fu = Cu/C \qquad 15$$

is of greater utility than fraction bound. Obviously, only if fu is constant is total plasma concentration a good measure of changes in unbound drug concentration. Approximate values of fu usually associated with therapy for representative drugs are shown in Fig. 10–5.

Binding is a function of the affinity of the protein for the drug. The affinity is characterized by an association constant, K_a. Because the number of binding sites on a protein is limited, binding also depends on the molar concentrations of both drug and protein. For a single binding site on the protein, the association is simply summarized by the following reaction:

$$\text{Drug} + \text{Protein} \rightleftharpoons \text{Drug-protein complex} \qquad 16$$

Equilibrium may lie either to the right or to the left. High affinity, of course, implies that equilibrium lies far to the right. This is a relative statement, however, as the greater the protein concentration for a given drug concentration, the greater the bound drug concentration and the converse. From mass law considerations, the equilibrium is expressed in terms of the concentrations of unbound-drug, Cu, unoccupied protein, P, and bound drug, Cbd, thus

$$K_a = \frac{Cbd}{Cu \cdot P} \qquad\qquad 17$$

The unoccupied protein concentration depends on the total protein concentration, P_t. These two concentrations are related by $fu_p = P/P_t$, where fu_p is the fraction of the total number of binding sites unoccupied. Furthermore, the unbound concentration is $fu \cdot C$ and the bound concentration is $(1 - fu) \cdot C$. Appropriately substituting into Eq. 17, it therefore follows upon rearrangement that

$$fu = \frac{1}{1 + K_a \cdot fu_p \cdot P_t} \qquad\qquad 18$$

From this relationship the value of fu is seen to depend on the total protein concentration, as illustrated in Fig. 10–6 for the binding of propranolol to α_1-acid glycoprotein. When fu is small (<0.1), Eq. 18 is approximately $1/(K_a \cdot fu_p \cdot P_t)$. By taking the ratio of this equation for normal and altered conditions, the value of fu (fu') when the concentration of binding protein is altered (P_t') is,

$$fu' = \frac{P_t}{P_t'} \cdot fu \qquad\qquad 19$$

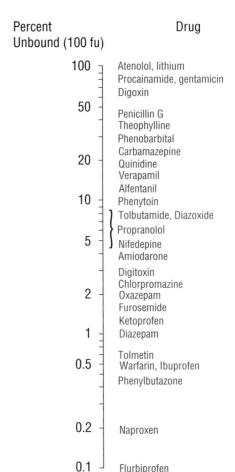

Fig. 10–5. The fraction of drug in plasma not bound to protein varies widely among drugs.

Percent Unbound (100 fu)	Drug
100	Atenolol, lithium / Procainamide, gentamicin / Digoxin
50	Penicillin G / Theophylline / Phenobarbital / Carbamazepine
20	Quinidine / Verapamil / Alfentanil
10	Phenytoin / Tolbutamide, Diazoxide / Propranolol
5	Nifedepine / Amiodarone
2	Digitoxin / Chlorpromazine / Oxazepam / Furosemide / Ketoprofen
1	Diazepam
0.5	Tolmetin / Warfarin, Ibuprofen / Phenylbutazone
0.2	Naproxen
0.1	Flurbiprofen

Consider, for example, the change in *fu* expected for ibuprofen (*fu* = 0.005), a drug bound primarily to albumin, when the albumin concentration is decreased from 43 g/L to 28 g/L. The fraction unbound is expected to increase to 0.0077.

Usually, only a small fraction of the available sites on binding proteins is occupied (fu_p ≃ 1) at the therapeutic concentrations of most drugs; the fraction unbound is then relatively constant at a given protein concentration and independent of drug concentration. Occasionally, therapeutic concentrations are sufficiently high so that most of the available binding sites are occupied. Then both *fu* and fu_p are concentration-dependent (see Chap. 22, Dose and Time Dependencies).

In subsequent chapters, it will be helpful to remember that pharmacologic activity relates to the unbound concentration. Plasma protein binding, then, is often only of interest because the total plasma concentration is measured. The total plasma concentration depends on both the extent of protein binding and the unbound concentration, i.e.,

$$C = Cu/fu \qquad\qquad 20$$

When conceptualizing dependency and functionality, this equation should not be rearranged.

Tissue Binding. The fraction of drug in body located in plasma depends on its binding to both plasma and tissue components, as shown schematically in Fig. 10–7. A drug may have a great affinity for plasma proteins, but may still be located primarily in tissue if the

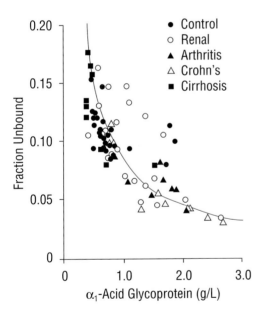

Fig. 10–6. The fraction unbound of propranolol varies with the plasma concentration of α_1-acid glycoprotein in 78 patients with various diseases and in healthy volunteers. The line drawn through the data represents the relationship expected from Eq. 18, using a value of 11 L/g (4.84×10^5 L/mole) for K_a. This relationship appears to account for most of the observed variability in the fraction unbound. In all cases, the protein is not saturated; the molar concentration of propranolol is below that of α_1-acid glycoprotein (1 mg/L = 22.7 μM). (Redrawn from Tozer, T.N.: Implications of altered plasma protein binding in disease states. *In*: Pharmacokinetic Basis for Drug Treatment. Edited by L.Z. Benet, N. Massoud, and J.G. Gambertoglio. Raven Press, New York, 1983, pp. 173–193. Original data from Piafsky, K.M., Borga, O., Odar-Cederlof, I., Johansson, C., and Sjoqvist, F.: Increased plasma protein binding of propranolol and chlorpromazine mediated by disease-induced elevations of plasma α_1-acid glycoprotein. N. Engl. J. Med., 299:1435–1439, 1978. Reproduced with permission of Raven Press.)

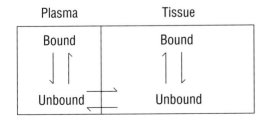

Fig. 10–7. At equilibrium, the distribution of a drug within the body depends on binding to both plasma proteins and tissue components. In the model, only unbound drug is capable of entering and leaving the plasma and tissue compartments.

tissue has an affinity even greater than that of plasma. Unlike plasma binding, tissue binding of a drug cannot be measured directly. The tissue must be disrupted, resulting in the loss of its integrity. Even so, tissue binding is important in drug distribution.

Tissue binding may be inferred from measurement of drug binding in plasma. Consider, e.g., the following mass–balance relationship,

$$V \cdot C = V_P \cdot C + V_{TW} \cdot C_{TW}$$

$$\underset{\substack{\text{Amount} \\ \text{in body}}}{} \quad \underset{\substack{\text{Amount} \\ \text{in plasma}}}{} \quad \underset{\substack{\text{Amount} \\ \text{outside plasma}}}{} \qquad 21$$

in which V_{TW} is the aqueous volume outside of plasma into which the drug distributes and C_{TW} is the corresponding total drug concentration.

Dividing by C,

$$V = V_P + V_{TW} \cdot \frac{C_{TW}}{C}$$

$$\underset{\substack{\text{Apparent} \\ \text{volume of} \\ \text{distribution}}}{} \quad \underset{\substack{\text{Volume} \\ \text{of} \\ \text{plasma}}}{} \quad \underset{\substack{\text{Apparent} \\ \text{volume of} \\ \text{tissue}}}{} \qquad 22$$

Recall that $fu = Cu/C$. Similarly, for the tissue, $fu_T = Cu_T/C_{TW}$. Given that distribution equilibrium is achieved when the unbound concentrations in plasma, Cu, and in tissues, Cu_T, are equal, then

$$\frac{C_{TW}}{C} = \frac{fu}{fu_T} \qquad 23$$

which on substituting into Eq. 22 yields

$$V = V_P + V_{TW} \cdot \frac{fu}{fu_T} \qquad 24$$

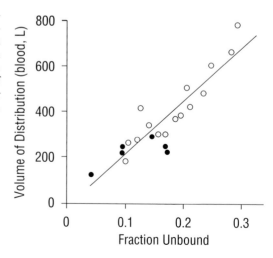

Fig. 10–8. The volume of distribution of (+)-propranolol varies with the fraction unbound. The observation was made in 6 control subjects (●) and in 15 patients (○) with chronic hepatic disease after an i.v. bolus (40 mg) of (+)-propranolol. (Data from Branch, R.A., Jones, J., and Read, A.E.: A study of factors influencing drug disposition in chronic liver disease, using the model drug (+)-propranolol. Br. J. Clin. Pharmacol., 3:243–249, 1976.)

From this relationship it is seen that the apparent volume of distribution increases when fu is increased and decreases when fu_T is increased.

To appreciate the relationship in Eq. 22–24, consider the data for propranolol shown in Fig. 10–8. The linear relationship between V and fu not only indicates that V_{TW}/fu_T is constant, but also that differences in binding of propranolol in plasma account for most of the variation observed in its volume of distribution.

The relationship expressed in Eq. 24 explains why, because of plasma and tissue binding, V rarely corresponds to a real volume, such as plasma volume (3 L), extracellular space (15 L), or total body water (42 L). Even if V corresponds to the value of a physiologic space, one cannot conclude unambiguously that the drug distributes only into that volume. Binding of drugs in both plasma and tissues complicates the situation and often prevents making any conclusion about the actual volume into which the drug distributes. An exception is when drug is restricted to plasma; the volumes of distribution, apparent and real, are then the same, about 3 L in an adult. This last situation is expected for small molecular weight drugs that are highly bound to plasma proteins but not bound in the tissues. However, this apparent volume cannot be an equilibrium value, because plasma proteins equilibrate slowly between plasma and other extracellular fluids. The apparent volume of plasma proteins, about 7.5 L for albumin, is perhaps a better estimate of the minimum value for such drugs.

For drugs of high molecular weight (greater than approximately 70,000 g/mole), extravascular distribution is very slow to nonexistent. For such drugs, the volume of distribution then tends to approximate that of plasma, 3 L. An exception can occur if the macromolecular drug binds to endothelial linings within the vascular system.

For drugs that are bound in neither tissue nor plasma, the volume of distribution varies between the extracellular fluid volume (16 L) and the total body water (42 L), depending on the degree to which the drug gains access to the intracellular fluids. Examples of drugs that distribute in total body water are caffeine and alcohol, both small molecules that pass freely through membranes.

SMALL VOLUME OF DISTRIBUTION

Model

The model expressed by Eq. 24 is conceptually useful, but it does not take into account that plasma proteins distribute throughout extracellular fluids, as shown for albumin in Table 10–3. A model is therefore needed to distinguish, in tissues, between binding to plasma protein and binding to other constituents. This need is particularly great for drugs that bind to a plasma protein and that have small (less than 0.2 L/kg; 14 L/70 kg) volumes of distribution. Much of the drug in the body is then bound to the plasma protein and any change in binding or in the distribution of the protein can substantially influence the distribution of unbound drug within the body. A model to describe such distribution is derived in Appendix I–F.

For a drug bound to albumin, the approximate relationship between V and binding to albumin and other sites is

$$V = 7.5 + \left(7.5 + \frac{V_R}{fu_R}\right) fu \qquad\qquad 25$$

where fu is the fraction unbound, V_R is the aqueous volume of the intracellular fluids into which drug distributes (total available volume = 27 L), and fu_R is the apparent fraction unbound in the intracellular fluids. The virtue of this model is that it provides a means of analyzing the distribution of both drug and the plasma protein to which it binds. Representative drugs with volumes of distribution less than 0.2 L/kg and to which this model is specifically applicable are given in Table 10–5.

To illustrate the utility of the proposed model, consider the data in Fig. 10–9. Shown is a linear relationship between V and fu for a series of cephalosporins. This dependence might have been explained by the general model, $V = V_P + V_{TW} \cdot fu/fu_T$, assuming fu_T does not vary among the cephalosporins. A major problem would have been noticed here, however. The observed volume intercept when fu approaches zero is 7 L/70 kg (0.11 L/kg), a value much larger than the plasma volume, V_P, of 3 L. The observations are much better explained by the proposed model. The discrepancy between the two models lies in the distribution of the plasma protein. The proposed model suggests that albumin is the major binding protein for these antibiotics in that those cephalosporins that are tightly bound have distribution characteristics in common with albumin.

The volumes of distribution of the cephalosporins at higher fractions unbound, however, indicate that the drugs must partially enter cells or be bound to some extravascular structures. The extent of this distribution outside the extracellular fluids, on average, must be relatively small in that by extrapolation to $fu = 1$, corresponding to a cephalosporin with no binding to plasma albumin, the volume is 0.29 L/kg (20 L/70 kg), a value greater than

Table 10–5. Representative Drugs With Volumes of Distribution of 0.2 L/kg or Less[a]

Acetylsalicylic acid	Cefotetan	Dicloxacillin	Piperacillin
Bumetanide	Ceftriaxone	Diflunisal	Piroxicam
Carbenicillin	Cefuroxime	Flurbiprofen	Probenecid
Cefamandole	Chlorothiazide	Furosemide	Salicylic acid
Cefazolin	Chlorpropamide	Ibuprofen	Sulfisoxazole
Cefonicid	Clofibric acid	Ketoprofen	Tolbutamide
Cefoperazone	Cloxacillin	Naproxen	Tolmetin
Ceforanide	Diclofenac	Oxyphenbutazone	Valproic acid
Cefotaxime	Dobutamine	Phenylbutazone	Warfarin

[a]Binding to albumin is known or assumed.

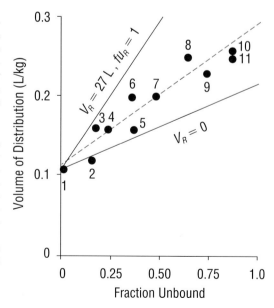

Fig. 10–9. The volumes of distribution of a series of cephalosporin antibiotics increase with the fraction unbound to plasma proteins. The slope of the line of best fit (---) lies between the expected relationships for drugs that do not enter tissue cells, $V_R = 0$, and those that do, $V_R = 27$ L (Eq. 25), but do not bind to tissue components ($fu_R = 1$). The cephalosporins shown are: 1 = cefonicid, 2 = cefazolin, 3 = ceforanide, 4 = cefamandole, 5 = cefotaxitin, 6 = cephalothin, 7 = moxalactam, 8 = cefotaxime, 9 = ceftazidime, 10 = cephalexin, and 11 = cephradine. (Drawn from data compiled by Dudley, M.N., and Nightingale, C.H.: Effects of protein upon activity of cephalosporins: New beta-lactam antibiotics: A review from chemistry to clinical efficacy of the new cephalosporins. Edited by H.C. Neu, Philadelphia, Francis Clark Wood Institute for the History of Medicine, College of Physicians of Philadelphia, 1982, pp. 227–239.)

the extracellular volume (15 L/70 kg), but considerably less than total body water (42 L/70 kg).

The unbound volumes of distribution within the series of cephalosporins Fig. 10–10 in contrast to the total volume of distribution, dramatically decrease as the fraction unbound is increased. For those cephalosporins that are highly bound (low fu), the binding protein effectively ties up the drug. The consequence of plasma protein binding here is that a much larger amount of drug must be in the body to give the same antimicrobial effect for those drugs with the same minimum inhibitory unbound concentration.

Location in Body

The fractions of drug in the body that are in plasma (bound and unbound), in or outside extracellular fluids, and bound in plasma or throughout extracellular fluids can be useful pieces of information, particularly with those conditions, examples listed in Table 10–6, in

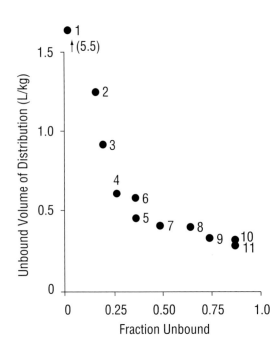

Fig. 10–10. The unbound volumes of distribution of the same cephalosporins shown in Fig. 10–9 decrease dramatically with an increase in the fraction unbound. For those cephalosporins with unbound volumes much greater than the extracellular space ($V_E = 0.22$ L/kg) or the total body water (0.6 L/kg), binding to plasma proteins clearly reduces the concentration of the active form for a given dose. (See Fig. 10–9 for identification of the cephalosporins and the source of the information.)

Table 10–6. Examples of Conditions in Which the Plasma Concentration of the Two Major Plasma Proteins to Which Drugs Bind Are Altered

PLASMA PROTEIN	CONDITION	CHANGE IN CONCENTRATION OF PLASMA PROTEIN
Albumin	Hepatic cirrhosis	Decrease
	Burns	Decrease
	Nephrotic syndrome	Decrease
	End-stage renal disease	Decrease
	Pregnancy	Decrease
α_1-Acid glycoprotein	Myocardial infarction	Increase
	Surgery	Increase
	Crohn's disease	Increase
	Trauma	Increase
	Rheumatoid arthritis	Increase

which there are changes in the distribution of plasma proteins. Relationships to calculate these fractions are given in Table 10–7. Their derivations are given in Appendix I–F.

When the apparent volume of distribution of a drug is large (greater than 50 to 100 L), Eq. 25 approximately reduces to

$$V \approx V_R \cdot \frac{fu}{fu_R} \qquad\qquad 26$$

which is virtually the same as that predicted by Eq. 24. The major practical application of Eq. 25, however, is for drugs with small volumes of distribution, i.e., with values approaching 7.5 L/70 kg (0.11 L/kg) for a drug bound to albumin.

Altered Binding and Loading Dose

Loading doses are given to rapidly achieve a therapeutic response, putatively by rapidly producing a desired unbound concentration. With variations in both plasma and tissue binding, the question arises whether or not the loading dose needs to be adjusted.

For many drugs volume of distribution is greater than 50 L, i.e., much greater than the apparent volume of the binding protein, implying that only a small fraction of drug in body resides on the plasma protein. Therefore, ignoring the first two terms in Eq. 25 and realizing that $fu \cdot C = Cu$, it follows that

$$\text{Amount in body} \approx \frac{V_R}{fu_R} \cdot Cu \qquad\qquad 27$$

This equation indicates that Cu is independent of plasma binding and thus no adjustment in loading dose is needed. The total plasma concentration does, of course, change with altered plasma binding, but this is of no therapeutic consequence with respect to loading dose requirements. If, however, tissue binding (fu_R) were to change, so would the initial value(s) of Cu (and C), necessitating a decision to change the loading dose.

Table 10–7. Approximate Relationships for Analyzing Distribution of a Drug That Binds to Albumin and Distributes Throughout Total Body Water

FRACTION OF DRUG IN BODY	RELATIONSHIPS[a]
In plasma	$3/V$
Outside plasma	$\dfrac{V - 3}{V}$
Unbound in body water	$\dfrac{42 \cdot fu}{V}$
Unbound in extracellular fluids	$\dfrac{15 \cdot fu}{V}$
In extracellular fluids	$\dfrac{7.5(1 + fu)}{V}$
Outside extracellular fluids	$\dfrac{V - 7.5(1 + fu)}{V}$
Bound to proteins in plasma	$\dfrac{3(1 - fu)}{V}$
Bound to extracellular proteins	$\dfrac{7.5(1 - fu)}{V}$
Bound outside the extracellular fluids (in tissues)	$\dfrac{V - 35 \cdot fu - 7.5}{V}$

[a]Derivations are given in Appendix I–F.

STUDY PROBLEMS

(Answers to Study Problems are in Appendix II.)

1. Define the terms apparent volume of distribution, fraction unbound, tissue-to-blood equilibrium distribution ratio, and perfusion-rate and permeability-rate limitations in drug distribution.

2. The volume of distribution of quinacrine, a drug bound to albumin in plasma, is about 40,000 L. The fraction unbound in plasma is 0.08.
   a. The plasma concentration when 1 g of drug is in the body would therefore be _____ mg/L.
   b. The amount of drug in the body when the plasma concentration is 0.015 mg/L is _____ mg.
   c. The percentage of drug in the body that is:
      1. outside the plasma
      2. in extracellular fluids.
      3. bound outside extracellular fluids

3. The volume of distribution of a drug (molecular weight = 351 g/mole) in a 70-kg subject is observed to be 8 L. Indicate which one (or more) of the following statements is (are) consistent with this observation. The drug is:
   a. Highly bound to plasma proteins.
   b. Bound to components outside plasma and is highly bound to proteins in plasma.
   c. Not bound to plasma proteins.

4. The total (left) and unbound (right) concentrations of Drug A following single i.v. doses are shown in the Figs. 10–11 and 10–12. Sketch on each of the same figures the anticipated corresponding concentrations of the drug when administered:
   a. In the presence of Drug B, which significantly (two-fold change) displaces Drug A (500-mg dose) from tissue binding sites only.

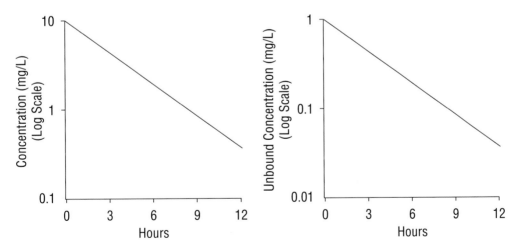

Fig. 10–11.

   b. At a subsequent time (1000-mg dose) when the patient's serum albumin, the protein to which the drug binds, is reduced from 42 to 21 g/L (e.g., when the patient develops nephrotic syndrome). Binding to other constituents in the body is unaffected.

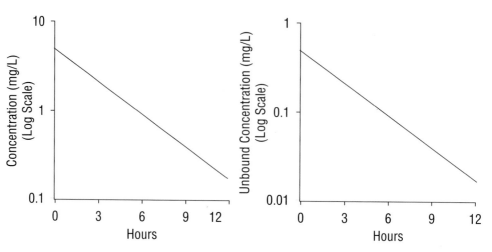

Fig. 10–12.

5. Briefly comment on the validity of each of the following statements.
   a. The equilibrium distribution ratio for a drug between liver and plasma is 50; there-fore, its volume of distribution must be at least 75 L in a man weighing 70 kg.
   b. A drug that reaches distribution equilibrium within 30 min, yet whose volume of distribution in a 70-kg man is 200 L, must distribute primarily into highly perfused organs.
6. Using the information in Table 10–8, calculate the time required for the amounts in each of the tissues listed to reach 50% of the equilibrium value for a drug with perfusion rate-limited distribution when the arterial blood concentration is kept constant with time (by giving a bolus and an appropriate infusion). Rank the times and the corre-sponding tissues.

Table 10–8.

ORGAN	EQUILIBRIUM DISTRIBUTION RATIO	PERFUSION RATE (mL/min/mL of tissue)
Lungs	1	10
Kidneys	4	4
Heart	3	0.6
Liver	15	0.8
Skin	12	0.024

7. Digitoxin has a volume of distribution of 38 L in a 70-kg man and is 97% bound in plasma. Given that the unbound drug distributes evenly throughout total body water, what fraction of drug is unbound in the intercellular fluids?
8. Digoxin has a volume of distribution of about 550 L in a 70-kg subject and is 23% bound in plasma. Using the information provided in problem 7, determine if digoxin is more or less extensively bound in intracellular fluids than digitoxin?
9. Ganeval et al. studied the pharmacokinetics of warfarin in 11 patients with the ne-phrotic syndrome (daily urinary protein excretion = 10.2 ± 4.5 g; serum creatinine = 105 ± 32 μM) versus 11 controls (no proteinuria; serum creatinine = 96 ± 20 μM). Table 10–9 illustrates the differences in warfarin kinetics in the two populations. No data on differences in weight between the two groups were given. For this problem, both groups averaged 70 kg.

Table 10-9. Mean Pharmacokinetic Parameters and Serum Albumin Concentrations in 11 Control and 11 Nephrotic Patients After Oral Administration (8 mg) of Warfarin[a]

PARAMETERS	CONTROL GROUP	NEPHROTIC PATIENTS
V (L)	9.4 ± 2.7	13.7 ± 6.6
CL (L/hr)	0.20 ± 0.07	0.58 ± 0.26
$t_{1/2}$ (hr)	36 ± 14	18 ± 11
Serum albumin (g/L)	43 ± 5	12.5 ± 6.5

[a]From Ganeval, D., Fischer, A.M., Berre, J., Pertuiset, N., Dautzenberg, M.D., Jungers, P., and Houin, G.: Pharmacokinetics of warfarin in the nephrotic syndrome and effect on vitamin K-dependent clotting factors. Clin. Nephrol., 25:78–80, 1986.

a. Given a fraction unbound of 0.005 in the control group, estimate the value expected in the nephrotic group.

b. Warfarin has a small volume of distribution. Calculate the expected volume of distribution if fu is increased to the value calculated in "a." Hint: determine the value of fu_R in the control group, and assume it is the same in the nephrotic patients.

c. Had the half-life data not been given, could you have predicted the observed shortening of the value in the nephrotic patients? This condition usually suggests induction of metabolism.

ELIMINATION

This chapter is concerned with elimination processes and particularly with the concept of clearance. In Chap. 3, 6, and 7, the methods of quantifying clearance were presented. Here its physiologic meaning is given.

ELIMINATION

Elimination occurs by excretion and metabolism. Some drugs are excreted via the bile. Others, particularly volatile substances, are excreted in the breath. For most drugs, however, excretion occurs predominantly via the kidneys.

Metabolism is the major mechanism for elimination of drugs from the body. Some drugs are eliminated almost entirely unchanged by the kidneys, but these drugs are relatively few.

The most common routes of drug metabolism are oxidation, reduction, hydrolysis, and conjugation. Frequently, a drug simultaneously undergoes metabolism by several competing pathways. The fraction going to each metabolite depends on the relative rates of each of the parallel pathways. Metabolites may undergo further metabolism. For example, oxidation, reduction, and hydrolysis are often followed by a conjugation reaction. These reactions occur in series or are said to be *sequential*. Because they often occur first, oxidation, reduction and hydrolysis are commonly referred to as Phase I reactions, and conjugations as a Phase II reactions.

Generally, the liver is the major and sometimes only, site of drug metabolism. Occasionally, however, a drug is extensively metabolized in one or more other tissues, such as the kidneys, skin, lungs, blood, and gastrointestinal wall. Nitroglycerin is such an example.

Table 11–1 illustrates patterns of biotransformation (metabolism) of representative drugs. The pathways of metabolism are classified by chemical alteration. Several of the transformations occur in the endoplasmic reticulum of the liver and of certain other tissues. On homogenizing these tissues, the endoplasmic reticulum is disrupted with the formation of small vesicles called *microsomes*. For this reason, metabolizing enzymes of the endoplasmic reticulum are called *microsomal enzymes*. Drug metabolism, therefore, may be classified as microsomal and nonmicrosomal.

Table 11-1. Patterns of Biotransformation[a] of Representative Drugs[b]

PRODRUG	DRUG	ACTIVE METABOLITE	INACTIVE METABOLITE[c]
	Acetylsalicylic acid —(H)→	Salicylic acid	(C)→ Salicyl (acid) glucuronide (C)→ Salicyl (phenolic) glucuronide (C)→ Salicyluric acid (O)→ Gentisic acid
	Glutethimide —(O)→	Hydroxyglutethimide —(C)→	Hydroxyglutethimide glucuronide
	Morphine —(C)→	Morphine-6-glucuronide	(C)→ Morphine-3-glucuronide
	Phenytoin		(O)→ p-Hydroxyphenytoin
Prednisone —(R)→	Prednisolone		
	Succinylcholine		(H)→ Succinylmonocholine
	Theophylline		(O)→ 1-Methylxanthine (O)→ 1,3-Dimethyluric acid

[a]Classification: (O), oxidation; (R), reduction; (H), hydrolysis; (C), conjugation.
[b]For some drugs only representative metabolic pathways are indicated.
[c]Inactive at concentrations obtained following the therapeutic administration of the parent drug.

The major enzymes responsible for the oxidation and reduction of drugs belong to the superfamily of cytochrome P450 enzymes. The isozymes of this family display a relatively high degree of structural specificity; a drug is often a good substrate for one enzyme but not another (see also Chap. 14).

The consequences of drug metabolism are manifold. Biotransformation provides a mechanism for ridding the body of undesirable foreign compounds and drugs; it also provides a means of producing active compounds. Numerous examples are now recognized in which the administered drug is really an inactive prodrug, which is converted into a pharmacologically active species. Often both the drug and its metabolite(s) are active. The duration and intensity of the responses vary with the time courses of these substances in the body. The pharmacokinetics of active metabolites, as well as that of the compound administered, is therefore of therapeutic concern. The common pathways of biotransformation and the kinetics of metabolites are presented in Chap. 21, Metabolite Kinetics. The elimination processes are emphasized here.

CONCEPT OF CLEARANCE

Of the concepts in pharmacokinetics, *clearance* has the greatest potential for clinical applications. It is also the most useful parameter for the evaluation of an elimination mechanism.

Loss Across an Organ of Elimination

Recall from Chap. 3 that clearance is defined as the proportionality factor relating rate of drug elimination to the plasma (drug) concentration. That is, rate of elimination $= CL \cdot C$. Clearance may be viewed in another way, namely from the loss of drug across an organ of elimination. This latter physiologic approach has a number of advantages, particularly in predicting and in evaluating the effects of changes in blood flow, plasma protein binding, enzyme activity, or secretory activity on the elimination of a drug. Fig. 11–1 summarizes the various ways of viewing mass balance across an eliminating organ. In this scheme, drug in the eliminating organ is assumed to have reached distribution equilibrium; thus, the sole reason for any difference between the arterial and venous concentrations is elimination. For all but the earliest moments, this assumption is reasonable for the kidneys and the liver, which are among the most highly perfused and hence most rapidly equilibrating organs in the body.

The rate of presentation of a drug to an organ of elimination is the product of blood flow, Q, and concentration in blood entering the arterial side, C_A, that is, $Q \cdot C_A$. Similarly, the rate at which drug leaves on the venous side is $Q \cdot C_V$, where C_V is the concentration in the returning venous blood. The difference between these rates is the rate of drug extraction (elimination) by the organ,

$$\text{Rate of extraction} = Q(C_A - C_V) \qquad 1$$

If the rate of drug extraction is related to the rate at which it is presented to the organ, $Q \cdot C_A$, a useful parameter, the *extraction ratio, E,* is derived:

$$E = \frac{\text{Rate of extraction}}{\text{Rate of presentation}} = \frac{(C_A - C_V)}{C_A} \qquad 2$$

The extraction ratio lies between zero, where no drug is eliminated, and 1, where no drug escapes past the organ.

If the rate of drug extraction is related to the incoming concentration in blood, one obtains, by definition, the value of clearance (Chap. 3),

$$\text{Clearance} = \frac{Q(C_A - C_V)}{C_A}$$

3

in this instance, blood clearance, CL_b, since the concentration in blood is measured. On substituting Eq. 2 into Eq. 3, the following important relationship is obtained:

$$\begin{array}{ccc} CL_b & = & Q & \cdot & E \\ \text{Blood} & & \text{Blood} & \text{Extraction} \\ \text{clearance} & & \text{flow} & \text{ratio} \end{array}$$

4

That is, blood clearance may be regarded as the volume of blood from which all the drug would appear to be removed per unit time. For example, if the extraction ratio of a drug across an organ is 0.5 and organ blood flow is 1 L/min, then all drug in 0.5 L of the incoming blood is effectively removed each minute as blood passes through the organ. Furthermore, if the arterial concentration is 1 mg/L, then the rate of elimination is 0.5 L/min times 1 mg/L, or 0.5 mg/min.

Blood clearance cannot be any value. Examination of Eq. 4 shows that if the extraction ratio approaches 1.0, then blood clearance approaches a maximum, organ blood flow. For

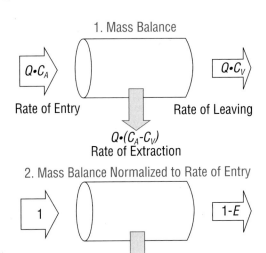

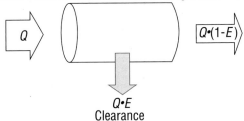

Fig. 11–1.   The extraction of a drug by an eliminating organ under steady-state conditions may be considered from the fundamental concepts of mass balance: I, The extraction of drug may be accounted for from its rates in and out of the organ. II, Normalizing to the rate of entry provides a means of determining the fraction extracted, the extraction ratio. III, Normalizing to the entering concentration allows one to account for the drug in terms of clearance and blood flow. The symbols are defined in Eqs. 1 through 4.

kidneys and liver, the average organ blood flows are 1.1 and 1.35 L/min (Table 10–1), respectively.

Before considering clearance of drug by specific organs, several comments are in order.

Description of Clearance by Organ, Process, or Site of Measurement

Clearance can be described in terms of the eliminating organ, e.g., hepatic clearance, renal clearance, or pulmonary clearance. It can also be described by the difference between renal excretion and elimination by all other processes, e.g., renal clearance and extrarenal clearance. How an organ clears the blood of drug may also be described by the nature of the elimination process, e.g., metabolic clearance or excretory clearance. Furthermore, the clearance value depends on the reference fluid. Thus, to be specific, the clearance of a drug eliminated, e.g., by metabolism in the liver, using plasma concentration measurements would then be hepatic metabolic plasma clearance. Similarly, "clearance by excretion of drug" in the kidneys would be renal excretory plasma clearance. In practice, the term *plasma* is dropped, as plasma is the common site of measurement. In addition, one often drops *metabolic* or *excretory* when describing clearance by the liver and kidneys, respectively, because these processes generally occur in these respective organs. However, metabolism does occur in the kidneys, and excretion (into bile) does occur in the liver. Therefore, the assumptions underlying the clearance nomenclature for a specific drug should always be questioned.

Plasma Versus Blood Clearance

For many applications in pharmacokinetics, it matters little whether clearance measurements are based on drug in plasma or in blood. The exception is when a clearance value is used to estimate extraction ratio. Then the blood clearance value must be used, because it is this parameter that directly relates to organ blood flow and extraction ratio (see Eq. 4).

Plasma clearance is more frequently reported than blood clearance. Thus, if one wishes to estimate extraction ratio, one needs to convert this clearance value based on drug concentration in plasma to one based on the concentration in blood. This conversion is accomplished by experimentally determining the blood-to-plasma concentration ratio. Since, by definition, the products of the respective clearance and concentration terms, based on measurements in blood and plasma, are equal to the rate of elimination, it follows that:

$$\frac{\text{Plasma clearance}}{\text{Blood clearance}} = \frac{\text{Blood concentration } (C_b)}{\text{Plasma concentration } (C)} \qquad 5$$

The concentration ratio is a function of the hematocrit and of the binding of drug to both plasma proteins and blood cell components. The relationship is derived in Appendix I–G. Strong binding to plasma proteins produces a ratio less than 1.0 with a lower limit of (1-hematocrit), when drug is restricted to plasma. When binding to blood cells is extensive, the ratio may be much greater than 1.0.

Additivity of Clearance

The anatomy of the human body dictates that the clearance of a drug by one organ adds to clearance of another. This is a consequence of the circulation. Consider, for example, a drug that is eliminated by both renal excretion and hepatic metabolism. Then

$$\text{Rate of elimination} = \text{Rate of renal excretion} + \text{Rate of hepatic metabolism} \qquad 6$$

Dividing the rate of removal associated with each process by the incoming drug concentration (blood or plasma), which for both organs is the same (C), gives the clearance associated with that process:

or

$$\frac{\text{Rate of elimination}}{C} = \frac{\text{Rate of renal excretion}}{C} + \frac{\text{Rate of hepatic metabolism}}{C}$$

$$\text{Total clearance} = \text{Renal clearance} + \text{Hepatic clearance} \qquad 7$$

Thus, total clearance is the sum of the clearances by each of the eliminating organs.

Because of the additivity of clearance, the relative contribution of any organ to drug elimination is readily calculated. For example, the fraction of drug excreted unchanged (designated fe, see Chap. 3), being the fraction of total elimination that occurs via renal excretion, is just renal clearance divided by total clearance.

One exception to the additivity of clearance is pulmonary clearance. This is due in part to the blood supply to the lungs being in series, rather than in parallel, with other organs of elimination and in part to the total cardiac output passing through the lungs before reaching the site of measurement, usually blood in a peripheral vein. The concentration measured is that leaving, rather than entering, the lungs. The use of this concentration to calculate clearance is inconsistent with its definition (see Eq. 3). Indeed, if the pulmonary extraction ratio is high, clearance values calculated in the usual manner may even exceed cardiac output, making interpretation problematic.

Clearances of drugs by the liver and the kidneys are now examined. Each organ has special anatomic and physiologic features that require its separate consideration.

HEPATIC CLEARANCE

Although drug metabolism can take place in many organs, the liver frequently has the greatest metabolic capacity and consequently has been the most thoroughly studied. The most direct quantitative measure of the liver's ability to eliminate a drug is hepatic clearance. Hepatic clearance includes biliary excretory clearance, which is subsequently discussed, and hepatic metabolic clearance.

As with other organs of elimination, the removal of drug by the liver may be considered from mass balance relationships. That is,

$$\text{Hepatic blood clearance} = \underset{\substack{\text{Hepatic} \\ \text{blood} \\ \text{flow}}}{Q_H} \cdot \underset{\substack{\text{Hepatic} \\ \text{extraction} \\ \text{ratio}}}{E_H} \qquad 8$$

Here Q_H is the sum of hepatic portal and hepatic arterial blood flows, for which average values are 1050 and 300 mL/min, respectively.

Perfusion, Protein Binding, and Enzyme Activity

The following principles, relating changes in clearance and extraction ratio to alterations in perfusion, plasma protein binding, or inherent elimination characteristics, apply in general to all organs of elimination. These principles are exemplified here with hepatic extraction.

Perfusion. At least five processes, as shown in Fig. 11–2, may affect the ability of the liver to extract drug from blood. However, when the hepatic extraction ratio approaches 1.0, the drug must have had sufficient time while in the liver to partition out of the blood cell, dissociate from the plasma protein, pass through the hepatic membranes, and be either metabolized by an enzyme or transported into the bile, or both. Also blood clearance approaches its maximum value, hepatic blood flow. Under this condition, elimination is rate-limited by perfusion and not by the speed of any of the processes depicted in Fig. 11–2. Changes in blood flow produce corresponding changes in clearance and rate of elimination, but the extraction ratio is virtually unaffected. In contrast, elimination of a drug with a low extraction ratio (approaching zero) must be rate-limited somewhere else in the overall scheme (Fig. 11–2).

When the extraction ratio of a drug is low, the venous drug concentration is virtually identical with the arterial concentration, by definition. Therefore, changes in blood flow should produce no change in the drug concentration within the organ, in rate of elimination

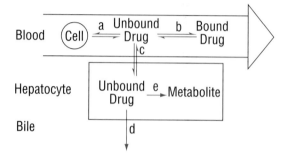

Fig. 11–2. Drug in blood is bound to blood cells (process *a*) and to plasma proteins (process *b*); however, it is the unbound drug that diffuses (process *c*) into the hepatocyte. Within the hepatocyte, the unbound drug is subject to secretion into bile (process *d*) or to enzymatic biotransformation (process *e*). The metabolite leaves the hepatocyte via blood or bile or it is subjected to further transformation.

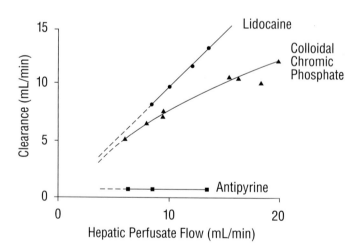

Fig. 11–3. Composite data showing that the sensitivity of the clearance of a compound to changes in blood flow varies. When extraction ratio is low, as occurs with antipyrine (■), clearance is low and independent of blood flow. Clearance varies in direct proportion to flow rate for lidocaine (●), a drug with an extraction ratio close to 1.0. Between these extremes is colloidal chromic phosphate (▲), the clearance of which moves away from a perfusion-rate limitation at higher flows. All data, obtained in an isolated, perfused rat liver, have been normalized to a 10-g liver. The lines are drawn by eye. (Data abstracted from: Antipyrine and lidocaine—Pang, K.S. and Rowland, M.: Hepatic clearance of drugs I. J. Pharmacokin. Biopharm., 5:655–680, 1977; Colloidal chromic phosphate—Brauer, R.W., Leong, G.F., McElroy Jr., R.F., and Holloway, R.J.: Circulatory pathways in the rat liver as revealed by ^{32}P chromic phosphate colloid uptake in the isolated, perfused liver preparation. Am. J. Physiol., 184:593–598, 1956.)

or by definition in clearance. From Eq. 8, however, it is seen that the hepatic extraction ratio varies inversely with blood flow when clearance is constant. These expectations regarding perfusion for drugs of high and low extraction ratios are illustrated in Fig. 11–3. Representative drugs and metabolites with low (less than 0.3), intermediate (0.3 to 0.7), and high (greater than 0.7) extraction ratios in the liver are listed in Table 11–2.

A word of caution is needed here. Although mass-balance principles state that changes in blood flow are not expected to alter the clearance of drugs of low extraction ratio, there are physiologic mechanisms that may secondarily produce such an effect. Examples are the presence of homeostatic control mechanisms and a perfusion-limited supply of cofactors such as oxygen or sulfate.

Binding Within Blood. For a drug with a high extraction ratio, the liver is clearly capable of removing all the drug presented to it in spite of binding to blood cells and to plasma proteins. Rate of elimination depends on total concentration in blood. Certainly, a decrease in binding aids in removing a drug; but in this case, it is essentially all removed anyway. Therefore, neither extraction ratio nor clearance is materially affected by changes in binding.

For a drug with a low extraction ratio, clearance depends on plasma protein binding because only unbound drug penetrates membranes and is available for elimination and because the drop in drug concentration across the liver is small. The unbound concentration in plasma leaving the liver is almost identical to that in the circulating plasma, Cu. Then the rate of drug elimination in the liver is directly related to the concentration of drug unbound in the circulating plasma. Accordingly,

$$\text{Rate of elimination} = \underset{\substack{\text{Clearance}\\\text{based on}\\\text{unbound}\\\text{concentration}}}{CLu} \cdot \underset{\substack{\text{Unbound}\\\text{concentration.}}}{Cu} \qquad 9$$

Table 11–2. Hepatic and Renal Extraction Ratios of Representative Drugs and Metabolites

	Extraction Ratio		
	Low (<0.3)	Intermediate (0.3–0.7)	High (>0.7)
Hepatic[a] extraction	Carbamazepine Diazepam Indomethacin Naproxen Nitrazepam Phenobarbital Phenytoin Procainamide Salicylic Acid Theophylline Valproic Acid Warfarin	Aspirin Quinidine Codeine Nifedipine Nortriptyline	Alprenolol Cocaine Desipramine Lidocaine Meperidine Morphine Nicotine Nitroglycerin Pentazocine Propoxyphene Propranolol Verapamil
Renal[a] extraction	Amoxicillin Atenolol Cefazolin Ciprofloxacin Digoxin Furosemide Gentamicin Lithium Tetracycline	Amiloride Cimetidine Cephalothin Ranitidine	(Many) Glucuronides Hippurates (Some) Penicillins (Many) Sulfates

[a]At least 30% of the drug is eliminated by this route.

Expressing the rate of hepatic elimination relative to the plasma concentration, it is apparent that the hepatic plasma clearance varies proportionally with changes in the fraction unbound.

$$\text{Hepatic clearance} = \underset{\substack{\text{Clearance}\\\text{based on}\\\text{unbound}\\\text{concentration}}}{Cl_u} \cdot \underset{\substack{\text{Fraction}\\\text{in plasma}\\\text{unbound}}}{f_u} \qquad\qquad 10$$

For example, if f_u varies twofold, so does hepatic clearance; the unbound clearance remains unchanged.

The data in Fig. 11–4 obtained in the isolated, perfused rat liver, illustrate the points made above. In this preparation, protein binding can be readily altered by changing the concentration of the binding protein, and perfusion can be held constant. Consider first tolbutamide, a drug of low extraction even in the absence of binding ($f_u = 1.0$). As expected, the extraction ratio (and clearance) of tolbutamide is directly proportional to f_u.

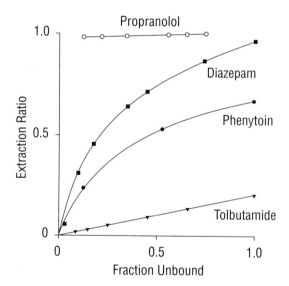

Fig. 11–4. Composite mean data, obtained in an isolated, perfused rat liver, showing that the sensitivity of hepatic extraction ratio to changes in fraction of drug unbound varies. Extraction ratio is proportional to fraction unbound only when the extraction ratio is low, as observed over the entire range of binding for tolbutamide (▼) but only over a limited range for diazepam (■) and phenytoin (●). When the extraction ratio is high, as occurs with phenytoin and diazepam at low binding and with propranolol (○) at all degrees of binding studied, extraction ratio is relatively insensitive to changes in fraction unbound. Notice that in this preparation, in which the fraction unbound is varied over a wide range by modifying the concentration of albumin, the binding protein, a drug such as diazepam can be changed from one of high to one of low extraction. The solid lines are drawn by eye. (Data abstracted from: Phenytoin—Shand, D.G., Cotham, R.H., and Wilkinson, G.R.: Perfusion-limited effects of plasma drug binding on hepatic extraction. Life Sci., *19*:125–130, 1976; Diazepam—Rowland, M., Leitch, D., Fleming, G., and Smith, B.: Protein binding and hepatic clearance: Discrimination between models of hepatic clearance with diazepam, a drug of high intrinsic clearance, in the isolated, perfused rat liver preparation. J. Pharmacokinet. Biopharm., *12*:129–147, 1984; Tolbutamide—Schary, W.L. and Rowland, M.: Protein binding and hepatic clearance: Studies with tolbutamide, a drug of low intrinsic clearance, in the isolated, perfused rat liver preparation. J. Pharmacokin. Biopharm., *11*:225–244, 1983; Propranolol—Jones, D.B., Ching, M.S., Smallwood, R.A., and Morgan, D.J.: A carrier-protein receptor is not a prerequisite for avid hepatic elimination of highly bound compounds: A study of propranolol elimination by the isolated, perfused rat liver. Hepatology, 5:590–593, 1985.)

The observations with diazepam are illuminating. The extraction ratio (and clearance) changes from a value close to 1.0 (in the absence of binding, $fu = 1.0$) to one close to zero on decreasing the fraction unbound. Clearly, protein binding can limit extraction if binding is high enough. However, this situation is nonphysiologic in that the fraction unbound is varied between 1.0 and 0.05, a 20-fold change. In practice, a threefold change in fu would be considered particularly large for a drug bound to albumin. Under these more restricted conditions, the expected relationship between clearance and fu holds. Thus, for diazepam, in the region where extraction ratio is low (low fu), clearance is directly proportional to fu. At the other extreme, in the region where the extraction ratio is high, clearance varies little with a moderate change in fu.

Enzyme Activity. As stated above, when clearance is perfusion rate-limited, there is so much hepatocellular activity that modest changes in this activity cause little or no change in clearance. Almost all the drug is extracted anyway. Conversely, if enzyme activity is the rate-limiting step, then clearance is low and directly proportional to activity, e.g., when changed by induction or inhibition by another drug.

Most of our present knowledge of enzyme kinetics is derived from studies *in vitro* in which substrate, enzyme, and cofactor concentrations are controlled. Correlation of such studies with those performed *in vivo* has been difficult. Many factors are involved *in vivo* that cannot be isolated. Nevertheless, the basic principles of enzyme kinetics have application in pharmacokinetics.

The upper curve in Fig. 11–5 is characteristic of metabolism by a given enzyme both *in vitro* and *in vivo*. The behavior displayed, typical of Michaelis-Menten kinetics if the approach toward the maximum rate, Vm, follows the relationship:

$$\text{Rate of metabolism} = \frac{Vm \cdot Cu}{Km + Cu} \qquad\qquad 11$$

in which Km is a constant, the Michaelis-Menten constant. In enzyme kinetics the value of Vm is directly proportional to the total concentration of enzyme, and Km is an inverse function of the affinity between drug and enzyme. Note in Eq. 11 that a value of Cu equal to Km gives a rate that is one-half the maximum; this is a convenient way of defining the constant. An estimate of the true Km requires measurement of the unbound drug concentration at the metabolizing enzyme site. Lacking this capability *in vivo*, the unbound plasma concentration is conventionally used. At unbound plasma concentrations well below Km, which apply to most drugs used therapeutically, rate and concentration vary in direct proportion. At concentrations above Km, the rate approaches the value of Vm. Since unbound metabolic clearance is defined as the rate of metabolism relative to the unbound plasma concentration,

$$\text{Unbound metabolic clearance} = \frac{Vm}{Km + Cu} \qquad\qquad 12$$

Its value decreases at drug concentrations approaching and exceeding the value of Km. This is shown in the lower part of Fig. 11–5. Note that the highest clearance is the ratio Vm/Km, a value often called the *intrinsic metabolic clearance*. The value may be so high that elimination *in vivo* is perfusion rate-limited. Because of the complexities introduced, the administration of drugs showing saturable metabolism at therapeutic concentrations is difficult. Throughout the rest of the book, except Chap. 22 on Dose and Time Dependencies, drug metabolism is assumed not to show saturability.

A Memory Aid. The general principles just discussed can be difficult to remember. Models of hepatic elimination have been developed to quantify changes in clearance when perfusion, plasma protein binding, and enzyme activity are altered. One of these models, the *well-stirred model*, in which instantaneous and complete mixing occurs within the liver, is particularly attractive because it can readily be used to summarize these principles. Even though it may not be quantitative, the model allows one to predict those situations in which either clearance or extraction ratio is affected and the expected direction of change.

The well-stirred model states that

$$CL_{b,H} = \frac{Q_H \cdot fu_b \cdot CL_{int}}{Q_H + fu_b \cdot CL_{int}} \qquad 13$$

where Q_H is the hepatic blood flow; CL_{int} is the intrinsic clearance that relates rate of metabolism to unbound concentration at the enzyme site, and fu_b is the fraction unbound in plasma. The hepatic extraction ratio, $CL_{b,H}/Q_H$, is then

$$E_H = \frac{fu_b \cdot CL_{int}}{Q_H + fu_b \cdot CL_{int}} \qquad 14$$

These two equations have the desired properties at the limits. Thus, when E_H approaches 1.0 (the perfusion rate-limited condition), $fu_b \cdot CL_{int}$ is much greater than Q_H,

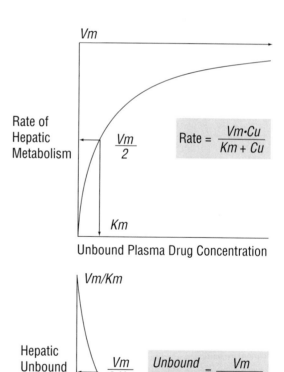

Fig. 11–5. When hepatic metabolism follows Michaelis-Menten kinetics, the rate of metabolism increases (top graph) toward a maximum value, *Vm*, as the plasma drug concentration is increased. The concentration at which the rate is one-half the maximum is the *Km* value. The unbound metabolic clearance (bottom graph) falls with increasing drug concentration. The concentration at which the clearance is one-half the maximum is also the *Km* value. The equations for the relationships are shown.

and clearance approaches Q_H (Eq. 13). Changes in CL_{int} and fu here are not expected to influence CL_H and E_H much. Conversely, when E_H is small, Q_H must be much greater than $fu_b \cdot CL_{int}$. Now E_H and $CL_{b,H}$ are approximated by $fu_b \cdot CL_{int}/Q_H$ and $fu_b \cdot CL_{int}$, respectively; the value of the extraction ratio depends on all three factors, whereas clearance depends only on fu_b and CL_{int}.

Equation 14 offers an explanation for why the extraction ratios of most drugs appear to be either low ($E_H < 0.3$) or high ($E_H > 0.7$). Suppose, e.g., that the hepatocellular activity (intrinsic clearance) varied evenly from 0.01 to 100 L/min among a large group of compounds, i.e., over a 10,000-fold range, and that none is bound in plasma ($fu_b = 1.0$). Then substitution of these values into Eq. 14 shows that only those drugs with an intrinsic clearance in the narrow range of $0.43 \cdot Q_H$ to $2.3 \cdot Q_H$ have an intermediate extraction ratio, i.e. values between 0.3 and 0.7.

Strictly, as whole blood delivers drug to the liver, the fraction unbound in Eqs. 13 and 14 should refer to that in blood, not plasma. For didactic purposes, however, here and throughout remainder of the book where Eqs. 13 and 14 are applied, the two terms are equivalent. A major discrepancy occurs when the blood-to-plasma concentration ratio is much greater than 1.

First-Pass Considerations

To reach the general circulation, a drug given orally must pass through the liver via the portal system. The fraction escaping elimination by the liver, F_H, is the upper limit of the oral bioavailability. It may be calculated from the hepatic extraction ratio, E_H, since

$$\text{Maximum oral bioavailability} = 1 - \text{Hepatic extraction ratio} \qquad 15$$

Hepatic extraction ratio can be estimated if the hepatic (blood) clearance and hepatic blood flow are known or can be approximated.

For illustrative purposes, consider the following data obtained after an intravenous (i.v.) dose (500 mg) of a drug: Cumulative amount excreted unchanged (Ae_∞) = 152 mg, AUC = 385 mg-min/L, and the blood-to-plasma concentration ratio (C_b/C) = 1.2. Extrarenal elimination is assumed to occur only in the liver. The clearance (Dose/AUC) is then 1.3 L/min, and the blood clearance [$CL/(C_b/C)$] is 1.08 L/min. The fraction excreted unchanged (Ae_∞/Dose) is 0.304. Accordingly, the renal blood clearance ($fe \cdot CL_b$) is 0.32 L/min, and by difference, the hepatic blood clearance [$(1 - fe)CL_b$] is 0.76 L/min. Dividing by hepatic blood flow to obtain the hepatic extraction ratio, the maximum oral bioavailability is

$$F \simeq F_H = 1 - (1 - fe)\, CL_b/Q_H \qquad 16$$

which, in this example, is 0.56 for a hepatic blood flow of 1.35 L/min. Being physiologically determined, no amount of pharmaceutical manipulation can improve on this value for an oral dosage formulation. Any drug with a high hepatic extraction ratio (see Table 11–2) has a low oral bioavailability. There may be other factors that limit drug reaching the portal vein and so further decrease bioavailability, as described in Chap. 9, Absorption.

First-Pass Predictions

The effects of changing blood flow, intrinsic clearance, or protein binding on first-pass extraction can be predicted using the *well-stirred* model by substituting Eq. 14 into the relationship $F_H = 1 - E_H$. That is,

$$F_H = \frac{Q_H}{Q_H + fu_b \cdot CL_{int}} \qquad\qquad 17$$

It should be re-emphasized that the prediction here, for changes in CL_H, E_H, and F_H with changes in Q_H, CL_{int}, or fu_b, are based on modest alterations. A low extraction ratio drug can become a high extraction ratio drug if CL_{int} or fu_b is increased or if Q_H is decreased by a sufficiently large factor (Fig. 11–4). The principles here refer to the relative tendencies that modest changes in these factors are likely to produce.

The effect on first-pass extraction can also be visualized by regarding perfusion and protein binding to be in competition with enzymatic activity; perfusion and protein binding help to move drug through the organ, making drug available to the general circulation, whereas enzyme activity removes drug from the perfusing blood.

Consider first the case of a drug with an E_H near zero, that is, Q_H much greater than $fu_b \cdot CL_{int}$. Then F_H is independent of changes in Q_H, CL_{int} or fu_b. This is not surprising as the extraction is so small that everything presented gets past the liver anyway. Consider next the condition in which $fu_b \cdot CL_{int}$ is much greater than Q_H, so that E_H approaches 1.0. In this case, $F_H = Q_H/(fu_b \cdot CL_{int})$, that is, bioavailability is low and dependent on all three factors. An increase in blood flow increases bioavailability by decreasing the time drug spends in the liver, where elimination occurs. An increase in either enzymatic activity or in fu_b (which raises the unbound concentration for a given incoming total concentration) decreases bioavailability by increasing the rate of elimination for a given rate of presentation to the liver.

Biliary Excretion and Enterohepatic Cycling

Small molecular weight drugs are found in bile; whereas protein drugs tend to be excluded. Drug in bile enters the intestine after storage in the gallbladder. In the intestine it may be reabsorbed to complete an enterohepatic cycle. Drug may also be metabolized in the liver, e.g., to a glucuronide. The glucuronide is then secreted into the intestine, where the β-glucuronidase enzymes of the resident flora may hydrolyze it back to the drug, which is then reabsorbed. Enterohepatic cycling of drugs directly and indirectly through a metabolite is represented schematically in Fig. 11–6. Recall from Chap. 2 that enterohepatic cycling is a component of distribution not elimination.

Any drug in bile not reabsorbed, either directly or indirectly via a metabolite, is excreted from the body via the feces. The efficiency of biliary excretion can be expressed by biliary clearance.

$$\text{Biliary clearance} = \frac{(\text{Bile flow}) \cdot (\text{Concentration in bile})}{(\text{Concentration in plasma})} \qquad\qquad 18$$

Bile flow is a relatively steady 0.5 to 0.8 mL/min. Thus, for a drug with a concentration in the bile equal to or less than that in plasma, the biliary clearance is small. A drug that concentrates in the bile, however, may have a relatively high biliary clearance. Indeed, the bile-to-plasma concentration ratio can approach 1000. Therefore, biliary clearances of 500 mL/min or higher can be achieved. Eventually, of course, biliary clearance is limited by hepatic perfusion.

Bile is not a product of filtration, but rather of secretion of bile acids and other solutes. The pH of bile averages about 7.4. The biliary transport of drugs, however, is similar to active secretion in the kidneys (p. 172) in that it may be competitively inhibited.

A few generalizations can be made regarding the characteristics of a drug needed to ensure high biliary clearance. First, the drug must be actively secreted; separate secretory mechanisms exist for acids, bases, and un-ionized compounds. Second, it must be polar, and, last, its molecular weight must exceed 250 g/mole. The latter two requirements may be a consequence of the apparent porous as well as lipophilic nature of bile cannaliculae. Both nonpolar and small molecules may be reabsorbed. These arguments do not aid in predicting the nature and specificity of the secretory mechanisms, but they do aid in predicting the likelihood of a high biliary clearance. For example, glucuronide conjugates of drugs are polar, ionized, pKa about 3, and have molecular weights exceeding 300 g/mole. They are often highly cleared into bile.

RENAL CLEARANCE

When the rate of urinary excretion is directly proportional to the plasma drug concentration,

$$\text{Rate of excretion} = CL_R \cdot C \qquad\qquad 19$$

renal clearance is constant. This constancy forms the basis for the use of urine data to determine the time course of a drug in the body (Chap. 3). Interpretation of urine data with respect to plasma concentration is clearly complicated for drugs whose renal clearance varies. Factors that influence renal clearance include plasma drug concentration (see Chap. 22, Dose and Time Dependencies), plasma protein binding, urine flow, and urine pH. How these factors influence renal clearance is explained by the anatomy and physiology of the kidneys.

The Nephron: Anatomy and Function

The basic anatomic unit of renal function is the nephron (Fig. 11–7). Basic components are the glomerulus, proximal tubule, loop of Henle, distal tubule, and collecting tubule. The glomerulus receives blood first and filters about 120 mL of plasma water each minute. The filtrate passes down the tubule. Most of the water is reabsorbed; only 1 to 2 mL/min

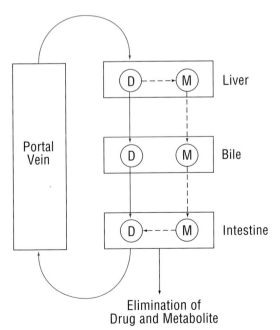

Fig. 11–6. When a drug (D) is absorbed from intestine, excreted in bile, and reabsorbed from intestine, it has undergone enterohepatic cycling (colored arrows), a component of distribution. Similarly, when a drug is converted to a metabolite (M) that is secreted in bile, converted back to drug in the intestine, and drug is reabsorbed (dashed arrows), the drug has also undergone enterohepatic cycling, in this case indirectly through a metabolite.

leave the kidneys as urine. On leaving the glomerulus, the same blood perfuses both proximal and distal portions of the tubule through a series of interconnecting channels.

Appearance of drug in the urine is the net result of filtration, secretion, and reabsorption. The first two processes add drug to the proximal part of the lumen of the nephron; the last process involves the movement of drug from the lumen back into the bloodstream. The excretion rate is, therefore,

$$\text{Rate of Excretion} = (1 - F_R) \left[\text{Rate of Filtration} + \text{Rate of Secretion} \right] \qquad 20$$

where F_R is the fraction reabsorbed from the lumen. A schematic representation of these processes and their approximate location in the nephron are given in Fig. 11–8. Let us look at each process in turn.

Glomerular Filtration

Approximately 20 to 25% of cardiac output, or 1.1 L of blood per minute goes to the kidneys. Of this volume, about 10% is filtered at the glomerulus. Small molecules (molecular weight less than 2000 g/mole) pass through the sieve with ease, and even for small proteins such as insulin and myoglobulin, the ultrafiltrate concentration is close to that in

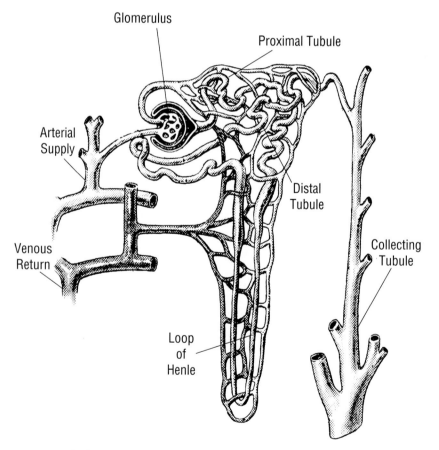

Fig. 11–7. The functional nephron, an anatomical view. (Modified from Smith, H.W.: The Kidney: Structure and Function in Health and Disease. New York, Oxford University Press, 1951.)

plasma (see Table 11–6). Only when the molecular weight of the protein exceeds 20,000 does filtration fall off sharply. Indeed, virtually no albumin (molecular weight 69,000 g/mole) is normally found in the ultrafiltrate. Accordingly, as the binding of most drugs in plasma is to albumin or other proteins of similar or higher molecular weight, as a general rule, only unbound drug in plasma water (concentration Cu) is filtered (see Table 10–4).

The rate at which plasma water is filtered, 120 mL/min in a 70-kg 20-year-old man, is conventionally called the glomerular filtration rate, GFR. It follows that

$$\text{Rate of filtration} = GFR \cdot Cu \qquad 21$$

Recall that fu is the ratio of the unbound to total plasma drug concentration; therefore,

$$\text{Rate of filtration} = fu \cdot GFR \cdot C \qquad 22$$

If a drug is only filtered and all filtered drug is excreted into the urine, then the rate of excretion is the rate of filtration. Since renal clearance, CL_R, by definition is

$$CL_R = \frac{\text{Rate of excretion}}{\text{Plasma concentration}} \qquad 23$$

it follows that for such a drug its renal clearance (by filtration) is $fu \cdot GFR$. The extraction ratio of such a drug is low. For example, even if the drug is totally unbound in blood ($Cu = C_b$), the extraction ratio is still only 0.11. This follows because

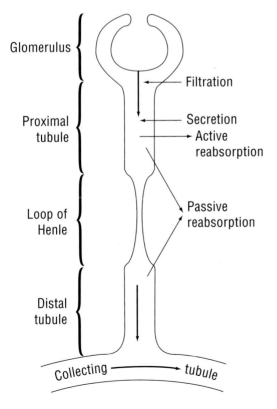

Fig. 11–8. Drug is added to the lumen of the nephron by filtration and secretion. Filtration occurs in the glomerulus; secretion is primarily restricted to the proximal tubule. Reabsorption occurs all along the nephron. Active reabsorption, when present, usually occurs in the proximal tubule.

$$\text{Extraction ratio} = \frac{\text{Rate of extraction}}{\text{Rate of presentation}} = \frac{GFR \cdot Cu}{\text{Renal blood flow} \cdot C_b} = \frac{120 \text{ mL/min}}{1100 \text{ mL/min}} = 0.11$$

Inulin, an exogenous polysaccharide, is neither bound to plasma proteins nor secreted, and all the filtered load of each substance is excreted into the urine. Accordingly, the renal clearance is a measure of *GFR*. Under normal conditions, *GFR* is relatively stable and insensitive to changes in renal blood flow.

Active Secretion

Filtration always occurs, but as shown above, extraction of a drug by this mechanism alone is low, especially if drug is highly bound within blood. Secretion facilitates extraction.

Mechanisms exist for secreting acids (anions) and bases (cations), including quaternary ammonium compounds, from the plasma into the tubular lumen. The secretory processes are located predominantly in the proximal tubule. Although active, these transport systems appear to lack a high degree of specificity, as demonstrated by the wide variety of substances transported by them. As expected, however, substances transported by the same system compete with each other.

Secretion is inferred when rate of excretion $(CL_R \cdot C)$ exceeds the rate of filtration $(fu \cdot GFR \cdot C)$. Stated differently, secretion is apparent when $CL_R > fu \cdot GFR$. Some reabsorption may still occur, but it must be less than secretion.

Protein Binding and Perfusion

The influence of protein binding on secretion depends on the efficiency of the secretion process and on the contact time at the secretory sites. These conclusions are similar to those drawn for hepatic elimination.

Blood resides at the proximal secretory sites for approximately 30 sec. When a drug is secreted, but poorly, this contact time is insufficient to transport much drug into the lumen, and accordingly, the drop in drug concentration across the region is small. Then, the unbound concentration at the secretion site is almost identical to the unbound concentration in plasma, *Cu*. Since the rate of secretion depends on the unbound drug concentration, or $fu \cdot C$, it follows that clearance due to secretion, obtained by dividing rate of secretion by *C*, is directly proportional to *fu*. As variation in renal blood flow does not cause any change in the plasma drug concentration, no change in renal clearance with perfusion is expected under these circumstances. Furthermore, the sum of clearances associated with filtration $(fu \cdot GFR)$ and secretion, must also be directly proportional to *fu*. Obviously, the extraction ratio of such a drug is low. Figure 11–9 supports these predictions for furosemide in an isolated rat kidney preparation. Furosemide is secreted and is bound to albumin. In this preparation the fraction unbound could be varied over a wide range.

Some drugs are such excellent substrates for the secretory system that they are virtually completely removed from blood within the time they are in contact with the active transport site, even when they are bound to plasma proteins or located in blood cells. In such cases, evidently dissociation of the drug–protein complex and movement of drug out of the blood cells is sufficiently rapid so as to not limit the secretory process. Para-aminohippuric acid (PAH) is handled in this manner and is not reabsorbed. Accordingly, the extraction ratio of PAH is close to 1.0, and hence its renal blood clearance is a measure of renal blood flow. Obviously, under these circumstances, clearance is perfusion rate-limited. Examples of drugs with a variety of renal extraction ratios are listed in Table 11–2.

Reabsorption

Reabsorption is the third factor controlling the renal handling of drugs. Reabsorption must occur if the renal clearance is less than the calculated clearance by filtration

$(CL_R < fu \cdot GFR)$. Some secretion may still occur, but it must be less than reabsorption. Reabsorption varies from being almost absent to being virtually complete. Active reabsorption occurs for many endogenous compounds, including vitamins, electrolytes, glucose, and amino acids. However, for the vast majority of exogenous compounds, reabsorption occurs by a passive process. The degree of reabsorption depends on the properties of the drug, e.g., its polarity, state of ionization, and molecular weight. As with many membranes throughout the body, the lipoidal membranes of the cells that form the tubule act as a barrier to water-soluble and ionized substances. Thus, lipophilic molecules tend to be extensively reabsorbed, polar molecules do not. Reabsorption also depends on physiologic variables such as urine flow and urine pH.

Reabsorption occurs all along the nephron, associated with the reabsorption of water filtered at the glomerulus. The majority, 80 to 90%, of the filtered water is reabsorbed in the proximal tubule. Most of the remainder is reabsorbed in the distal tubule and collecting tubules, where urine flow is controlled. If no water is reabsorbed in the distal tubule, urine flow is about 15 to 20 mL/min. Normally, however, water is reabsorbed to the extent that urine flow is 1 to 2 mL/min or lower.

Consequently, with water reabsorption, drugs concentrate in the filtrate. In fact, if a drug were neither reabsorbed (generally polar) nor secreted, with approximately 99% water reabsorption the concentration in the urine would be about 100 times as great as that unbound in plasma. Thus, reabsorption of water favors the reabsorption of a drug that diffuses across tubular membranes.

Urine Flow and Protein Binding. Urine flow can only have a substantial effect on renal clearance if a drug is mostly reabsorbed. Certainly, the effect is most dramatic when reabsorption approaches equilibrium.

As only unbound drug diffuses through membranes, equilibrium is reached when the concentration in urine and that unbound in plasma, Cu, are equal. Consequently, since

$$CL_R = \frac{\text{Urine flow} \cdot \text{Urine concentration}}{\text{Plasma concentration}} \qquad 24$$

and since $Cu = fu \cdot C$, it follows that

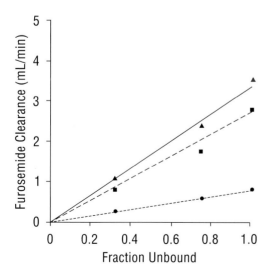

Fig. 11–9. Contribution of glomerular filtration (●) and tubular secretion (■) to the total renal clearance (▲) of furosemide at different values of fraction unbound. (Hall, S.: Doctoral dissertation, University of Massachusetts.)

$$\text{Renal clearance} = fu \cdot \text{Urine flow} \qquad 25$$

This last relationship is a simple test of how close reabsorption is to equilibrium. A drug may have a renal clearance below this value if it is actively reabsorbed. Moreover, if drug is highly bound to plasma proteins, renal clearance (and extraction ratio) would be extremely small since urine flow is normally only 1 to 2 mL/min. Note also that renal clearance is directly proportional to fu, when urine flow is constant.

Ethyl alcohol is an example of a compound that is not significantly bound to plasma proteins and is reabsorbed to the extent that its concentration in urine is virtually the same as that in the plasma regardless of urine flow. Consequently, it follows from Eqs. 24 and 25 that renal clearance of alcohol is approximately equal to urine flow and, therefore, urine-flow dependent.

Urine pH. For weak acids and weak bases, urine pH is an additional factor affecting reabsorption. The extremes of urine pH are 4.5 and 7.5 under forced acidification and alkalinization, respectively. These extremes contrast with the narrow range of plasma pH, 7.3 to 7.5. On the average, urine pH is close to 6.3. Thus, a large pH gradient may exist between plasma and urine.

Urine pH is altered by diet, drugs, and the clinical state of a patient. It also varies during the day. Respiratory and metabolic acidosis produces acidification, and respiratory and metabolic alkalosis produces alkalinization. When metabolic acidosis is of renal origin, for example, renal tubular acidosis, the urine is alkaline. Drugs such as the carbonic anhydrase inhibitor, acetazolamide, produce an alkaline urine.

Equilibrium Considerations. Renal clearances of several weak acids and bases, listed in Table 11–3, were calculated using Eq. 24. The urine-to-plasma concentration ratio was calculated using the Henderson-Hasselbalch equation (Chap. 8), given that these compounds do not bind to plasma proteins, that equilibrium is achieved between un-ionized drug in urine and plasma, and that the ionized form is not diffusible. It appears that the renal clearance of some acids, pKa less than 6.0, can be much less than urine flow (1 mL/min), whereas that of any base cannot, because urine pH is never much higher than plasma pH.

An interesting observation may be made about weak bases. At low urine pH, renal clearance, by calculation, approaches renal blood flow, which usually suggests active secretion. It is unlikely, however, that such a high clearance value can be obtained by passive diffusion—for three reasons. First, the fraction of renal blood flow that reaches the end of the distal tubule and collecting tubule, where the major change in pH occurs, is small. Second, the calculation of renal clearance in Table 11–3 is based on the ratio of urine concentration to plasma concentration leaving, rather than entering, the kidneys. The ve-

Table 11–3. Calculated Renal Clearances (mL/min) of Selected Nonpolar Weak Acids and Weak Bases at Various Values of Urine pH Under Equilibrium Conditions[a]

DRUG	NATURE	pKa	URINE pH		
			4.4	6.4	7.9
A	Acid	2.4	0.001	0.1	3
B		6.4	0.1	0.2	3
C		10.4	1.0	1.0	1.0
D	Base	2.4	1.0	1.0	1.0
E		6.4	90	2	0.9
F		10.4	1000	10	0.3
G		12.4	1000	10	0.3

[a]Conditions: no binding of drug to plasma proteins; $fu = 1.0$; urine flow of 1 mL/min; plasma pH, 7.4.

nous concentration here is less than that entering the kidneys, particularly when the extraction ratio of the drug is high—a perfusion rate-limited condition. Third, the high values of calculated clearance apply to those bases, which at blood pH values tend to be almost completely ionized; thus the rate of movement through the membranes, which depends on the concentration of un-ionized drug, is reduced. A similar argument applies to weak acids. Accordingly, a renal clearance value greater than $fu \cdot GFR$ for either on acid or a base at normal urine pH probably suggests active secretion.

A Rate Process in Reality. The foregoing discussion was based primarily on equilibrium concepts, but passive reabsorption may not approach equilibrium. The primary consideration is how rapidly equilibrium is approached. In reality, then, reabsorption should be considered from a kinetic rather than from an equilibrium point of view, as was true for absorption of drugs from the gastrointestinal tract (Chap. 9).

The rate at which reabsorption occurs depends on the ability of the un-ionized drug to diffuse across membranes, its polarity, and the fraction un-ionized in the lumen. The percentages un-ionized for the same drugs listed in Table 11–3 are given in Table 11–4. The calculation is based on the Henderson-Hasselbalch equation (Chap. 8).

Weak Bases. The effect of urine pH on the cumulative amount of unchanged methamphetamine (pKa 10) that is excreted in the urine is shown in Fig. 11–10. After 16 hrs about 16% of the dose is excreted unchanged when the urine pH is not controlled. On alkalinizing the urine, e.g., by ingesting sodium bicarbonate, only 1 to 2% of the dose is in

Table 11–4. Percent Un-ionized of Selected Weak Acids and Weak Bases at Various Values of Urine pH^a

DRUG	NATURE	pKa	URINE pH 4.4	URINE pH 6.4	URINE pH 7.9
A	Acid	2.4	1.0	0.01	0.0003
B		6.4	99	50	3
C		10.4	100	100	99.7
D	Base	2.4	99	100	100
E		6.4	1.0	50	97
F		10.4	0.0001	0.01	0.3
G		12.4	10^{-6}	0.0001	0.003

^{a}Same drugs as in Table 11–3.

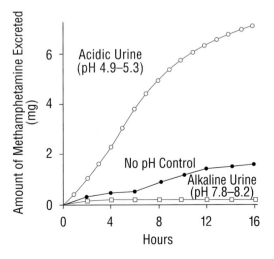

Fig. 11–10. The cumulative urinary excretion of methamphetamine (11 mg orally) in man varies with the urine pH. (Adapted from Beckett, A.H., and Rowland, M.: Urinary excretion kinetics of methylamphetamine in man. Nature, *206*:1260–1261, 1965.)

the urine, while acidification by ingesting ammonium chloride results in 70 to 80% recovery in the urine. Clearly, for this drug, urine pH is important in determining the contribution of the renal route to total elimination. Under conditions of no pH control, urine pH varies throughout the day, and the excretion of methamphetamine fluctuates accordingly. The explanation for these observations is contained in Tables 11–2 and 11–3. At low urine pH, both equilibrium and kinetic considerations favor high renal clearance of a basic drug of *pKa* 10. In particular, the percent un-ionized, and hence the un-ionized concentration in the renal tubule, is so small that there is little opportunity for reabsorption within the time that the drug resides in the nephron. At high urine pH with a greater percent of drug un-ionized in the tubule, both equilibrium and rate considerations favor reabsorption. Drugs that show these substantial changes in renal clearance are said to be pH sensitive.

The effect of urine pH on the reabsorption of basic drugs, in general, can be summarized as follows:

1. A basic drug that is polar in its un-ionized form is not reabsorbed, regardless of its degree of ionization in the urine, unless actively transported. The aminoglycoside gentamicin is an example; its renal clearance is independent of urine pH.

2. A very weakly basic nonpolar drug, whose *pKa* is around 6.0 or below, such as propoxyphene, is extensively reabsorbed at all values of urine pH because the percent of drug in the diffusible un-ionized form is sufficient to have no limiting effect on its rate of reabsorption, regardless of urine pH. Furthermore, equilibrium favors reabsorption. The renal clearance of such a drug may vary with urine pH but its value is low, especially if the drug is highly bound to plasma proteins.

3. For a strong base with a *pKa* value approaching 12 or greater, such as guanethidine, little or no reabsorption is expected throughout the range of urine pH because ionization is so extensive that it limits the rate of reabsorption. Accordingly, renal clearance is independent of urine pH and generally high.

4. For a basic nonpolar drug with a *pKa value between 6.0 and 12*, the extent of reabsorption varies from negligible to almost complete (equilibration) with changes in urine pH. The renal clearance of such a drug (e.g., methamphetamine) varies markedly with urine pH.

Weak Acids. The principles developed for weak bases also apply to weak acids. However, for acids, an increase in pH causes more ionization, not less. Consequently, acids are reabsorbed less and have larger renal clearances at higher urine pH.

Again, the effect of *pKa* on reabsorption is seen by inspecting Tables 11–3 and 11–4. An acid with a *pKa* value of 2.0 or less, e.g., chromoglycic acid, is so completely ionized at all urine pH values that it is simply not reabsorbed; its renal clearance is generally high and insensitive to pH. At the other extreme, a very weak acid with a *pKa* value above 8.0, such as phenytoin, is mostly un-ionized throughout the range of urine pH; its renal clearance is always low and insensitive to pH. Only for a nonpolar acid whose *pKa lies between 3.0 and 7.5* is renal clearance expected to be pH sensitive. Note in Table 11–3 that for all nonpolar acids equilibrium favors reabsorption.

Data supporting the expected urine pH sensitivity in renal clearance of nonpolar weak acids with a pKa between 3 and 7.5 and nonpolar weak bases with a *pKa* between 6 and 12 are provided by salicylic acid, *pKa* 3 (Fig. 11–11), and the anthelmintic diethylcarbamazine, *pKa* 10 (Table 11–5), respectively.

Weak acids and bases that show pH-sensitive reabsorption also generally show flow-rate dependence. Again, however, the degree to which renal clearance is changed by urine flow depends on the extent of reabsorption. If 50% of that filtered and secreted is reabsorbed at normal urine flow, 50% is excreted. Increased urine flow decreases reabsorption toward zero, but renal clearance cannot be increased by more than a factor of 2. Figure 11–12

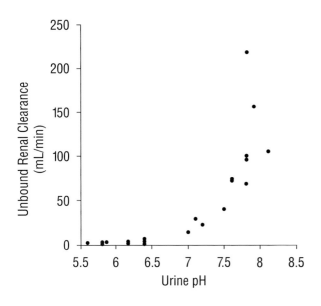

Fig. 11–11. The unbound renal clearance of salicylic acid increases dramatically with an increase in urine pH above 6.5. (Adapted from Smith P.K., Gleason, H.L., Stall, C.G., and Ogorzalek, S.: Studies on the pharmacology of salicylates. J. Pharmacol. Exp. Ther., 87:237–255, 1946.)

Table 11–5. Sensitivity of Diethylcarbamazine Renal Clearance to Change in Urine pH[a]

URINE pH	RENAL CLEARANCE (L/hr)
Not controlled (~6.3)[b]	8.6
Acidic, <5.5	38.0
Alkaline, >7.5	1.0

[a]From Edwards, G., Breckenridge, A.M., Adjepam-Yamoah, K.K., Orme, M.L.E., and Ward, S.A.: The effect of variations in urinary pH on the pharmacokinetics of diethylcarbamazine. Br. J. Clin. Pharmacol., 12:807–812, 1981.
[b]Typical pH of urine.

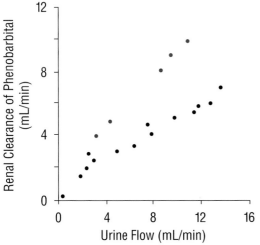

Fig. 11–12. Renal clearance of phenobarbital varies with urine flow in man. It is also a function of urine pH: without alkalinization (black circles), with alkalinization (colored circles). (Redrawn from Linton, A.L., Luke, R.G., and Briggs, M.D.: Methods of forced diuresis and its application in barbiturate poisoning. Lancet, 2:377–380, 1967.)

shows how the renal clearance of phenobarbital (*pKa* 7.2) varies with urine flow. As expected, the renal clearance of this drug is pH sensitive as well as urine flow-rate dependent.

Forced Diuresis and Urine pH Control. Increased urine flow by forced intake of fluids and, in some cases, the coadministration of mannitol or another diuretic, can increase the excretion of some drugs. More rapid elimination is, of course, desirable for the purpose of detoxifying a patient who is overdosed. Several criteria must be met for forced diuresis to be of value:

1. Renal excretion under conditions of forced diuresis must become the major route of drug elimination. Increasing the renal clearance of a drug 10-fold, for example, does little to hasten drug elimination from the body if renal clearance normally is only 1% of total clearance.

2. The compound must normally be extensively reabsorbed in the renal tubule.

3. If the reabsorption is pH sensitive, both forced diuresis and pH control may be of value. This applies if forced diuresis or pH control alone only partially prevents reabsorption.

The last point bears further discussion. Suppose that, on alkalinizing the urine, the reabsorption of a weak acid is decreased from 90 to 10% of that filtered and secreted. The addition of forced diuresis will be of little additional value; the excretion rate can only be increased by a further 10%. The converse applies to the use of pH control when forced diuresis almost completely prevents reabsorption.

Renal Handling of Protein Drugs

As shown in Table 11–6, many, especially low molecular weight, proteins are substantially filtered in the glomerulus, yet little of these are usually found in urine. This low renal clearance of proteins arises from their metabolism in the proximal tubule. Low molecular weight proteins are metabolized by enzymes located in the brush border of the lumen, whereas high molecular weight proteins of the size of albumin are transported into the proximal tubular cells by endocytosis and metabolized there by lysozomal enzymes. Generally, catabolism of proteins continues until the constituent amino acids are formed. The amino acids are then conserved by reabsorption into the vasculature. Although quantitative data are sparse, it appears that for some proteins, and probably also protein drugs, the kidney is a, if not *the*, major organ of elimination (see Disease, Chap. 16; Turnover Concepts, Chap. 23).

DEPENDENCE OF ELIMINATION KINETICS ON CLEARANCE AND DISTRIBUTION

The physiology of the body dictates that several pharmacokinetic parameters are related to and dependent on one another. Perhaps the most fundamental dependency in clinical

Table 11–6. Molecular Size and Glomerular Filtration of Proteins[a]

PROTEIN	MOLECULAR WEIGHT (g/mole)	ULTRAFILTRATE CONCENTRATION / PLASMA CONCENTRATION
Insulin	6,000	0.89
Myoglobulin	16,900	0.75
Growth hormone	20,000	0.72
Superoxide dismutase	32,000	0.33[b]
Bence Jones	44,000	0.08
Albumin	69,000	0.001[c]

[a]Mostly abstracted from Maack, T., Johnson, V., Kau, S.T., Figueiredo, J., and Sigulem, D.: Renal filtration, transport and metabolism of low-molecular-weight proteins: A review. Kidney Int., 16:251–290, 1979.
[b]Calculated from data in Tsao, C., Green, P., Odlind, B., and Brater, C: Pharmacokinetics of recombinant human superoxide dismutase in healthy volunteers. Clin. Pharmacol. Ther., 50:713–720, 1991.
[c]From Oaken, D.E., Cotes, S.C., and Mende, C.W.: Micropuncture study of tubular transport of albumin in rats with aminonucleoside nephrosis. Kidney Int., 1:3–11, 1972.

pharmacokinetics is that of half-life on (total) clearance and volume of distribution. This dependency is derived as follows.

Half-Life in Plasma

Recall from Chap. 3 that the elimination rate constant (i.e., fractional rate of drug elimination), k, is related to total clearance, CL, and volume of distribution, V, by the expression

$$k = \frac{\text{Rate of elimination}}{\text{Amount in body}} = \frac{CL}{V} \qquad 26$$

Because clearance is the volume of plasma cleared of drug per unit of time and V is the volume that drug appears to occupy at a concentration equal to that in plasma, it is apparent from Eq. 26 that fractional rate of drug elimination can be thought of as the fraction of the volume of distribution from which drug is removed per unit time.

Furthermore, recall that half-life, $t_{1/2}$, is related to k, or to V and CL through the expressions

$$t_{1/2} = \frac{0.693}{k} = \frac{0.693\ V}{CL} \qquad 27$$

To appreciate the dependence of half-life on clearance and volume of distribution, consider a drug that undergoes complete enterohepatic cycling yet distributes to bile and subsequently to the intestines in significant amounts as a result of slow intestinal reabsorption. The consequence of biliary obstruction would be a decreased volume of distribution, but no change in total clearance, and therefore a shorter half-life. On the other hand, if there is no enterohepatic cycling, the bile and the intestines are not part of the volume of distribution. Biliary obstruction, by decreasing clearance without affecting distribution, would then cause the half-life to increase.

Figure 11–13 illustrates half-lives of drugs with various combinations of clearance and volume of distribution. When clearance is low and volume of distribution is large, the half-life can be weeks or months. There is a paucity of drug examples with these characteristics. This is not surprising, as drug accumulation would be extensive and occur slowly on daily dosing. Furthermore, detoxification of a patient who exhibits toxicity while on such a drug would be slow without intervention.

Half-Life in Blood and Plasma Water

The interrelationships expressed in Eqs. 26 and 27 are just as readily derived from clearance and volume parameters based on measurements of drug in blood (CL_b, V_b) or in plasma water (CLu, Vu). Thus, by definition,

$$\begin{aligned} \text{Rate of elimination} &= CL \cdot C \\ &= CL_b \cdot C_b = CLu \cdot Cu \end{aligned} \qquad 28$$

and

$$\begin{aligned} \text{Amount in body} &= V \cdot C \\ &= V_b \cdot C_b = Vu \cdot Cu \end{aligned} \qquad 29$$

Note that each clearance or volume term can be related to the other using the definitions

$fu = Cu/C$ and $fu_b = Cu/C_b$. For example, $CL = fu \cdot CLu$. Dividing each term in Eq. 28 by the respective term in Eq. 29 gives

$$k = \frac{CL}{V} = \frac{Cl_b}{V_b} = \frac{Clu}{Vu}$$

30

and on substituting Eq. 30 into Eq. 27, it follows that

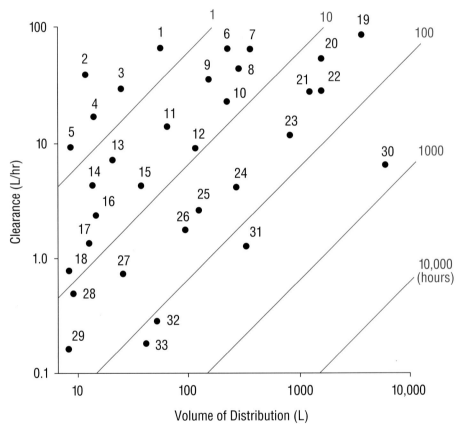

Fig. 11–13. Clearance (ordinate) and volume of distribution (abscissa) of selected drugs vary widely. The diagonal lines show the combinations of clearance and volume with the same half-life (hours). Note that drugs with low clearances and large volumes (right lower quadrant of graph) are difficult to find: their half-lives are often too long for these drugs to be used practically in drug therapy. (Adapted from Tozer, T.N.: Concepts basic to pharmacokinetics. Pharmacol. Ther., *12*, 109–131, 1981. Used with permission of author and publisher.) The drugs are as follows:

1. Penicillin V	12. Tetracycline	23. Digoxin
2. Aspirin	13. Gentamicin	24. Clonazepam
3. Penicillin G	14. Amikacin	25. Diazepam
4. Oxacillin	15. Theophylline	26. Carbamazepine
5. Furosemide	16. Acetazolamide	27. Sulfamerazine
6. Morphine	17. Sulfisoxazole	28. Valproic Acid
7. Meperidine	18. Tolbutamide	29. Warfarin
8. Propranolol	19. Desmethylimipramine	30. Amiodarone
9. Procainamide	20. Doxepin	31. Amphotericin B
10. Quinidine	21. Chlorpromazine	32. Phenobarbital
11. Chloramphenicol	22. Nortriptyline	33. Digitoxin

$$t_{1/2} = \frac{0.693\ V}{CL} = \frac{0.693\ V_b}{CL_b} = \frac{0.693\ V_u}{CL_u} \qquad 31$$

Thus, the value of the elimination rate constant, k, or the half-life, $t_{1/2}$, is independent of the site of measurement in blood.

The clearance parameter based on measurement of drug in blood is useful in considerations of drug extraction in the eliminating organs. Volume and clearance parameters based on the unbound drug concentration are particularly useful in therapeutics, because it is the unbound drug that is thought to relate most closely to the effects of a drug. Both sets of parameters are of value in anticipating and evaluating the pharmacokinetic and therapeutic consequences of alterations in protein binding, blood flow, and other physiologic variables. In practice, plasma drug concentrations are usually measured, but the application of the volume and clearance parameters so obtained is limited.

STUDY PROBLEMS

(Answers to Study Problems are in Appendix II.)

1. The renal clearances and the fractions unbound in plasma of three drugs in a 70-kg subject are as follows:

	Renal Clearance (mL/min)	Fraction Unbound
Theophylline	10	0.50
Phenytoin	0.15	0.10
Cefonicid	20	0.02

State the likely involvement of filtration, secretion, and reabsorption in the renal handling of each of these drugs, when *GFR* is 120 mL/min and urine flow is 1.5 mL/min.

2. For each of the following multiple choice questions indicate the letters of all (one or more) of the correct answers. Briefly comment on why the others are not correct.
   a. The conditions that indicate the probability of renal clearance of a weakly acidic drug being sensitive to urine pH are
      1. It is secreted and not reabsorbed.
      2. It has a pKa value of 5.0.
      3. It has a small volume of distribution.
      4. All of the drug is renally excreted unchanged, $fe = 1.0$.
   b. Forced diuresis is likely to enhance significantly the elimination kinetics of a drug
      1. Which is both polar and slowly removed from the body.
      2. For which most of the filtered and secreted drug is reabsorbed and fe is greater than 0.5.
      3. Which is neutral, polar, and has a value of fe greater than 0.9.
      4. Which is not secreted and for which the ratio of its unbound renal clearance to creatinine clearance is 1.0.
   c. A renal blood clearance of 567 mL/min for oxacillin indicates that:
      1. It is secreted into the luminal contents of the nephron.
      2. Its renal extraction ratio is 0.1.
      3. The majority of drug entering the body is excreted in the urine unchanged.
      4. It is not bound to plasma proteins.
   d. The renal clearance of a drug is constant with time if
      1. Its value exceeds 300 mL/min.
      2. The concentration in urine is independent of urine flow.

3. A constant fraction of filtered and secreted drug is reabsorbed.
3. Payne et al. (Payne, J.P., Foster, D.V., Hill, D.W., and Wood, D.G.L.: Observations on interpretation of blood alcohol levels derived from analysis of urine. Br. Med. J., 3:819, 1967) were interested, for legal reasons, in determining if the concentration of alcohol in urine could be related to its blood concentration. Table 11–7 summarizes their findings.
   a. Knowing that alcohol is not bound to components in blood, what explanation(s) can you offer for the very close correlation between concentrations of alcohol in blood and in urine?
   b. Would you expect the excretion rate of alcohol to correlate with the blood alcohol concentration? Discuss briefly.

Table 11–7. Frequency Distribution of the Ratio of Alcohol Concentrations, Urine/Blood

Percent of observations	9	51	32	8
Urine Concentration / Blood Concentration	<1.2	1.2–1.4	1.4–1.6	>1.6

4. Three drugs are listed in Table 11–8 together with some of their physical properties and disposition characteristics in a 70-kg man.

Table 11–8.

PROPERTY OR CHARACTERISTIC	NAFCILLIN	TOCAINIDE	CYCLOSPORINE
Polarity of un-ionized form	Polar	Non-polar	Non-polar
pKa	3.0	9.0	Not an acid
	(weak acid)	(amine)	or a base
Usual dose (mg)	250	400–600	350
Volume of distribution (L)	25	210	245
Fraction unbound (fu)	0.1	0.9	0.06
Half-life (hr)	1	14	8
Fraction excreted unchanged (fe)	0.27	0.14	<0.01

   a. Indicate the drug(s) for which each of the following statements is probably most applicable:
      1. The renal clearance of this drug is the most sensitive to changes in urine pH.
      2. This drug has the highest renal clearance of the three listed.
      3. This drug most likely shows the greatest diffusion limitation in crossing the placenta to the fetus.
      4. Forced diuresis is most likely to be of value for this drug in a case of drug overdose.
      5. For 100 mg in the body, the plasma concentration is highest for this drug after distribution equilibrium is achieved.
      6. This drug has the lowest total clearance.
   b. Circle the most appropriate word, term, or value (of those shown in italics) for the following statements:
      1. The renal clearance of nafcillin will *increase, decrease, show little change* if the drug is significantly displaced from plasma protein binding sites.

2. For the drug with a renal clearance that is most sensitive to changes in urine pH, *alkalinization, acidification* of the urine should decrease the renal clearance.

3. Nafcillin *is, is not* distributed evenly throughout and accounted for within the extracellular fluids.

4. Cyclosporine is primarily eliminated by *metabolism, renal excretion.*

5. Cyclosporine *can, cannot* be highly bound (*fu* less than 0.1) to plasma proteins since it has such a large apparent volume of distribution.

6. *51, 97, 99, 99.9* % of tocainide in the body is located outside the plasma.

c. Indicate the drug(s) for which each of the following statements is most applicable.

1. After an i.v. bolus dose, 30% remains in the body at 24 hrs.

2. Given every 8 hr, this drug will show the greatest degree of accumulation.

3. This drug will achieve the lowest plasma concentration at plateau following a constant-rate i.v. infusion of 10 mg/hr.

4. When the usual dose is administered intravenously, this drug will have the largest *AUC*.

5. Following a constant rate infusion of 20 mg/hr, this drug is expected to achieve the highest plasma concentration at 8 hr.

5. Recall from analysis of the data of problem 5, Chapter 6, that the systemic bioavailability of the drug droperidol from a rectal drug delivery device was 0.50. Given that the blood-to-plasma concentration ratio of this drug is 1.0, and negligible unchanged drug is found in urine following i.v. administration, to what extent could hepatic first-pass elimination account for the loss of bioavailability?

6. In Table 11–9 are listed some pertinent pharmacokinetic data, following administration orally (tablet) and intravenously of a 100-mg dose of a drug to a 68-kg subject. The blood-to-plasma concentration ratio of the drug is 0.77.

Table 11–9.

ROUTE	AUC (mg-hr/L)	Ae_∞ (mg)
Intravenous	1.93	10.5
Oral	0.22	1.22

a. Calculate the oral bioavailability of the drug.

b. By appropriate calculation, estimate to what extent the observed bioavailability might be attributed to first-pass hepatic elimination.

INTEGRATION WITH KINETICS

OBJECTIVES

The reader will be able to:

1. List examples of physiologic variables that may alter the primary pharmacokinetic parameters: absorption rate constant, bioavailability, hepatic clearance, renal clearance, and volume of distribution.
2. Given plasma (or blood) concentration versus time data in normal and altered states, determine the changes that have occurred in the primary and secondary pharmacokinetic parameters and list the possible physiologic mechanism(s) involved.
3. Predict and graphically demonstrate the effects of an alteration in plasma protein or tissue binding, perfusion, or metabolic activity on the time course of drug in blood when the appropriate primary pharmacokinetic parameters are known.
4. Predict the pharmacologic consequences of each of the alterations given in objective 3.

Reference is frequently made to *the* value of half-life or clearance of a drug. The pharmacokinetic parameters of a drug can, however, change—with disease, with concomitant drug therapy, and even within the same individual with time. An ability to assign likely physiologic and pathologic mechanisms to these observed changes in the kinetics of a drug is important, as is the prediction of the kinetic consequences of an alteration in a physiologic variable. Both approaches are taken in this chapter in order to integrate and practice the physiologic and pharmacokinetic concepts learned to this point. No attempt is made to examine situations involving all possible changes of physiologic variables as the theoretical possibilities are too numerous. In subsequent chapters, especially Chaps. 17 (Interacting Drugs) and 22 (Dose and Time Dependencies), additional examples that demonstrate and require integration of physiologic and kinetic concepts are given.

Frequently, conditions that produce a change in one physiologic parameter cause changes in others as well. For example, renal disease appears not only to decrease the renal clearance of digoxin, but to decrease its tissue binding and extrarenal clearance as well (see Chap. 16). The interaction of quinidine and digoxin is another example. Similar to renal disease, quinidine decreases tissue binding and both renal and extrarenal clearances of digoxin. Thus, neither of these situations is a good example of the kinetic consequences of any *one* of the alterations that occur. Yet, these kinds of observations occur frequently. The first step in analyzing them is to examine the expectations for an alteration in each physiologic variable involved. The overall picture is then gained by integrating these expectations.

INTERRELATIONSHIPS AMONG PHARMACOKINETIC PARAMETERS AND PHYSIOLOGIC VARIABLES

A summary of the interrelationships among pharmacokinetic parameters and physiologic variables is appropriate here.

Primary Parameters and Physiologic Variables

The processes of absorption and disposition depend on many physiologic variables. Gastrointestinal absorption may be affected by blood flow at the absorption site, gastric emptying, and gastrointestinal motility. Distribution is influenced by binding to both plasma proteins and tissue components and by body composition. Renal excretion may depend on secretion (active transport), urine pH, and urine flow. Each of these physiologic variables is affected by numerous factors. Thus, rubbing increases subcutaneous and muscle blood flow, food slows gastric emptying, and diseases and drugs produce many effects.

The pharmacokinetics of a drug often can be described by relatively few parameters. Recall that absorption can be characterized by bioavailability and by an absorption rate constant, when absorption is first order; distribution can be characterized by the volume of distribution; and elimination can be characterized by hepatic and renal clearances. As discussed in Chaps. 8 through 11, each of these parameters may be directly affected by changes in physiologic variables. Because of this direct relationship, these parameters are referred to in this book as *primary pharmacokinetic parameters*. Physiologic variables that affect primary pharmacokinetic parameters are listed in Table 12–1.

Secondary Pharmacokinetic Parameters and Derived Values

Half-life, elimination rate constant, and fraction excreted unchanged in urine are examples of *secondary pharmacokinetic parameters*, in that their values depend on those of the primary pharmacokinetic parameters. Furthermore, there are several derived values, such as *AUC*, that depend not only on the primary pharmacokinetic parameters but also on either dose or rate of administration. These dependencies are summarized briefly in Table 12–2.

The equations in Table 12–2 plus a few previous equations provide the basic relationships for interpreting and predicting alterations in kinetic behavior. Particularly useful are the memory aids of Eqs. 13 and 17 in Chap. 11, namely

$$CL_H = \frac{Q_H \cdot fu_b \cdot CL_{int}}{Q_H + fu_b \cdot CL_{int}} \qquad 1$$

and

$$F_H = \frac{Q_H}{Q_H + fu_b \cdot CL_{int}} \qquad 2$$

Table 12–1. Dependence of Primary Pharmacokinetic Parameters on Physiologic Variables

PRIMARY PHARMACOKINETIC PARAMETER	PHYSIOLOGIC VARIABLES
Absorption rate constant	Blood flow at absorption site, gastric emptying (oral), intestinal motility (oral)
Bioavailability	Gastric emptying, secretion of acid in stomach and hydrolytic enzymes in bile, intestinal motility
Hepatic clearance; bioavailability[a]	Hepatic blood flow, binding in blood, intrinsic hepatocellular activity
Renal clearance	Renal blood flow, binding in blood, active secretion, active reabsorption, urine pH, urine flow, glomerular filtration rate
Volume of distribution	Binding in blood, binding in tissues, partitioning into fat, body composition, body size

[a]Hepatic elimination is assumed to be the only cause of a decrease in oral bioavailability.

Volume of distribution depends on binding to both plasma proteins and tissue constituents. For a drug with a large volume (> 50 L),

$$V \approx \frac{V_R \cdot fu}{fu_R} \qquad\qquad 3$$

while for a low molecular weight (< 500 g/mole) drug with a small volume of distribution (< 0.2 L/kg), V tends to be independent of changes in fu (Chap. 10).

The subsequent examples are analyzed using these relationships. They exemplify alterations in intrinsic hepatocellular activity (induction and inhibition), hepatic blood flow, active tubular secretion, and plasma protein binding.

Induction of Metabolism

Some drugs can induce the metabolism of others by increasing the rate of synthesis of the enzyme(s) involved. The kinetic and therapeutic consequences depend on whether the affected drug initially has a low or a high extraction ratio in the eliminating organ in which induction occurs and on the route of administration.

Low Extraction Ratio. Figure 12–1 demonstrates the kinetic effect of induction of warfarin metabolism by the antitubercular agent rifampin. Warfarin is predominantly metabolized in the liver; little is excreted in urine unchanged. Warfarin is also completely and rapidly absorbed when given orally.

The data in Fig. 12–1 support warfarin having a low hepatic extraction ratio. This conclusion is based on a rough calculation of clearance. Thus, during the control phase clearance, obtained by dividing dose (1.5 mg/kg) by AUC [1360 mg-hr/L, calculated from $C(0)/k$], is 0.0011 L/hr/kg. The blood/plasma concentration ratio is 0.6, so that the corresponding blood clearance is 0.0018 L/hr/kg. This value is low compared to the hepatic blood flow of 81 L/hr/70 kg or 1.2 L/hr/kg. In the presence of rifampin, the AUC of warfarin is decreased compared to that of the control value, reflecting a higher clearance. This observation is consistent with induction of hepatic enzymes; the clearance of a drug of low hepatic extraction ratio is expected to be sensitive to changes in hepatocellular enzymatic activity. The data suggest no effect of rifampin on warfarin distribution. The estimated volumes of distribution, obtained from CL/k, are 0.079 and 0.068 L/kg during the control and rifampin phases, respectively. These values are probably not significantly different.

Table 12–2. Dependence of Secondary Pharmacokinetic Parameters and Derived Values on Primary Pharmacokinetic Parameters

	EQUATIONS
Secondary Pharmacokinetic Parameters	
Elimination half-life	$0.693 \cdot \dfrac{\text{Volume of distribution}}{\text{Clearance}}$
Elimination rate constant	Clearance/(Volume of distribution)
Fraction excreted unchanged	(Renal clearance)/(Total clearance)
Derived Values	
Area under curve (i.v.)	Dose/Clearance
Steady-state concentration (i.v.)	(Infusion rate)/Clearance
Area under curve (oral)	$\dfrac{\text{Dose} \cdot (\text{Oral bioavailability})}{\text{Clearance}}$
Average plateau concentration (oral)	$\dfrac{\text{Dose} \cdot (\text{Oral bioavailability})}{\text{Clearance} \cdot (\text{Dosing interval})}$

The therapeutic consequence of induction can be appreciated from the difference in the response-time curves, shown in the bottom graph of Fig. 12–1. *Response* here is defined as the elevation in prothrombin time above a baseline value of 14 sec. The overall response, given by the area under the response-time curve after the single oral dose, is substantially reduced in the presence of rifampin. Consequently, one would expect under steady-state conditions that the dosage of warfarin must be increased in the presence of rifampin to maintain the same prothrombin time. The reason for the apparently poor correlation between response and plasma warfarin concentration during the first 48 hr after warfarin administration, when response is increasing and concentration is falling, is discussed in Chap. 23, Turnover Concepts.

Rifampin is a known inducer of hepatic drug metabolism, and the data provided in Fig. 12–1 are generally consistent with induction of warfarin metabolism by rifampin. However, there are problems with respect to the interpretation of these data, in addition to the above mentioned problem of relating warfarin concentration to response. Warfarin is marketed as a racemate. Its enantiomers have different anticoagulant potencies and different kinetic properties. Furthermore, the change in prothrombin time is a consequence of changes in several clotting factors. Racemates are commonly used today, instead of a pure enantiomer. One isomer may potentiate or inhibit the kinetics or dynamics of the other. As long as racemates are administered, kinetic and dynamic data on the pure enantiomers, while helpful to define mechanisms involved, are of questionable value without corresponding data following the racemate as well. Clearly, chirality is a major issue in therapeutics.

High Extraction Ratio. Induction of metabolism of a drug with a high hepatic extraction ratio has kinetic consequences very different from those of a drug with a low hepatic extraction ratio, as illustrated in Fig. 12–2. Pretreatment with the inducer pentobarbital appears to have little effect on the pharmacokinetics of alprenolol after its intravenous (i.v.) administration. Following oral administration, however, both the peak concentration (C_{max}) and *AUC* are dramatically reduced, although there is little apparent change in the half-life. These observations, at first glance, appear to be inconsistent. Knowing that this drug is metabolized only in the liver and on calculating (from dose and *AUC* following i.v. admin-

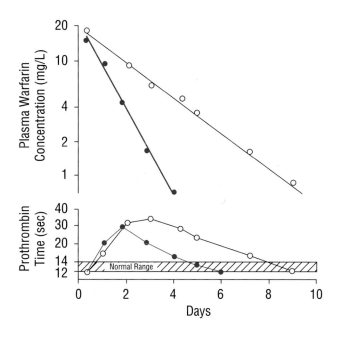

Fig. 12–1. The half-life of warfarin, a drug with a low extraction ratio, is shortened and clearance is increased when it is given (open circles) as a single dose (1.5 mg/kg) before (black line) and while (colored circles and line) the inducer, rifampin, is being administered as a 600-mg dose daily for 3 days prior to warfarin administration. The peak and duration of the elevation in the prothrombin time (response) are decreased when rifampin is coadministered (lower graph) (1 mg/L = 3.3 μM). (Reproduced, with permission, from O'Reilly, R.A.: Interaction of sodium warfarin and rifampin. Ann. Intern. Med., *81*:337–340, 1974.)

istration) a clearance of 1.2 L/min in this individual, an explanation can be offered. Pentobarbital induces alprenolol metabolism, which manifests itself as a decrease in alprenolol oral bioavailability. The argument for this conclusion follows.

The hepatic extraction ratio of alprenolol is high; its clearance approaches hepatic blood flow, approximately 1.35 L/min, and its oral bioavailability (F), calculated by comparing the dose-corrected AUC after oral and i.v. administrations, is 0.22. Given that the low bioavailability is due solely to hepatic extraction, the hepatic extraction ratio $(1 - F_H)$ is 0.78. Bioavailability reflects the balance between perfusion, which forces drug through the organ, and enzymatic activity, which removes drug. After induction, which increases enzyme activity, oral bioavailability (based on comparison of AUC values) decreases to 0.06, almost a fourfold change, and hence the hepatic extraction ratio increases to 0.94. Because clearance is perfusion rate-limited and because there is no evidence in humans that pentobarbital alters hepatic blood flow, there is only a small increase in clearance. The increase in hepatic extraction ratio, and hence clearance, is only 20% (from 0.78 to 0.94). The lack of change in terminal half-life after induction also indicates that pentobarbital has no effect on the volume of distribution of alprenolol. Thus, induction of the metabolism of this drug, or any other drug with a high hepatic extraction ratio, has therapeutic implications when administered orally, but not when given intravenously. A larger oral dose, or more frequent administration, is needed in the presence of the inducer to produce the same effect, assuming all activity resides with the drug.

Alprenolol, like warfarin, is also administered as a racemate. With little difference in the kinetics of the isomers, the conclusions here for the mixture apply as well to each of the isomers. Indeed, if there are virtually no pharmacologic, toxicologic, or pharmacokinetic differences between the isomers, a benefit in using the racemate is that it does not incur the often considerable cost of separating the isomers.

Decreased Hepatocellular Activity

Examples of drugs that inhibit the metabolism of other drugs are given in Chap. 17, Interacting Drugs. Reduced metabolism can also be a consequence of hepatic disease (Chap. 16), dietary deficiencies, and other conditions. Whatever the cause of decreased metabolic activity, the kinetic consequences depend on the hepatic extraction ratio of the drug.

Low Extraction Ratio. The effect of decreasing hepatocellular activity for a drug of low hepatic extraction ratio is illustrated by data for chlorzoxazone and chlordiazepoxide.

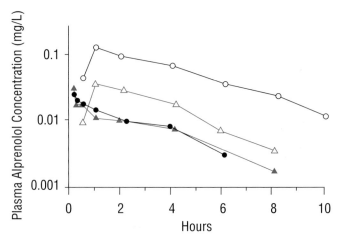

Fig. 12–2. Induction of alprenolol metabolism by pentobarbital treatment produces marked differences in the plasma concentration when the drug is given orally (200 mg), but not when given i.v. (5 mg). Alprenolol was administered before (black lines: ●, i.v.; ○, oral) and 10 days into (colored lines: ▲, i.v.; △, oral) a pentobarbital regimen of 100 mg at bedtime (1 mg/L = 4.0 μM) (From Alvan, G., Piafsky, K., Lind, M., and von Bahr, C.: Effect of pentobarbital on the disposition of alprenolol. Clin. Pharmacol. Ther., 22:316–321, 1977.)

The concentration-time profile of the muscle relaxant chlorzoxazone in a subject after a 750-mg oral dose is very different from that seen 10 hr after a single 500-mg oral dose of disulfiram (Fig. 12–3). The mean clearance and half-life values were 3.3 ml/min/kg and 1.2 hr in the absence and 0.5 ml/min/kg and 5.1 hr in the presence of disulfiram, a selective inhibitor of oxidative metabolism. The changing concentration of the inhibitor (and its metabolites following the single 500-mg dose) and the limited time of sampling in the presence of the inhibitor preclude being highly quantitative. Nonetheless, the effect of decreased hepatocellular activity is clear for a drug with a low extraction ratio; clearance decreases and half-life increases.

Another example is that of the anxiolytic drug chlordiazepoxide (Fig. 12–4). Its half-life is increased and its clearance is decreased in patients with hepatic cirrhosis. Oral bioavailability and volume of distribution (not shown) are unaffected.

That chlordiazepoxide has a low hepatic extraction ratio even in healthy subjects can be deduced from the data in the figure if one also knows that the drug is eliminated primarily

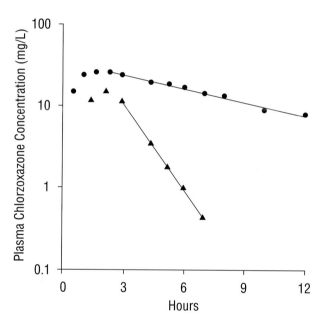

Fig. 12–3. The plasma concentration-time profile of chlorzoxazone after a single 750-mg oral dose (▲) is dramatically increased after disulfiram treatment (●). Disulfiram (500 mg orally) was given 10 hr before the chlorzoxazone. The increase in half-life and decrease in clearance are expected for a low extraction ratio drug when metabolic activity is decreased. (Redrawn from Kharasch, E.D., Thummel, K.E. Mhyre, J., and Lillibridge, J.H.: Single-dose disulfiram inhibition of chlorzoxazone metabolism: A clinical probe for P450 2E1. Clin. Pharmacol. Ther. 53:643–650, 1993. Reproduced with permission of C.V. Mosby.)

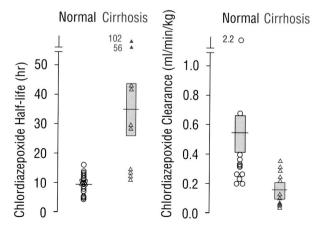

Fig. 12–4. Chlordiazepoxide's half-life is increased and total clearance is decreased in patients with hepatic cirrhosis compared to normal subjects. Mean (±SEM) and individual values are shown. (Redrawn from Sellers, E.M., Greenblatt, D.J., Giles, H.G., Naranjo, C.A., Kaplan, H., and Mac-Leod, S.M.: Chlordiazepoxide and oxazepam disposition in cirrhotics. Clin. Pharmacol. Ther., 26:240–246, 1979. Reproduced with permission of C.V. Mosby.)

by hepatic metabolism, the blood-plasma concentration ratio is close to 1.0, and average hepatic blood flow is 20 mL/min/kg. In subjects with normal hepatic function, the hepatic extraction ratio $[CL_H/Q_H = (0.55 \text{ mL/min/kg})/(20 \text{ mL/min/kg})]$ is then expected to be only about 0.03 or less.

High Extraction Ratio. The kinetic consequences of inhibition of metabolism of a drug with a high hepatic extraction ratio are illustrated by the coadministration of cimetidine and labetolol (Fig. 12–5). That labetolol is a drug of high hepatic extraction ratio is deduced from its clearance, 1.06 L/hr (estimated by dividing the i.v. dose by the corresponding AUC given in the article), approaching hepatic blood flow and from the knowledge that labetolol is eliminated almost exclusively by hepatic metabolism. The i.v. dose of labetolol is much smaller than the oral dose, because the drug is highly extracted in the liver, and hence subject to extensive first-pass hepatic loss, and because the pharmacologic activity primarily resides with the drug, rather than with its metabolites.

There is a large increase in AUC for labetolol when administered orally, but not when given intravenously, in the presence of cimetidine. This observation is expected following inhibition of the elimination of a drug with a high hepatic extraction ratio. The lack of change in area following i.v. administration reflects the minor decrease caused by cimetidine in the hepatic extraction ratio and hence in clearance. Evidently, blood flow continues to limit the hepatic elimination of labetolol even when inhibition occurs. This would not be so if the degree of inhibition were such as to reduce labetolol to a drug of low hepatic extraction ratio. The large increase in AUC following oral administration is a consequence of increased bioavailability; here the increment is about 56%, while only a minor decrease (20%) was seen in the hepatic extraction ratio. The therapeutic corollary of the kinetic changes in the presence of cimetidine is heightened activity of labetolol when given orally, but not when given intravenously.

Altered Blood Flow

As presented in Chap. 11, changes in organ blood flow affect clearance only when extraction ratio is high. This conclusion is based on the concept of a perfusion-rate limitation. It should be borne in mind, however, that effects secondary to an altered blood flow, particularly when decreased, may supersede perfusion considerations alone. For example, a decreased blood flow may produce anoxia, which in turn may affect hepatocellular activity and hence the extraction ratio. The extraction ratio may also be altered by a decreased blood flow

Fig. 12–5. Bioavailability increased, but clearance showed no significant (N.S.) change, when 6 healthy volunteers were given labetolol either as a 200-mg dose orally or as a 0.5-mg/kg dose i.v. before and on the fourth day of cimetidine treatment (400 mg every 6 hr). This conclusion is based on a significant change in AUC after oral, but not after i.v. administration. (Adapted from Daneshmend, T.K., and Roberts, C.J.C.: The effects of enzyme induction and enzyme inhibition on labetolol pharmacokinetics. Br. J. Clin. Pharmacol., *18*:393–400, 1984.)

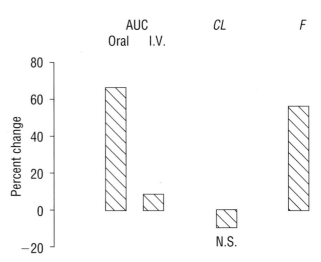

because every blood vessel in the organ may not provide the same exposure of the drug to hepatic parenchymal cells, and the pattern of distribution of blood flow within the eliminating organ may change. This alteration in the degree of shunting or bypassing of the parenchymal cells may occur in certain hepatic diseases and under a variety of conditions.

Good examples of the kinetic consequences of altered blood flow are hard to find. This is not because they are uncommon, but because a number of additional complications always seem to occur concurrently. For example, conditions such as congestive cardiac failure, in which cardiac output is decreased, are often associated with increased third-spacing (build-up of fluid in intestinal spaces and body cavities), diminished hepatic and renal functions; and slowed distribution to the tissues. A decrease in hepatic blood flow, brought about by cirrhosis, chronically leads to portal hypertension and extrahepatic shunting of portal blood. Thus, the kinetic consequences of altered blood flow are subsequently examined alone, with the realization that in therapeutic scenarios the effects of changes in more than one physiologic variable need to be considered.

For this theoretical presentation, consider the two drugs given in Table 12–3. Drug L is eliminated in both the liver and the kidneys; its major property is low extraction in both organs. Drug H has a high hepatic extraction ratio and is almost exclusively eliminated by the liver.

Low Hepatic Extraction Ratio. Figure 12–6 shows the effect of a doubling of hepatic blood flow for the poorly cleared drug, drug L. Because drug L has a low hepatic extraction ratio, altered blood flow has little or no effect on the pharmacokinetics of this drug.

High Hepatic Extraction Ratio. The events following i.v. administration of a drug with a high hepatic extraction ratio, drug H, when hepatic blood flow is increased, are readily apparent. Not so apparent are the likely events that follow when drug H is given orally. Recall that $F \cdot Dose = CL \cdot AUC$ or $AUC = F \cdot Dose/CL$. Although the half-life is shortened, clearance and oral bioavailability are increased simultaneously; oral bioavailability is elevated because drug in blood remains in the hepatic sinusoids for a shorter period of time with an increased blood flow, and therefore there is less chance of drug being eliminated. Accordingly, the result may be little or no change in AUC (last graph of Fig. 12–6). The outcome depends on whether or not the increase in bioavailability is exactly matched by that of clearance when blood flow is increased. The memory aids of Eqs. 2 and 3 predict equal effects, in that the ratio of these equations ($CL_b/F_H = CL_{int} \cdot fu_b$) is independent of blood flow. Unfortunately, there is a lack of good quantitative information to be specific here.

An example of a change in kinetics with a change in blood flow is given with lidocaine in Fig. 12–7. Lidocaine is a drug with a high hepatic extraction ratio and whose clearance is perfusion rate limited. Here, as expected, the concurrent administration of either β-blocker, propranolol or metoprolol produces a decrease in the clearance of lidocaine. β-Blockers reduce cardiac output and hepatic blood flow. The change in lidocaine clearance following propranolol administration is larger than that expected for the change in hepatic blood flow, suggesting that one or more other mechanisms may also be operating.

Table 12–3. Pharmacokinetic Parameters of Two Hypothetical Drugs

DRUG	BIOAVAILABILITY[a]	VOLUME OF DISTRIBUTION (L)	CLEARANCE[b] (L/hr)	FRACTION EXCRETED UNCHANGED	EXTRACTION RATIO HEPATIC	RENAL
L	0.97	26	6	0.60	0.03	0.05
H	0.05	430	77	0.05	0.95	0.06

[a]Bioavailability is fully accounted for by first-pass metabolism in the liver.
[b]Clearance is based on measurement of drug in blood.

Altered Active Tubular Secretion

Figure 12–8 shows the effect of inhibiting the renal tubular secretion of amoxicillin by probenecid. An increased *AUC* of amoxicillin is obvious; it reflects a decrease in clearance. The prolongation of elimination half-life is also due primarily to reduced clearance; the volume of distribution (*CL/k*) is changed relatively little, indicating that probenecid does not affect the distribution of amoxicillin. The inhibition of renal excretion of this penicillin by probenecid becomes apparent when this pathway is isolated. Renal clearance, that is, the excretion rate relative to the plasma concentration, is clearly reduced by probenecid. The substantial renal excretion of amoxicillin explains why a reduced renal clearance has such a pronounced effect on total clearance.

The decrease in renal clearance occurs by inhibition of the tubular secretory mechanism for amoxicillin, a drug that is virtually unbound to plasma proteins. The degree of inhibition of this process is masked by the contribution of filtration at the glomerulus. If secretion is

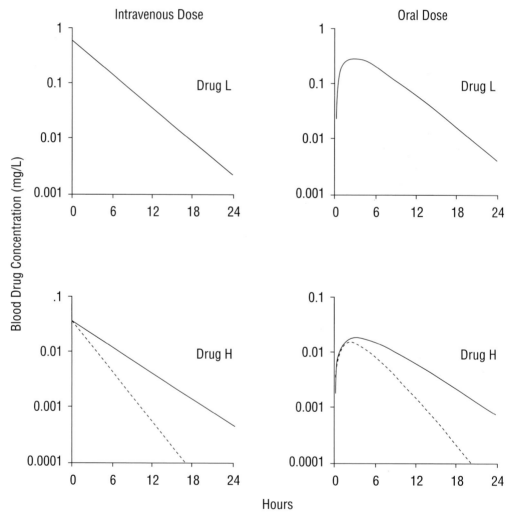

Fig. 12–6. Increased blood flow to the liver has very little effect on the time course of Drug L, a poorly extracted drug, after either an oral or i.v. 15-mg dose but has a pronounced effect on Drug H, a highly cleared drug, following single i.v. (15-mg) and oral (300-mg) doses. Altered condition (----); normal condition (———). The absorption rate constant of both drugs is 1.4 hr. See Table 12–3 for other pharmacokinetic properties of these two drugs.

completely blocked, renal clearance of this polar antibiotic is expected to have a lower limit of $fu \cdot GFR$ because it is not reabsorbed in the tubule.

Altered Plasma Protein Binding

Knowledge of conditions in which the binding to plasma proteins is altered is critical to plasma drug concentration monitoring (Chap. 18). When activities, desired and undesired, relate to the unbound concentration, changes in binding directly affect the interpretation of total concentration data. This problem applies to drugs of both low and high extraction. Whether or not the altered binding affects the unbound plasma concentration, and therefore the concentration at the active site is therapeutically important. These aspects are now addressed in turn.

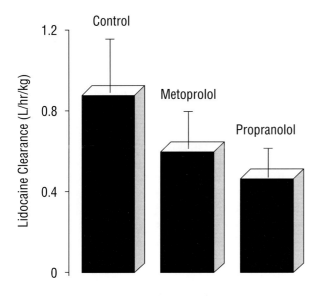

Fig. 12–7. The clearance of lidocaine following a 4-min i.v. infusion (3 mg/kg) is reduced during metoprolol (50 mg) or propranolol (40 mg) administration (every 6 hr beginning 24 hr before the test dose and continuing for 8 hr thereafter). These drugs decrease cardiac output and hepatic blood flow, the primary mechanism by which the clearance of lidocaine is thought to be reduced. (1 mg/L = 4.3 µM) (Adapted from Conrad, K.A., Byers, J.M., Finley, P.R., and Burnham, L.: Lidocaine elimination: Effects of metoprolol and of propranolol. Clin. Pharmacol. Ther., 33:133–138, 1983.)

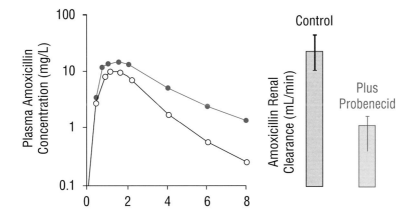

Fig. 12–8. The plasma concentration (on left), and hence the *AUC*, for amoxicillin is increased when 500 mg are administered orally in solution to fasting subjects in the presence (colored curve) and absence (black curve) of probenecid (1 g, 12 hr and then 1 hr before the antibiotic). The effect is due to probenecid decreasing the renal clearance of amoxicillin (on right), the major component of total clearance (1 mg/L = 2.7 µM) (Data from Staniforth, D.H., Jackson, D., Clarke, H.L., and Horton, R.: Amoxicillin/clavulanic acid: The effect of probenecid. J. Antimicrob. Chemother., *12*:273–275, 1983.)

Low Extraction Ratio. Changes in the therapeutic window of phenytoin as a function of serum creatinine concentration, an index of renal function, is shown in Fig. 12–9. The higher the creatinine concentration, the lower is the renal function. The window falls because fu, normally about 0.1, increases to about 0.25 to 0.3 in patients with severe renal function impairment.

For example, given that the unbound concentration required to produce a given response in the presence of renal disease is the same as that in the absence, it follows that

$$fu \cdot C = fu' \cdot C' \qquad\qquad 4$$

where fu' and C' are the unbound fraction and total drug concentration in the presence of the disease, respectively. On rearrangement

$$C' = \frac{fu}{fu'} \cdot C \qquad\qquad 5$$

Concentrations of 10 and 20 mg/L in normal conditions thus become equivalent to 4 and 8 mg/L when fu and fu' are 0.1 and 0.25, respectively.

Phenytoin is a low extraction drug eliminated by hepatic metabolism. Consequently, elimination is related to its unbound concentration (Chap. 11). Total clearance $(fu \cdot CLu)$ increases in renal disease, but there is no requirement for dosing rate adjustment because unbound clearance, the proportionality constant between rate of input and unbound concentration at steady state, is not affected by the binding change.

High Extraction Ratio. Figure 12–10 shows how blood clearance, volume of distribution, and half-life of propranolol vary with the fraction unbound in six healthy male volunteers. Clearance appears to be independent of protein binding. The volume of distribution (blood) and half-life both increase with an increase in fu. This is the behavior expected for a drug with a large volume of distribution and for which elimination is perfusion rate-limited. The drug is primarily eliminated by hepatic metabolism, and the met-

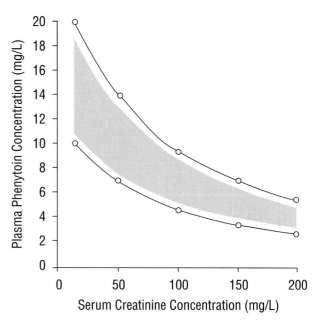

Fig. 12–9. The therapeutic range of phenytoin based on total plasma concentration decreases with the degree of renal function impairment, as measured by serum creatinine, from the usual values of 10 to 20 mg/L. This decrease is a consequence of reduced binding, which is related to the severity of the renal disease (1 mg/L = 4.0 μM). (Redrawn from Reidenberg, M.M., and Affrime, M.: Influence of disease on binding of drugs to plasma proteins. Ann. N.Y. Acad. Sci., 226:115–126, 1973.)

abolic (blood) clearance approaches hepatic blood flow (1.35 L/min on average). The increase in volume of distribution with fu is anticipated, as is the increase in half-life.

With the increase in fu and no change in clearance, there must be a corresponding decrease in unbound clearance, since $CL_b = fu_b \cdot CL_{int}$. This means that the unbound concentration under constant-rate i.v. infusion conditions is increased when binding is decreased and the converse; an effect with potentially important therapeutic consequences. An alternative view of this situation is to remember that when clearance approaches blood flow in the eliminating organ, total steady-state concentration is not expected to change with altered plasma binding. An increase in fu thereby raises the unbound concentration and the drug's effects. Although there are many drugs with a high hepatic extraction ratio, they are fortunately seldom given chronically by the parenteral route under conditions in which binding is altered.

The oral bioavailability of a drug with a high extraction ratio is expected to decrease with an increase in fu, as seen from Eq. 17 of Chap. 11, when CL_{int} is much greater than Q/fu. Here $CLu/F = CL_{int}$. The memory aid model of Chap. 11 predicts little or no change in the steady-state unbound concentration or the therapeutic response after oral administration, because CL_{int} is unchanged.

Small Volume of Distribution. The consequence of altering binding to plasma proteins is illustrated by clofibrate. The half-life of clofibric acid (the active material formed by hydrolysis of the administered ethyl ester, clofibrate) shortens from the usual 16.5 hr to 8.7 hr in patients with the nephrotic syndrome (Table 12–4). It is tempting to conclude that metabolism (only 6% of clofibric acid is excreted unchanged) is induced and that dosage requirements need to be increased in these patients. From a pharmacokinetic point of view, these conclusions are incorrect, as the following shows.

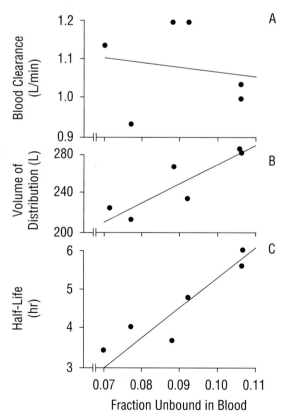

Fig. 12–10. The clearance of propranolol (Graph A), based on its concentration in blood, does not appear to correlate with the fraction unbound in blood of six healthy male volunteers after intravenous administration of 20 mg. On the other hand, the volume of distribution (graph B) and the half-life (graph C) are observed to increase with an increase in the fraction unbound. This kinetic behavior is anticipated for a drug, such as propranolol, that is highly extracted in the liver. Clearance here is perfusion rate-limited. Binding to plasma proteins does not influence clearance but does affect the volume of distribution and, therefore, the half-life. The lines are the best fits by linear regression. (1 mg/L = 3.9 μM) (Data from Evans, G.H., and Shand, D.G.: Disposition of propranolol. VI: Independent variation in steady-state circulating drug concentrations and half-life as a result of plasma drug binding in man. Clin. Pharmacol. Ther., *14*:494–500, 1973. Reproduced with permission of C.V. Mosby.)

In the nephrotic syndrome, there is an extensive loss of plasma proteins into the urine, which results in a twofold drop in serum albumin, as shown in Table 10–7. The influence of this drop in serum albumin on fu can be estimated from rearrangement of Eq. 18 (Chap. 10). The normal serum albumin concentration reported is 4.3 g/dL and for clofibric acid fu is 0.03. Given that fu_p, the fraction of available binding sites unoccupied, is equal to 1, the value of Ka is 7.5 dL/g. At a serum albumin concentration of 2.3 g/dL, the calculated fraction unbound in nephrotic patients is then

$$fu = \frac{1}{1 + 7.5 \times 2.3} = 0.055 \qquad\qquad 6$$

Clofibric acid has a low extraction ratio in that its clearance (calculated from $k \cdot V$) is 0.32 L/hr in healthy subjects, a value much smaller than hepatic blood flow, 81 L/hr. Although one might argue that blood clearance is much larger than plasma clearance (also $C/C_b >$ 1), this is impossible. Virtually all drug in the body is bound to albumin ($V = 0.11$ L/kg). Thus, plasma drug concentration can only be greater than blood drug concentration by a factor of 1.7 [1/(1 − hematocrit); see Appendix I–F.

With clofibric acid being a low extraction ratio drug, clearance is expected to increase in nephrotic patients. The value of unbound clearance, CL/fu, is 10.7 L/hr in healthy subjects. If one assumes the same unbound clearance in nephrotic patients, then clearance, $fu \cdot CLu$, in this group is 0.59 L/hr.

The volume of distribution of clofibric acid, given in the footnote to Table 12–4, is 7.7 L/70 kg. This value depends little on changes in plasma protein binding. This is seen from the relationship between V and fu for a drug with a small volume of distribution (Eq. 25, Chap. 10), namely,

$$V = 7.5 + \text{Constant} \cdot fu$$

With an apparent volume of 7.7 L, the constant is 6.7. If fu is increased to 0.055, then the apparent volume becomes 7.9 L. The volume unbound (V/fu), however, decreases from 257 to 143 L. The calculated half-life ($0.693 \cdot V/CL$ or $0.693 \cdot Vu/CLu$) in the nephrotic patients is then about 9.3 hr, a value very close to that observed, 8.7 hr.

The two questions originally posed are now answered. The half-life is shortened in the nephrotic patients because of decreased binding to albumin; metabolism was not induced. Unbound clearance was not changed, and therefore no change in the usual dosing rate of 1.5 to 2.0 g/day is needed in nephrotic patients to produce the same average unbound concentration in plasma, as achieved in patients with normal serum albumin. A shorter

Table 12–4. Renal Function Measures, Serum Albumin, Daily Protein Excretion, and Half-Life of the Active Form of Clofibrate, Clofibric Acid, in Patients With and Without the Nephrotic Syndrome[a]

	SERUM CREATININE (mg/dL)[b]	CREATININE CLEARANCE (mL/min)	SERUM ALBUMIN (g/dL)	CLOFIBRIC ACID HALF-LIFE (hr)	PROTEIN EXCRETION (g/day)
Nephrotic group (N = 5)	1.3 ± 0.1	100 ± 24	2.3 ± 0.5	8.7 ± 3.5	13 ± 12
Control group (N = 8)[c]	1.2 ± 0.2	98 ± 20	4.4 ± 0.4	16.5 ± 4.7	0

[a]From Goldberg, A.P., Sherrard, D.J., Haas, L.B., and Brunzell, J.D.: Control of clofibrate toxicity in uremic hypertriglyceridemia. Clin. Pharmacol. Ther., 21:317–325, 1977.
[b]One mg/dL = 88 μM.
[c]In healthy subjects, the volume of distribution of clofibric acid is 0.11 L/kg, the fraction unbound in plasma is 0.03, and the fraction excreted unchanged is 0.06. (Data from Benet, L.Z., and Williams R.L.: Appendix II. In The Pharmacologic Basis of Therapeutics. 8th ed. Edited by A.G. Gilman, T.W. Rall, A.S. Nies, and P. Taylor. New York, Macmillan, 1993.)

Table 12-5. Anticipated Effects of Alterations in Selected Physiologic Variables on Various Parameters and Observations for Drugs Eliminated Solely by the Liver

ADMINISTRATION	PARAMETERS OR OBSERVATIONS	PHYSIOLOGIC VARIABLE ALTERED			
		INCREASED ENZYME ACTIVITY[b]	INHIBITION OF METABOLISM	DECREASED BLOOD FLOW	INCREASED FRACTION UNBOUND IN BLOOD
		Low Hepatic Extraction Ratio Drug			
Intravenous	Half-life	↓[c]	↑	↔	↔
	AUC (blood)	↓	↑	↔	↓
Oral	Bioavailability	↔	↔	↔	↔
	AUC (blood)	↓	↑	↔	↓
		High Hepatic Extraction Ratio Drug			
Intravenous	Half-life	↔	↔	↑	↑
	AUC (blood)	↔	↔	↑	↔
Oral	Bioavailability	↓	↑	↓	↓
	AUC (blood)	↓	↑	↔[d]	↓

[a]$V > 50$ L for all drugs.
[b]Enzyme activity is increased by one of several mechanisms, such as enzyme activation, induction, or increased availability of cofactors, if rate-limiting.
[c]↑ Increased; ↓ decreased; ↔ little or no change.
[d]The decrease in bioavailability is assumed to be equally matched by a decrease in clearance.

dosing interval (and correspondingly smaller maintenance dose) might be considered because of the shortened half-life.

The combinations of conditions and scenarios in drug therapy are multitudinous. This chapter has presented approaches and examples toward integrating kinetic principles and physiologic concepts. To complete this integration, Table 12–5 summarizes the effects expected from increased enzyme activity, inhibition of metabolism, decreased blood flow, and increased fu in blood for a drug eliminated exclusively in the liver. Conditions involving drugs of both low and high extraction ratios are considered. The expectations are similar for a drug eliminated only by the kidneys; however, increased active tubular secretion rather than increased enzyme activity applies. Also, oral bioavailability of a drug highly extracted in the kidneys is unaffected by changes in the physiologic variables considered here.

STUDY PROBLEMS

(Answers to Study Problems are in Appendix II.)

1. List 10 examples of physiologic variables that alter pharmacokinetic parameter values.
2. Complete Table 12–6 below to show tendencies by marking: ↑ for increase, ↓ for decrease, and ↔ for little or no change in the empty spaces. The drug is only eliminated in the liver, and its volume of distribution is greater than 100 L. There is no change in intrinsic clearance.

Table 12-6.

HEPATIC EXTRACTION RATIO	HEPATIC BLOOD FLOW	FRACTION IN BLOOD UNBOUND	FRACTION IN TISSUE UNBOUND	TOTAL CLEARANCE[a]	VOLUME OF DISTRIBUTION[a]	HALF-LIFE	ORAL BIOAVAILABILITY
High	↑	↔	↔				
High	↔	↓	↔				
High	↔	↔	↑				
Low	↑	↔	↔				
Low	↔	↔	↑				
Low	↔			↑	↔		

[a]Based on drug concentration in blood.

3. Figure 12–11 shows plasma drug concentration-time profiles following oral administration of two drugs (both drugs are eliminated exclusively by hepatic metabolism)
under the following conditions:

 Top Graph. Low extraction ratio. Plasma protein binding is: normal (case A); halved
(case B, twofold increase in fu); and doubled (case C, twofold decrease in fu).

 Bottom Graph. High extraction ratio. Tissue binding is: normal (case A); halved (case
B, twofold increase in fu_T); and doubled (case C, twofold decrease in fu_T).

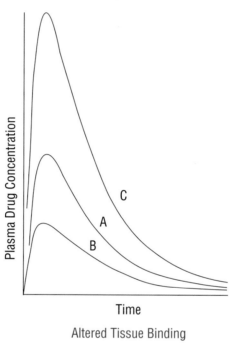

Altered Binding to Plasma Proteins

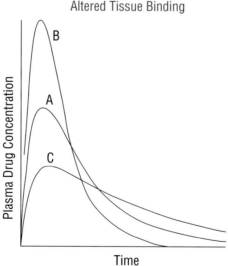

Altered Tissue Binding

Fig. 12–11.

Draw the corresponding time profiles of the unbound concentrations for the three
situations given for each of the two drugs. Be sure that each graph shows the salient

features including relative areas under the curve, peak times, and half-lives. The volumes of distribution of both drugs are greater than 100 L.

4. Although recognized for many years, the interaction between allopurinol, used in the treatment of gout, and 6-mercaptopurine, an antineoplastic agent, was not well understood until the kinetics of the interaction was elucidated. The AUC values of 6-mercaptopurine before and after pretreatment with allopurinol (100 mg orally three times a day for 2 days) following oral and i.v. administrations of 0.8 mmole of 6-mercaptopurine are given in Table 12–7. Both drugs are mostly eliminated by metabolism in the liver.

Table 12–7. Average Areas Under the Plasma 6-Mercaptopurine Concentration-Time Curves (μM–min) Before and After Allopurinol Pretreatment[a]

	Before	After
Oral	142	716
Intravenous	1207	1405

[a]Adapted from data in Zimm, S., Collins, J.M., O'Neill, D., Chabner, B.A., and Poplack, D.G.: Inhibition of first-pass metabolism in cancer chemotherapy: Interaction of 6-mercaptopurine and allopurinol. Clin. Pharmacol. Ther., 34:810–817, 1983.

The half-life of 6-mercaptopurine was not significantly changed by allopurinol treatment. For the purpose of this problem, use a blood/plasma concentration ratio of 0.6.

a. Calculate the clearance and bioavailability of 6-mercaptopurine before and after allopurinol.

b. Provide a logical kinetic explanation for the enhanced efficacy of 6-mercaptopurine in the presence of allopurinol.

5. The pharmacokinetics of DL-threo-methylphenidate (Ritalin) shows enantioselectivity. Table 12–8 summarizes the observations after i.v. (10 mg) and oral (40 mg, immediate release) doses of (+)- and (−)-isomers.

Table 12–8. AUC and Half-Lives of Methylphenidate Isomers After Separate Intravenous and Oral Administrations[a]

	INTRAVENOUS (10 mg)		ORAL (40 mg)	
	(+)-ISOMER	(−)-ISOMER	(+)-ISOMER	(−)-ISOMER
AUC (μg-hr/L)	148	89	120	15
Half-life (hr)	6.0	3.6	5.7	3.9

[a]Adapted from Srinivas, N.R., Hubbard, J.W., Korchinski, E.D., and Midha, K.K.: Enantioselective pharmacokinetics of dl-threo-methylphenidate in humans. Pharm. Res., 10:14–21, 1993.

a. Calculate the following for each isomer
   1. Clearance
   2. Oral bioavailability
   3. Volume of distribution

b. Methylphenidate is given orally. Briefly discuss the differences in absorption and disposition of these two isomers.

c. Given that the kinetics of each of the isomers is not affected by the other, estimate the approximate isomeric composition (ratio of amounts of (−) and (+)) of absorbed material entering the systemic circulation. Do you expect the ratio of the isomers in plasma to change with time? Comment briefly.

6. A drug highly bound to plasma proteins ($fu = 0.01$) has a volume of distribution of 240 L/70 kg. The liver is the only organ of elimination. The hepatic extraction ratio is 0.95 despite the fact that the fraction in blood that is unbound, fu_b is only 0.005. The hepatic blood flow is 81 L/hr.

a. Estimate the values of the following parameters for this drug: blood clearance (CL_b), clearance (CL), volumes of distribution based on drug concentrations in plasma water (Vu) and in blood (V_b), and half-life.

b. In uremic patients the volume of distribution and the fraction unbound in plasma, fu, average 140 L and 0.03, respectively. Is there any evidence that the uremic state affects the tissue binding? If so, in what direction and by what factor is tissue binding altered?

c. When this drug is infused intravenously at the same constant rate to a patient who is and has been receiving another drug, the value of fu_b is now found to be 0.03. Under steady-state conditions for both drugs, predict the ratio of the unbound concentrations of the drug in the presence and absence of the other drug.

7. Ampicillin has the following average pharmacokinetic parameter values in a 70-kg subject:

$$F(\text{oral}) = 0.6 \qquad V = 20 \text{ L}$$

$$CL = 160 \text{ mL/min} \quad fe = 0.8$$

Determine the minimum oral maintenance dose of ampicillin, to be given every 6 hr, to keep the urinary drug concentration (in ureters) above 50 mg/L. This value is the minimum inhibitory concentration against an antibiotic-resistant organism believed to be producing the patient's urinary tract infection. Use an average urine flow of 1 mL/min. Instantaneous absorption and distribution of ampicillin and steady-state conditions apply.

8. The effects of food on the oral bioavailability, systemic clearance, and AUC of propranolol are summarized in Table 12–9. Propranolol is eliminated by hepatic metabolism.

Table 12-9. Effect of Food on Bioavailability, Systemic Clearance, and Oral *AUC* of Propanolol[a]

PARAMETERS	FASTING	HIGH-PROTEIN MEAL
Bioavailability (%)	27 ± 2[b]	46 ± 4[c]
Clearance[d] (L/min)	1.00 ± 0.06	1.38 ± 0.12[c]
Oral AUC[e] (mg·hr/L)	21.8 ± 2.6	27.8 ± 10.0[f]

[a]Data from Olanoff, L.S., Walle, T., Cowart, T.D., Walle, U.K., Oexmann, M.J., and Conradi, E.C.: Food effects on propranolol systemic and oral clearances: Support for a blood flow hypothesis. Clin. Pharmacol. Ther., *40*:408–414, 1986.
[b]Mean ± SEM; N = 6.
[c]Significantly different; P < 0.05.
[d]Dose$_{i.v.}$/$AUC_{i.v.}$ (blood).
[e]$AUC_{p.o.}$ (blood) of deuterated propranolol given concurrently with the i.v. dose.
[f]Not significant; P > 0.05.

The authors suggest that an increase in hepatic blood flow is, in large part, responsible for the observations. Do you agree with the authors or not? Justify your position.

INDIVIDUALIZATION

13

VARIABILITY

OBJECTIVES

The reader will be able to:

1. List six major sources of variability in drug response.
2. Evaluate whether variability in drug response is caused by a variability in pharmacokinetics, pharmacodynamics, or both, given response and pharmacokinetic data.
3. State why variability around the mean and shape of the frequency distribution histogram of a parameter are as important as the mean itself.
4. Explain how variability in hepatic enzyme activity manifests itself in variability in both pharmacokinetic parameters and plateau plasma drug concentrations for drugs of high and low hepatic extraction ratios.
5. Suggest an approach for initiating a dosage regimen for an individual patient, given patient population pharmacokinetic data and the individual's measurable characteristics.

Thus far, the assumption has been made that all people are alike. True, as a species, humans are reasonably homogeneous, but differences among people do exist including their responsiveness to drugs. Accordingly, there is a frequent need to tailor drug administration to the individual patient. A failure to do so can lead to ineffective therapy in some patients and toxicity in others.

This section of the book is devoted to individual drug therapy. A broad overview of the subject is presented in this chapter. Evidence for and causes of variation in drug response, and approaches toward individualizing drug therapy are examined. Subsequent chapters deal in much greater detail with genetics (Chap. 14), age and weight (Chap. 15), disease (Chap. 16), interactions between drugs within the body (Chap. 17), and monitoring of plasma concentration of a drug as a guide to individualizing drug therapy (Chap. 18).

Before proceeding, a distinction must be made between an individual and the population. Consider, e.g., the results of a study designed to examine the contribution of an acute disease to variability in drug response. Suppose, of 30 patients studied during and after recovery, only 2 showed a substantial difference in response; in the remainder the difference was insignificant. Viewed as a whole, the disease would not be considered as a significant source of variability, but to the two affected patients it would. Moreover, to avoid toxicity, the dosage regimen of the drug may need to be reduced in these two patients during the disease. The lesson is clear: Average data are useful as a guide; but ultimately, information pertaining to the individual patient is all-important.

On a similar but broader point, substantial differences in response to most drugs exist among patients. Such *inter*individual variability is often reflected by a variety of marketed dose strengths of a drug. Because variability in response within a subject (*intra*individual) is generally much smaller than *inter*individual variability, once well-established, there is usually little need to subsequently adjust an individual's dosage regimen. Clearly, if *intra*individual variability were large and unpredictable, trying to titrate dosage for an individual would be an extremely difficult task, particularly for drugs with narrow therapeutic windows. Stated differently, a drug that exhibits a high *intra*individual variability in pharmacokinetics can be prescribed only if it has a wide therapeutic window.

EXPRESSIONS OF INDIVIDUAL DIFFERENCES

Evidence for interindividual differences in drug response comes from several sources. Variability in the dosage required to produce a given response is illustrated in Figure 1–5 (Chap. 1), which shows the wide range in the daily dose of warfarin needed to produce a similar degree of anticoagulant control. Variability in the intensity of response with time to a set dose is seen with the neuromuscular agent doxacurium (Fig. 13–1). As illustrated in Figs. 13–2, and 13–3, which show frequency distribution histograms of the plateau plasma concentration of the antidepressant drug nortriptyline, to a defined daily dose of the drug and the plateau unbound plasma concentration of warfarin required to produce a similar degree of anticoagulant control, variability exists in both pharmacokinetics and pharmacodynamics. Variability in pharmacokinetics was also illustrated by the wide scatter in the plateau plasma concentration of phenytoin seen following various daily doses of this drug (see Fig. 1–6, Chap. 1).

The Need for Models

The magnitude and relative contribution of pharmacokinetics and pharmacodynamics to variability in response to a given dosage within a patient population vary with the drug and, to some extent, the condition being treated. For example, with a nonsteroidal anti-inflammatory drug, the relative contribution of pharmacodynamic variability may be different when the endpoint is the relief of a headache than when it is the relief from chronic aches and pains associated with inflamed joints. In clinical practice, attempts to assign the relative contribution to pharmacokinetics and pharmacodynamics may be made based on direct observations of plasma concentration and response. The assignment could be strongly influenced, however, by the timing of the observations and the magnitude of the response,

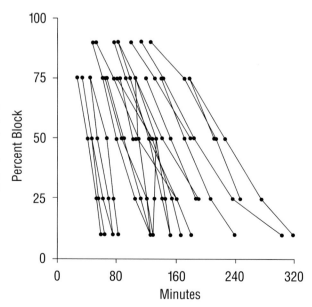

Fig. 13–1. The degree of neuromuscular blockage with time after an i.v. bolus dose of 0.04 mg/kg doxacurium to patients varies widely. (1 mg/L = 0.97 μM) (Modified from Schmith, V.D., Fiedler-Kelly, J., Abou-Donia, M., Huffman, C.S., and Grasela, T.H.: Population pharmacodynamics of doxacumin. Clin. Pharmacol. Ther., 52:528–536, 1992.)

as illustrated in Fig. 13–4. Here, a drug that displays little interpatient variability in C_{max}, t_{max} and in maximum effect, but large variability in half-life and concentration needed to produce 50% maximum response, is given orally at two doses, one that achieves close to maximal response in all patients and one that does not. At the higher dose, observations made at C_{max} would suggest little variability in either concentration or pharmacodynamics, with perhaps a greater assignment of variability to the former, as variation in plasma concentration produces relatively little change in response. At later times after this higher dose, substantial variability is observed in both concentration and response. In contrast, for

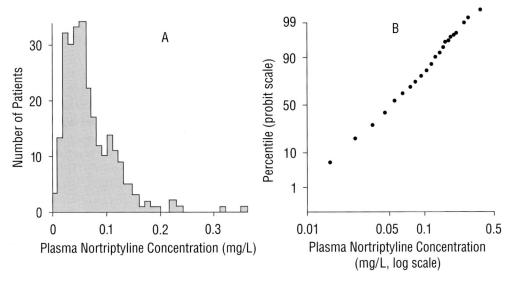

Fig. 13–2. *A,* The plateau plasma concentration of nortriptyline varies widely in 263 patients receiving a regimen of 25 mg nortriptyline orally three times daily. *B,* The concentrations are log-normally distributed, as seen from the straight line, when the percentiles of the cumulative number of patients are plotted on probit scale against the logarithm of the concentration. (1 mg/L = 3.8 µM) (Redrawn and calculated from Sjoqvist, F., Borga, O., and Orme, M.L.E.: Fundamentals of clinical pharmacology. *In* Drug Treatment. Edited by G.S. Avery. Edinburgh, Churchill Livingstone, 1976, pp. 1–42.)

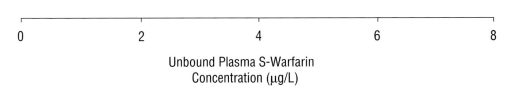

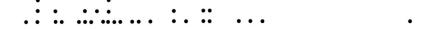

Fig. 13–3. The unbound plateau concentration of the predominately active S-warfarin associated with a similar degree of anticoagulation, varies widely among a group of 38 patients receiving racemic warfarin. (1 mg/L = 3.3 µM) (Adapted from Chan, E., McLachlan, A.J., Pegg, M., Mackay, A.D., Cole, R. B., and Rowland, M.: Disposition of warfarin enantiomers and metabolites in patients during multiple dosing. Br. J. Clin. Pharmacol., 37:563–569, 1994.

the lower dose, at t_{max} there is still little interpatient variability in C_{max}, but now there is considerable variability in response. This dependence on dose and time in the assignment of variability is minimized by expressing variability not in terms of observations but rather in terms of the parameter values defining pharmacokinetics and pharmacodynamics, that is, in F, ka, CL, and V for pharmacokinetics, and in maximal response, concentration to achieve 50% of the maximum response, and the factor defining the steepness of the concentration–response relationship for pharmacodynamics (Chap. 20, Pharmacologic Response). Once variability in these parameters is defined, the expected variability in concentration and response within the patient population associated with given dosage regimens can be estimated. The accuracy of the models defining pharmacokinetics and pharmacodynamics is obviously critical to an understanding of variability in patient response. Where appropriate, these models should incorporate such factors as protein binding, active metabolites, and tolerance.

DESCRIBING VARIABILITY

Knowing how a particular parameter varies within the patient population is important in therapy. To illustrate this statement consider the frequency distributions in clearance of

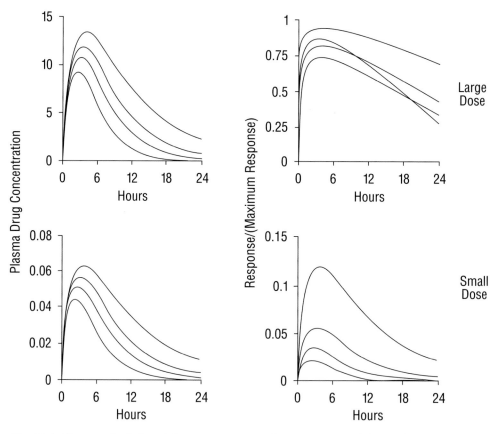

Fig. 13–4. The interindividual variability in concentration and response varies with dose and time of observation. Shown are plasma concentrations (left) and responses (right) following large and small doses of a drug that displays little interpatient variability in C_{max}, t_{max} and maximum response, but large interpatient variability in half-life and concentration needed to produce 50% maximum response. High dose (top): at t_{max}, the maximum response in all patients is produced with little variability in either C_{max} or response. Greater variability in concentration and response is seen at later times. Low dose (bottom): at t_{max}, variability in C_{max} is still low, but that in response is now considerable.

the three hypothetical drugs shown in Fig. 13–5. The mean, or central tendency, for all three drugs is the same, but the variability about the mean is very different. For Drugs A and B, the distribution is unimodal and normal; here the mean represents the typical value of clearance expected in the population. As variability about the mean is much greater for Drug B than for Drug A, one has much less confidence that the mean of Drug B applies to an individual patient. For Drug C, distribution in clearance is bimodal, signifying that there are two major groups within the population: those with high and low clearances. Obviously, in this case, the mean is one of the most unlikely values to be found in this population.

Generally, distributions of pharmacokinetic parameters or observations are unimodal rather than polymodal, and they are often skewed rather than normal, as seen, e.g., in the frequency distribution of plateau plasma concentrations of nortriptyline (Fig. 13–2A). A more symmetrical distribution is often obtained with a logarithmic transformation of the parameter; such distributions are said to be log-normal. A common method of examining for log-normal distribution is to plot the cumulative frequency, or percentile, on a probit scale against the logarithm of the variable. The distribution is taken to be log-normal if the points lie on a straight line. As can be seen in Fig. 13–2B, this is the case for the plateau plasma concentration of nortriptyline. In such cases the median, or value above and below which there are equal numbers, differs from the mean. For nortriptyline, examination of Fig. 13–2B indicates that the median concentration is 0.05 mg/L, which is less than the average value of 0.069 mg/L.

A comment on the quantitation of variability is needed here. Variance is a measure of the deviations of the observations about the mean; it is defined as the sum of the squares of these deviations. While useful to convey variability within a particular set of observations, variance does not allow ready comparison of variability across sets of observations of different magnitude. Suppose, e.g., clearance in an individual is 50 mL/min and the mean is 100 mL/min; the squared deviation is 2500 $(mL/min)^2$. If instead clearance had been quoted in L/min, the squared deviation would be $(0.05 - 0.1)^2$, or 0.0025 $(L/min)^2$. Coefficient of variation, which expresses variability with respect to the mean value, overcomes this problem. Specifically, it is the square root of variance (the standard deviation) normalized to the mean. In the example above, the deviation normalized to the mean is 0.5 and is independent of the units of clearance. Furthermore, a large coefficient of variation now always signifies a high degree of variability. Subsequently, in the book, *high* and *low variability* refer to distributions that have high and low coefficients of variation, respectively.

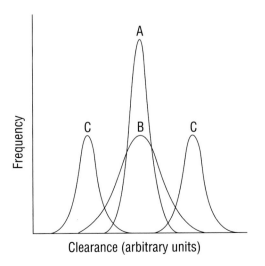

Fig. 13–5. As the frequency distributions for the clearance of three hypothetical drugs (A, B, C) show, it is as important to define variability around the mean and the shape of the frequency distribution curve as it is to define the mean itself.

WHY PEOPLE DIFFER

The reasons why people differ in their responsiveness to drugs in medicinal products are manifold and include, in general order of importance, genetics, disease, age, drugs given concomitantly, and a variety of environmental factors. Although inheritance accounts for a substantial part of the differences in response among individuals, much of this variability is largely unpredictable. Increasingly, however, this source of variability, particularly that related to drug metabolism, is being understood and made more predictable using the tools of molecular biology (Chap. 14, Genetics).

Disease can be an added source of variation in drug response. Usual dosage regimens may need to be modified substantially in patients with renal function impairment, hepatic disorders, congestive cardiac failure, thyroid disorders, gastrointestinal disorders, and other diseases. The modification may apply to the drug being used to treat the specific disease but may apply equally well to other drugs the patient is receiving. For example, to prevent excessive accumulation and so reduce the risk of toxicity, the dosage of the antibiotic gentamicin used to treat a pleural infection of a patient must be reduced if the patient also has compromised renal function. Similarly, hyperthyroidic patients require higher than usual doses of digoxin, a drug used to improve cardiac efficiency. Moreover, a modification in dosage may arise not only from the direct impairment of a diseased organ but also from secondary events that accompany the disease. Drug metabolism, e.g., may be modified in patients with renal disease; plasma and tissue binding of drugs may be altered in patients with uremia and hepatic disorders.

Age, weight, and concomitantly administered drugs are important because they are sources of variability that can be taken into account. Gender-linked differences in hormonal balance, body composition, and activity of certain enzymes manifest themselves in differences in both pharmacokinetics and responsiveness, but overall, the effect of gender is small.

Table 13–1 lists examples of additional factors known to contribute to variability in drug response. Perhaps the most important factor is noncompliance. Noncompliance includes the taking of drug at the wrong time, the omission or supplementation of prescribed dose, and the stopping of therapy, either because the patient begins to feel better or because of development of side-effects that the patient considers unacceptable. Whatever the reason, these problems lie in the area of patient counselling and education. Occasionally, plasma concentration data are used as an objective measure of noncompliance.

Pharmaceutical formulation and the process used to manufacture a product can be important as both can affect the rate of release, and hence entry, into the body (Chap. 9).

Table 13–1. Additional Factors Known to Contribute to Variability in Drug Response

FACTORS	OBSERVATIONS AND REMARKS
Noncompliance	A major problem in clinical practice; solution lies in patient education.
Route of administration	Patient response can vary on changing the route of administration. Not only pharmacokinetics of drug but also metabolite concentrations can change.
Food	Rate and occasionally extent of absorption are affected by eating. Effects depend on composition of food. Severe protein restriction may reduce the rate of drug metabolism.
Pollutants	Drug effects are often less in smokers and workers occupationally exposed to pesticides; a result of enhanced drug metabolism.
Time of day and season	Diurnal variations are seen in pharmacokinetics and in drug response. These effects have been sufficiently important to lead to the development of a new subject, chronopharmacology.
Location	Dose requirements of some drugs differ between patients living in town and in the country.

A well-designed formulation diminishes the degree of variability in the release character-istics of a drug *in vivo*. Good manufacturing practice, with careful control of the process variables, ensures the manufacture of a reliable product. Drugs are given enterally, topi-cally, parenterally, and by inhalation. Route of administration not only can affect the con-centration locally and systemically but also can alter the systemic concentration of metab-olite compared with that of drug (Chap. 21). All these factors can profoundly affect the response to a given dose or regimen.

Food, particularly fat, slows gastric emptying and so decreases the rate of drug absorp-tion. Oral bioavailability is not usually affected by food, but there are many exceptions to this statement. Food is a complex mixture of chemicals, each potentially capable of inter-acting with drugs. Recall from Chap. 9, e.g., that the oral bioavailability of tetracycline is reduced when taken with milk, partly because of the formation of an insoluble complex with calcium. Recall also that a slowing of gastric emptying may increase the oral bioavail-ability of a sparingly soluble drug, such as griseofulvin. Diet may also affect drug metab-olism. Enzyme synthesis is ultimately dependent on protein intake. When protein intake is severely reduced for prolonged periods, particularly because of an imbalanced diet, drug metabolism may be impaired. Conversely, a high protein intake may cause enzyme induc-tion.

Chronopharmacology is the study of the influence of time on drug response. Many endogenous substances, e.g., hormones, are known to undergo cyclic changes in concen-tration in plasma and tissue with time. The amplitude of the change in concentration varies among substances. The period of the cycle is often diurnal, approximately 24 hr, although there may be both shorter and longer cycles upon which the daily one is superimposed. The menstrual cycle and seasonal variations in the concentrations of some endogenous substances are examples of cycles with a long period. Drug responses may therefore change with time of day, day of the month, or season of the year. Particular note of this phenom-enon is taken in cancer chemotherapy. Many chemotherapeutic agents have very narrow margins of safety and are given in combination. Appropriate phasing in the timing of ad-ministration of each drug during the day can improve the margin of safety.

Cigarette smoking tends to reduce clinical and toxic effects of some drugs, including chlordiazepoxide, diazepam, and theophylline. The drugs affected are extensively metab-olized by hepatic oxidation; induction of the drug-metabolizing enzymes is the likely cause. Many environmental pollutants exist in higher concentrations in the city than in the country; they can also stimulate synthesis of hepatic metabolic enzymes.

Identifying the Sources of Variability

In practice, all the above-mentioned factors can contribute to observed variability in re-sponse, and care must be taken to ensure an appropriate conclusion is reached when trying to assign causes of variability. Consider, e.g., the data displayed in Fig. 13–6 which show the half-lives of phenylbutazone, a once widely used drug, in healthy subjects and in patients with hepatic disease (primarily cirrhosis). Initially, no difference was revealed between the two groups, except for a greater variability in the half-life among the patients with hepatic disease (Fig. 13–6A). When, however, both groups were further subdivided on the basis of whether they received other drugs, a clearer picture emerged (Fig. 13–6B). Of those receiving no other drugs, patients with hepatic disease handled phenylbutazone more slowly than did healthy subjects. Evidently, some of the other drugs received hasten phen-ylbutazone elimination.

Various strategies can be employed to identify sources of variability in response. The classic design is one in which as many of the variables as possible are fixed, apart from the one of interest. For example, to test if renal disease affects the pharmacokinetics of a drug, all other factors such as age, gender, other drugs, and diet should be held constant. The ideal would be a longitudinal cross-over design in which each patient acts as his or her own control. This design is often not possible, however. The patient with renal disease is generally not available for study prior to the disease, and renal disease is generally irreversible. The penalty for deviating from such a design is greater variability with loss of efficiency, such that many more patients are needed to allow a firm conclusion to be made about the contribution of a factor to variability. The benefit of loosening the design, however, is that many patients who might otherwise be excluded can be a part of the study. In this category, e.g., are elderly patients suffering from several diseases and requiring many drugs, including the one of interest. Care must still be taken, however, to ensure that a sufficient number of patients are included with each of the attributes or conditions of interest.

DEFINING THE DOSE–RESPONSE RELATIONSHIP

Variability has an important bearing on the *estimation* of dose–response relationships in clinical trials. A common procedure is to divide patients into several groups, each group receiving a different dose of drug such as 5, 10, or 20 mg. An attempt to establish a dose–response relationship is then made on the mean data for each group, using variability within groups to test for levels of statistical significance. A problem arises when much of the variability between dose and response resides in pharmacokinetics such that there is considerable overlap in the plasma concentrations among the groups. Thus, individuals from

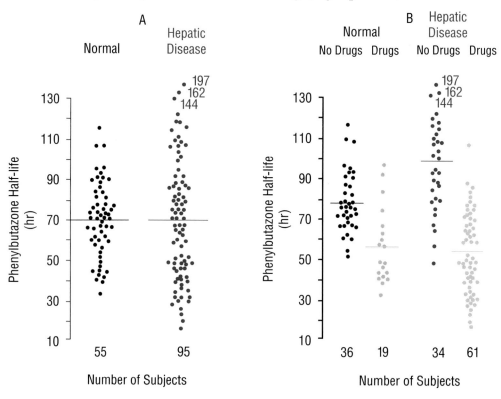

Fig. 13–6 *A*, No difference is seen between the average half-life of phenylbutazone (horizontal line) in normal subjects (black points) and that in patients with hepatic disease (colored points). *B*, After separating those who take other drugs (light points) from those who do not (dark points), the prolonged elimination of phenylbutazone in patients with hepatic disease becomes evident. In both groups the half-life tends to be shorter when other drugs are taken concurrently. (Redrawn from Levi, A.J., Sherlock, S., and Walker, D.: Phenylbutazone and iso-niazid metabolism in patients with liver disease in relation to previous drug therapy. Lancet, *1*:1275–1279, 1968.)

the high- and low-dose groups can have the same plasma concentration (and response), namely, those in the low-dose group with a low clearance and those in the high-dose group with a high clearance of the drug. The overall effect, by increasing variability within each group, is to weaken the ability to detect a dose–response relationship.

One solution is to increase the number of subjects in each group to reduce the uncertainty of estimating the mean response at each dose level. Here, the problem is often one of not knowing in advance how many subjects would be needed in the trial, as well as the added expense of an increased number of subjects. Another solution is to expose each patient to several dose levels of the drug. This last solution has the distinct advantage of not only increasing the chances of establishing a dose–response relationship, but also of providing an estimate of interpatient variability in the relationship. Unfortunately, in practice, this design is not always possible, especially for drugs for which the full effect only occurs after several months or longer into drug administration. A third solution is the concentration-controlled clinical trial. In this approach, the pharmacokinetics of the drug is first evaluated in the patient cohort and then, based on this information, doses are adjusted so that the plasma concentration in each patient lies in one of several tightly defined bands. This more elaborate, and sometimes more expensive, design enables much clearer statements to be made about the concentration–response relationship and about interpatient variability in pharmacokinetics. However, it may have limited utility for dose recommendations, if a poor correlation is found between plasma drug concentration and response. Many other designs, varying in complexity, each with advantages and disadvantages, can be envisaged. In all cases, variability is a central issue.

KINETIC MANIFESTATIONS

Considerable variability in enzymatic activity and, to a lesser extent, in plasma and tissue binding exists even among healthy individuals. How such variability manifests itself, in pharmacokinetic parameters and in such measurements as plateau plasma concentration, depends on the hepatic extraction ratio and route of administration of the drug. For example, the large interindividual variability in half-life of theophylline (Fig. 13–7) can be explained primarily by variations in hepatic enzyme activity, probably associated with variations in the amounts of the enzymes responsible for metabolism of this compound. This conclusion is based on theophylline being predominantly metabolized in the liver, having a low extraction ratio, and being only moderately bound to plasma and tissue components. In contrast, such a high degree of variability in enzymatic activity is expected to be masked in the clearance of a drug having a high hepatic extraction ratio, because clearance tends to be perfusion rate-limited and hepatic blood flow is relatively constant among healthy individuals. Moreover, unless plasma and tissue binding are highly variable, volume of distribution, and hence disposition kinetics, of such a drug are much the same for all healthy individuals. This is so for propranolol (Fig. 13–8) a drug of high hepatic clearance.

As described in Chap. 11, when considering induction and inhibition, changes in hepatic enzyme activity result in variations in oral bioavailability for a drug with a high hepatic extraction ratio. Accordingly, with subsequent disposition being controlled by hepatic perfusion, a series of similarly shaped plasma drug concentration-time profiles, but reaching different peak concentrations, should be seen among individuals with varying enzyme activity receiving the same oral dose of drug. This is indeed seen with propranolol (Fig. 13–8). In contrast, for a drug with a low hepatic extraction ratio, such as theophylline, variation in enzymatic activity is reflected by variation in clearance (and half-life) rather than in oral bioavailability (and maximum plasma concentration), which is always high (Fig. 13–7).

The impact of variability in oral bioavailability, because of a high first-pass effect, depends on the intended use of a drug. It may result in patients' needing different single oral doses to produce the same effect, as might be the case if the drug is to be used as a sedative hypnotic or to relieve a headache. However, if the drug is intended for chronic use, the degree of variability in average plateau concentration should not be inherently different from that which exists for a drug of low hepatic clearance and having the same degree of variability in enzymatic activity. (Fig. 13–9). This statement is based on the following reasoning. At plateau, the average concentration ($C_{ss,av}$) is given by

$$C_{ss,av} = \frac{F \cdot \text{Dose}}{CL \cdot \tau} \qquad 1$$

where τ is the dosing interval. For a drug of high hepatic clearance, variability in $C_{ss,av}$ reflects variability in enzyme activity through F; whereas, for a drug of low hepatic clearance, variability in $C_{ss,av}$ reflects variability in enzyme activity through CL (with $F \approx 1$). In both cases the oral dosing rate (Dose/τ) would need to be adjusted by the same degree to maintain a common $C_{ss,av}$ within subjects. This is achieved by adjusting the dose for the high-clearance drug (as half-life is relatively constant) and perhaps by a mixture of adjusting dose and dosing interval (given that half-life varies) for the low-clearance drug. Of major importance is the underlying variation in enzyme activity, which differs from one enzyme system to another. Obviously, to minimize variation in pharmacokinetics, molecules would need to be selected which, if metabolized, are substrates of enzyme systems that show the least variability among subjects. Unfortunately, current information is insufficient to make this selection.

Fig. 13–7. Five healthy subjects each received 350 mg theophylline orally, in solution as an elixir. Large differences in *AUC* are seen, but in contrast to propranolol (Fig. 13–8), the peak concentrations are almost identical. These observations are as expected for theophylline, a drug of low hepatic extraction that is extensively metabolized in the liver. Variability in hepatic enzyme activity is manifested primarily in variability in clearance, and hence half-life; the weight-corrected volume of distribution of theophylline is relatively constant. Oral bioavailability is close to 100% in all subjects, and because absorption occurred much faster than elimination, peak concentrations are similar. Each symbol refers to a different subject. (Data provided by S. Toon, personal observations.)

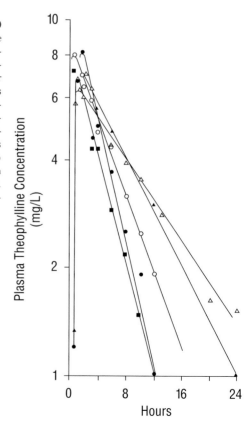

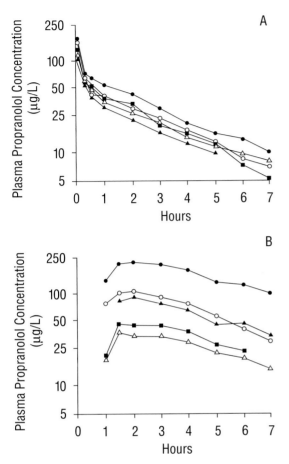

Fig. 13–8. Five healthy subjects each received propranolol i.v. (10 mg over 10 min) and orally (80 mg) on separate occasions. The plasma concentration-time profiles were very similar following i.v. administration (*A*), but showed large differences, particularly in peak concentration and *AUC*, following oral administration (*B*). Such differences in variability with the two routes of administration are expected for propranolol, a drug of high hepatic extraction. Variability in hepatic enzyme activity among the group is manifested primarily in variability in oral bioavailability (16–60%), rather than in differences in clearance (1 L/min) which is perfusion rate-limited, or hence in half-life (1 mg/L = 3.9 µM). (Redrawn from Shand, D.G., Nuckolls, E.M., and Oates, J.A.: Plasma propranolol levels in adults, with observations in four children. Clin. Pharmacol. Ther., *11*:112–120, 1970. Reproduced with permission of C.V. Mosby.)

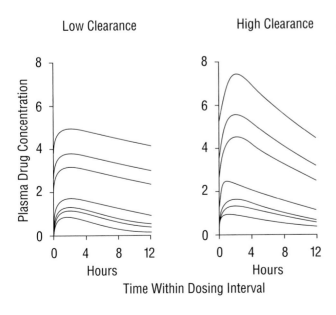

Fig. 13–9. Expected plasma drug concentration-time profiles during a dosing interval at steady state following chronic oral administration of a drug; changes in hepatic enzyme activity for a drug of low extraction ratio (left) and high extraction ratio (right). In this simulation both drugs are substrates for the same enzyme, the concentration (and intrinsic clearance) of which varies ninefold. The result is a corresponding ninefold variation in the average concentration. Prediction is based on the well-stirred model of hepatic elimination.

It follows from the foregoing that there is no inherent reason to believe that a set variation in enzyme activity (caused by a variation in concentration of enzymes, inhibitors, or inducers) should cause a greater *intra*individual variation in pharmacokinetic parameters, or in $C_{ss,av}$, for a drug of high hepatic extraction than for one of low hepatic extraction.

DOSE STRENGTHS

Products are frequently marketed as unit doses of defined strength, such as 50 or 100 mg. Obviously, if the therapeutic index is sufficiently wide, all patients can receive the same dose strength almost irrespective of any differences in pharmacokinetics among the patient population. A narrow therapeutic index necessitates the manufacture of several dose strengths, however. Although the final number of strengths chosen depends on many practical issues, a rough estimate of the number can be calculated in the following manner for drugs intended for chronic maintenance therapy.

Suppose that the maximum and minimum clearance values that encompass 95% of the patient population, designated CL_{max} and CL_{min}, respectively, differ by a factor of six. That is, $CL_{max} = 6 \cdot CL_{min}$. It would then follow from the familiar relationship

$$\frac{F \cdot \text{Dose}}{\tau} = CL \cdot C_{ss,av} \qquad\qquad 2$$

that the range of dosing rates needed would be sixfold if the object was to obtain the same $C_{ss,av}$ in all patients. In practice, the therapeutic index is sufficiently wide to allow some tolerance. Let average plateau concentrations within 20% of the optimal value be acceptable. Accordingly, the highest dosing rate that could be given to a patient with a clearance value of CL_{min} is one that produces a $C_{ss,av}$ that is 1.2 times the optimal value; the lowest dosing rate that could be given to a patient with a clearance of CL_{max} is one that produces a $C_{ss,av}$ that is 0.8 times the optimal value. The range of associated dosing rates (and hence amounts, if the dosing interval is kept constant) is fourfold. Now, usually, adjacent dose strengths differ by a factor of 2. Therefore, in the current example, if the smallest dose strength is 50 mg, it would be reasonable to market three dose strengths, 50-mg, 100-mg, and 200-mg products, which would suffice for 95% of the population. Of the outstanding 5%, those with a particularly high clearance may be accommodated with a larger-than-usual maintenance dose, comprising a combination of the marketed unit dose strengths, or they may receive a marketed dose strength more frequently. Those with a particularly low clearance value may be accommodated by taking the lowest available dose strength less frequently than usual, because the half-life in this group is likely to be the longest in the population.

ACCOUNTING FOR VARIABILITY

It remains to be seen how information on variability can be used to devise an optimal dosage regimen of a drug for treatment of a disease in an individual patient. Obviously, the desired objective would be most efficiently achieved if the individual's dosage requirements could be calculated *before administering the drug*. While this ideal cannot be totally met in practice, some success may be achieved by adopting the following type of approach, which applies when all patients require the same (unbound) plasma concentration range. The approach is to move from the population pharmacokinetic parameter estimates to the individual patient's values.

The first step is to identify the most variable parameter within the patient population. Variability in the various pharmacokinetic parameters within the patient population differs widely among drugs, as shown in Table 13–2 for a number of representative drugs. For some drugs, such as digoxin and propranolol, there is substantial variability in absorption, but for different reasons. With digoxin the variability is caused primarily by differences in pharmaceutical formulation, but with propranolol it is caused by differences in the extent of first-pass loss, as mentioned previously (Fig. 13–8). For other drugs, such as theophylline, the only substantial variability is in clearance. With others, amiodarone and phenytoin included, significant variability exists in all parameters. Finally, for some, considerable variability exists in plasma protein binding.

The next step is to try to accommodate as much of the variability as possible with measurable characteristics. If the characteristic is discrete and independent, this can be achieved by partitioning the population into subpopulations. For example, as illustrated for clearance in Fig. 13–10, if the discrete characteristics are hepatic disease and smoking, then the population would be divided into four categories: those who smoke and have no hepatic disease; those who smoke and have hepatic disease; those who have hepatic disease

Table 13–2. Degree of Variability in the Oral Absorption, Disposition, and Specific Distribution of Representative Drugs Within the Patient Population[a]

DRUG	F	V	Cl	fu
Amiodarone	+	+ +	+	+ +
Cyclosporine	+	−	+	+
Digoxin	+	+	+ +	−
Ibuprofen	−	−	+	+
Interferon Alfa	N/A	+	+	?
Lithium	−	−	+	−
Phenobarbital	−	−	+ +	−
Phenytoin	+	+	+ +	+ +
Propranolol	+ +	+ +	+	+ +
Quinidine	+	+ +	+	+
Salicylic acid	−	+	+ +	+ +
Theophylline	−	−	+ +	−

[a]Symbols: − = little variability; + = moderate variability; + + = substantial variability; NA = not applicable.

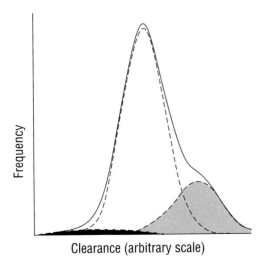

Clearance (arbitrary scale)

Fig. 13–10. The frequency distribution of clearance within the total patient population (——) is a function of the shape of the frequency distribution within the various subpopulations that comprise the total patient population and the relative sizes of each of these subpopulations. In this simulation the variables are smoking and hepatic disease, and the subpopulations are: (- - -)—those who neither have hepatic disease nor smoke (78.4%), the majority; (shaded gray)—those who smoke but have no hepatic disease (19.6%); (shaded black)—those who have hepatic disease but do not smoke (1.6%); and those who both smoke and have hepatic disease. The size of the last subpopulation is too small (0.4%) to be seen in this figure. The average values for clearance in the four subpopulations were set at 1, 1.5, 0.5, and 0.75 units, respectively, assuming that smoking increases clearance by induction and that clearance is reduced in hepatic disease.

but do not smoke; and those who neither have hepatic disease nor smoke. The relative size and shape of the distribution curve of each subpopulation determine the frequency distribution for the entire population. If, on the other hand, the measurable characteristic is continuous, such as age, weight, or degree of renal function, it may be possible to find a functional relationship with one or more pharmacokinetic parameters, as seen, e.g., between the renal clearance of the cephalosporin, ceftazidime (and many other drugs), and creatinine clearance, a graded measure of renal function (Fig. 13–11).

To envisage how the entire strategy would work, consider the data in Fig. 13–12 for a drug, partly metabolized in the liver and partly excreted unchanged, for which population pharmacokinetics are: oral bioavailability, 0.82; volume of distribution, 10.3 L; renal clearance, 6.7 L/hr; and metabolic clearance, 16.2 L/hr. Depicted are four tablets, representing

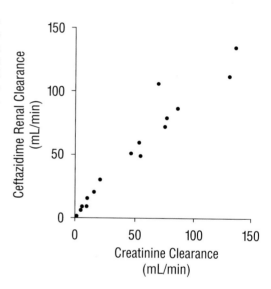

Fig. 13–11.   The renal clearance of the cephalosporin, ceftazidime, varies in direct proportion to creatinine clearance in a group of 19 patients with varying degrees of renal function. (Drawn from the data of van Dalen, R., Vree, T.B., Baars, A.M., and Termond, E.: Dosage adjustment for ceftazidime in patients with impaired renal function. Euro. J. Clin. Pharmacol., *30*:597–605, 1986.)

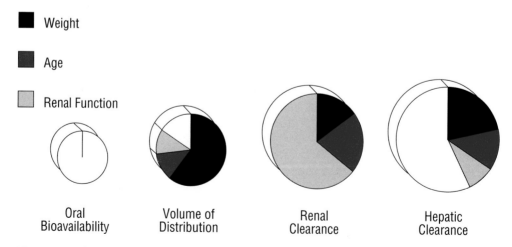

Fig. 13–12.   Schematic representation of variability in various pharmacokinetic parameters within a population. The size of each tablet is related to the degree of variability in the parameter. The portion of the tablet labeled weight, age, or renal function reflect the fractions of the total variability accounted for by each of these factors.

oral bioavailability, volume of distribution, renal clearance, and metabolic clearance. The size of each tablet is a measure of variability of that parameter within the patient population. For this drug, oral bioavailability is the least and hepatic clearance is the most variable. Stated differently, greatest confidence exists in assigning the population value of oral bio-availability to the patient; least confidence exists in assigning the population value of hepatic clearance to the patient. Moreover, as the population value for hepatic clearance is much greater than that for renal clearance, variability in total clearance within the population is also high.

Not unexpectedly, weight accounts for most of the variability in volume of distribution and for some of the variability in hepatic clearance. Age, separated from its influence on body weight, accounts for some of the variability in hepatic clearance and, to a lesser extent, in volume of distribution. Renal function also accounts for almost all the variability in renal clearance. Surprisingly perhaps, renal function helps to explain some of the variability in metabolic clearance and volume of distribution, but drug distribution and metabolism can be altered in patients with renal function impairment (see Chap. 16). None of the variability in oral bioavailability is accounted for but, as mentioned, it is small and acceptable.

Finally, the inability to account for most of the variability in metabolic clearance should be noted. None of the characteristics included could adequately account for the influence of genetics, disease, and other drugs on this parameter. Markers of genetic control of drug metabolism have been developed that help to explain much of the inherited interindividual differences in metabolic clearance of certain drugs (Chap. 14). Few, however, are employed clinically.

Returning to the individual patient, correcting the population pharmacokinetics for the patient's weight, age, and renal function should give reasonable individual estimates of F, V, and CL_R but little confidence in the estimate of CL_H and hence total clearance. As the ratio F/V strongly influences the peak plasma concentration after a single dose, reasonable confidence can be expected in estimating the patient's loading dose, if required. However, since the ratio F/CL controls the average plateau concentration, less confidence can be expected in estimating the patient's maintenance dose requirements. If the therapeutic index of the drug is sufficiently narrow, there may be a case for monitoring the plasma concentration to aid in adjusting the maintenance dosing rate through feedback as de-scribed in Chap. 18 (Concentration Monitoring). Nonetheless, the estimate of maintenance dose based on the information provided in Fig. 13–12 should be better than using the mean parameter values for the whole population. Clearly, if the drug had just been excreted unchanged, the probability of being able to estimate the correct dosage regimen for the patient would have been much higher.

The approach presented above for predicting an individual's dosage regimen before administering the drug is based on the assumption that little interindividual variability in pharmacodynamics exists. This is not always so. Sometimes, most of the variability in re-sponse is due to differences in pharmacodynamics. Although knowing the mean pharma-cokinetic parameters of the drug may help to explain the time course in response, quan-tifying pharmacokinetic variability adds little to the ability to predict individual dosage. Nonetheless, the basic strategy still holds: to determine the relative contribution of measur-able characteristics, such as age and weight, to response within the patient population, and then use the individual's characteristics to predict his or her initial dosage regimen. Fre-quently, however, age, weight, and other measurable characteristics fail to account for much of the variability in pharmacodynamics. Then, there is little choice but to start the individual patient on the typical dosage regimen, which may be far from the individual's requirement. Subsequent adjustment in the regimen is made based on response produced. Here, as with feedback based on plasma concentration, the use of a model helps in dose adjustment (Chap. 18, Concentration Monitoring).

STUDY PROBLEMS

(Answers to Study Problems are in Appendix II.)

1. a. List three major sources of variability in response to drugs.
   b. What pharmacokinetic parameters vary the most in the patient population for digoxin, phenytoin, theophylline, and ibuprofen?
2. Discuss briefly why mean pharmacokinetic parameters alone are not sufficient to characterize how a drug is handled in the patient population.
3. Suggest which pharmacokinetic parameter is most likely to explain the variation in the plateau concentration of nortriptyline shown in Fig. 13–2. The drug is lipophilic, stable in the gastrointestinal tract, and little is excreted unchanged.
4. By coincidence, the weight, age, and renal function of the patient, discussed under the section "Accounting for Variability" corresponded to the patient population values. Yet, when the pharmacokinetics of the drug was studied in the patient, the values of F, 0.42, and V, 22 L, were considerably different (outside the 99% confidence intervals) from the population values of F, 0.82, and V, 10.3 L. Briefly discuss how this could arise.
5. Lithium, used in the treatment of patients with manic depression, is administered chronically. The therapeutic window of this drug is narrow (0.4 to 1.4 milliequivalents/L), its fe is 1, its and dosage requirements vary widely among patients.
   a. What is a major cause of this variability in dosage?
   b. What characteristic of a patient should help to tailor his or her dosage requirement?
6. In a group of healthy subjects, the average pharmacokinetic parameters of the β-adrenergic blocking agent alprenolol, which is eliminated almost exclusively by hepatic metabolism, were found to be volume of distribution, 230 L; clearance, 1.06 L/min; and half-life, 2.5 hr. After i.v. administration, values of these parameters differed little within this group; yet, when the drug was ingested orally, both peak plasma concentration and AUC varied over a fivefold range. Suggest why variability in the observed plasma concentration-time curve is much greater after oral than after i.v. administration.
7. The following data (Table 13–3) were obtained in a study of the pharmacokinetic variability of a drug that is predominantly excreted unchanged, $fe = 0.98$. The drug was infused intravenously in five subjects at a constant rate of 20 mg/hr for 48 hr. The fraction unbound was found to be independent of drug concentration but did vary among the subjects.

Table 13-3.

Subject	1	2	3	4	5
Steady-state plasma concentration (mg/L)	2.5	1.6	3.0	1.5	2.3
Postinfusion Half-life (hr)	14.4	5.9	4.7	9.9	8.2
Fraction unbound	0.1	0.15	0.09	0.16	0.01

   a. Analyze the data to identify the most and the least variable (use the *range/mean* as your index of variability) of the following parameters:
   Clearance based on unbound drug (CLu), fraction unbound in plasma (fu), and fraction unbound in tissue (fu_T). Use a V_{TW} of 39 L.
   b. Discuss briefly the therapeutic implications of these data with regard to the rate of attainment and maintenance of a "therapeutic" concentration in the various subjects.

8. The 95% confidence interval of clearance of a drug within a patient population is 1.5 to 7.5 L/hr, a difference of fivefold. Other pharmacokinetic parameters, F and V, vary much less. Therapeutic activity resides exclusively with the drug, and not the metabolites. Discuss the potential impact of this variability in clearance on the attempt to define a dose–response relationship within a patient population, using a design in which patients are randomly assigned to one of three groups receiving a multiple-dose regimen of either 50, 100, or 200 mg daily of the drug.

GENETICS

OBJECTIVES

The reader will be able to:

1. Give examples of inherited variability in pharmacokinetics and pharmacodynamics.

2. Define the terms: pharmacogenetics, genotype, phenotype, genetic polymorphism, idiosyncrasy, allele, homozygous, and heterozygous.

3. Demonstrate how population studies and studies in twins can be used to indicate the existence of genetic polymorphism.

4. State under what circumstances phenotype status is of therapeutic value.

5. Describe at least two ways, other than twin studies, in which genetic polymorphism can be demonstrated and list two examples of each.

Inheritance accounts for a large part of both the striking and subtle differences among individuals, including much of the variation in response to an administered drug. *Pharmacogenetics* is the study of hereditary variations in drug response. Before proceeding to consider specific examples, some definitions are important to an understanding of the subject.

The basic biological unit of heredity is the gene. *Genotype* is the fundamental assortment of genes of an individual, the blueprint, while *phenotype* is the outward characteristic expression of an individual. The mode of inheritance is either monogenic or polygenic depending on whether it is transmitted by a gene at a single locus or by genes at multiple loci on the chromosomes. Tables 14–1 and 14–2 list genetic conditions that affect the pharmacokinetics and pharmacodynamics of some drugs. All of these conditions are transmitted monogenically. Many are expressed as polymorphisms, others as rare phenotypes. Genetic polymorphism defines monogenic traits that exist in the normal population in at least two phenotypes, neither of which is rare (less than 1%). Monogenically controlled conditions are often detected as a dramatic and, abnormal drug response, that is, *a drug idiosyncrasy*. They may also be detected in population studies by a polymodal frequency distribution of the characteristic or some measure of it. Polygenically controlled variations give rise to a unimodal frequency distribution and are usually detected in studies of twins.

An *allele* is one of two or more different genes containing specific inheritable characteristics that occupy corresponding positions (loci) on paired chromosomes. An allele is dominant if it expresses itself and recessive if it does not. An individual possessing a pair of identical alleles, either dominant or recessive is *homozygous* for the gene. A union of a dominant with a recessive allele produces a *heterozygous* individual for that characteristic. Both homozygous individuals with dominant alleles and heterozygous individuals may show the same phenotype, and homozygous individuals with recessive alleles may show another.

Table 14–1. Some Genetically Determined Variations in Pharmacokinetics

CONDITION/ ARCHETYPE	CLINICAL CONSEQUENCE WITH ARCHETYPE	ENZYME INVOLVED	FREQUENCY OF POOR METABOLIZER	DRUG SUBSTRATES
Poor and extensive hydroxylation of debrisoquine	Poor metabolizers may show toxicity	CYP2D6	5–10% Caucasians 3.8% Blacks 0.9% Orientals 1% Arabs	Encainide, flecainide bufurolol, timolol, codeine, nortriptyline, metoprolol, dextromethorpan, sparteine, and perhexiline
Poor and extensive hydroxylation of S-mephenytoin	Poor metabolizers may show increased sedation	CYP2C(18?)	3–5% Caucasians, 16% Orientals	Diazepam
Poor and extensive S-methylation of 6-mercaptopurine	Rapid methylators may show high risk of treatment failure	?	14% Caucasians, slow methylation	Azathioprine
Slow and fast acetylation of isoniazid	Slow acetylators may show toxicity	N-Acetyltransferase (NAT2)	60% Caucasians 10–20% Orientals and Eskimos	p-Aminosalicylic acid, amrinone, aminoglutethimide, clonazepam, dapsone, hydralazine, phenelzine; procainamide, promizole, sulfamethazine, sulfasalazine
Slow hydrolysis of succinylcholine	Prolonged apnea	Cholinesterase in plasma	Several abnormal genes; most common disorder 1 in 2500	Succinylcholine

Table 14–2. Some Genetically Determined Variations in Pharmacodynamics

CONDITION	CLINICAL CONSEQUENCE	RECEPTOR/ ENZYME INVOLVED	FREQUENCY	DRUGS THAT PRODUCE THE RESPONSE
Warfarin resistance	Resistance to anticoagulation	Altered receptor or enzyme in liver with increased affinity for vitamin K	2 large pedigrees	Warfarin
Favism or drug-induced hemolytic anemia	Hemolysis in response to certain drugs	Glucose-6-phosphate dehydrogenase (G6PD deficiency)	Approximately 100 million affected in world; occurs in high frequency where malaria is endemic; 80 biochemically distinct mutations	Variety of drugs, e.g., acetanilide, primaquine, nitrofurantoin, and chloramphenicol
Glaucoma	Abnormal response of intraocular pressure to steroid eye drops	Unknown	Approximately 5% USA population	Corticosteroids
Malignant hyperthermia	Uncontrolled rise in body temperature with muscular rigidity	Ca^{2+} binding protein	Approximately 1 in 15,000 anesthetized patients	Various anesthetics, especially halothane

More than one inheritable characteristic may be present on the same pair of alleles. For example, the genes for blood types A, B, and O are in the same position on alleles.

INHERITED VARIATION IN PHARMACOKINETICS

Examples of inherited variability in pharmacokinetics have been almost exclusively restricted to drug metabolism. Renal excretion of drugs does not appear to show genetic polymorphism; the renal clearance for any drug tends to be similar in age- and weight-matched, healthy subjects. As a corollary, drugs that are predominantly excreted unchanged tend to show much less interindividual variability in disposition kinetics than extensively metabolized ones. The degree to which variability in drug absorption and distribution is under genetic control is poorly defined. Certainly, there are several variants of α_1-acid glycoprotein expressed polymorphically, with each variant having a different affinity for basic compounds.

Metabolism has remained one of the last major unaccounted sources of variability in pharmacokinetics. Although there has long been a strong awareness of the influence of genetics on metabolism, it is only recently, with advances in molecular biology, that the basic mechanisms involved are being understood.

Several genetic polymorphisms of drug metabolism have now been identified, involving oxidation, S-methylation, and acetylation (Table 14–1). Most were detected by adverse reactions occurring in a distinct group within the population termed poor metabolizers, following normal doses of the archetypic drugs. A rare phenotype is seen with succinyl-choline. Typically, muscle paralysis wears off within minutes of discontinuing this neuro-muscular blocking agent, because it is rapidly hydrolyzed to inactive products, choline and monosuccinylcholine, by plasma and hepatic pseudocholinesterases. In an occasional patient, however, neuromuscular blockade may last several hours after stopping the infusion, because hydrolysis is much slower than usual. The reason is the existence of an atypical enzyme rather than a lower concentration of the typical cholinesterase; the atypical cholin-esterase has only 1/100th of the usual affinity for succinylcholine, and it behaves differently from the typical cholinesterase to various enzyme inhibitors. Many aberrant forms of the enzyme are now known to exist, each determined by a different gene.

Oxidation

Most small lipophilic drugs are subject to oxidation by the cytochrome P-450 mixed function oxidation system, primarily located within the liver but also found elsewhere, such as the gut wall. This superfamily, which comprises many enzymes, is divided in humans into three major distinct families, designated CY(cytochrome)P(450)1, 2 and 3, each further divided into subfamilies, A through E. Arabic numerals are used to refer to individual enzymes (gene products) within each subfamily. This nomenclature is based on the divergent evolution of the genes. The CYP3A3-5 subfamily of enzymes, particularly CYP3A4, is the most abundant.

Debrisoquine, an antihypertensive agent now no longer in use, was the first drug shown to exhibit genetic polymorphism in oxidation. There is a deficiency in the metabolism of this drug in 5 to 10% of Caucasians, with wide differences in other ethnic groups (Table 14–1). It is a recessive trait, caused by a defect on a single chromosome, that affects a particular oxidative enzyme, debrisoquine hydroxylase (CYP2D6). Since this discovery, a whole host of drugs, including metoprolol (Fig. 14–1) and the antiarrhythmic drug encain-ide (Table 14–1) have been found to be substrates for this enzyme.

Many drugs are oxidized with widely differing efficiencies by the different forms of cytochrome P-450 that exist in addition to debrisoquine hydroxylase. The clearance values associated with the oxidation of certain drugs cosegregate, indicating that they are substrates for the same enzyme (Fig. 14–2). There is also considerable overlap in the structural specificity of some of these enzymes, such that a drug may be a substrate for more than one of them. Evidence favoring genetic control of many of these processes is gained from studies with twins. Fig. 14–3 illustrates such an investigation with the antidepressant drug nortriptyline. Variability in the plateau plasma nortriptyline concentration after oral administration among identical twins is much less than among fraternal twins or, indeed, among any randomly selected, age-matched group. Similar data exist for other drugs. Although the evidence presented in Figs. 14–1 and 14–3 are striking, analysis based solely on the unchanged drug in plasma may be misleading. Consider, for example, a drug that is eliminated by several metabolic pathways of which only a minor one is under genetic control. Examining only half-life or total clearance may fail to detect this genetically controlled source of variability. Yet, if the affected metabolite is very potent or toxic, identifying this source of variation may be therapeutically important. The need to measure both drug and metabolites under these circumstances and to calculate clearance associated with formation of each metabolite is self-evident.

Acetylation

Individuals vary widely in their elimination kinetics of the antitubercular drug isoniazid. The bimodality of the frequency distribution histogram of the 6-hr plasma isoniazid concentration following a single oral dose (Fig. 14–4) was taken as evidence of polymorphism under monogenic control. Although subsequent evidence confirmed that polymorphic isoniazid elimination exists, the use of a single time-point measurement could have been misleading. One does not know, a priori, whether a low concentration reflects poor bioavailability, slow absorption, with perhaps the concentration still rising, or rapid elimination, with the concentration falling. Moreover, if the measurements had been taken at 2 hr, when the concentration primarily reflects absorption rather than elimination, one might have obtained a unimodal frequency distribution and excluded monogenic control.

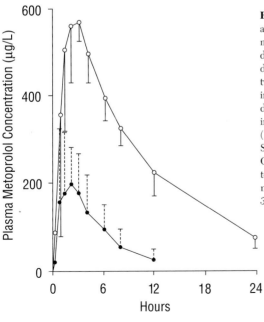

Fig. 14–1. Plasma metoprolol concentrations after a single oral dose of 200 mg metoprolol tartrate were much higher in poor (○) than in extensive (●) hydroxylators of debrisoquine. Because metoprolol is a drug of high hepatic clearance, the difference between poor and extensive metabolizers is expressed in the large difference in oral bioavailability, due to differences in first-pass hepatic loss. The vertical lines indicate the standard deviation (1 mg/L = 3.7 μM). (Redrawn from Lennard, M.S., Silas, J.H., Freestone, S., Ramsay, L.E., Tucker, G.T., and Woods, H.F.: Oxidative phenotype—a major determinant of metoprolol metabolism and response. Reprinted by permission of The New England Journal of Medicine, *307*:1558–1560, 1982.)

Isoniazid is primarily acetylated in the liver to N-acetylisoniazid, a precursor of a hepatotoxic compound; differences in the elimination kinetics of isoniazid reflect polymorphism of a particular N-acetyltransferase NAT2, a cytosolic enzyme. As shown in Table 14–3, large genetically controlled ethnic differences exist in the distribution of acetylator status. Both Caucasians and blacks have approximately equal numbers of slow and fast acetylators, but in Oriental and Eskimo populations the percent of slow acetylators is much smaller. Slow acetylators are genetically homozygous with a recessive allele pair, and because acetylator status is under monogenic control, it is possible to calculate the frequency of heterozygous and homozygous fast acetylators from gene frequencies. The results displayed in Table 14–3 for each ethnic group are calculated in the following manner: if p and q are the frequencies of two alleles, so that $p + q = 1$, then the frequencies of the genotypes (consisting of a combination of the alleles) are $p^2 + 2pq$, and q^2. The sum of these frequencies is 1.0. For example, in the data in Table 14–3 for Caucasians, p^2 (for the homozygous slow acetylators) is 0.586, so that $p = 0.766$, that is, 76.6% of Caucasians have one slow acetylator allele. Hence, the frequency for the fast acetylator allele is 0.234, which leads to distributions for heterozygous and homozygous fast acetylators of 0.359 ($2pq$) or 35.9% and 0.055 (q^2) or 5.5%, respectively.

SUBSTRATES:

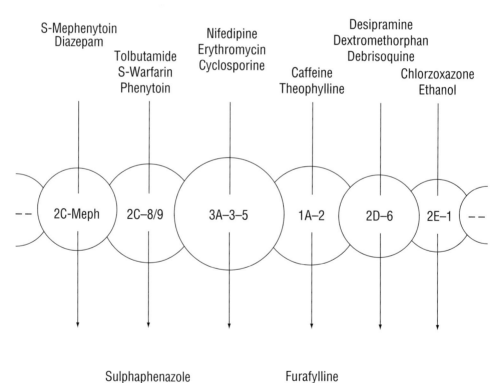

Fig. 14–2. Graphic representation of the different forms of cytochrome-P450 (circles) in humans with different but some overlapping substrate and product specificities. The arrows indicate single metabolic pathways. Representative substrates are listed above for each enzyme. Also listed are relatively selective inhibitors of the enzymes. (From Pelkonen, O. and Breimer, D.D.: Role of environmental factors in the pharmacokinetics of drugs: Considerations with respect to animal models, P-450 enzyme, and probe drugs. *In* Handbook of Experimental Pharmacology. Vol. 110. Pharmacokinetics of Drugs. Edited by P.G. Welling and L.P. Balant. Berlin, Springer-Verlag, 1994, pp. 289–332.)

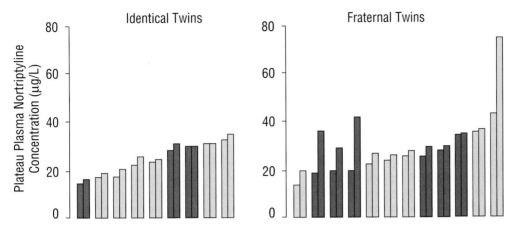

Fig. 14–3. The much smaller intrapair variability in plateau plasma concentration of nortriptyline between (9) identical twins than between (12) fraternal twins indicates that genetics plays a major role in nortriptyline pharmacokinetics. Female (dark color); male (light color). (From Alexanderson, B., Price-Evans, D.A., and Sjöqvist, F.: Steady-state plasma levels of nortriptyline in twins: Influence of genetic factors and drug therapy. Br. Med. J., 4:764–768, 1969.)

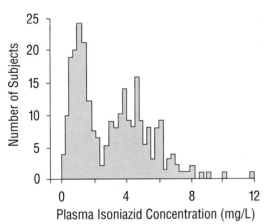

Fig. 14–4. The bimodal distribution of the 6-hr plasma isoniazid concentration in 483 subjects after 9.8 mg/L isoniazid orally results from acetylation polymorphism (1 mg/L = 7.3 µM). (Redrawn from Evans, D.A.P., Manley K.A., and McKusick, V.A.: Genetic control of isoniazid metabolism in man. Br. Med. J., 2:485–491, 1960.)

Table 14–3.   Distribution of Acetylators of Isoniazid in Different Populations

POPULATION	NUMBER	SLOW ACETYLATORS (%)	FAST ACETYLATORS (%) HETEROZYGOTES	HOMOZYGOTES
South Indians (Madras)	1477	59	35.6	5.4
Caucasians	1958	58.6 (52–68)	35.9	5.5
Blacks	531	54.6 (49–65)	38.6	6.8
Eskimos	485	10.5 (5–21)	43.8	45.7
Japanese	2141	12.0 (10–15)	45.3	42.7
Chinese	682	22	49.8	28.2

From Kalow, W.: Ethnic differences in drug metabolism. Clin. Pharmacokinet., 7:373–400, 1982. Reproduced with permission of ADIS Press Australasia Pty Limited.

Isoniazid is an exception. In most cases the frequency of occurrence of an allele is linked with other factors, such as gender. Also, several subgroups within the general population are often of a given ethnicity. These effects make it difficult to calculate the genotype frequency. However, notwithstanding the difficulties in making precise calculations, knowledge of the existence of large ethnic differences in pharmacokinetics, such as seen with isoniazid and some other drugs including desipramine (see below), is clearly important for the optimal use of drugs. This is particularly true for drugs prescribed worldwide or used in a multiracial society.

Interest in acetylation polymorphism is not just academic. Peripheral neuropathy, associated with elevated concentrations of isoniazid, occurs more prevalently in slow acetylators unless an adjustment is made in the dosage of isoniazid or vitamin B_6 is concomitantly administered. Awareness of the prevalence of homozygous and heterozygous rapid acetylators may also be clinically relevant, as they appear to differ in their susceptibility to adverse reactions, such as isoniazid-induced hepatic damage. Acetylation polymorphism also occurs and is important for several other drugs, such as hydralazine and procainamide (Table 14–2). For both drugs the N-acetyl derivative is the major metabolite. A systemic lupus erythematosus-like syndrome, a generalized inflammatory response, can limit the use of both drugs; it develops more rapidly in slow rather than rapid acetylators. The mechanism remains obscure, but does appear to be associated with elevated plasma concentrations of hydralazine and procainamide. Rapid acetylators also require higher doses of hydralazine to control hypertension.

Additional Clinical Considerations

Several points need to be made in addition to those made already. First, the clinical implications of genetic polymorphism in drug metabolism depend on whether activity lies with the affected substrate or the metabolite, as well as the importance of the pathway to overall elimination. For drugs such as debrisoquine, activity resides predominantly with the drug, and elimination is almost completely via the affected pathway. In such cases, unless the dose is reduced, more pronounced and sustained effects may occur together with potentially more frequent adverse reactions in poor metabolizers. A contrasting and interesting situation is seen with codeine. Part of its analgesic activity is due to morphine formed from codeine by debrisoquine hydroxylase (CYP2D6). Accordingly, subjects deficient in debrisoquine hydroxylase may derive less analgesic benefit from codeine. The conversion of the antitubercular drug dapsone to N-acetyldapsone by N-acetyltransferase exhibits genetic polymorphism. However, as acetylation is a minor pathway of dapsone elimination and N-acetyldapsone contributes little to activity, or toxicity, genetic polymorphism has no clinical consequence. Many other scenarios can be envisaged depending on the relative importance of the affected pathway to elimination and whether drug, metabolite, or both, contribute to activity and toxicity. Some of these scenarios are summarized in Table 4–4.

Second, part of the large interindividual variability in the degree of drug interactions involving inhibition and induction (increased synthesis) of drug metabolizing enzymes is under genetic control and increasingly predictable. Thus, quinidine is a potent inhibitor of debrisoquine hydroxylase and therefore inhibits the formation of all metabolites that are produced from substrates of this enzyme (see Table 14–1). Quinidine effectively converts a normally extensive metabolizer to an apparently enzyme-deficient one (poor metabolizer), with the attendant outcomes.

Last, genetic polymorphism has implications in clinical trials during drug development. Relatively few subjects are studied in the early phases of clinical evaluation of a potentially new therapeutic agent. Accordingly, if the frequency of an important drug-metabolizing enzyme deficiency is very low, an important source of interpatient variability in pharmacokinetics, and response, may be missed until the drug becomes widely prescribed, with potentially serious consequences. Fortunately, with the increasing availability of pure human drug-metabolizing enzymes, produced using biotechnology, preclinical *in vitro* screens are beginning to be used to characterize the enzymes primarily responsible for metabolism of a drug. If the enzyme involved is one known to display genetic polymorphism, the drug can be evaluated in a preselected group of subjects with the enzyme deficiency to examine whether serious problems might arise during its subsequent use.

INHERITED VARIATION IN PHARMACODYNAMICS

As previously noted, patients vary in the dosage requirements of warfarin needed to produce adequate anticoagulant control. At most, the variation in dosage requirements is five-fold. In several members of some families, however, massive doses of warfarin are needed to achieve a therapeutic response. Figure 14–5 illustrates the findings in two families. In common with other genetic traits, warfarin resistance is not found in all kindred. Analysis of the frequency of the resistance in several generations indicates that the resistance is a dominant characteristic transmitted in a single gene. A normal pharmacokinetic profile of warfarin in the resistant subjects points to a pharmacodynamically based resistance. A probable mechanism is increased affinity of the receptor for vitamin K, with which warfarin

Table 14–4. Potential Consequences of Genetic Polymorphism Involving Drug and Metabolite for Poor Metabolizers[a]

	DRUG IS ACTIVE	METABOLITE IS ACTIVE/TOXIC
D ⟶ [b]	Exaggerated response, Potential toxicity Example[c]: Metoprolol	Diminished response Example: Proguanil[d]
D ⟶ M	No change in response	Exaggerated response, potential toxicity Example: Imipramine[e]
D ⟶ M	No change in response Example: Dapsone	Diminished response Example: Codeine
D ⟶ M	No change in response Example: Caffeine[f]	Exaggerated response, potential toxicity

[a]Affected pathway shown in color.

[b]Major pathway, ⟹ ; minor pathway, ⟹ .
[c]Where known, examples are given and either discussed further in the text or presented in Table 14–1.
[d]Proguanil, a prodrug, is metabolized to the active antimalarial cycloquanil.
[e]Imipramine is N-dealkylated to desipramine. Both compounds are 2-hydroxylated by CYP2D6. As both imipramine and desipramine are active, the dose of imipramine may need to be reduced in poor metabolizers.
[f]Caffeine is converted to a minor metabolite, which then undergoes acetylation polymorphism.

Fig. 14–5. Reduction of the one-stage prothrombin activity (an index of anticoagulability) from 0 to 48 hr, after an oral dose of 1.5 mg/kg sodium warfarin, for 59 members of two warfarin-resistant kindreds. The dotted lines represent the 99% confidence limits for the response in 50 normal subjects given the same dose. The 34 members of both kindreds with a normal response are indicated by the white bars, and 25 of the 26 members with a resistant response are indicated by the colored bars. (Redrawn from O'Reilly, R.A.: Symposium on pharmacogenetics. Genetic factors in the response to the oral anticoagulant drugs in human genetics. Proceedings of the Fourth International Congress of Human Genetics, International Congress Series 250. Amsterdam, Excerpta Medica, 1972, pp. 428–438.)

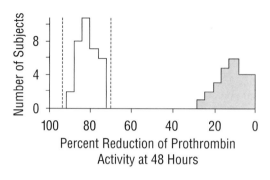

competes to produce its anticoagulant effect. The inability of approximately 30% of Caucasians to taste certain drugs such as propylthiouracil, which contains a thiocyanate group, illustrates how genetics also contributes to variability in the senses.

Other examples of genetically determined variation in pharmacodynamics are given in Table 14–2. Although the number of examples is currently small, the importance of such sources of variability in response should not be overlooked.

PHENOTYPING

Phenotyping patients for a particular metabolic pathway, such as acetylation or oxidation, prior to drug administration has been proposed based upon the ratio of drug and metabolite concentrations in urine following a single dose of a marker. Sulfamethazine has been used to phenotype for slow acetylation; and sparteine, for slow oxidation involving debrisoquine hydroxylase. This approach aims to better anticipate the dosage regimen of a drug required in an individual. Its appeal is greatest in those situations in which: the therapeutic index of the drug is low; the analyses of drug and its metabolites in plasma are difficult; the marker is relatively safe, easy to measure, and its phenotypic characteristic is highly correlated with that of the drug.

Despite its appeal, metabolic phenotyping is not widely employed in clinical practice, for many reasons. One is the inconvenience associated with taking of the marker and collecting urine; another is assay costs; and yet another is the possibility of false positives that are due to other currently administered drugs, such as quinidine, inhibiting the enzyme. Genotyping, based on DNA analysis of a small sample of blood or any other tissue, holds the promise of providing a more direct approach toward predicting metabolic phenotype. Currently, DNA tests have predicted the phenotypes for both N-acetylation and debrisoquine hydroxylation in 95 to 97.5% of healthy volunteers, which clearly indicates the importance of genetics as the major source of variability here. The application of phenotyping to predict dosage depends on the relative contribution of other factors, such as disease and concurrent drugs, to the overall variability in drug metabolism in the patient population.

STUDY PROBLEMS

(Answers to Study Problems are in Appendix II).

1. Give two examples each of inherited variation in pharmacokinetics and pharmacodynamics.

2. Define the terms: genotype, phenotype, and genetic polymorphism.
3. Discuss briefly how an inherited source of variation in pharmacokinetics can be iden-tified within the patient population.
4. A drug developed for worldwide use is metabolized by N-acetyltransferase. What are the potential implications of this finding?
5. Subjects phenotyped according to their debrisoquine oxidation status (poor or extensive metabolizers) ingested one of the following four β-adrenergic blocking drugs: atenolol, metoprolol, propranolol, and timolol. Table 14–5 lists the mean values of various phar-macokinetic parameters for each drug and whether the correlation with debrisoquine status was weak or strong. Discuss briefly possible reasons for the observed correlations.

Table 14–5.

	PHARMACOKINETIC PARAMETERS (MEAN VALUE)			CORRELATION WITH DEBRISOQUINE OXIDATION PHENOTYPE
DRUG	Cl (L/hr)	V (L)	Cl_R (L/hr)	
Atenolol	5.0	38	4.3	Weak
Metoprolol	63.0	290	6.0	Strong
Propranolol	50.0	280	<0.3	Weak
Timolol	31.0	150	4.7	Strong

6. a. Give two examples, in addition to metoprolol and timolol, of drugs that are oxidized and that exhibit genetic polymorphism in their clearance.
   b. Briefly discuss each of the following statements:
      1. Flecainide, an antiarrythmic agent (fe = 0.43), is a substrate for debrisoquine hydroxylase (CYP2D6), yet only in patients with severe renal dysfunction is ge-netic polymorphism in clearance readily apparent.
      2. Dapsone and codeine are two examples of drugs that form minor metabolites via pathways that exhibit genetic polymorphism, but only for codeine is there a po-tential therapeutic implication.
      3. Quinidine converts extensive metabolizers of substrates of debrisoquine hydrox-ylase to poor metabolizers.
7. The frequency within the population of an allele associated with slow oxidation of a drug is 0.15. If slow oxidizers are homozygous with a recessive allele pair, what are the expected frequencies of slow and fast oxidizers in the population? Assume that oxida-tion status is under monogenic control and that all the variability in oxidation within the population is of genetic origin.

AGE AND WEIGHT

OBJECTIVES

The reader will be able to:

1. Determine those drugs for which loading dose, normalized for body weight, is likely to be independent of age, given the volume of distribution and fraction unbound.

2. Describe the likely changes in the pharmacokinetics of a drug predominantly excreted unchanged, from neonate to elderly patients.

3. Adjust, based on age and weight, the usual adult dosage regimen for an individual older than one year of age.

Aging, characterized by periods of growth, development, and senescence, is an additional source of variability in drug response and, as a result, the usual adult dosage regimen may need to be modified, particularly in the young and the old, if optimal therapy is to be achieved. Furthermore, it is the very young and the aged who often are in most critical need of drugs. It is against this background in which an attempt is made in this chapter to develop a framework for making dosage adjustments for age.

The life of a human is commonly divided into various stages. In this book the various stages are defined as follows: *neonate*, up to one month *post utero; infant*, between the ages of one month and two years; *child*, between two years and 12 years of age; *adolescent*, between the ages of 13 and 19 years; *adult*, between 20 and 70 years; and *elder*, older than 70 years of age. It is recognized, however, that this stratification of human life is arbitrary. Life is a continuous process with the distinction between one period and the next often ill-defined. It is also recognized that chronologic age does not necessarily define functional age, and accordingly, statements made in this chapter pertain to the average person within the age bracket rather than to the individual.

Expediency and practicality dictate against the wide use of longitudinal studies in individuals to examine the influence of age on pharmacokinetics. Rather, single observations are made in individuals of differing ages. The information obtained therefore pertains to the population and does not necessarily reflect how an individual may change with age.

A POINT OF REFERENCE

Throughout this chapter reference is made to the "(usual) adult dosage regimen." Before proceeding, this phrase needs to be defined. The word *adult* refers here to the typical adult patient with the disease or condition requiring the drug. The "(usual) adult dosage regimen" is defined as that regimen which when given to this typical patient achieves therapeutic success. Clearly, the characteristics of the adult patient population differ with the disease being treated. Age is certainly one of these characteristics.

The data in Fig. 15–1 show different age trends for the use of two drugs. Thus, patients taking digoxin, used to treat cardiac disorders, are generally older than those taking nitrofurantoin, used to treat urinary tract infections, a condition more evenly affecting people of all ages. Patients with incontinence are generally even older, 70 to 80 years, than those with cardiac disorders. However, there are few drugs for which extensive pharmacokinetic data are obtained at the mean age of the adult patient population. Since most patients taking drugs tend to be middle-aged, for the purposes of subsequent calculations, an adult age of 55 years is assumed.

The data in Table 15–1 illustrate a point about age and disease. Listed are estimates of the population pharmacokinetics of digoxin in a group of young healthy adults and in a

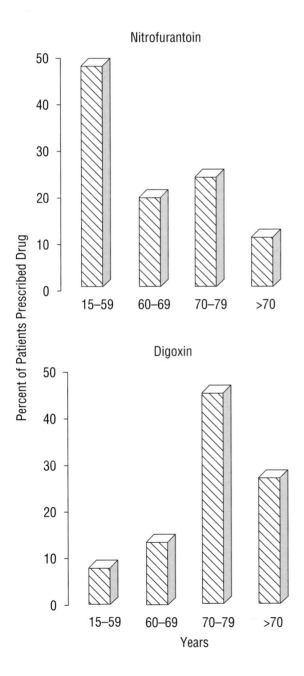

Fig. 15–1. Age distribution of drug consumption. Outpatients in the county of Jämtland, Sweden, taking digoxin are generally older than those taking nitrofurantoin. (Abstracted from Boethius, G. and Sjöqvist, F.: Doses and dosage intervals of drugs—clinical practice and pharmacokinetic principles. Clin. Pharmacol. Ther., 24:255–263, 1978.)

group of inpatients receiving digoxin for treatment of severe congestive cardiac failure. Notice the differences in the values of the estimates, particularly for renal clearance, between the two groups. Evidently, estimates in the young healthy group are of little therapeutic value.

Part of the difference in renal clearance of digoxin between the two groups is accounted for by the disease. Part, however, is accounted for by age. One objective of this chapter is to suggest means of correcting values of pharmacokinetic parameters for age. The intent thereby is to permit a better estimate to be made of the initial dosage required to treat a disease in an individual patient or in a patient population whose age differs substantially from the mean age of the patient population in which the usual adult dosage regimen was established. The influence of all other factors—such as disease being treated, concurrent diseases, and other drugs—on pharmacokinetics are assumed to be independent of age, or it is assumed that the age-related effects can be accounted for independently.

PHARMACODYNAMICS

Throughout this chapter, the range of unbound plasma drug concentrations associated with successful therapy is assumed to be independent of age. For antiepileptic drugs and digoxin, effective plasma drug concentrations appear to be the same in both children and adults, although children appear to tolerate a higher concentration of these drugs before any toxic manifestations become apparent. Differences in response with age are likely to exist for certain drugs. For example, the observed increased sensitivity of elderly patients to the central nervous effects of benzodiazepines cannot be explained on the basis of differences in pharmacokinetics of this group of drugs.

ABSORPTION

Drug absorption does not appear to change dramatically with age. Nonetheless, all the factors discussed in Chap. 9 that affect drug absorption, including gastric pH, gastric emptying, intestinal motility, and blood flow, do change with age. Thus, in the neonate, a condition of relative achlorhydria persists for the first week of life, and only after 3 years of age does gastric acid secretion approach the adult value. Gastric emptying is also prolonged and peristalsis is irregular during the early months of life. Skeletal muscle mass is also much reduced, and muscle contractions, which tend to promote both blood flow and spreading of an intramuscularly administered drug, are relatively feeble. An elevated gastric pH, a delay in gastric emptying, and both diminished intestinal motility and blood flow are also seen in the elderly. Differences in drug absorption among adults, the very young and the elderly, are therefore expected. Generally, changes in rate rather than in extent of absorption are found. These changes tend to be less apparent in the elderly than in the

Table 15–1. Population Pharmacokinetic Parameters of Digoxin in Young Healthy Subjects and Inpatients With Severe Congestive Cardiac Failure

	AGE (Years)	WEIGHT (kg)	ORAL BIOAVAILABILITY (%)	VOLUME OF DISTRIBUTION (l)	RENAL CLEARANCE (L/hr)	EXTRARENAL CLEARANCE (L/hr)
Young healthy subjects[a]	28	71	40–70	760	8.5	3.5
Inpatients, severe congestive cardiac failure[b]	54	68	60	476	3.5	1.4

[a]Abstracted from the data of Koup, J.R., Greenblatt, D.J., Jusko, W.J., Smith, T.W., and Koch-Weser, J.: Pharmacokinetics of digoxin in normal subjects after intravenous bolus and infusion dose. J. Pharmacokinet. Biopharm., 3:181–192, 1975.
[b]Abstracted from the data of Sheiner, L.B., Rosenberg, B., and Marthe, V.V.: Estimation of population characteristics of pharmacokinetic parameters from routine clinical data. J. Pharmacokinet. Biopharm., 5:445–479, 1977.

very young. Children often appear to absorb drugs as completely and, if anything, more rapidly than adults. Accordingly, in subsequent calculations of dosage, extent of absorption is assumed not to vary with age. A major exception is for some high first-pass drugs given to the elderly. Here oral bioavailability increases with age.

BODY WEIGHT

One aspect of aging is body weight. Weight, 3.5 kg at birth, increases rapidly in childhood and adolescence and then declines slowly in the elderly (Fig. 15–2). Because body water spaces, muscle mass, organ blood flow, and organ function are related to body weight, so too should volume of distribution, clearance, and hence dosage regimens of drugs. Owing to large variability, however, a weight adjustment is generally thought necessary only if the weight of an individual differs by more than 30% from the average adult weight (70 kg). In practice, then, adjustments for weight are made only for the child and for the adult who is petite, emaciated, big, or obese.

LOADING DOSE

Clinically, correcting the adult loading dose proportionately for body weight appears reasonable. The volume of distribution based on unbound drug, Vu, is frequently both directly proportional to body weight and independent of age, but not always so. Much depends on the physicochemical properties of the drug and on the reason for the difference in weight.

Shown in Table 15–2 are values for degree of plasma protein binding, volume of distribution (V), unbound volume of distribution (Vu), and percent of drug in the body unbound, for a number of drugs in neonates and adults. The last two parameters were calculated

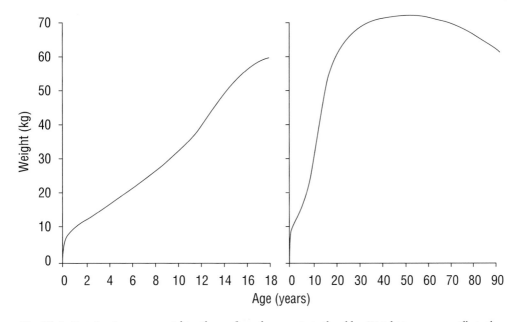

Fig. 15–2. Variation in average weight with age, from the neonate to the elder. Weight increases rapidly in the young, particularly during the first year of life, and during puberty. It declines slowly after 50 years of age. (Data from: 0–20 years, Documenta Geigy. 5th Ed., Basel, Karger, 1959, pp. 255–256; 20–75 years, 2nd National Health and Nutrition Examination Survey, 1976–80. Maryland, U.S. National Center for Health Statistics; 75–94 years, CRC Handbook of Nutrition in the Aged. Edited by R.R. Watson, Florida, CRC Press, 1985, p. 18.)

from *fu* and V (see Chap. 10). As commonly found, plasma binding is lower in neonates than adults. Yet, for the first three drugs, phenobarbital and the two sulfonamides, *Vu*, corrected for body weight, is the same because most of the drug is unbound in the body. Clearly, for these drugs a weight-normalized dose produces the same unbound drug concentration in both neonates and adults or in any other age group. In contrast, little of either digoxin or phenytoin is unbound in the body. Even so, a difference in binding only occurs to plasma protein (*Vu* is virtually the same), and so a weight-corrected loading dose, if required, should suffice.

During adulthood the value of *fu* remains unchanged or tends to rise for those drugs bound to albumin, the concentration of which falls slightly with advancing years. The change in binding is generally too small, however, to warrant any consideration of dose adjustment.

Body composition is important. A dose correction must be considered for emaciated and obese patients. The difference in loading dose may not be as great as anticipated from body weight alone. However, as with age-related changes in distribution, much depends on the physicochemical properties of the drug. Digoxin and polar drugs, for example, do not partition well into fat. Accordingly, for these drugs, *Vu* correlates better with lean body mass, which is similar in obese and average persons of the same height and frame, than with total body weight.

DISPOSITION KINETICS

Figure 15–3 shows changes with age in half-life and clearance of creatinine expressed per kilogram of body weight. Creatinine distributes into total body water spaces, is negligibly bound to tissue or plasma constituents, is eliminated almost entirely by renal excretion, and has a clearance equal to the glomerular filtration rate. The example of creatinine is chosen because changes in total body water and glomerular filtration rate with age are well understood. To the extent that creatinine mimics other drugs, the data displayed in Fig. 15–3 further our understanding of age-related changes in pharmacokinetics and suggest a means of individualizing dosage regimens for age. Let us consider the various parts of Fig. 15–3 in some detail.

Clearance, if normalized for body weight, is depressed in the neonate, but increases rapidly to reach a maximum value at 6 months, when it is almost twice that in the adult. Thereafter, weight-normalized clearance falls but still remains, throughout childhood, considerably above the adult value. Also, an often forgotten point is that throughout adulthood many functions decrease (Fig. 15–4). This is certainly so for creatinine clearance (glomerular filtration rate), which diminishes at a rate of about 1% per year.

Taking into account differences observed in males and females, the change in creatinine clearance beyond 20 years of age can be approximated by

Table 15–2. Plasma Protein Binding and Distribution Data for Some Drugs in Neonates and Adults[a]

DRUG	FRACTION UNBOUND IN PLASMA (fu)		VOLUME OF DISTRIBUTION (V, L/kg)		UNBOUND VOLUME OF DISTRIBUTION (Vu, L/kg)		PERCENT OF DRUG IN BODY UNBOUND[b]	
	NEONATE	ADULT	NEONATE	ADULT	NEONATE	ADULT	NEONATE	ADULT
Phenobarbital	0.68	0.53	1.0	0.55	1.4	1.0	56	58
Sulfisoxazole	0.32	0.16	0.38	0.16	1.2	1.0	65	58
Sulfamethoxypyrazine	0.43	0.38	0.47	0.24	1.1	0.63	72	92
Digoxin	0.80	0.70	5–10	7.0	6–12	10	6–12	6
Phenytoin	0.2	0.10	1.3	0.63	6.5	6.3	12	9

[a]Adapted from the data collected by Morselli, P.L.: Clinical pharmacokinetics in neonates. Clin. Pharmacokinet., 1:81–98, 1976.
[b]Calculated from third equation in Table 10–7, assuming that the unbound drug distributes evenly throughout total body water.

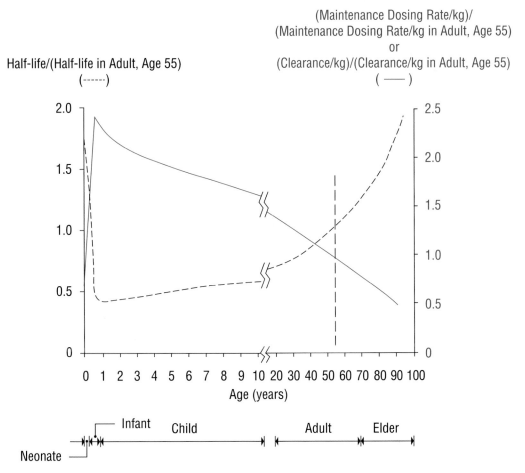

Fig. 15–3. How half-life (left scale, dashed line) and both clearance and maintenance dosing rate (right scale, colored line) of a drug might vary with age. The values were calculated from data on creatinine. The drug, like creatinine, distributes into total body water, is not bound in plasma or tissues, and is eliminated entirely by renal excretion with a clearance equal to the glomerular filtration rate. Half-life is expressed as a fraction of the average value for a typical 55-year-old adult patient; the dosage regimen is calculated assuming that the desired average plateau unbound concentration remains constant throughout life. Notice that, because of poor renal function, elimination is slow in the neonate, but improves rapidly such that, by 1 year, half-life is about one-half the adult value. During childhood and adolescence, the half-life becomes longer because clearance, a function of surface area, increases more slowly with growth than does volume of distribution, a function of body weight. Although body weight and therefore volume of distribution change only slightly beyond 30 years, half-life is longer in the aged, because renal function and therefore clearance progressively diminish. By 95 years half-life is twice the typical adult value. These changes in clearance and weight with age explain why the maintenance dose per kilogram of body weight is higher in the child and lower in both the neonate and the aged than in the adult.

The data used in the calculations were obtained as follows: Half-life—Calculated from volume of distribution and clearance. Half-life in an average adult, 55 years, is 5.9 hr. Volume of distribution—Taken as 78% of body weight at birth, 67% of body weight at 6 months, and 60% of body weight thereafter (Friis-Hansen, B.: Changes in body water compartments during growth. Acta Paediatr., (Supp.) *110*:1–68, 1956). Clearance—at birth, taken as inulin clearance, 3 mL/min (Weill, W.B.: The evaluation of renal function in infancy and childhood. Am. J. Med. Sci., 229:678–694, 1955); between 6 months and 20 years, calculated by multiplying creatinine clearance, 120 mL/min/per 1.8 square meters in an average, healthy, young adult of 21–29 years, by body surface area; between 30 and 99 years, taken from the data of Siersbaek-Nielsen (Siersbaek-Nielsen, K., Hansen, J.M., Kampmann, J., and Kristensen, M.: Rapid evaluation of creatinine clearance. Lancet, *1*:1133–1134, 1971). Surface Area—Calculated from body weight using the relationship: Surface area = 1.8 square meters • [Weight (kg)/70]$^{0.7}$.

Males

$$\text{Creatinine Clearance (mL/min)} = (140 - \text{Age}) \cdot \frac{\text{Weight}}{70} \qquad 1$$

Females

$$\text{Creatinine Clearance (mL/min)} = (140 - \text{Age}) \cdot \frac{\text{Weight}}{85} \qquad 2$$

where age is expressed in years and weight in kg. Thus, in an average 90-year-old, 60-kg adult, clearances (43 mL/min, males; 35 mL/min, females) are 0.5 times those of the typical 55-year-old patients, while the values in a 20-year-old, 70-kg adult (120 mL/min, males; 102 mL/min, females) are 1.4 times these values. More global relationships that incorporate serum creatinine, a reflector of both creatinine production and renal excretion, as well as age, weight, and gender, are given in Chap. 16.

Because total body water as a percent of body weight, and hence distribution, changes relatively little during life, the change in creatinine half-life inversely reflects the change in clearance. That is, the half-life is shortest around 1 year of age; it is longest in both newborn and elderly patients. Although extensive data are lacking, similar age-related changes in disposition of drugs seem to occur.

In *premature* newborns, creatinine clearance is even more depressed per kilogram of body weight than in full-term neonates. Creatinine clearance appears to increase exponentially by a factor of 8 between 28 and 40 weeks, as shown in Fig. 15–5. The data indicate that creatinine clearance during the first few weeks after birth is predicted by conceptional

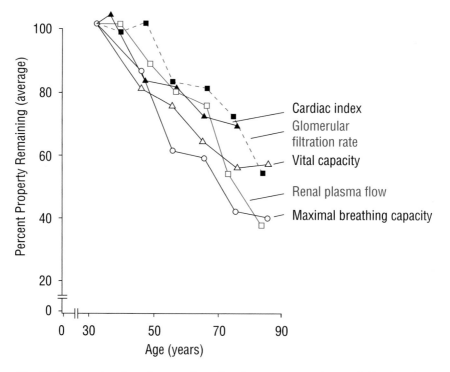

Fig. 15–4. Many physiologic functions diminish with increasing age during adulthood. (Adapted from Shock, N.W.: Age changes in physiological functions in the total animal: The role of tissue loss. Edited by B.L. Strehler. The biology of aging. Washington, D.C., American Institute of Biological Sciences, 1960, pp. 250–264.)

age, (time since conception). Dosing requirements for a drug that is primarily excreted unchanged during this period may be approximated from knowledge of the conceptional age; but the requirements, as reflected by creatinine clearance, are rapidly changing and must be continually updated.

Next, consider the data on diazepam, a drug metabolized primarily in the liver. As seen in Fig. 15–6, diazepam half-life is longest in the neonate, particularly within the first few days, and in adults older than 55 years of age. Infants eliminate the drug most rapidly. With creatinine, the long half-life in the neonate is caused by depressed renal function, which

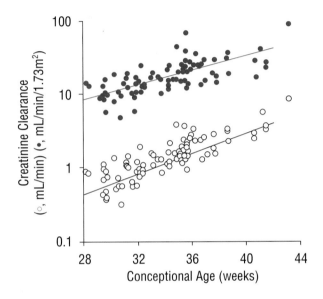

Fig. 15–5. Creatinine clearance, corrected (colored circles) and uncorrected (open black circles) for body surface area, plotted versus conceptional age. The lines represent the best fit of an exponential equation to the data. For the upper and lower curves, the equations are $CL_{cr}(\text{mL/min}/1.73\ \text{m}^2) = 0.373\ e^{0.111\ \cdot\ Age}$ and $CL_{cr}(\text{mL/min}) = 0.00462\ e^{0.161\ \cdot\ Age}$, respectively. Even after correcting for surface area, clearance is greatly depressed in neonates, especially those of earlier conceptional age. Recall that creatinine clearance from 6 months to 20 years is about 120 mL/min/1.73 m^2. (Adapted from Al-Dahhan, J., Haycock, G.B., Chantler, C., and Stimmler, L.: Sodium homeostasis in term and preterm neonates. Arch. Dis. Child., 58:335–342, 1983.)

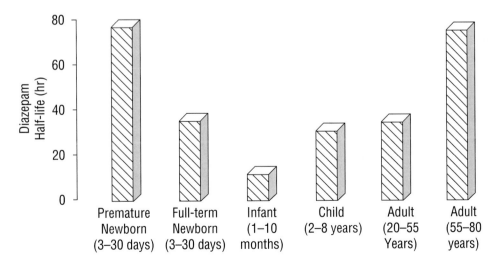

Fig. 15–6. Half-life of diazepam is shortest in the infant and longest in the newborn and the aged. (Adapted from the data of Morselli, P.L.: Drug Disposition During Development. New York, Spectrum Publications, 1977, pp. 311–360 and p. 456; and from the data of Klotz, U., Avant, G.R., Hoyumpa, A., Schenker, S., and Wilkinson, G.R.: The effect of age and liver disease on the disposition and elimination of diazepam in adult man. J. Clin. Invest., 55:347–359, 1975.)

takes several months to mature. With diazepam the long half-life in the neonate reflects an undeveloped drug-metabolizing activity. Metabolic activity may take months to mature; the time required for full maturation varies with the enzyme system. That the premature neonate has the longest half-life of diazepam is not surprising and stresses a point made earlier: chronologic and functional age must be distinguished, especially in neonates.

The shorter half-life of diazepam in the infant than in the 20- to 55-year-old adult reflects differences in clearance per kilogram, because volume of distribution of this drug is approximately the same (1.2 L/kg) in both groups. The further prolongation in half-life in the most elderly group, clearly shown to be age-related (Fig. 15–7), requires some discussion. Clearance remains essentially constant, and volume of distribution is increased with age from 20 to 80 years, but only because of the tendency for lower plasma binding of drug. Diazepam is a drug of low extraction and large volume of distribution, and both its clearance and volume of distribution are dependent on protein binding. The unbound volume of distribution changes relatively little with age. However, the all-important unbound clearance is reduced (Fig. 15–8), probably reflecting diminished capacity for hepatic metabolism, which occurs primarily by oxidation.

A decrease in unbound metabolic clearance in the elderly patient has been demonstrated for an increasing number of drugs, especially those eliminated principally by oxidation. For example, the clearance (predominantly metabolic) of antipyrine, a model compound used to assess the status of oxidative metabolism in the liver, decreases by approximately 1% per year (Fig. 15–9). However, the overall variability in oxidative clearance of drugs is usually large, and as with antipyrine, age may capture only a small percent of the total variance in clearance. Conjugative capacity also decreases but by a lesser extent than oxidative capacity. These changes may be associated, in part, with the decrease in the size of the liver, as a proportion of body weight, from 2.5% in the young adult to 1.6% at 90 years of age.

For some metabolized drugs, no change in clearance or half-life has been observed in the elderly. Until more data become available, the best current prediction is that metabolism is either decreased or not changed in the elderly. To be on the conservative side and

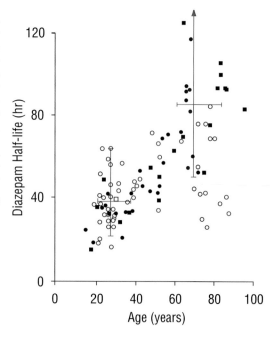

Fig. 15–7. The half-life of diazepam increases with age, from 20 to 80 years. (Composite data from (●)—Klotz, U., Avant, G.R., Hoyumpa, A., Schenker, S., and Wilkinson, G.R.: The effects of age and liver disease on the disposition and elimination of diazepam in adult man. J. Clin. Invest., 55:347–359, 1975: (colored bars, mean and range)—Greenblatt, D.J., Allen, M.D., Harmatz, J.S., and Shader, R.I.: Diazepam disposition determinants. Clin. Pharmacol. Ther., 23:301–312, 1979; (○)—Macleod, S.M., Giles, H.G., Bengert, B., Lui, F.F., and Sellers, E.M.: Age and gender-related differences in diazepam pharmacokinetics. J. Clin. Pharmacol., 19:15–19, 1979; (■)—Macklow, A.F., Barton, M., James, O., and Rawlins, M.D.: The effect of age on the pharmacokinetics of diazepam. Clin. Sci. 59:479–483, 1980.)

as a rough approximation, the decline for unbound metabolic clearance with age should be considered to be the same as that for renal clearance, 1% per annum.

Next consider the increasing ratio of plateau plasma concentration to dosing rate per kilogram, determined after chronic oral dosing of several antiepileptic drugs with increasing age in children (Fig. 15–9). All these drugs are completely bioavailable and since

$$\frac{C_{ss,av}}{(Dose/kg)/\tau} = \frac{1}{Clearance/kg} \qquad\qquad 3$$

it follows that the weight-corrected clearance must be higher in a younger and smaller child. All these antiepileptic drugs are extensively metabolized, and in none studied does protein binding appear to change substantially between the different age groups. Greater hepatic metabolic capacity per unit body weight is therefore implicated in the younger group.

Finally, there is some evidence that hormonal status in woman may also influence, or be a component of, changes in drug kinetics with age. Figure 15–10 shows the relationship between plasma clearance of alfentanil, a potent opioid, and age. A significant decrease in

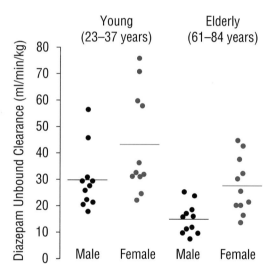

Fig. 15–8. The unbound clearance of diazepam is reduced in elderly patients compared with young adults. Differences also exist between males and females. The reduced unbound clearance is the primary reason for a prolonged half-life of diazepam in the elderly patient. (Redrawn from Greenblatt, D.J., Allen, M.D., Harmatz, J.S., and Shader, R.I.: Diazepam disposition determinants. Clin. Pharmacol. Ther., 27:301–312, 1980. Reproduced with permission of C.V. Mosby.)

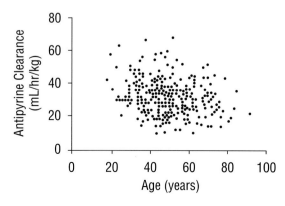

Fig. 15–9. The clearance of antipyrine, an extensively metabolized drug, declines but marginally with age when studied in 307 healthy subjects, each of whom received 1 g antipyrine i.v. Age accounts for little of the variability in clearance within this population. (Adapted from Vestal, R.E., Norris, A.H., Tobin, J.D., Cohen, B.H., Shock, N.W., and Andres, R.: Antipyrine metabolism in man: Influence of age, alcohol, caffeine, and smoking. Clin. Pharmacol. Ther., 18:425–432, 1975.)

clearance occurs in women but not in men. The decrease in women may be related to their menopausal status. Further work is needed to determine the influence of hormones and other factors on the general tendency for metabolism to decrease with age.

MAINTENANCE DOSE THERAPY

Adult

For most patients, there is generally no need to adjust dosage for age. A need may exist when the difference between the individual and the typical patient exceeds 20 years, for example, in young adults less than 35 years of age and in those individuals beyond 75 years of age, when the typical patient is 55 years old.

Generally, dosage is not changed based on gender. The "usual" adult dose is derived from clinical studies in a mixed population. Consideration of adjusting for gender becomes more important at the extremes, i.e., for elderly women and young men. As shown in Table 15–3, creatinine clearances of male and female 55-year-old patients are fairly close, but a 90-year-old woman and a 20-year-old man differ by threefold in their creatinine clearances. A 20-year-old woman, however, differs only two-fold from that of a 90-year-old man. Weight is also a factor here, as the average 20-year-old man may be close to 70 kg in weight, while the average 90-year-old woman is probably only 60 kg in size. The difference may

Fig. 15–10. Plasma clearance of alfentanil decreases with age. The decrease is more pronounced in females (colored circles) than in males (open black circles). The decrease in females may be related to their pre- or postmenopausal status. (Redrawn from Gustavson, L.E., and Benet, L.Z.: Menopause: Pharmacodynamics and pharmacokinetics. Exp. Gerontol., 29:437–444, 1994. With permission. Original data from Lemmens, H.J.M., Burm, A.G.L., Hennis, P.J., Gladines, M.P.P.R., and Bovill, J.G.: Influence of age on the pharmacokinetics of alfentanil. Gender difference. Clin. Pharmacokinet., 19:416–422, 1990.)

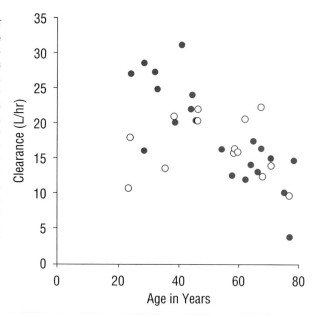

Table 15–3. Expected Creatinine Clearances for Male and Female 70-kg Adults at Three Selected Ages[a]

AGE	CREATININE CLEARANCE (mL/min)	
	MALE	FEMALE
20	120	102
55	85	72
90	50	43

[a]Calculation based on Eqs. 1 and 2.

then be even greater than noted in Table 15–3. Thus, added attention might be given to reducing maintenance dosage in elderly women and increasing dosage in young men.

Dosage in obese and emaciated patients must also be adjusted to maintain the same average unbound plasma concentration. Usually, drug elimination (e.g., renal clearance) is not increased because of added adipose tissue. An exception may be in drugs undergoing glucuronidation, in which case there is an increase with obesity. People with larger body frames (height and build) probably have higher clearances. To a first approximation (based on height alone) such increases can be estimated from *ideal body weight*. Ideal body weight in kilograms (from life insurance actuarial studies) can be estimated from the following relationships with body height.

$$\text{Ideal body weight (men)} = 50 + 0.91 \, (\text{height in cm} - 152)$$

$$\text{Ideal body weight (women)} = 45 + 0.91 \, (\text{height in cm} - 152)$$

The expected clearance of creatinine can then be calculated from Eqs. 1 and 2 for adults.

For emaciated patients, estimation of dosage requirements is even more complex. Dosage requirements depend on the cause of the emaciation. Malnourishment and various disease states may affect renal and hepatic elimination. In most of such patients, however, dosage requirements are not commensurately reduced with body weight. Ideal body weight may then be a better approximation of unbound clearance and maintenance dosing rate. Clearly, more definitive information is needed for both obese and emaciated patients.

Neonate

The lack of maturation of renal and hepatic function necessitates that the rate of administration of drugs to both neonates and young infants be reduced, even on a body weight basis, if toxicity is to be avoided. Unfortunately, changes occur so rapidly in these early stages of life that it is impossible to predict with confidence clearance and hence the required dosage regimen. Caution must clearly be exercised in administering drugs to this patient population. Besides carefully noting response, monitoring of the plasma concentration of drugs with a narrow therapeutic index should be helpful.

In passing, noteworthy here is the incidental exposure of fetus and suckling infant to drugs. For those drugs that can pass the placenta, the unbound plateau concentration in the fetus is likely to equal that in the pregnant mother in chronic therapy. With eliminating capacity generally poorly developed, the fetus acts for the most part as an additional "tissue" of distribution, with half-life in the fetus being the same as that in the mother. A drastic change occurs, however, on delivery. Deprived of access to the fully developed eliminating organs of the mother, elimination of drug from the newborn child can be very slow indeed.

The suckling infant is exposed to those drugs taken by the mother. As suckling occurs regularly, of concern are events at plateau. The risks are greatest for drugs, particularly lipophilic ones, that concentrate in breast milk, that are poorly cleared by the infant, and that have a narrow therapeutic index.

Child

The evidence in Figs. 15–3 and 15–11 suggests that a maintenance regimen, calculated by correcting the adult dosage for body weight, would prove inadequate for children, especially for the very young. Dosage requirements, cardiac output, hepatic and renal blood flow, and glomerular filtration rate in children and in young adults of widely differing sizes have been found to correlate better with *body surface area* than body weight. Because clearance relates dosing rate to plateau plasma concentration and because renal clearance is proportional to glomerular filtration rate (see Fig. 13–11), the choice of surface area over weight as the method of calculating maintenance therapy has some justification. Taking a 55-year-old as the typical patient receiving the drug, the clearance expected for a 70-kg, 20-year-old is 1.4 times that for the reference patient (Eq. 2). According to this concept a child's maintenance dosage is calculated from the formula:

$$\frac{\text{Child's}}{\text{maintenance dosage}} = 1.4 \cdot \left[\frac{\text{Surface area of child} \ (\text{m}^2)}{1.8 \ \text{m}^2}\right] \cdot \frac{\text{Typical adult}}{\text{maintenance dosage}} \qquad 4$$

where 1.8 m^2 is the surface area of an average 70-kg adult. The surface area of a child can

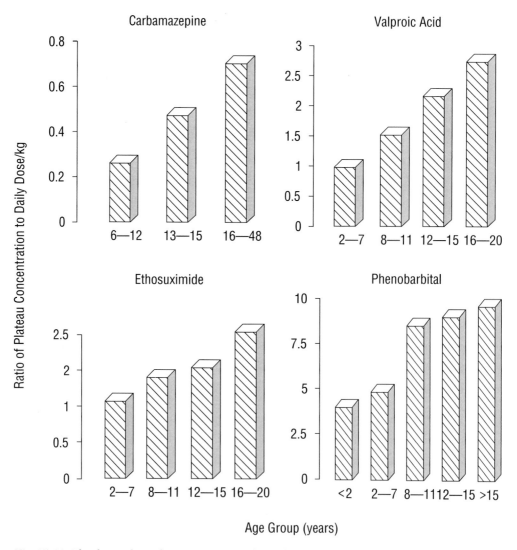

Fig. 15–11. The plateau plasma drug concentrations of several antiepileptic drugs were measured after chronic oral medication in children. An increased clearance per kilogram of body weight explains the lower ratio of concentration to daily dose per kilogram in the youngest children. (Adapted from the data of Morselli, P.L.: Antiepileptic drugs. *In* Drug Disposition During Development. Edited by P.L. Morselli. New York, Spectrum Publications, 1977, Chap. 11, pp. 311–360.)

be determined from its body weight using the observation that surface area is proportional to body weight to the 0.7 power (weight$^{0.7}$). Using this last relationship, Eq. 4 may be rewritten as

$$\text{Child's maintenance dosage} = 1.4 \cdot \left[\frac{\text{Weight of child (kg)}}{70 \text{ kg}}\right]^{0.7} \cdot \text{Typical adult maintenance dosage} \qquad 5$$

To illustrate the use of the relationship expressed in Eq. 5, consider the example of the antibiotic tobramycin; the usual adult maintenance dose is 3 mg/kg daily given in three divided doses. Question: What is the daily tobramycin dosage needed in a 15-kg child? Answer: 100 mg daily. This answer can be estimated from the ratio of surface areas (estimated from body weight) using Eq. 5.

$$\text{Child's dosage of tobramycin} = 1.4 \times \left(\frac{15}{70}\right)^{0.7} \cdot 70 \text{ kg} \times 3 \text{ mg/kg}$$

$$= 100 \text{ mg/day}$$

Notice that the weight-normalized daily dose of tobramycin in the child, 6.7 mg/kg, is much higher than that in the adult. The reason is that clearance is proportional to surface area and surface area per kilogram *increases* disproportionately with decreasing weight. The need for a higher maintenance dose per kilogram body weight, the smaller and hence usually the younger the child, is seen in Fig. 15–3 for children between 6 months and 12 years. Note the complementary decrease in the half-life with decreasing size and age. Thus, not only may a 1-year-old child require a larger maintenance dose per kilogram body weight than an adult, but because of a shorter half-life, the drug may also need to be given more frequently. This is especially so if the drug has a low therapeutic index and large fluctuations around the average plateau concentration are to be avoided.

The Elder

The elderly constitute an increasingly greater proportion of the total population. They also consume more prescription drugs per capita than do people at any other age. As a broad generalization, dosage should be reduced in elderly patients, reflecting the general decline in body function with age (Fig. 15–4). A reduction in dosage is needed particularly in the weak and infirm elderly patient. Such a patient often suffers from several diseases, receives multiple drug therapy, and has body functions that have decreased sharply with advancing years.

Certainly, the marked and progressive decrease in renal function implies that the dosage regimens of drugs that are predominantly excreted unchanged should be reduced in the elderly population. For example, an 80-year-old patient requires, on average, only 70% of the usual adult dosage expressed relative to 70 kg of body weight. The dose required may be even less because the elderly patient is, on average, lighter. A depressed clearance without dose adjustment probably explains, in part, the increased frequency and degree of adverse drug effects often noted in elderly patients.

General Equation

To return to the example of creatinine and similarly handled drugs, from 1 year to 20 years of age, the relationship between renal clearance and age is expressed in Eq. 5; beyond 20 years, this relationship is expressed in Eqs. 1 and 5. Because the value of 140-Age changes little between 1 and 20 years of age, these equations can be combined to give the general equation:

$$\frac{\text{Maintenance}}{\text{dosage}} = \frac{[140 - \text{Age (years)}] \cdot [\text{Weight (kg)}]^{0.7}}{1660} \cdot \frac{\text{Usual adult}}{\text{maintenance}} \qquad 6$$

that permits the rough approximation of a maintenance dosage for a patient of any age, except the infant and the neonate, when maintenance of the same average unbound plateau concentration is needed. No distinction in gender requirements is made. The value of the denominator, 1660, in Eq. 6 is the product of the age-related decline in renal clearance for a 55-year-old: 85 $(140 - 55)$ and $70^{0.7}$ or 19.5.

Figure 15–12 summarizes the dosage changes with age beyond 1 year required to maintain the same average unbound concentration. The maintenance dosing rate increases almost linearly between 1 and 12 years of age. These predictions are based on changes in body surface area with age, which are estimated from average weights, and the general correlation observed between clearance and body surface area in children. Because clearance increases up to 20 years of age and then declines thereafter, there are pairs of age values for which the same rate of administration is required. For example, on average, a 4-year-old child (16 kg) requires the same rate of drug administration as a 90-year-old person (60 kg). Similarly, a 12-year-old child (39 kg) requires the same daily dose as the reference 70-kg patient, namely, the usual maintenance dose.

These equations can serve to facilitate and improve the initial estimate of the dosage regimen needed for a patient of any age beyond 1 year. In general, a correction in the

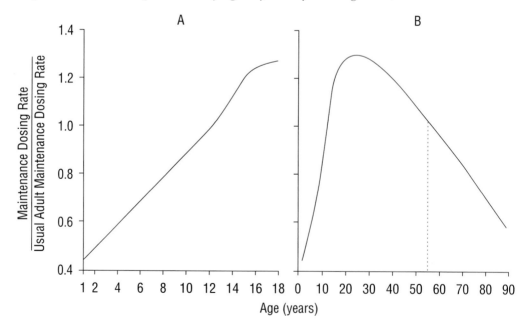

Fig. 15–12. Variation in the maintenance dosing rate expressed as a fraction of the maintenance dosing rate in a 55-year-old adult (dotted vertical line) as a function of age, from 1 year to 90 years. Note the almost linear increase in maintenance dosing rate with age from 1 to 12 years (*A*), associated primarily with an increase in body size, and the almost linear decline between 30 and 90 years (*B*), associated primarily with diminished organ function with advancing years. Also note that the dosing rates as a function of age differ by no more than about 2.5-fold from the usual adult dosing rate. Values are calculated using Eq. 6 and the weight-for-age relationships given in Fig. 15–2.

usual adult dosage is worthwhile when administering drugs to the very young, to the child, and to the aged. A correction is also worthwhile in emaciated and obese patients.

A final note is in order with regard to changes in physiologic parameters concerning age. Physiologic parameters such as cardiac output, hepatic blood blow, renal blood flow, and glomerular filtration rate decrease with age (Fig. 15–4). The values most widely quoted, e.g., glomerular filtration rate = 120 mL/min, and hepatic blood flow = 1.35 L/min, are typical for young healthy adults, not the typical patient who may be 55 or 70 years of age. Whenever comparisons are made in typical patients they should be done carefully. For example, an hepatic blood clearance of 0.7 L/min for a drug may indicate high hepatic extraction in a 70-year-old patient population in whom the hepatic blood flow may be 0.8 L/min instead of 1.35 L/min. Similarly, a renal clearance/fu of 70 ml/min may be equal to the GFR of an elderly patient population.

STUDY PROBLEMS

(Answers to Study Problems are in Appendix II.)

1. Comment on whether each of the following statements is true or false. Qualify your answer when you think it appropriate.
   a. Oral bioavailability increases with increasing body weight.
   b. Volume of distribution varies in direct proportion to body weight.
   c. In children, clearance/body weight decreases with increasing age.
   d. Beyond 20 years of age, renal function decreases by approximately 0.3% per year.
   e. The half-life of a drug is shortest in young adults.
2. Simons et al. studied the pharmacokinetics of the antihistamine diphenhydramine in children and both young and elderly adults after i.v. administration. Their findings are listed in Table 15–4.

Table 15–4. Average Demographic and Pharmacokinetic Data for Diphenhydramine[a]

	CHILDREN	YOUNG ADULTS	ELDERLY ADULTS
Age (year)	8.9	32	69
Weight (kg)	32	70	71
Clearance (L/hr)	93	98	50
Volume of distribution (L)	690	1223	966

[a]Abstracted from Simons, K.J., Watson, T.A., Martin, T.J., Xue, Y.C., and Simons, F.E.R.: Diphenhydramine: Pharmacokinetics and pharmacodynamics in elderly adults, young adults and children. J. Clin. Pharmacol. 30:665–671, 1990.

     a. Are the differences in volume of distribution across the age groups those expected?
     b. Are the differences in clearance across the age groups those expected?
3. The usual adult dosage regimen of a drug is 20 mg once a day. What daily dose would you recommend for a 3-year-old, 10-kg child?
4. Calculate a maintenance dosage regimen of gentamicin to treat a severe infection caused by *Pseudomonas aeruginosa* with the objective of maintaining the same average concentration in:
   a. A child, age 4 years, weight 15 kg, with normal renal function for its age.

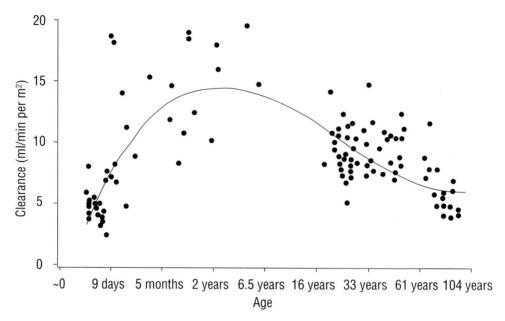

Fig. 15–13. Clearance of ceftriaxone in subjects from 1 day to 92 years of age. Each symbol represents a value in an individual. Note the scale for age, which is age raised to the power of 0.25 ($age^{0.25}$). (Redrawn from Hayton, W.L. and Stoeckel, K.: Age-associated changes in ceftriaxone pharmacokinetics. Clin. Pharmacokinet., *11*:76–86, 1986. Reproduced with permission of ADIS Press Australasia Pty Limited.)

    b. An elderly female patient, age 87 years, weight 63 kg, with normal renal function for her age.

    c. A premature infant of conceptional age 36 weeks.

The adult dose of gentamicin usually recommended (for a typical 55-year-old, 70-kg patient) is 1 mg/kg administered intramuscularly every 8 hr. This antibiotic is almost completely renally excreted unchanged.

  5. Figure 15–13 shows the variation in clearance per square meter (m²) of body surface area of the cephalosporin antibiotic ceftriaxone in individuals from 1 day to 92 years of age. Renal and biliary excretion are about equally involved in the elimination of this drug in normal adults.

    a. Discuss briefly the changes observed.

    b. Given that no change in drug distribution with age is observed, superimpose on the figure the expected trend of half-life with age.

    c. What are the general implications of the finding for the administration of ceftriaxone?

  6. Blychert et al. studied the pharmacokinetics of the calcium antagonist felodipine, used in the management of hypertension, in a group of 140 subjects. All subjects received either 5 or 10 mg orally twice daily for 6 to 30 days. Forty-two of them also received the drug intravenously (either 0.04 or 1.5 mg). The subjects were divided into three age groups: 20 to 39 years, 40 to 59 years, and 60 to 80 years. Table 15–5 summarizes the demographic data and pharmacokinetic findings. Clear age dependencies in AUC_{ss} (0 to 12 hr), clearance and half-life are seen.

Table 15–5. Mean Demographic Data and Felodopine Pharmacokinetic Parameters and Measures[a]

AGE GROUP (Years)	NUMBER	AGE (Years)	WEIGHT (kg)	NUMBER RECEIVING i.v. DOSE	CL (L/min)	$t_{1/2}$ (hr)	ORAL DOSING AUC_{ss} (0–12 hr)[b] (mg·hr/L)
20–39	70	26	76	17	0.82	18	0.028
40–59	30	52	88	12	0.64	24	0.041
60–80	40	68	77	13	0.45	29	0.052

[a]Abstracted from Blychert, E., Edgar, B., Elmfeldt, D., and Hedner, T.: A population study of the pharmacokinetics of felodipine. B. J. Clin. Pharmacol., 31:15–24, 1991.
[b]AUC data normalized to a 10-mg twice daily oral dose.

In answering the questions below, the clearance values estimated from the i.v. data in the three subgroups apply to all those in each of the respective age groups.

a. With activity residing in the parent drug, comment on the need to adjust the dose of felodipine for age.
b. Comment on whether the distribution of felodopine varies with age.
c. Estimate the corresponding oral bioavailabilities for each group.
d. Given that little felodipine is found in urine after i.v. administration and that the drug undergoes extensive hepatic metabolism, comment on the likely reason for the oral bioavailability values.
e. Which parameter, F or CL, most likely explains the increase in AUC_{ss} (0 to 12 hr) with increasing age?
f. What mechanism might explain your answer to part "e"?

7. When administering drugs to obese patients, a concern exists whether or not dose should be weight-corrected. Table 15–6 lists information on the volume of distribution of three drugs in control and obese patients; an individual was classified as obese if his or her weight for height was in excess of 150% of ideal body weight. Neither theophylline nor digoxin, relatively polar drugs, showed a difference in the volume of distribution between normal and obese individuals; the weight-corrected values were lower in the obese individuals. In contrast, the volume of distribution of diazepam, a nonpolar drug, was much greater in the obese group, even after correcting for differences in body weight. No significant difference in plasma binding of these three drugs has been found between obese and normal weight subjects.

Table 15–6.[a]

DRUG	VOLUME OF DISTRIBUTION (L)		WEIGHT-CORRECTED VOLUME OF DISTRIBUTION (L/kg)		AVERAGE RATIO OF WEIGHT TO IDEAL BODY WEIGHT (%)	
	OBESE	CONTROL	OBESE	CONTROL	OBESE	CONTROL
Theophylline	29	27	0.32	0.47	165	91
Digoxin	981	937	10.7	14.3	162	98
Diazepam	292	91	2.81	1.53	164	95

[a]Abstracted from Abernethy, D.R., and Greenblatt, D.: Drug disposition in obese humans, an update. Clin. Pharmacokinet., 11:199–213, 1986.

a. What explains the difference in the effect of obesity on the volume of distribution for each of the drugs?
b. What impact do such findings have on the dosage regimens of these drugs?

DISEASE

Disease is a major source of variability in drug response. For many diseases this variability is due primarily to differences in pharmacokinetics, the area of principal focus in this chapter. The chapter begins with a general discussion of diseases known to affect drug kinetics and concludes with extensive details on adjusting drug administration in patients with renal insufficiency.

DISEASE STATES

The pharmacokinetics, as well as the pharmacodynamics, of some drugs has been shown to be influenced by the presence of concurrent diseases other than the one for which a drug is used. Examples of concurrent diseases that increase variability in drug response are listed in Table 16–1. The subsequent discussion centers on the first three groups of disease listed, namely hepatic, cardiovascular, and renal diseases.

There are occasions when the pharmacokinetics of a drug is altered in the disease for which it is used. An example is immunoglobulin, used in bone marrow transplant patients for the prevention of cytomegalovirus complications. In these patients the half-life is about 6.2 days, while in normal subjects it is 22 days.

Table 16–1. Examples of Increased Variability in Drug Response Associated with Concurrent Disease States

CONDITION	DRUG	CLASS	OBSERVATION	VARIATION IN		COMMENTS
				PHARMACO-KINETICS	PHARMACO-DYNAMICS	
Hepatic Diseases						
Cirrhosis	Theophylline	Bronchodilator	Slower fall in plasma concentration	+	−	Clearance reduced; reduce dosage to avoid toxicity
Acute viral hepatitis	Warfarin	Anticoagulant	Excessive anticoagulant response	−	+	Reduce dosage to lessen risk of hemorrhage
Cardiovascular disease						
Congestive cardiac failure	Lidocaine	Antiarrhythmic agent	Elevated plasma concentration after usual dosage	+	−	Clearance and volume of distribution diminished; reduce dosage to lessen risk of toxicity
Renal disease						
Uremia	Gentamicin	Gram-negative antibiotic	Increased toxicity with usual dosage	+	−	Renal clearance diminished; reduce dosage to lessen risk of toxicity
Uremia	Thiopental	Anesthetic	Prolonged anesthesia	+/−	+	Reduce dose to avoid excessive sleeping time
Gastrointestinal diseases						
Celiac disease	Fusidic acid	Antibacterial agent	Elevated plasma concentration after usual oral dose	+	−	Bioavailability increased and/or clearance diminished
Crohn's disease	Propranolol	β-Blocker	Elevated plasma concentration after an oral dose	+	NS	Increased plasma binding, elevated α_1-acid glycoprotein suspected cause; observed only in active phase
Respiratory diseases						
Asthma	Tolbutamide	Hypoglycemic agent	More rapid fall in plasma concentration	+	−	Therapeutic consequences uncertain
Emphysema	Morphine	Analgesic	Increased sensitivity to respiratory depressant effect	NS	NS	Reduce dose to diminish risk of respiratory complications
Cystic fibrosis	Dicloxacillin	Antibiotic	Reduced area under plasma drug concentration-time curve	+	−	Renal clearance increased
Pneumonia	Theophylline	Bronchodilator	Elevated plasma concentration	+	−	Metabolic clearance decreased; reduce dose to lessen risk of toxicity
Endocrine disease						
Thyroid disease	Digoxin	Cardioactive agent	Diminished response in hyperthyroidism; increased response in myxedema	−	+	Adjust dosage according to thyroid activity
Fever						
	Quinine	Antimalarial agent	Plasma concentration of drug elevated, of metabolite depressed, after usual dosage	+	NS	Impaired metabolism suspected; may need to reduce doses in severe febrile states

+, established source of variability.
−, no evidence that variability is increased due to disease.
NS, not studied.

Hepatic Disorders

Because the liver is the major site for drug metabolism, an impression prevails that special care should be taken in administering drugs to patients with disease states modifying hepatic function. Objective data, while generally supporting this impression, are occasionally in conflict.

One reason for the conflict arises from an attempt to classify hepatic disorders as a single entity. However, disorders of the liver, local or diffuse, are caused by many diseases; each disease affects various levels of hepatic organization to a different extent. With few exceptions, the hepatic clearance of drugs is, on average, decreased in cirrhosis. In contrast, in acute viral hepatitis, there appears to be a fairly even division between those drugs for which clearance is decreased, or half-life prolonged, and those for which no change is detected. Existing data suggest that drug elimination is diminished in obstructive jaundice. The effect is expected to be more extensive for those drugs eliminated predominantly by biliary excretion.

Another potential pitfall is to equate prolongation of half-life with diminution of hepatic drug-metabolizing activity. Half-life is controlled by both total clearance and volume of distribution, two independent parameters (Chap. 11). To assess clearance and volume of distribution, the drug should be given intravenously to ensure complete bioavailability. When so studied, the volumes of distribution of some drugs remain unaltered in hepatic disease, but those of others are increased. An increase in volume of distribution is found particularly with drugs bound to albumin in patients with cirrhosis. The explanation lies in the depressed synthesis of albumin and many proteins, including various enzymes and clotting factors, in these patients. The resultant fall in albumin concentration is responsible for a decreased plasma binding, an associated increase in volume of distribution, and an associated increase in clearance for a drug of low extraction. A fall in hepatic enzymes is responsible, in large part, for a diminished hepatic unbound clearance of many drugs. Oxidized drugs appear to be more affected than those eliminated by conjugation.

The influence of hepatic disease on drug absorption is poorly understood. The problem is complicated by the need to separate disposition from absorption when analyzing plasma concentration-time data. It is likely, though, that the oral bioavailability of drugs highly extracted by the liver is increased in cirrhosis, e.g., Fig. 16–1. There are two reasons for this increase. One is a diminished first-pass hepatic loss due to depressed hepatocellular activity. The other is that many cirrhotic patients develop portal bypass, a condition in which a significant fraction of the portal blood bypasses parenchymal tissue in the liver or enters directly into the superior vena cava via esophageal varices. These portacaval shunts can greatly increase oral bioavailability; an increase of greater than 200% has been reported for some drugs with extensive first-pass metabolism.

From the foregoing discussion, it is apparent that drug dosage may need to be reduced in patients with hepatic function impairment as a result of both decreased clearance and increased oral bioavailability. An adjustment in dosage is particularly warranted when the usual regimen results in the unbound drug concentration at plateau approaching or exceeding the upper limit of the therapeutic concentration window. This condition arises when the clearance based on unbound drug is substantially depressed, because it is this clearance that controls the unbound drug concentration at plateau (see Chaps. 11 and 12).

Hepatic dysfunction is a graded phenomenon, and theoretically a correlation should exist between changes in the pharmacokinetic parameters of drugs, especially hepatic clearance, and an appropriate measure of hepatic function. Attempts to establish such relationships, although encouraging, have not been too successful. This failure probably arises because, unlike drug excretion, there are numerous pathways of drug metabolism, each with a different set of cofactor requirements and each affected to a different degree in hepatic disorders. The contribution of each pathway to total drug elimination also varies with the drug. This variability is apparent from the activities of four hepatic enzymes responsible for conjugation reactions (Fig. 16–2). The enzyme activities were measured in liver samples obtained by biopsy. Glucuronyltransferase appears to be unaffected by hepatic disease. Supporting this observation, the pharmacokinetics of the benzodiazepine oxazepam, which is eliminated almost entirely by glucuronidation, is unaffected in hepatic disease. It is also apparent that while the activities of the other three enzymes are on average decreased, there are some individuals with normal activity and others in whom very little activity remains. Altered metabolism in chronic persistent hepatitis, chronic active hepatitis, and cirrhosis is therefore a function of the enzyme involved, the substrate, and the activity remaining in the individual patient.

In cirrhosis, a correlation between the severity of the condition and the likelihood of depressed metabolism by oxidative and some conjugation reactions has often been reported. In severe cirrhosis, signified by the combination of a low albumin (less than 3 g/dL), an elevated clotting time (prothrombin time greater than 130% of normal), and the presence of encephalopathies, drug metabolism is often decreased. The decreased metabolism frequently requires reducing the dose and monitoring the patient for adverse reactions.

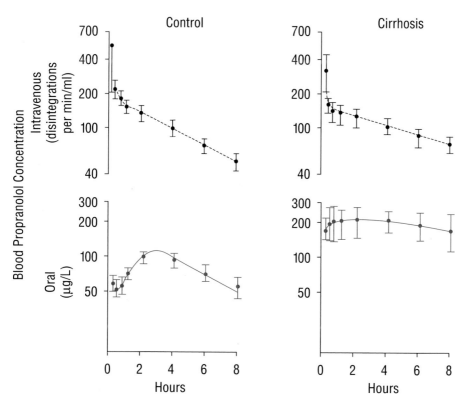

Fig. 16–1. In cirrhosis, the oral bioavailability of propranolol is greatly increased, as evidenced by comparison of the blood concentration of unlabeled drug after oral administration (colored line) with that of tritiated drug after i.v. administration (dashed black line), following simultaneous determination of the kinetics of propranolol during the seventh dosing interval of an oral 8 hr dosing regimen in 9 normal subjects and 7 patients with cirrhosis (mean ± SE). (1 mg/L = 3.9 μM) (Redrawn from Wood, A.J.J., Kornhauser, D.M., Wilkinson, G.R., Shand, D.G., and Branch, R.A.: The influence of cirrhosis on steady-state blood concentrations of unbound propranolol after oral administration. Clin. Pharmacokinet., 3:478–487, 1978. Reproduced by permission of ADIS Press Australasia Pty Limited.)

Indeed, one needs to consider if an extensively metabolized drug is truly needed or if an alternative (renally excreted) drug is available.

Circulatory Disorders

Circulatory disorders, which include shock, malignant hypertension, and congestive cardiac failure, are generally characterized by diminished vascular perfusion to one or more parts of the body. Since blood flow may influence drug absorption, distribution, and elimination, it is not surprising that the pharmacokinetics of drugs may be altered in circulatory disorders.

A diminished perfusion of absorption sites, e.g., gastrointestinal tract and muscle, with an associated protracted and erratic drug absorption, tends to be seen in patients with depressed cardiovascular states; it may be necessary to give the drug intravenously if a prompt response is desired. However, in these conditions the kinetics of distribution is also affected, with perfusion to many organs diminished. Exceptions are the brain and the myocardium, which consequently receive an increased fraction of an i.v. bolus dose, particularly in the earlier moments. For centrally acting and cardioactive agents, the rate of administration of a bolus dose to patients with circulatory depression must be tempered if the risk of toxicity is to be reduced. In these depressed circulatory states, cardiac output

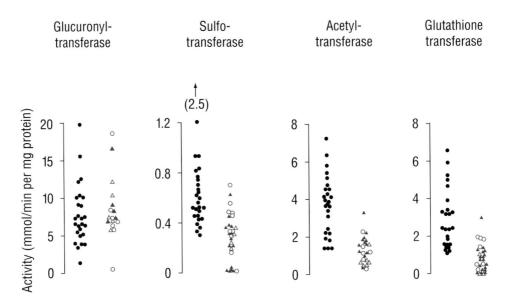

Fig. 16–2. Activities of the conjugating enzymes, glucuronyltransferase, sulfotransferase, acetyltransferase, and glutathione transferase, in normal (black) and abnormal (color) human livers vary widely. Stars, circles, and triangles refer to biopsied samples from patients with chronic persistent hepatitis, chronic active hepatitis, and cirrhosis, respectively. The substrates were: 2-naphthol for glucuronyltransferase and sulfotransferase; p-aminobenzoic acid for acetyltransferase; and benzo(a)pyrene-4,5-oxide for glutathione transferase. In contrast to the other enzymes, glucuronyltransferase does not appear to be affected by any of the hepatic conditions. Also apparent is a virtual lack of activity of the last three enzymes in some patients. The implications for drugs primarily eliminated by the conjugation pathways are great. (Adapted from Pacifici, G.M., Viani, A., Franchi, M., Santerini, S., Temillini, A., Giuliani, L., and Carrai, M.: Conjugation pathways in liver disease. Br. J. Clin. Pharmacol., *30*:427–435, 1990.)

and therefore hepatic blood flow and, to a much lesser extent, renal blood flow are also reduced. Thus, a decrease in clearance of highly extracted drugs is expected. Evidence supporting this concept is illustrated in Fig. 16–3 by a strong positive correlation between the clearances of lidocaine and indocyanine green in patients both without and with varying degrees of congestive cardiac failure. Both indocyanine green, used as a dynamic test of hepatic function, and lidocaine are high hepatic extraction ratio drugs whose clearances should therefore reflect a diminished hepatic blood flow. Notice in Fig. 16–3 the almost 16-fold variation in clearance of both lidocaine and indocyanine green. This range is almost certainly greater than the range of hepatic blood flows in these patients. The hepatic flow, usually about 18 mL/min/kg, is unlikely to fall to a value as low as 2 mL/min/kg because severe anoxia is expected to result at even higher flow rates. Hepatocellular enzyme activity is most probably also depressed when perfusion is severely diminished: this would further depress the clearances of both lidocaine and indocyanine green. As lidocaine has a narrow therapeutic window (see Table 15–2), dosage should be reduced in patients with congestive cardiac failure if the risk of toxicity is to be kept low.

RENAL DYSFUNCTION

In patients with compromised renal function, urinary excretion of drugs is diminished. The degree of reduction in renal elimination depends on the reduction in renal function, as shown in Fig. 16–4 for cefepime, a fourth-generation cephalosporin antibiotic.

When the usual i.m. regimen of amikacin is administered to a patient with renal function that is only 17% of normal, the drug accumulates excessively, as shown in curve B of Fig. 16–5. The figure also reminds us that the extent of accumulation depends on both frequency of administration and half-life, and that the time required to approach plateau is a function of half-life only (Chap. 7). Having a much longer half-life than usual, the time to reach steady state is much longer in this patient than in a patient with normal renal function. Obviously, to avoid excessive accumulation, dosage must be reduced in the patient with renal dysfunction.

The clinician needs information on which drugs accumulate excessively in renal dysfunction and, more importantly, how to adjust drug administration to achieve an optimal therapeutic response. The basic principles that permit this calculation follow. They are developed with the view that drug effect and therefore drug concentration need to be maintained.

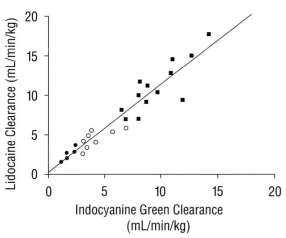

Fig. 16–3. A strong positive correlation exists between the clearance of lidocaine and indocyanine green in patients without (■) and with both mild (○) and severe (●) congestive cardiac failure. (From Zito, R.A. and Reid, P.R.: Lidocaine kinetics predicted by indocyanine green clearance. Reprinted, by permission of The New England Journal of Medicine, 298:1160–1163, 1978.)

Decrease in Clearance

The elements of the problem of renal dysfunction are shown in Fig. 16–6. Ceftazidime clearance, unbound clearance here because the drug is not bound to plasma proteins, is low when renal function, measured by creatinine clearance, is low and increases linearly with renal function. Note that some clearance remains (y-intercept) even when there is no renal function. This represents clearance by nonrenal pathways. The magnitude of change in unbound clearance depends on the renal function remaining and the fraction excreted unchanged.

In what follows, emphasis is placed on unbound rather than total clearance. This is not only because the all-important unbound concentration is related to unbound clearance but also because, for many drugs, fu varies in renal disease, making interpretation based on total plasma concentration uncertain. The goal is to devise a relationship that allows estimation of the maintenance regimen in a patient with renal dysfunction. The first step is to relate unbound renal clearance in the patient with renal dysfunction(d) impairment, $CLu_R(d)$, to unbound renal clearance in the typical(t) 55-year-old, 70-kg patient, $CLu_R(t)$.

$$CLu_R(d) = RF \cdot CLu_R(t) \qquad\qquad 1$$

Fig. 16–4. The mean plasma concentration-time profiles of cefepime, a cephalosporin antibiotic, are different in patients with varying degrees of renal function after i.v. infusion of a 1000-mg dose over 30-min. The subjects were grouped according to their measured creatinine clearance values (in mL/min). (Adapted from Barbhaiya, R.H., Knupp, C.A., Fargue, S.T., Matzke, G.R., Guay, D.R.P., and Pittman, F.A.: Pharmacokinetics of cefepime in subjects with renal insufficiency. Clin. Pharmacol. Ther., *48*:268–276, 1990.)

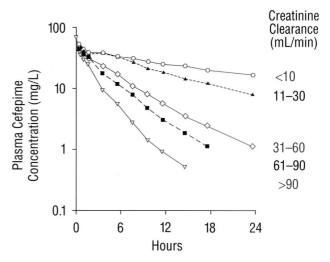

Fig. 16–5. Sketch of the amount of amikacin sulfate in the body with time following a regimen of 500 mg every 12 hr in a patient whose renal function is normal, curve *A*, and in a patient whose age and weight are the same but whose renal function is 17% of normal, colored curve *B*. Intravenous bolus administration is simulated. The normal half-life is assumed to be 2 hr. The dashed lines are the average plateau values.

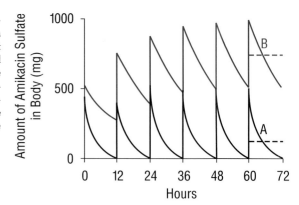

The ratio of the two is the renal function (RF) in the patient relative to that in the typical patient. In the typical patient, $CLu_R(t)$ is a fraction, $fe(t)$, of unbound (renal + nonrenal) clearance, $CLu(t)$.

$$CLu_R(t) = fe(t) \cdot CLu(t) \qquad\qquad 2$$

By combining Eqs. 1 and 2, the unbound renal clearance in the patient can be related to $CLu(t)$, by

$$CLu_R(d) = RF \cdot fe(t) \cdot CLu(t) \qquad\qquad 3$$

The next step is to consider the unbound clearance by nonrenal routes, CLu_{NR}. In the typical patient, it is

$$CLu_{NR} = [1 - fe(t)] \cdot CLu(t) \qquad\qquad 4$$

On the assumption that CLu_{NR} is not changed in renal disease, its value can be estimated for the patient by taking into account his or her age and weight.

Using the approximation $\dfrac{(140 - \text{Age}) \cdot wt(d)^{0.7}}{1660}$ for the factor by which nonrenal clearance deviates from that in the typical patient (Chap. 15), its value in the individual patient becomes

$$CLu_{NR}(d) = [1 - fe(t)] \cdot CLu(t) \cdot \frac{[140 - \text{Age}] \cdot wt(d)^{0.7}}{1660} \qquad\qquad 5$$

where age and weight are in years and kilograms, respectively. Now, under any condition,

$$CLu(d) = CLu_R(d) + CLu_{NR}(d) \qquad\qquad 6$$

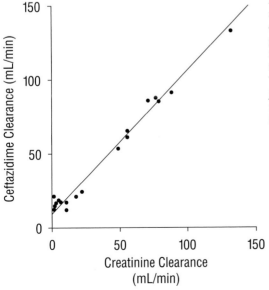

Fig. 16–6. The total clearance of the cephalosporin, ceftazidime, varies linearly with creatinine clearance in a group of 19 patients with varying degrees of renal function. Note that some clearance remains (y-intercept) when there is no renal function. (Drawn from the data of van Dalen, R., Vree, T.B., Baars, A.M., and Termond, E.: Dosage adjustment for ceftazidime in patients with impaired renal function. Europ. J. Clin. Pharmacol., 30:597–605, 1986.)

For a given age and weight, $CLu_{NR}(d)$ is expected to be constant, independent of renal function; while $CLu_R(d)$ is expected (Eq. 4) to change in direct proportion to renal function (RF). Thus, the unbound clearance in the patient, $CLu(d)$, increases linearly with RF. The extent of the increase depends on $fe(t)$, the contribution of the renal route to all routes of elimination in the typical patient. This relationship is shown in Fig. 16–7 for a drug with an $fe(t)$ of 0.8.

On substituting Eqs. 1 to 5 into Eq. 6, the following useful relationship is derived for R_d, the unbound clearance ratio, $CLu(d)/CLu(t)$.

$$R_d = \frac{CLu(d)}{CLu(t)} = RF \cdot fe(t) + [1 - fe(t)] \cdot \frac{[(140 - Age) \cdot wt(d)^{0.7}]}{1660} \qquad 7$$

The first term, $RF \cdot fe(t)$, does not incorporate age and weight directly, because RF is estimated from creatinine clearance in the dysfunctional patient relative to that of the typical patient. Age and weight, of course, play a role in determining the value.

Fig. 16–8A illustrates the relationship between R_d and renal function for values of $fe(t)$ in a 55-year-old, 70-kg patient. It is apparent that R_d changes the most with renal function when $fe(t) = 1$ and is unchanged when $fe(t) = 0$. The value of $fe(t)$ is, by definition,

$$fe(t) = \frac{CLu_R(t)}{CLu(t)} = \frac{CL_R(t)}{CL(t)} \qquad 8$$

where $CL_R(t)$ and $CL(t)$ are the renal and total clearances of the drug in the typical patient for whom the usual regimen is intended. Experimentally, $fe(t)$ is the fraction of an intravenous (i.v.) dose recovered unchanged in urine in a typical patient.

Recall that $t_{1/2} = 0.693 \, Vu/CLu$. The half-life in a patient with renal dysfunction, $t_{1/2}(d)$, compared to that in a patient with fully functioning kidneys, $t_{1/2}(t)$, is then

$$\frac{t_{1/2}(d)}{t_{1/2}(t)} = \frac{Vu(d)}{Vu(t)} \cdot \frac{1}{R_d} \qquad 9$$

Fig. 16–7. Renal, nonrenal, and total unbound clearances, expressed relative to the total unbound clearance of a typical patient, versus renal function (RF) for a drug with an $fe(t)$ value of 0.8. Unbound nonrenal clearance remains constant and independent of renal function. In contrast, unbound renal clearance increases in direct proportion to renal function. The resulting (total) unbound clearance (colored dashed line) increases in parallel with renal clearance from a value of 0.2, represented by nonrenal clearance, to a value of 1.0, when the renal function is that of the typical patient. In this illustration, renal function varies in a group of 55-year-old, 70-kg patients. Nonrenal clearance is, of course, expected to change with age and weight (Chap. 15).

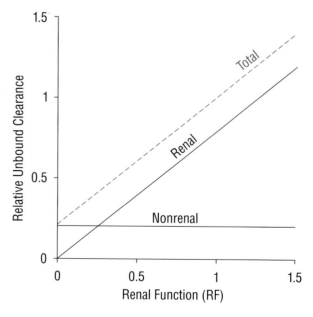

where $Vu(d)$ and $Vu(t)$ are the unbound volumes of distribution in the patient with renal disease and in the typical patient, respectively.

Also, recall that Vu tends to vary in direct proportion to body weight. If renal function does not affect Vu, then

$$\frac{t_{1/2}(d)}{t_{1/2}(t)} = \frac{wt(d)}{wt(t)} \cdot \frac{1}{R_d}$$

10

Figure 16–8B illustrates the dependence of half-life on both renal function and fraction excreted unchanged. Notice that for a drug excreted entirely unchanged, half-life changes the most when renal function approaches zero.

An additional point needs to be made with respect to data acquired in the different individuals in Figure 16–6. The x-axis, creatinine clearance, is a function of age, weight, and renal disease. One might expect that nonrenal clearance may also be related to age and weight. Higher values of nonrenal clearance occur in younger and larger patients, who have higher creatinine clearances, and smaller values are expected in older and smaller patients. This positive correlation of nonrenal clearance with creatinine clearance may distort the regression so that the y-intercept is lower and the slope is greater than expected. Ideally, renal clearance should be correlated with creatinine clearance, and the nonrenal clearance should be examined separately for its dependence on age, weight, and perhaps renal disease.

Estimation of Renal Function

Commonly employed measures of renal function are based on creatinine. Its usefulness lies in its clearance varying in direct proportion to the renal clearance of many drugs (e.g., Fig. 13–11).

In clinical practice, creatinine clearance is usually estimated from serum creatinine alone rather than from measurements in both plasma and urine. Apart from the extra analysis

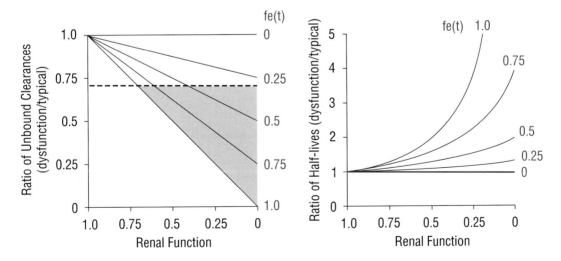

Fig. 16–8. The extent of decrease in unbound clearance, (left), and corresponding increase in half-life, (right), caused by renal dysfunction also depend on the fraction of bioavailable drug typically excreted in urine unchanged, $fe(t)$. Note that generally dose adjustment would not be considered unless the unbound clearance in the patient fell below 70% of the value for a typical patient, that is, below the horizontal dotted line. The calculations have been made for a 70-kg patient of comparable age to a typical patient. The unbound volume of distribution of the drug is kept constant. The screened area shows the combinations of $fe(t)$ and renal function for which a decrease in rate of administration becomes therapeutically prudent.

involved, incomplete urine collection is a major problem resulting in the underestimation of creatinine clearance. Serum creatinine alone can be used because its daily production is matched by its elimination under normal circumstances. Consequently, serum creatinine is related to creatinine clearance by

$$\text{Serum creatinine} = \frac{\text{Rate of creatinine production}}{\text{Creatinine clearance}} \qquad 11$$

Table 16–2 summarizes some of the relationships currently found to approximate creatinine clearance from serum creatinine. These relationships include corrections of creatinine production for age, weight, and gender. It should be emphasized that they are most accurate for individuals with an average muscle mass (source of creatinine) for their age, weight, and height. For emaciated, highly muscular, or obese adult patients, poor estimates are obtained. For these patients a creatinine clearance measurement may be more appropriate than an estimate of its value from serum creatinine alone. Finally, on passing, it should be noted that rates of both production and clearance of creatinine tend to decline in parallel with age. Consequently, serum creatinine remains relatively constant (about 1 mg/dL) from age 20 years onward for patients with normal renal function for their age.

Renal function in the individual patient remains to be calculated. This value is given by

$$RF = CL_{cr}(d)/CL_{cr}(t) \qquad 12$$

where $CL_{cr}(d)$ and $CL_{cr}(t)$ are the creatinine clearances in this patient and in the typical patient, respectively.

Adjustment of Dosage Regimens

The alternatives for adjustment of maintenance and loading doses in patients with renal function impairment apply, in principle, to all disease conditions in which drug elimination is altered. For no other condition, however, is the adjustment required as readily predicted and assessed.

Maintenance Rate. The simplest way of conceiving the adjustment of a maintenance regimen for a patient with renal insufficiency is to maintain the same average unbound concentration at steady state, $Cu_{ss,av}$:

Table 16–2. Estimation of Creatinine Clearance in Adults[a] and Children[b]

POPULATION	CREATININE CLEARANCE (mL/min)	
	SERUM CREATININE (mg/dL)	SERUM CREATININE (μM)
Adults (20–100 years of age)[c]		
Males	$\dfrac{(140 - \text{Age}) \times \text{Weight}}{72 \times \text{Serum creatinine}}$	$\dfrac{1.23 \times (140 - \text{Age}) \times \text{Weight}}{\text{Serum creatinine}}$
Females	$\dfrac{(140 - \text{Age}) \times \text{Weight}}{85 \times \text{Serum creatinine}}$	$\dfrac{1.04 \times (140 - \text{Age}) \times \text{Weight}}{\text{Serum creatinine}}$
Children (1–20 years of age)[d]		
	$\dfrac{0.48 \times \text{Height}}{\text{Serum creatinine}} \times \left(\dfrac{\text{Weight}}{70}\right)^{0.7}$	$\dfrac{42.5 \times \text{Height}}{\text{Serum creatinine}} \times \left(\dfrac{\text{Weight}}{70}\right)^{0.7}$

[a]Adults 20 years of age and older. Poor estimates are obtained for obese and emaciated patients. Adapted from the review by Lott, R.S., and Hayton, W.L.: Estimation of creatinine clearance from serum creatinine concentration. Drug Intell. Clin. Pharm., *12*:140–150, 1978.
[b]Children 1 to 20 years of age. Adapted from Traub, S.L., and Johnson, C.E.: Comparison of methods of estimating creatinine clearance in children. Am. J. Hosp. Pharm., *37*:195–201, 1980.
[c]Age in years; body weight in kg.
[d]Height in cm; body weight in kg. The equation given by the authors has been modified to adjust for body surface area. A child of normal weight for height is assumed.

$$F \cdot \frac{D_M}{\tau} = Cl_u \cdot Cu_{ss,av} \qquad\qquad 13$$

Rate of administration in renal insufficiency, $(D_M/\tau)(d)$, compared to the usual rate of administration to the typical patient, $(D_M/\tau)(t)$, is then

$$\frac{(D_M/\tau)(d)}{(D_M/\tau)(t)} = \frac{Cl_u(d)}{Cl_u(t)} \cdot \frac{F(t)}{F(d)} \qquad\qquad 14$$

where $F(d)$ and $F(t)$ are the bioavailabilities of drug in the patient with renal insufficiency and in the typical patient, respectively. When bioavailability does not change, the required rate of administration in a patient with renal dysfunction is

$$(D_M/\tau)(d) = R_d \cdot (D_M/\tau)(t) \qquad\qquad 15$$

The reduction in dosing rate is therefore seen to depend only on the ratio of unbound clearances R_d. Associated with the reduction in renal function is a prolongation in half-life, which means that the time to achieve the desired plateau is longer the more severe the dysfunction (Eq. 10). This last feature is illustrated in Fig. 16–9 for constant-rate administration. In practice, administration is by discrete doses and adjustment of a maintenance regimen may be made by decreasing the frequency of administration, decreasing the maintenance dose, or a combination of both. The outcomes of these approaches are different. To appreciate the differences consider the adjustment of the usual regimen of amikacin sulfate 7.5 mg/kg injected intramuscularly every 12 hr, to a 23-year-old, 68-kg patient with an estimated creatinine clearance of 13 mL/min.

As the expected creatinine clearance in a typical 55-year-old, 70 kg patient is 77 mL/min (Chap. 15), the value of RF in the 23-year-old patient is 0.17. Using Eq. 15, it is apparent that the maintenance dosing rate of amikacin sulfate should be decreased by a factor of 6. Thus, the maintenance regimen might be one of the following: (1) dosing interval increased sixfold, regimen: 500 mg (7.5 mg/kg × 68 kg) every 72 hr. (2) The maintenance dose may

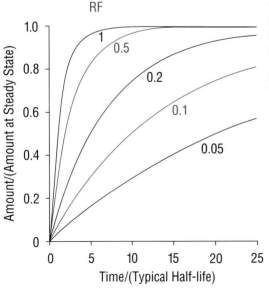

Fig. 16–9. It takes longer to reach plateau following constant-rate administration of a drug as renal function (RF) falls because half-life is correspondingly increased. The effect of renal insufficiency is particularly marked if $fe(t) = 1$. No effect is expected if $fe(t) = 0$. Note that time is expressed in units of half-life for a typical patient.

be reduced by a factor of 6, regimen: 83 mg every 12 hr. (3) Both dosing interval and maintenance dose may be adjusted to reduce the average dosing rate sixfold, regimen: e.g., 167 mg every 24 hr.

The typical half-life of amikacin is 2 hr, so for the patient under consideration the half-life is prolonged sixfold to 12 hr (Eq. 10). Fig. 16–10A is a sketch of the amount in the body with time for the three maintenance regimens considered, given that absorption from the i.m. site is complete and instantaneous. Although both time to reach plateau and average amount in body at plateau are the same for all three regimens, the picture is very different for each one. Clearly, changing the interval to three days (dashed curve) results in the greatest fluctuation, with many hours at both high and low levels. Changing the maintenance dose (colored curve) reduces fluctuation but suffers from the inconvenience of frequent i.m. injections. Finally, changing both maintenance dose and dosing interval (dotted curve) reduces both fluctuation and inconvenience to the patient and as such may be preferred for this drug and for many others.

In this example with amikacin, administration of the usual dosage regimen to the patient with renal dysfunction results in a twofold increase in the maximum amount in the body and a sixfold increase in the average amount at plateau (Fig. 16–5). It is important, however, to consider whether the maximum amount (or concentration) or the average amount is more closely related to efficacy and toxicity of the drug. Only a twofold reduction in the maintenance dose would be required (Chap. 7) if the former were true.

Loading Dose. Particularly large differences in the amount of amikacin in the body exist following the first dose of the three regimens just considered (Fig. 16–10a). With the regimen of 500 mg given every 72 hr to a patient with renal dysfunction, as with the regimen of 500 mg given every 12 hr to a typical patient, there is little accumulation because the dosing interval is much longer than the half-life. Accordingly, effective levels are reached after the first dose. In contrast, appreciable accumulation occurs with the relatively frequent regimens of once every 12 or 24 hr in patients with renal dysfunction. The initial dose is now much less than the average amount in the body at plateau. Under these circumstances, a case may be made for a loading dose. Giving a usual dose of 500 mg can lead to high levels in the body for an extended period after initiating therapy (Fig. 16–8B), which may increase the chance of an adverse effect. A smaller loading dose might be prudent. In the

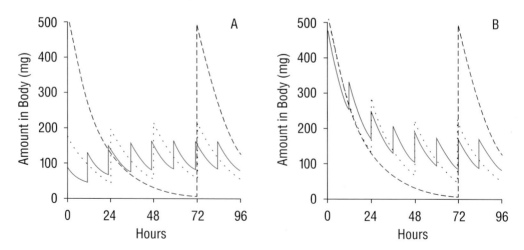

Fig. 16–10. Sketch of the amount of amikacin sulfate equivalents in the body with time in a patient whose renal function is 16.5% of the typical value. Shown are regimens without (A) and with (B) a 500-mg loading dose. The maintenance regimens are: (---)—500 mg every 72 hr; (colored line)—83 mg every 12 hr; (···)—167 mg every 24 hr. Note: i.v. bolus administration is simulated.

particular case of amikacin, based on experience, the manufacturer recommends not changing the usual loading dose.

General Guidelines and Limitations

Except for drugs with very low therapeutic indices, a reduction of less than 30% in the dosing rate, based on a change in renal function alone, is probably unwarranted for individuals in the usual patient population. For a variety of reasons variability in absorption, distribution, and extrarenal elimination is usually at least of this magnitude, and the therapeutic range is often sufficiently large to make adjustment here unnecessary. Consequently, as long as the fraction excreted unchanged in typical patients, $fe(t)$, is 0.30 or less and the metabolites are inactive, no change in a regimen is called for, based on renal function, regardless of the function. Similarly, regardless of the contribution of the renal route, if renal function is 0.70 of the typical value, no change is needed (see Eq. 15). These recommendations are summarized in Figure 16–8A.

As renal function approaches zero, the importance of nonrenal clearance increases. However, nonrenal clearance usually varies widely within the population, making prediction of the optimal dosage difficult for an individual with marginal renal function. When $fe(t)$ approaches one and RF approaches zero, total clearance is small, and the dosing rate must be drastically reduced. Three particularly difficult problems are encountered here. One is a relatively large change in the chronic requirements for a drug with only a small change in renal function, e.g., a change from 0.20 to 0.05 in renal function reduces the required rate of administration fourfold. The second problem is associated with accuracy of measurement of renal function. The third relates to the stability of renal function with time. The function may be improving during convalescence or deteriorating. All three problems create uncertainty in predicting dosage requirements.

A further complication in patients with severe renal disease is the concurrent and regular use of a dialysis technique to remove unwanted endogenous toxic substances, which would otherwise accumulate and cause problems. Unfortunately, dialysis sometimes also hastens elimination of drugs, complicating drug therapy in these patients, a topic covered in Chapter 24 (Dialysis).

The foregoing recommended adjustments are based on a number of assumptions. The method falters if bioavailability changes in renal dysfunction, which is relatively uncommon; compromised renal function alters the ability to metabolize drug, which occurs when the kidney is an organ of metabolism as well as excretion; or metabolism or renal excretion exhibits concentration-dependent kinetics, as the relationship between total clearance and renal function then becomes extremely complex. A problem also exists if renal function varies with time or renal clearance is not directly proportional to the measure of renal function.

Amplifying on the last qualification, regardless of whether the drug is excreted by glomerular filtration or active secretion, renal clearance is assumed to decrease in direct proportion to creatinine clearance. This assumption appears to be valid as a first approximation in chronic renal disease. Para-aminohippuric acid, procainamide, carbenicillin, and penicillin are all examples of actively secreted compounds with renal clearances directly proportional to endogenous creatinine clearance. Finally, interpatient differences in absorption, distribution, and metabolism, the response to a given plasma concentration, and concurrent disease states have not been considered.

Renal function is only one of several sources of variability. Adjustment of drug administration based on renal function alone must be put into perspective.

Further Considerations

Renal disease often affects more than just renal clearance. Furthermore, concurrent diseases may alter dosage requirements. Digoxin binds much less to tissues in uremia, resulting in a smaller volume of distribution and a shorter half-life than that predicted from loss of renal function. This decreased tissue binding reduces the loading dose required but has little or no effect on the maintenance dose. However, the presence of severe congestive cardiac failure, a condition for which the drug is used, is associated with decreased metabolic clearance and with a daily maintenance dosage requirement reduced beyond that expected for renal function impairment alone. The changes in digoxin clearance and volume of distribution with renal function and congestive cardiac failure, obtained from population pharmacokinetic studies, are summarized in Table 16–3.

Phenytoin and many other acidic drugs are two to three times less well-bound to plasma proteins in uremic than in normal subjects (Fig. 12–10). Part of this change is due to a decreased concentration of plasma albumin. The mechanism accounting for the rest of the change is uncertain, although displacement by an endogenous compound(s) that accumulates in renal impairment has been suggested. Even so, the unbound values of both clearance and volume of distribution of these principally metabolized drugs remain essentially unchanged, and no change in dosage regimen is anticipated in renal function impairment. The total plasma clearance, however, increases two- to threefold, giving rise to a corresponding drop in the steady-state plasma concentration. This change must be carefully considered when interpreting plasma concentrations of these drugs in patients with renal disease.

Another uncommon but potential complication to adjusting drug administration in renal disease is metabolism in the kidney. An example is that of imipenem, an antibiotic that undergoes hydrolysis during excretion by a renal brush border dehydropeptidase. Patients with renal disease have a decreased ability to metabolize as well as renally excrete the drug. The changes in both total and renal clearances are shown in Fig. 16–11 for adult patients with varying degrees of renal function. The expectation, as noted in Fig. 16–7, is that total plasma clearance and renal clearance increase in parallel when nonrenal clearance remains constant. Instead, it is apparent that the difference between them becomes smaller in patients with lower renal function. Here, a component of the so-called nonrenal clearance occurs in the kidney even though it involves metabolism. Furthermore, the intercept value, presumably where no kidney function is present, shows that nonrenal metabolism must occur as well.

Perhaps, the *most* commonly invalid assumption is that metabolites are pharmacologically and toxicologically inactive. For example, the metabolite of morphine, morphine-6-glucuronide, is also active. Prediction of the total activity of the drug and of the dosage adjustment needed in renal failure can be much more complex. Nonetheless, there are ways of treating such situations, as given in Chap. 21, Metabolite Kinetics.

In this chapter, approaches have been presented for predicting changes in the clearance of drugs in various disease states. Rules for estimating renal clearance of a drug from

Table 16–3. Estimation of Clearance and Volume of Distribution of Digoxin in Patients With Mild and Severe Congestive Cardiac Failure[a]

CONGESTIVE CARDIAC FAILURE	CLEARANCE (L/hr per kg)	VOLUME OF DISTRIBUTION (L/kg)
Mild	$Cl_{cr}{}^{b} + 0.048^{c}$	$3.8 + 52\, Cl_{cr}$
Severe	$0.9 \cdot Cl_{cr} + 0.02$	$3.8 + 52\, Cl_{cr}$

[a]Adapted from Sheiner, L.B., Rosenberg, B., and Marathe, V.V.: Estimation of population characteristics of pharmacokinetic parameters from routine clinical data. J. Pharmacokinet., Biopharm., 5:445–479, 1977.
[b]Cl_{cr} = Creatinine clearance in L/hr/kg.
[c]Approximation of nonrenal (metabolic) clearance.

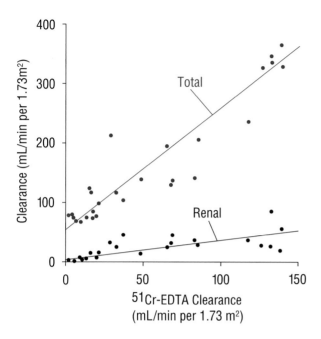

Fig. 16–11. Total plasma (color) and renal (black) clearances of the antibiotic imipenem increase with the renal clearance of ^{51}Cr-ethylene-diaminetetraacetic acid (normalized to 1.73 m^2 of body surface area), a marker of glomerular filtration rate. Surprisingly, the two clearances do not increase in parallel as expected (see Fig. 16–7), indicating that the "nonrenal" clearance of the drug must be decreasing with decreased renal function. The explanation is that the drug is metabolized by renal brush border dehydropeptidase and that this activity decreases with decreasing renal function. The intercept indicates that some nonrenal metabolism must be occurring. (Adapted from Verpooten, G.A., Verbist, L., Buntinx, A.P. Entwistle, L.A. Jones, K.H., and DeBroe, M.E.: The pharmacokinetics of imipenem (thienamycin-formamidine) and the renal dehydropeptidase inhibitor cilastatin sodium in normal subjects and patients with renal failure. Br. J. Clin. Pharmacol., *18*:183–193, 1984.)

creatinine clearance or serum creatinine have been given. This kind of information is useful for initiating drug therapy in an individual patient, but the variability remaining is often sufficiently large that monitoring of plasma concentration, the topic of Chap. 18, may be prudent for a drug with a narrow therapeutic window.

STUDY PROBLEMS

(Answers to Study Problems are in Appendix II.)

1. List and briefly discuss six diseases in which the pharmacokinetics of drugs is known to be altered.
2. a. Rank the situations in Table 16–4, from most important to least important, for considering a change in a dosage regimen of the cephalosporins listed in adult patients with varying degrees of renal function. Given that all these drugs have comparable therapeutic indices, use anticipated change in clearance as the basis of your ranking.
   b. Name the situations in Table 16–4 for which you would recommend that consideration be given to a change in the usual dosage regimen.

Table 16–4.

SITUATION	DRUG	PERCENT OF DOSE NORMALLY EXCRETED UNCHANGED (fe(f))	RENAL FUNCTION (Percent of Typical Patient)
A	Ceftizoxime	28	10
B	Cefonicid	98	5
C	Cefamandole	96	40
D	Ceforanide	80	20
E	Ceftazidime	84	60

3. Table 16–5 summarizes pharmacokinetic observations of two different opioid analgesics in patients with and without hepatic cirrhosis.

Table 16-5.[a]

	PENTAZOCINE		MEPERIDINE	
	CONTROL	CIRRHOTIC	CONTROL	CIRRHOTIC
Oral Bioavailability[b]	0.18	0.68	0.48	0.87
Blood clearance[c] (L/min)	1.25	0.68	0.90	0.57

[a]Average of data from Neal, E.A., Meffin, P.J., Gregory, P.B., and Blaschke, T.F.: Enhanced bioavailability and decreased clearance of analgesics in patients with cirrhosis. Gastroenterology, 77:96–102, 1979.
[b]From ratio of areas after oral and i.v. administrations on separate occasions.
[c]From Dose/AUC_b after an i.v. dose.

  a. Knowing that pentazocine and meperidine are eliminated primarily by hepatic metabolism, suggest a mechanism to explain the altered kinetics in hepatic cirrhosis.
  b. Explain why the oral bioavailability of pentazocine is affected much more than that of meperidine.

4. In Table 16–6, various data on four patients with varying degrees of renal function are listed. None of them is undergoing a dialysis procedure.

Table 16-6.

PATIENT:	S.W.	B.J.	D.A.	B.T.
Gender	M	F	F	M
Age (years)	25	82	3	15
Weight (kg)	84	60	15	68
Height (cm)	182	160	96	169
Serum Creatinine (mg/dL)	1.0	2.5	1.6	3.0

  a. Estimate the creatinine clearance in each of these individuals.
  b. Calculate the renal function in each of these patients. Express renal function as a ratio of creatinine clearance in the patient to the value expected in a typical 55-year-old, 70-kg patient.

5. Vancomycin is chosen for the therapy of a 17-kg, 4-year-old, 108-cm tall boy with staphylococcal pneumonia, which is refractory to other antibiotics. The child has moderately impaired renal function as indicated by a serum creatinine of 2.7 mg/dL. Approximately 95% of a dose of vancomycin is normally excreted unchanged. Its half-life and volume of distribution are 6 hr and 0.4 L/kg, respectively, in a typical 55-year-old patient.

  a. Estimate the maximum and minimum steady-state concentrations associated with therapy in a typical 55-year-old patient who receives a 1000-mg i.v. bolus dose every 12 hr.
  b. Determine a dosage regimen for the 4-year-old to attain and maintain the amount (or concentration) within the limits you derived in "a" above to minimize the likelihood of the child developing ototoxicity and a further decrease in renal function, both toxic manifestations of excessively high concentrations of vancomycin.
  c. Prepare sketches of the anticipated amount of vancomycin in the body with time had the usual maintenance dose been adjusted for:
    1. The child's age and weight only (no adjustment for renal disease).
    2. The child's age, weight, and renal function.
    No loading dose is given in either situation.

6. The kinetics of pentoxifylline, a hemorrheologic agent prescribed for the treatment of peripheral arterial disease and intermittent claudication, is affected by cirrhosis. Table 16–7 shows the changes in half-life and *AUC* following i.v. and oral (sustained-release tablet) administrations. Less than 1% is excreted unchanged in the urine. For the purpose of this problem, use only mean values.

Table 16–7. Half-Life and *AUC* of Pentoxifylline in Healthy Subjects and Cirrhotic Patients[a]

	HEALTHY SUBJECTS		CIRRHOTIC PATIENTS	
	HALF-LIFE (hr)	AUC (mg-hr/L)	HALF-LIFE (hr)	AUC (mg-hr/L)
Intravenous dose (100 mg)	0.8 ± 0.3	0.41 ± 0.08	2.1 ± 1.2	1.14 ± 0.51
Oral dose (400 mg) (sustained-release tablet)	—	0.52 ± 0.17	—	3.36 ± 1.76

[a]Abstracted from Rames, A., Poirier, J.-M, LeCoz, F., Midavaine, M., Lecocq, B., Grange J.-D., Poupon, R., Cheymol, G., and Jaillon, P.: Pharmacokinetics of intravenous and oral pentoxifylline in healthy volunteers and in cirrhotic patients. Clin. Pharmacol. Ther., 47:354–358, 1990.

a. Determine differences in pentoxifylline kinetic parameter values between healthy subjects and cirrhotic patients with respect to the following:
1. Absorption
2. Distribution
3. Elimination
b. Briefly discuss how hepatic cirrhosis is likely to produce the changes calculated for the absorption, distribution, and elimination parameters of this drug.

7. The pharmacokinetics of lorazepam, a benzodiazepine with demonstrated efficacy as an anxiolytic, anticonvulsant, antiemetic, and sedative hypnotic, was studied in patients with spinal cord injury. The drug (2-mg dose) was given as a single 1- to 2-min i.v. infusion. The results of the study in tetraplegics, paraplegics, and controls are summarized in Table 16–8. The drug is bound to albumin ($fu = 0.09$).

Table 16–8. Lorazepam Pharmacokinetic Parameters in Patients with Spinal Cord Injury and in Controls[a]

SUBJECTS	Cl (mL/min/m²)	V (L/kg)	$t_{1/2}$ (hr)
Tetraplegic (n = 9)	26 ± 6	1.6 ± 0.4	31 ± 13
Paraplegic (n = 6)	37 ± 11	1.6 ± 0.5	25 ± 9
Controls (n = 9)	42 ± 19	1.5 ± 0.5	20 ± 12

[a]Data from Segal, J.L., Brunnemann, S.R., Eltorai, I.M., and Vulpe M.: Decreased systemic clearance of lorazepam in humans with spinal cord injury. J. Clin. Pharmacol., 31:651–656, 1991.

a. When given orally, the bioavailability of lorazepam is 90%. Using the kinetic data in Table 16–8 and assuming instantaneous absorption, calculate the mean peak and trough concentrations expected on orally administering 2 mg twice daily (every 12 hr), a typical regimen for treatment of anxiety, in the tetraplegic and able-bodied (no spinal injury) patients. Use an average weight of 70-kg and $F = 0.9$ for all subjects.
b. Lorazepam is primarily eliminated by hepatic glucuronidation. Discuss each of the following mechanisms as a possible explanation for the decreased clearance of lorazepam in patients with spinal cord injury.
1. Decreased hepatic blood flow.
2. Decreased hepatocellular metabolic activity.

3. Enterohepatic cycling of drug through its glucuronide with less loss of drug or metabolite in feces.

4. Increased binding to plasma proteins.

8. The clearance and half-life values for flecainide, an antidysrhythmic agent, observed in six patients with hepatic cirrhosis and six healthy subjects, are listed in Table 16–9. The healthy subjects were, on average, matched in terms of age and weight with the cirrhotic group. The drug (2 mg/kg) was given by i.v. infusion over 15 min.

Table 16–9. Individual Values of Clearance and Half-life in Six Patients With Hepatic Cirrhosis and in Six Healthy Control Subjects[a]

	HEPATIC CIRRHOTICS	HEALTHY SUBJECTS
Clearance (mL/min/kg)	1.1, 1.6, 4.2, 4.6, 5.7, 5.8[b]	6.2, 8.2, 8.3, 9.5, 9.6, 11.7
Half-life (hr)	18, 28, 37, 43, 78, 107	9.1, 9.2, 9.4, 9.5, 9.5, 10.0

[a]Adapted from McQuinn, R.L., Pentikäinen, Chang, S.F., Conrad, G.J.: Pharmacokinetics of flecainide in patients with cirrhosis of the liver. Clin. Pharmacol. Ther., 44:566–572, 1988.
[b]Values are given in increasing order.

Do these observations support the notion that variability in clearance is greater in the presence of hepatic cirrhosis than in its absence? Briefly state the basis for your conclusions.

INTERACTING DRUGS

OBJECTIVES

The reader will be able to:

1. Discuss the graded nature of drug interactions.
2. Ascertain whether pharmacokinetics or pharmacodynamics of a drug, or both, is altered by another drug, given unbound plasma drug concentration-time data.
3. Anticipate the likely changes in plasma and unbound concentrations with time when the pharmacokinetics of a drug is altered by concurrent drug administration.
4. Show graphically the consequence of a pharmacokinetic drug interaction when the mechanism and the circumstances of its occurrence are given.

Patients commonly receive drugs two or more concurrently; indeed, inpatients on average receive five drugs during a hospitalization. The reasons for multiple drug therapy are many. One reason is that drug combinations have been found to be beneficial in the treatment of some conditions, including a variety of cardiovascular diseases, infections, and cancer. Another reason is that patients frequently suffer from several concurrent diseases or conditions, and each may require the use of one or more drugs. Furthermore, drugs are prescribed by different clinicians, and each clinician may be unaware of the others' therapeutic maneuvers.

Multiple drug therapy can give rise to a *drug interaction*. A drug interaction occurs when either pharmacokinetics or pharmacodynamics of one drug is altered by another. Drug interactions are of concern because, occasionally, the outcome of concurrent drug administration is diminished therapeutic efficacy or increased toxicity of one or more of the administered drugs. A *therapeutic drug interaction* has then occurred. The undesirable consequences of a drug interaction may arise from a lack of understanding of, or a failure to recall, the mode of action and the pharmacokinetics of each drug; many undesirable interactions are therefore potentially avoidable.

The possibilities for interactions among drugs within the body are almost limitless. Yet few of these interactions are of a type or of a sufficient magnitude to be clinically important. Many interactions between drugs within the body take place without affecting either the unbound drug concentration or the therapeutic activity of the drugs involved. Also, the dosage of many drugs needed to demonstrate a clinically significant drug interaction can exceed the median lethal dose. Furthermore, many affected processes and pathways of drug elimination are too minor to be of concern.

Implicit in the definition of drug interaction is the concept that, like essentially all responses of the body, they are graded. The degree of interaction depends on the concentration of the interacting species and hence on dose and time. That a given drug combination does not ensure the occurrence of a clinically significant interaction is illustrated by the data in Table 17–1. Chloral hydrate, a sedative hypnotic, is thought to potentiate transiently the anticoagulant effects of warfarin. Yet in only 22 of 237 patients, who were studied prospectively and who received chloral hydrate during warfarin therapy, was potentiation of warfarin's effect unambiguously demonstrated. The reasons for these differences in response are many. Included are individual differences in the dosage regimen and duration of administration of each drug, in the sequence of drug administration, and in patient compliance. Pharmacodynamic and pharmacokinetic differences due to genetics, to concurrent disease states, and to many other factors also contribute. Thus, the circumstances associated with a clinically significant interaction in an individual should always be carefully documented.

A final general comment needs to be made regarding the sequence of drug administration before considering specific mechanisms of drug interactions. A drug interaction is likely to be detected only when the interacting drug is initiated or withdrawn. For example, given the usual large degree of variability in patients' responses to drugs, it is unlikely that a drug interaction would be detected if the drug is administered to a patient stabilized on the drug causing the interaction. Certainly, the dosage regimen of the affected drug would be more different in *that* patient than would otherwise be the case, but the resulting regimen may still be within the normal range. In this case, only if the offending drug is withdrawn first, when the patient is stabilized on the drug combination, can the interaction be seen. The interaction would also have been detected if the interacting drug had been administered to the patient already stabilized on the original drug.

CLASSIFICATION

One system of classifying drug interactions is to note whether drug response is increased or decreased. While perhaps clinically useful, this classification does not help to define the mechanism of the interaction. In this book, interactions are classified on the basis of whether pharmacokinetics or pharmacodynamics is altered; occasionally, both are changed. Distinction between the two is made by relating response to the unbound plasma concentration of the pharmacologically active species. No change in the unbound concentration-response curve implies a pharmacokinetic drug interaction, which can arise either through a physical interaction, such as competition for protein binding sites, or through altered physiology, such as altered blood flow at an absorption site. The result is a change in one or more of the primary pharmacokinetic parameters, ka, F, V, CL_R, CL_H, which in turn alters the secondary pharmacokinetic parameters, such as half-life and fe.

Before proceeding, a discussion of what is meant by the word *interaction* is worthwhile. Strictly speaking, this word implies a *mutual effect*. The interaction between two drugs, A and B, might thus be denoted by A ↔ B. An example is the competition between two drugs for a common binding site on albumin: One drug displaces but is also displaced by the other. Generally, however, the term *interaction* is interpreted more broadly to indicate any situation in which one drug affects another. For example, phenobarbital appears to reduce the absorption of the diuretic, furosemide, but the renal clearance of phenobarbital

Table 17–1. Prospective Study of 237 Warfarin-Treated Patients for Detection of An Interaction Between Warfarin and Chloral Hydrate[a]

All patients who received chloral hydrate during warfarin therapy	237
Those patients who received chloral hydrate for at least 3 consecutive days	69
Impossible to evaluate interaction (clinically unstable or multiple drug changes)	28
Potentiation of hypoprothrombinemic action of warfarin	22
No demonstrable interaction	19

[a]Abstracted from Koch-Weser, J.: Hemorrhagic reactions and drug interactions in 500 warfarin-treated patients. Clin. Pharmacol. Ther., *14*:139–146, 1973.

is increased by the diuresis produced by furosemide. This might be regarded as a *bidirectional interaction* and may be denoted by A ⇌ B. Clearly, in the case of mutual and bidirectional interactions, the measured response of one drug cannot be considered without also defining the level of the other.

When given in sufficient quantities, two drugs almost always affect each other; this may not be the case, however, at concentrations achieved in therapy. For example, the antibiotic enoxacin inhibits the metabolism of theophylline, but theophylline, at doses normally given, does not affect the response or the pharmacokinetics of enoxacin. This interaction is *unidirectional* and may be denoted by A → B. In a unidirectional interaction, the unaffected Drug A, e.g., enoxacin, can be considered independently, but the change in response of the affected Drug B, e.g., theophylline, cannot be adequately defined without also considering the concentration-response curve of the effect of Drug A on Drug B. Examples of drug interactions are listed in Table 17–2.

The material in Chaps. 8 to 12 forms the basis for discussing many aspects of pharmacokinetic drug interactions. For convenience, in this chapter, the effect of one drug on another is examined under the separate headings of altered absorption, altered distribution, and altered clearance. However, it should be borne in mind that several pharmacokinetic parameters can be altered simultaneously.

ALTERED ABSORPTION

It was stated in Chaps. 4 and 7 that the more rapid the absorption process the higher and earlier is the peak plasma concentration and that neither total *AUC* after a single dose nor *AUC* within a dosing interval at plateau after chronic dosing changes unless the bioavailability of the drug is altered. Therapeutic consequences of a change in either rate or extent of drug absorption were discussed in Chap. 7.

Considered now are situations in which bioavailability is altered, with emphasis on changes in average plasma concentration with time; an altered rate of absorption changes only the degree of fluctuation around the average value. These situations are common in chronic drug therapy. The events are illustrated in Fig. 17–1.

Figure 17–1A depicts the situation in which a patient stabilized on Drug A, now receives Drug B, which reduces the bioavailability of Drug A. It is apparent that if no steps are taken to change the dosing rate of Drug A, its concentration falls to a lower plateau, the time being determined by the elimination half-life of this drug. Suppose that it is then noticed that the patient is no longer being treated effectively with Drug A, and that, having recognized the problem, the offending drug is withdrawn. The concentration of Drug A would then return to the previous plateau value in 3.3 elimination half-lives. Therapeutic control would again be restored. Alternatively, on another occasion, in anticipation of the problem but desiring to give the two drugs together, the dosing rate of Drug A is increased appropriately at the time that Drug B is introduced. As long as Drug B continues to be administered, therapeutic control is satisfactory. A problem arises, however, if Drug B is subsequently withdrawn, but the dosing rate of Drug A is not correspondingly reduced. Then, in 3.3 elimination half-lives, the concentration of Drug A reaches a higher plateau where toxicity is likely.

Another possible situation is one in which Drug A is added to the regimen of a patient stabilized on Drug B (Fig. 17–1B). Here, as before, optimal therapy with Drug A in the presence of Drug B is achieved only if the usual dosing rate of Drug A is appropriately increased. However, the danger of the concentration of Drug A rising too high, if the dosing rate of Drug A is not readjusted when Drug B is withdrawn, must always be kept in mind.

The situations just considered emphasize the dependence of time scale of events on the half-life of the affected drug. Thus, for affected drugs with very long half-lives, such as phenobarbital ($t_{1/2}$ of 4 days), changes in response are insidious, and the clinician may not associate the interaction with the causative drug, which was either initiated or stopped sometime previously.

ALTERED DISTRIBUTION

The most common explanation for altered distribution in a drug interaction is displacement. Displacement is the reduction in the binding of a drug to a macromolecule, usually a protein, caused by competition of another drug, the *displacer*, for common binding site(s). The result is a rise in the fraction of drug unbound in plasma or tissue, or both. Sometimes, binding is diminished through an allosteric effect. The second drug, binding at another site, induces a conformational change in the protein, thereby reducing the affinity of the first drug for the protein. Occasionally, an allosteric effect causes an enhanced affinity between drug and protein; drug binding is then increased.

Table 17–2. Classification and Examples of Drug Interactions

PHARMACODYNAMIC INTERACTIONS

RESPONSE	EXAMPLE	COMMENT
↑	Tranylcypromine →[a] Phenylpropano-lamine	By inhibiting monamine oxidase, tranylcypromine potentiates the sympathomimetic action of phenylpropanolamine.
	Chlorpheniramine ↔[b] Alcohol	Mutual sedative effects.
↓	Chlorpromazine → Guanethidine	Chlorpromazine blocks uptake of guanethidine at postganglionic adrenergic neuron.
	Warfarin ↔ Vitamin K	Each lowers the effectiveness of the other.

PHARMACOKINETIC INTERACTIONS

PARAMETER	RESPONSE	EXAMPLE	COMMENT
Absorption rate	↑	Metoclopramide → Acetaminophen	Metoclopramide hastens gastric emptying.
	↓	Epinephrine → Lidocaine	Epinephrine decreases blood flow to injection site of lidocaine.
Oral bioavailability	↑	Cimetidine → Metoprolol	Cimetidine inhibits metoprolol metabolism, expressed as diminished first-pass effect.
	↓	Calcium → Tetracycline	Calcium forms an insoluble complex with tetracycline.
Volume of distribution	↑	Phenytoin ← Valproic acid	Valproic acid displaces phenytoin from albumin.
	↓	Quinidine → Digoxin	Quinidine displaces digoxin from tissue binding sites
Hepatic clearance	↑	Rifampin → Warfarin	Rifampin induces microsomal enzymes.
	↓	Erythromycin → Theophylline	Erythromycin inhibits theophylline metabolism.
Renal clearance	↑	Cilastatin → Imipenem	Cilastatin inhibits the renal metabolism of imipenem. In this case, organ clearance is affected, not excretory clearance, the meaning of renal clearance by default.
	↓	Chlorothiazide → Lithium	Chlorothiazide diminishes secretion of lithium.

[a]Denotes a unidirectional interaction; the arrow points to affected drug.
[b]Denotes a mutual interaction.

Conditions Favoring Displacement

Two conditions must be met before substantial displacement occurs. First, in the absence of a displacer, the drug must be bound mostly to a protein, that is, its *fu* must be low. Obviously, if a drug is not bound, it cannot be displaced. Second, the displacer must occupy the majority of the binding sites, thereby substantially lowering the number of sites available to bind the drug. This second condition is likely to be met when the displacer occupies most of the binding sites.

Table 17–3 lists two groups of drugs that bind to albumin, a protein that exists abundantly in plasma (140 g/3 L; 0.6 mM) and in the interstitial fluids (210 g). Not all drugs bind

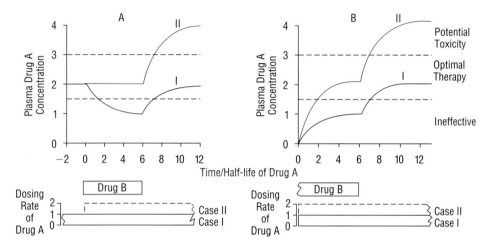

Fig. 17–1. Altered absorption. As long as Drug B is administered, the bioavailability of Drug A is reduced by one-half. For simplicity, Drug A is assumed to be given at a constant rate. The therapeutic concentration range of Drug A lies between 1.5 and 3 units/L.

A, Patient stabilized on Drug A. The plasma concentration of Drug A falls by one-half (case I), unless the dosing rate is doubled (case II, color), when Drug B is concurrently administered. A problem potentially arises if administration of Drug A is not reduced to its preexisting rate when Drug B is removed (case II, color).

B, Patient stabilized on Drug B. An adequate concentration of Drug A is not achieved (case I) unless the usual dosing rate of this drug is doubled (case II, color). When Drug B is withdrawn, there is a potential problem similar to that considered in *A.*

Table 17–3. Binding of Selected Drugs to Albumin

DRUGS THAT BIND TO AND COMPETE FOR ONE OF TWO SITES, DESIGNATED I AND II, ON ALBUMIN	
SITE I[a]	SITE II[b]
Chlorothiazide	Benzodiazepines
Furosemide	Cloxacillin
Indomethacin[c]	Dicloxacillin
Naproxen[c]	Glibenclamide
Phenytoin	Ibuprofen
Sulfadimethoxine	Indomethacin
Salicylic acid	Naproxen
Tolbutamide[c]	Oxacillin
Valproic acid	Probenecid
Warfarin	Tolbutamide

[a]Archetype: warfarin
[b]Archetype: diazepam
[c]These drugs bind to both sides

to and hence compete for the same primary binding site on albumin. Albumin and some other proteins have several binding sites, each exhibiting some degree of specificity; possessing an acidic function is not a sufficient criterion for predicting the ability of one acidic drug to displace another. Moreover, even though almost all those drugs that compete for the same site have a high affinity for albumin, only a few are generally listed as displacers, such as salicylic acid, valproic acid, and phenylbutazone. This list is limited because the plasma concentration achieved during therapy must approach or exceed 0.6 mM, the molar concentration of plasma albumin. For a substance with a molecular weight of 250, this concentration corresponds to 150 mg/L. This concentration is approached during salicylate and valproic acid therapy, because these drugs are commonly given in doses approaching 1 g and because they possess relatively small volumes of distribution, 10 to 15 L. With phenylbutazone the plasma concentration achieved with the usual dose, 100 mg ($V = 10$ L), is only 10 mg/L but because its clearance is low and half-life is long (3 days), the plateau concentration ultimately achieved is high when the usual maintenance regimen of 100 to 300 mg daily is administered.

Displacers share an expected common property; i.e., their *fu* values change with plasma concentration. With most sites occupied by the displacer, the fraction unoccupied is sensitive to a change in the concentration of displacer. Therefore, displacers must show concentration-dependent disposition kinetics (Chap. 22, Dose and Time Dependencies).

So far, distinction has been made between displacers and displaced drug, but it should be apparent that this classification is arbitrary. Phenylbutazone is said to displace warfarin from albumin, but only because the plasma concentration of phenylbutazone (100 mg/L; 0.3 mM) approaches the molar concentration of albumin (0.6 mM), whereas that of warfarin (1 to 4 mg/L; 0.003 to 0.01 mM) does not. Both drugs have similar affinities for the same site on albumin, and if the concentrations were reversed, warfarin would be called the displacer.

The conclusions drawn from the interactions between acidic drugs and albumin are generally applicable to all drug–protein interactions, bearing in mind the widely differing molar concentrations of the various binding proteins in plasma (Chap. 10, p. 143). For example, the molar concentration of α_1-acid glycoprotein, which avidly binds many basic drugs, is low (9–23 μM), and therefore displacement interactions can occur at plasma concentrations much lower than those required for displacement of acidic drugs from albumin (600 μM concentration).

Therapeutic Implications

Displacement interactions in plasma have been studied primarily *in vitro*. The potential displacer is added to a sample of plasma containing the drug, and changes in its binding are measured. Substantial displacement is frequently demonstrated *in vitro*; yet this may be of little therapeutic consequence. Much depends on whether the events are acute or occur at plateau during chronic therapy.

Acute Events. Two situations can be envisaged. One involves the administration of a loading dose of drug to a patient already stabilized on a displacer. The other involves the administration of a dose of displacer to a patient already stabilized on a drug. In both situations, the question of altering the usual dose of drug arises only if the unbound drug concentration increases above the therapeutic range, in the presence of the displacer. Stated differently, is the unbound volume of distribution (Vu) decreased significantly? Such a decrease in Vu occurs only if, in the absence of the displacer, the drug is substantially bound in the body and the displacer causes significant displacement of drug from the major binding sites. For example, the unbound concentration rises if displacement occurs from sites on a plasma protein for a drug with a small volume of distribution, around 10 L/70 kg, or if displacement occurs from tissue binding sites for a drug with a large volume of distribution. An example of the former situation is the displacement of warfarin from albumin binding sites by naproxen. An example of the latter situation is the displacement of digoxin from tissue binding sites by quinidine. These situations are relatively uncommon, however. More common is displacement, from plasma binding sites, of a drug with a large volume of distribution. Then, because so little drug resides in plasma only a minimal change in the unbound drug concentration occurs even when all the drug on the proteins is displaced, as discussed in Chap. 10, Distribution. For example, if the volume of distribution is 100 L and 99% of the drug in plasma is bound ($fu = 0.01$), then only 3% ($100 \times (1 - fu) \cdot$ (plasma volume)/V) of that in the body resides bound in plasma. Even if completely displaced, the small amount affected would redistribute throughout the rest of the body and so would only marginally increase the unbound body pool and hence unbound concentrations in plasma and tissue. Conceivably, if the displacer were injected rapidly enough, the unbound drug concentration in plasma would rise appreciably, but only momentarily, because displaced drug would move rapidly down the newly created unbound concentration gradient into the large tissue water space. In practice, this last situation is unlikely to arise because of adverse reactions often experienced when drugs are injected too rapidly.

Returning to the two examples above: With digoxin, quinidine causes a sufficiently large decrease in Vu to warrant considering a reduction in the loading dose of digoxin in the presence of quinidine. With warfarin, because the clinical response (prothrombin time) is so delayed and insensitive to acute changes in warfarin concentration (Fig. 5–7, Chap. 5), no adjustment in dosage of this oral anticoagulant would be contemplated in the event of acute displacement. A more important consideration for both of these drugs and most others is the effect of displacement on events at plateau, as most drugs, including displacers, are given chronically.

Events at Plateau. The influence of displacement on the unbound concentration at steady state (Cu_{ss}) depends on extraction ratio and route of administration of the affected drug.

Consider a drug with a *low extraction ratio*. Recall that clearance depends on fu, but unbound clearance (CLu) does not. Also recall the equalities (Eq. 28, Chap. 11)

$$\text{Rate of elimination} = CLu \cdot Cu = CL \cdot C \qquad 1$$

When drug is infused at a constant rate, R_o, and steady state is achieved,

$$R_o = CLu \cdot Cu_{ss} = CL \cdot C_{ss} \qquad 2$$

However, since unbound clearance, e.g., that of a glomerularly filtered drug, is unaffected by displacement, the same is true of the value of Cu_{ss}. Thus, although displacement by increasing fu increases clearance (and hence causes the total plasma concentration to fall), no change in response and therefore in dosing rate is anticipated at steady state. Neither is any change anticipated in $Cu_{ss,av}$, upon chronic oral dosing.

Now consider a drug with a *high extraction ratio*. Because clearance is unaffected by displacement, the steady-state blood concentration is also unaffected following a constant-rate intravenous (i.v.) infusion. However, as binding is diminished, Cu_{ss} and therefore response to the drug must be increased. The maintenance dosing rate of the drug may need to be reduced.

Prediction of the outcome when a drug with a high extraction ratio is given orally and when elimination occurs predominantly in the liver is difficult. In the presence of the displacer, both unbound drug clearance and oral bioavailability decrease (see Chap. 12); the effect of displacement on the unbound drug concentration at plateau is therefore likely to be relatively small. Irrespective of any effect of displacement, however, the unbound concentration at plateau is lower than that achieved following an equivalent i.v. infusion.

The events predicted at plateau before and after displacement for drugs of low and high extraction are shown in Fig. 17–2. Shown in Fig. 17–3 are the total and unbound plateau plasma concentrations of the antiepileptic drug phenytoin in patients before and after receiving valproic acid, another antiepileptic drug, which displaces phenytoin from albumin binding sites. As predicted for a drug of low extraction, the unbound concentration is unaltered, while the total plasma concentration is decreased. Accordingly, based on these observations, there is no need to alter the dosing rate of phenytoin in patients receiving valproic acid.

Kinetic Features. Both acute events and events at plateau have been discussed. Remaining to be discussed are the kinetic consequences of displacement on approach to plateau under the usual condition in which both drug and displacer are given chronically. To do so, consider the expected changes in disposition kinetics of a drug upon displacement.

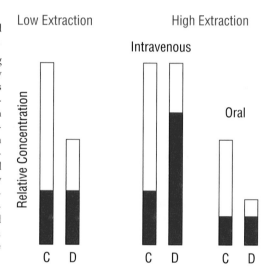

Fig. 17–2. Changes, at plateau, in the total (▨) and unbound (▮) concentrations (D = displaced; C = control) depend on the extraction ratio of the drug and route of drug administration. For a drug of low extraction ratio, diminished binding (fu ↑) reduces the total, but not the unbound, concentration regardless of the route of administration. For a drug of high hepatic extraction ratio, clearance, and so total concentration, is unaffected by diminished binding when the drug is given intravenously. The unbound concentration, however, is elevated. Because diminished binding decreases oral bioavailability of the highly cleared drug, the likely outcome of displacement after oral administration is a decrease in the total concentration and little or no change in the unbound concentration. The actual change depends on whether the effect on oral bioavailability or clearance predominates.

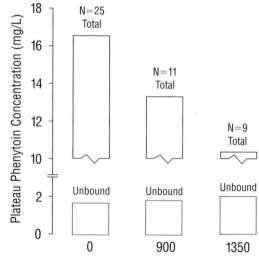

Fig. 17–3. The valproic acid–phenytoin interaction involves displacement only. Although plasma protein binding of phenytoin is decreased when sodium valproate is administered chronically to a group of patients stabilized on phenytoin, with a resultant fall in the steady-state plasma phenytoin concentration, there was no substantial change in the unbound phenytoin concentration (color). These observations are consistent with a displacement interaction of phenytoin by valproic acid. Note that the degree of phenytoin displacement depends on the dose of sodium valproate. Of the 25 patients stabilized on phenytoin, 11 received 900 mg sodium valproate per day; 9 received a 1350-mg daily dose; and some received both regimens (1 mg/L = 4.0 μM). (Taken from Mattson, R.H., Cramer, J.A., Williamson, P.D., Novelly, R.A.: Valproic acid in epilepsy: Clinical and pharmacological effects. Ann. Neurol., 3:20–25, 1978.)

Disposition Kinetics. The subsequent points summarize those made in Chapters 10 to 12. Because clearance of a drug with a high extraction ratio is unaffected by displacement, the half-life changes with volume of distribution. In contrast, for a drug of low extraction, because unbound clearance, CLu, does not change, half-life either remains constant (when Vu does not change) or shortens (if Vu decreases) with displacement from plasma proteins.

Plasma Concentration-Time Profile. Although there are many possible combinations of events, only one common situation is considered. In this case (Fig. 17–4) the displacer, which has a longer $t_{1/2}$ than that of the drug, is added to the regimen of a patient stabilized on a low extraction ratio drug. To simplify matters, both drug and displacer are administered by constant-rate infusion and both are assumed to always be at distribution equilibrium. While these conditions are somewhat restrictive, the situation chosen does illustrate the importance of both kinetics and the manner of drug administration on the likely therapeutic outcome.

Notice in Fig. 17–4 that slow accumulation and correspondingly slow elimination of the displacer results in insignificant changes in the unbound drug concentration and therefore response. This is a consequence of the kinetics of the displacer being slower than that of the drug. The concentration of the displacer is changing so slowly relative to that of the drug that at all times the drug is at a virtual steady state, with rate of elimination ($CLu \cdot Cu_{ss}$) matching the rate of administration. That is, although there is a tendency for the unbound drug concentration to rise above the concentration at steady state during accumulation of the displacer, there is an opposing tendency for the unbound concentration to fall because the rate of elimination ($CLu \cdot Cu$) would then exceed the rate of administration ($CLu \cdot Cu_{ss}$). The reverse tendencies occur on stopping the displacer, but once again they balance each other out. Accordingly, although the unbound concentration remains essentially unaltered, the total plasma drug concentration changes inversely with that of the displacer, reflecting the changing degree of displacement. A transient change in

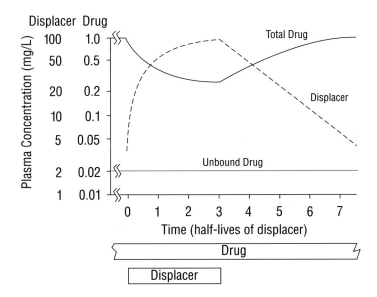

Fig. 17–4. When constantly infused, the unbound concentration (color) of a drug with a low extraction ratio remains virtually unchanged if a displacer with a long half-life, relative to the drug, is either infused or withdrawn. The change in total plasma drug concentration reflects the displacement.

unbound concentration might occur if the kinetics of the drug, rather than that of the displacer, had been the slower. However, this situation is relatively uncommon.

In the case just discussed, no change in effect and hence in the dosage regimen of the drug is anticipated even though displacement has occurred. Indeed, if only response were monitored, displacement would not have been suspected.

DIMINISHED UNBOUND CLEARANCE

A reduction in unbound clearance is potentially the most dangerous type of drug interaction. The unbound drug concentration can then rise to a toxic level, unless an adjustment in dosage is made. Consequently, it is extremely important to be able to identify, characterize, and where possible, avoid this type of interaction. Inhibition of drug metabolism is the major cause of reduced unbound clearance.

A Case Study

Some patients receiving theophylline develop nausea when enoxacin, an anti-infective quinoline, is added to the theophylline regimen. The nausea is associated with an elevated concentration of theophylline caused by enoxacin inhibiting the metabolism of theophylline.

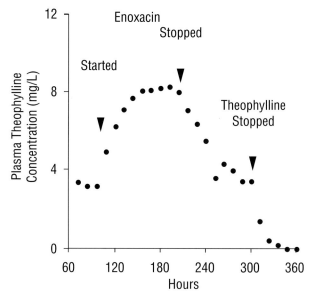

Fig. 17–5. Enoxacin inhibits theophylline elimination. Subjects received 150 mg theophylline (in a controlled-release dosage form) orally every 12 hr for 12 days (288 hr). By 72 hr, as expected, the trough had reached a plateau with an average concentration within a dosing interval of 4.8 mg/L (not shown). Enoxacin was given, 400 mg orally every 12 hr for 4 days, starting 96 hr into the theophylline regimen. On addition of enoxacin, the mean trough theophylline concentration rose to a new and higher plateau (average interdose concentration of 9 mg/L, not shown). The time course of the rise was determined by the half-life of theophylline in the presence of enoxacin (22 hr). Although, on withdrawal of enoxacin, the plasma theophylline concentration fell toward the pre-enoxacin value (average interdose concentration of 4 mg/L, not shown), the concentration of enoxacin must have been sufficient to maintain appreciable inhibition for some time. Otherwise, the return of theophylline to the pre-enoxacin concentration would have been much shorter, being determined by the normal half-life of theophylline, 8.8 hr (theophylline: 1 mg/L = 5.5 μM). (Modified from Rogge, M.C., Solomon, W.R., Sedman, A.J., Welling, P.G., Koup, J.R., and Wagner, J.G.: The theophylline-enoxacin interaction: II. Changes in the disposition of theophylline and its metabolites during intermittent administration of enoxacin. Clin. Pharmacol. Ther., *46*:420–428, 1989.)

The dramatic rise in the trough plasma concentration of theophylline when enoxacin is added to the regimen and the return to the pre-enoxacin value when enoxacin is withdrawn are illustrated in Fig. 17–5. Notice that it takes approximately 4 days of enoxacin administration for theophylline concentration to rise to the new plateau and a similar time for it to return to the pre-enoxacin value after enoxacin is withdrawn.

A more quantitative picture of the events may be gained from two equations. One, previously examined (Eq. 8, Chap. 7), defines the average concentration of drug at plateau

$$C_{ss,av} = \frac{F \cdot Dose}{CL \cdot \tau} \qquad\qquad 3$$

The other equation defines the new (and longer) half-life of theophylline ($t_{1/2,inhibited}$) in relation to the normal half-life ($t_{1/2,normal}$).

$$t_{1/2,inhibited} = t_{1/2,normal} \cdot \frac{CL_{normal}}{CL_{inhibited}} \qquad\qquad 4$$

where CL_{normal} and $CL_{inhibited}$ are the clearances of theophylline in the absence and presence of the inhibitor, respectively. Equation 4 follows from the equation $k = CL/V$ and from the knowledge that enoxacin does not affect the volume of distribution of theophylline, a drug only weakly bound in plasma and tissue.

The half-life of theophylline in the absence of enoxacin is 8.8 hr, estimated from the declining concentration when theophylline administration is stopped (day 13). As expected, with such a short half-life, the plateau concentration ($C_{ss,av}$), approximately 4 mg/L, is reached within about 2 days of starting the theophylline regimen.

Enoxacin is rapidly absorbed and immediately inhibits theophylline metabolism when administered on the fifth day into the theophylline regimen. With continual administration of the same dosage regimen of theophylline, its plasma concentration rises to a new plateau, approximately 9 mg/L, determined by the new, and lower, clearance value ($CL_{inhibited}$). Accordingly, by reference to Eq. 3,

$$\frac{CL_{inhibited}}{CL_{normal}} = \frac{C_{ss,av,normal}}{C_{ss,av,inhibited}} \qquad\qquad 5$$

and on substituting 4 mg/L and 9 mg/L for $C_{ss,av,normal}$ and $C_{ss,av,inhibited}$, one obtains $CL_{inhibited} = 0.44\, CL_{normal}$. That is, enoxacin reduces the clearance of theophylline by 56%. This calculation is based on the assumption that the bioavailability of theophylline, which is usually well absorbed, is unaffected by enoxacin.

The new half-life of theophylline in the presence of the inhibitor can now be calculated by appropriately substituting into Eq. 4; it is 22 hr (8.8 L × 1/0.44). This longer half-life explains why it takes 4 days, rather than the usual 2, to reach the new plateau. It is also consistent with the observation that the plasma concentration of theophylline (6.5 mg/L) midway between the previous and new plateaus occurs 1 day after administering enoxacin.

The slow return of the plasma theophylline concentration to the pre-enoxacin value on withdrawal of enoxacin remains to be explained. Although withdrawn, the concentration of enoxacin in plasma persists at a sufficiently high value to continue to inhibit the metabolism of theophylline for a considerable period of time. As such, the half-life of theophylline, which controls the return of theophylline to its pre-enoxacin concentration, remains elevated for some time. Had inhibition ceased immediately upon withdrawing enoxacin, the half-life of theophylline would have reverted back to its control value, 8.8 hr, and the return of theophylline concentration to the pre-enoxacin value would have been much quicker.

A Graded Effect

The last statement needs some amplification. The inhibition of theophylline by enoxacin is not an all-or-none response, but rather a graded one. The degree of inhibition varies with the plasma concentration, and hence dose, of enoxacin, as illustrated in Fig. 17–6. Shown are both the plasma concentration-time profiles and AUC of theophylline following a single dose of theophylline taken alone and at steady state during regimens of 25, 100, and 400 mg of enoxacin given every 12 hr. As expected for a drug of low clearance, both AUC and half-life of theophylline increase with inhibition. Notice that inhibition is evident even with the 25-mg enoxacin regimen and then increases, tending to approach an upper limit with the 400-mg regimen. Restated, even though the plasma enoxacin concentration falls after a 400-mg dose, inhibition persists, to varying degrees, for some time thereafter. Clearly, the longer the half-life of an inhibitor, the more persistent is inhibition on withdrawing it.

To appreciate more fully the graded nature of inhibition of metabolism, consider the following. Recall (Chap. 11) that for each metabolic pathway

$$\text{Rate of metabolite formation} = \frac{Vm}{Km} \cdot Cu \qquad\qquad 6$$

when the unbound drug concentration, Cu, is well below the Michaelis-Menten constant, Km. Or, expressed in terms of unbound clearance associated with metabolite formation, CLu_f.

$$\text{Rate of metabolite formation} = CLu_f \cdot Cu = fm \cdot CLu \cdot Cu \qquad\qquad 7$$

where fm is the fraction of the dose of drug that is converted to the metabolite. Inhibition decreases CLu_f of a metabolite. A common model to describe this effect is

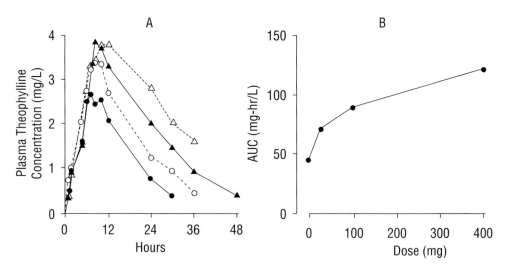

Fig. 17–6. The inhibition of theophylline elimination by enoxacin is graded, as evidenced by the prolongation in half-life of decline of plasma theophylline concentration (*A*) and increase in *AUC* (*B*) when a 200-mg dose of theophylline is administered alone (●) and during 7-day regimens of 25-mg (○), 100-mg (▲), and 400-mg (△) enoxacin given every 12 hr. Data are the means of 4 subjects (1 mg/L = 5.5 μM). (Data from Rogge, M.C., Solomon, W.R., Sedman, A.J., Welling, P.G., Toothaker, R.D., and Wagner, J.G.: The theophylline-enoxacin interaction: I. Effect of enoxacin dose size on theophylline disposition. Clin. Pharmacol. Ther., *44*:579–587, 1988.)

$$\text{Rate of metabolite formation} = \frac{CLu_f \cdot Cu}{1 + Cu_I/K_I} \qquad 8$$

where Cu_I is the unbound concentration of the inhibitor and K_I is the inhibition constant, given by the unbound concentration of inhibitor that decreases CLu_f by twofold. Clearly, the lower the K_I, the more potent is an inhibitor.

Two main conclusions may be drawn from Eq. 8. First, the degree of inhibition of a particular pathway depends on the unbound concentration of the inhibitor relative to its K_I. Many compounds have been shown to inhibit drug metabolism *in vitro* but fail to do so *in vivo*, because the unbound concentrations associated with therapeutic regimens of the inhibition are well below the K_I value.

Second, the impact of inhibition on drug elimination depends on *fm*. Inhibition has the most profound effect when the affected pathway is obligatory for the elimination of the drug, that is when *fm* $\approx$ 1. Often there are multiple pathways. Even at the highest dose, enoxacin is only able to reduce the (total) clearance of theophylline by approximately twofold with a corresponding doubling of theophylline half-life. Theophylline is eliminated by demethylation, ring oxidation, and renal excretion. Evidently, enoxacin inhibits only some of these pathways. The antidepressant desipramine, metabolized by the cytochrome P450 enzyme, CYP2D6 (see Chap. 13, Genetics) to form 2-hydroxydesipramine, is another example. Quinidine, a potent inhibitor of CYP2D6, effectively converts extensive metabolizers of desipramine, in whom this pathway is a major one, to poor metabolizers, with a pronounced reduction in clearance of approximately fourfold and corresponding prolongation in half-life. In such cases, the clinical consequences of an interaction depends on the relative contributions of drug and metabolite to efficacy and toxicity. With desipramine, the dose in extensive metabolizers should be reduced to avoid toxicity, if quinidine is co-administered. As might be expected, quinidine has little effect on the pharmacokinetics of desipramine in the already poor CYP2D6 metabolizer phenotype because the affected pathway is now a minor one.

A Multifaceted Interaction

Although the anti-inflammatory drug phenylbutazone is no longer widely used, its interaction with warfarin is well-documented. The interaction has caused serious bleeding episodes. Warfarin is highly bound in plasma to albumin. Phenylbutazone, devoid of inherent anticoagulant activity, displaces warfarin. Consequently, displacement has been advocated as the primary mechanism for this interaction.

Figure 17–7 shows the temporal effects of phenylbutazone administration on the plasma and unbound concentrations of warfarin in a subject who ingested 10 mg warfarin daily. The half-life of warfarin is approximately 2 days, and therefore, as anticipated, a steady state for this drug is reached within the first 12 days, when warfarin alone is administered. At this time the warfarin plasma concentration is approximately 4 mg/L and only 0.5% (0.02 mg/L) is unbound, i.e., *fu* = 0.005. Warfarin is completely absorbed, and therefore its clearance, estimated by dividing the daily dosing rate by the steady-state plasma concentration, is 0.1 L/hr. Thus, warfarin is a highly bound drug with a low extraction ratio.

Phenylbutazone is also poorly extracted, is highly bound (*fu* = 0.004 to 0.010), and has a half-life (approximately 3 days) even longer than that of warfarin. Accordingly, when on day 13 the subject commences the usually recommended dosage regimen of phenylbutazone, 100 mg three times a day, the plasma concentration of this drug rises and eventually reaches a plateau of approximately 100 mg/L, after approximately 10 days. During this period, the plasma warfarin falls steadily in half, to 2 mg/L, and the value of *fu* for warfarin rises approximately threefold.

At this point, the events in plasma appear remarkably similar to those depicted in Fig. 17–4 for a pure displacement interaction. However, there is one important difference. The unbound warfarin concentration rises and remains elevated during phenylbutazone administration. Because the effect of warfarin is related to its unbound concentration, this sustained elevation is in accord with the observed sustained augmentation of the effect as long as phenylbutazone is coadministered. Examination of Eq. 2 indicates that to account for the elevated values of unbound drug, either the rate of entry of drug into the body is increased or the value of CLu is decreased. As the dosage regimen of warfarin is unaltered and warfarin is fully bioavailable, CLu must have decreased.

Warfarin is almost exclusively metabolized in the liver to either weakly active or inactive metabolites. Thus, a lower value for CLu implies a decrease in the ability of the liver to metabolize warfarin. Analysis of several metabolites of warfarin in both plasma and urine subsequently confirmed that, indeed, phenylbutazone inhibits warfarin elimination, and it is this inhibition and not displacement that accounts for the clinical picture.

The interaction between phenylbutazone and warfarin is even more complex than portrayed above. Commercial warfarin is a racemate, that is, a 50:50 mixture of R(+)- and S(−)-warfarin, and the S(−) isomer is five times more active than the R(+)-isomer. Phenylbutazone primarily inhibits the formation of 7-(S)-hydroxywarfarin, the major metabolite of the more active isomer. The lesson is clear: Drug interactions can be complex; careful observations are required to unravel the facts.

Fig. 17–7. Warfarin–phenylbutazone interaction. A subject received 10 mg warfarin orally each day and 100 mg phenylbutazone three times a day on days 13 to 22. As the phenylbutazone concentration rose, bound warfarin was displaced, and the plasma warfarin concentration fell. The sustained elevation in the unbound warfarin during phenylbutazone administration implies inhibition of warfarin elimination (phenylbutazone, 1 mg/L = 3.2 μM; warfarin, 1 mg/L = 3.3 μM). (Modified from Schary, W.L., Lewis, R.J., and Rowland, M.: Warfarin-phenylbutazone interaction in man: A long term multiple-dose study. Res. Commun. Chem. Pathol. Pharmacol., 10:633–672, 1975.)

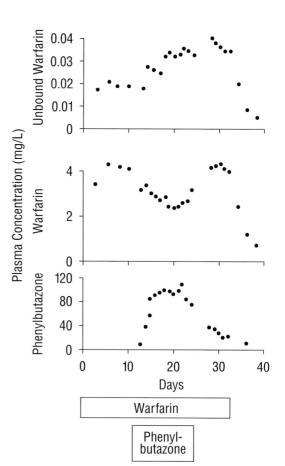

Other Causes of Reduced Clearance

Inhibition of metabolism and secretion are examples of chemically mediated pharmacokinetic interactions. The lower hepatic clearance of lidocaine when given together with propranolol, a β-adrenergic blocking drug, is an example of a physiologically mediated pharmacokinetic interaction. Propranolol diminishes cardiac output and hence hepatic blood flow, which, in turn, reduces the clearance of lidocaine, a drug highly extracted by the liver. Presumably, since the degree of β-adrenergic blockade is a graded response, the interaction with lidocaine is dependent on the plasma concentration of propranolol.

Beneficial Interactions

Penicillin–probenecid combination therapy is an example of the successful use of a drug interaction. Both of these acidic drugs are renally secreted by an anionic transport system. Probenecid competitively inhibits the renal secretion of penicillin thereby substantially reducing its renal clearance, the major component of total clearance. Consequently, in the presence of probenecid, higher than usual plasma concentrations of penicillin are achieved following a normal dosage regimen of the antibiotic. Of note is the lack of a major effect of penicillin on probenecid elimination. Although probenecid is also actively secreted into the kidney tubule; unlike penicillin, it is lipophilic and mostly reabsorbed. Consequently, the renal clearance of probenecid is low; metabolism is the major route of its elimination.

Another example of a beneficial interaction is that between cilastatin and the antibiotic imipenem. Imipenem is metabolized extensively in the kidney by a dehydropeptidase, located at the brush border of the proximal tubular cell. Consequently, the urinary excretion of intact imipenem is low and often insufficient to guarantee effective treatment of urinary tract infections. To improve the efficacy of imipenem, it is marketed in combination with cilastatin, a dehydropeptidase inhibitor, which markedly increases the urinary excretion of unchanged imipenem (Fig. 17–8).

ELEVATED UNBOUND CLEARANCE

The unbound clearance of a drug can be increased in numerous ways. Raising urine pH by giving acetazolamide or sodium bicarbonate increases the renal clearance of salicylic

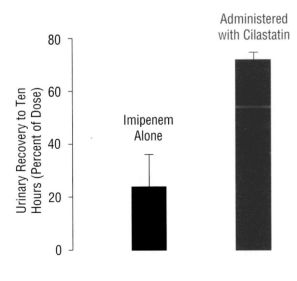

Fig. 17–8. Cilastatin markedly increases the urinary excretion of the antibiotic imipenem by inhibiting the dehydropeptidase in the kidney responsible for its metabolism. The urinary recovery of imipenem is shown after a 500-mg i.v. bolus dose administered alone (black) and together with an i.v. bolus of 500 mg cilastatin (color). (Redrawn from Norby S.R., Alestig, K., Björnegärd, B., Burman, L.A., Ferber, F., Huber, J.L., Jones, K.H., Kahan, F.M., Kahan, J.S., Kropp, H., Meisinger, M.A.P., and Sundelotf, J.G.: Urinary recovery of N-formimidoyl thienamycin (MK0187) as affected by coadministration of N-formimidoyl thienamycin dehydropeptidase inhibitors. Antimicrob. Agents Chemother., 23:300–307, 1983.)

acid and other acids whose renal clearance is pH sensitive. Giving ammonium chloride or ascorbic acid to make the urine more acidic increases the renal clearance of pH-sensitive basic drugs. Some drugs increase the metabolic clearance of other drugs. They do so most commonly by inducing the drug-metabolizing enzymes, but they may also activate enzymes or retard enzyme degradation. Occasionally, like glucagon, they increase hepatic blood flow and thereby increase the hepatic clearance of drugs that are highly extracted by the liver.

Kinetic consequences of an increased metabolic clearance were discussed in Chaps. 11 and 12. The implications of these changes on dosage requirements and the events that follow the addition or withdrawal of drug causing the altered clearance are now presented.

In general, a dosage regimen adjustment is required only when the clearance of the affected pathway is or becomes a significant fraction of total drug clearance. Thus, a need to change the dose is anticipated if the clearance associated with a particular pathway, previously 20% of total clearance, were to increase sixfold, because total drug clearance is then doubled. No change in the dose is anticipated, even if clearance associated with that pathway increased 20-fold, if this clearance contributes only 1% to total clearance. An exception arises when the metabolite formed is either the active species or is toxic, because its plasma concentration can be greatly increased.

The events depicted in Fig. 17–9 illustrate salient consequences of an increased clearance. In this illustration a patient stabilized on one drug (Drug A) also receives another (Drug B) that doubles the clearance of Drug A. If the dosing rate of Drug A is not changed, then its concentration falls by one-half, at a rate determined by the half-life of the drug *in the presence of Drug B* (Case I). The fall in concentration can be avoided by doubling the rate of administration of Drug A for as long as Drug B is given (Case II). However, a problem of excessive accumulation of Drug A exists if the higher dosing rate is maintained when Drug B is withdrawn. Because the half-life of Drug A is generally longer when given alone, especially for a drug of low extraction ratio, if follows that the time taken to reach a plateau is longer in the absence than presence of Drug B.

Two major assumptions were made in constructing the curves in Fig. 17–9, namely that the effect of Drug B is achieved instantly and remains constant as long as it is administered, and that the effect immediately disappears upon its withdrawal. In practice, both assumptions are invalid.

Fig. 17–9. When a patient stabilized on Drug A also receives Drug B, a drug that increases the clearance of Drug A twofold, the plasma concentration of Drug A falls (case I) unless the dosing rate is doubled (case II, color). The problem of excessive accumulation arises if administration of Drug A is not reduced to the previous rate when administration of Drug B is stopped. Note that the time to reach plateau is less in the presence, than in the absence, of Drug B. Note: the time scale in both the presence and absence of Drug B is expressed in half-lives of Drug A.

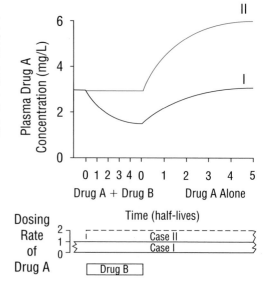

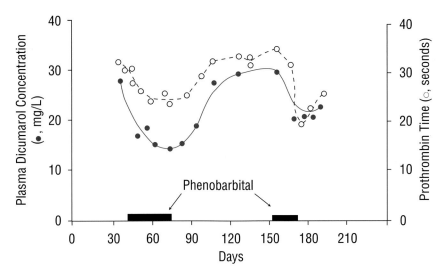

Fig. 17–10. Administration of phenobarbital (60 mg daily) to a patient receiving dicumarol chronically (75 mg daily) reduces the plasma concentration of the anticoagulant (●) and prothrombin time (○), a measure of its effect on the concentration of the vitamin K_1-dependent clotting factors) (1 mg/L = 3.0 μM). (Redrawn from Cucinell, S.A., Conney, A.H., Sansur, M.S., and Burns, J.J.: Lowering effect of phenobarbital on plasma levels of dicumarol and diphenylhydantoin. Clin. Pharmacol. Ther., 6:420–429, 1965.)

Enzyme induction was mentioned as the prime cause of increased metabolic clearance. However, a change in clearance is an indirect measure of the effect of an inducer; the direct effect is an increase in the synthesis rate of the drug-metabolizing enzyme. Accordingly, there is a delay between the direct effect and its reflection in the measured response. Thus, even if the plasma concentration of the inducer were attained instantly and then maintained constantly, the clearance of the affected drug would increase with time as the enzyme level rises from one plateau value to another. Similarly, there is a delay in the decrease in clearance of the affected drug on removing the inducer. The time delay depends, like other systems in the body, on the kinetics of the drugs and the enzyme involved.

When elimination of enzyme is the slowest process, then changes in clearance of the drug may continue to occur even though the concentration of the inducer is relatively constant. When, however, elimination of the inducer is slow, changes in the concentration of inducer are then reflected almost instantaneously by changes in the amount of enzyme and hence clearance of the affected drug. This last possibility may explain the effect of phenobarbital on the temporal changes in the plasma concentration of dicumarol and prothrombin time, a measure of its anticoagulant effect, in a patient receiving dicumarol chronically (Fig. 17–10). Both the fall in the concentration and effect of this drug following phenobarbital treatment have been attributed to the barbiturate inducing the enzymes responsible for dicumarol metabolism. It takes approximately 3 to 4 weeks for the plasma dicumarol both to fall to a minimum during phenobarbital administration and to return to the prebarbiturate value after phenobarbital is discontinued. Phenobarbital ($t_{1/2}$ of 4 days) also takes approximately the same period of time to reach a plateau in the body and to be eliminated. Thus, the observations are compatible with the hypothesis that the induced enzyme system responds relatively rapidly to changes in plasma phenobarbital concentration. For a further discussion of the kinetic aspects of induction, see Chap. 23, Turnover Concepts.

The data in Fig. 17–10 suggest that prothrombin time may be maintained at the pre-barbiturate value by raising the dose of dicumarol during phenobarbital administration. An increased risk arises, however, if the dose of anticoagulant is not reduced when phenobarbital is discontinued. The plasma dicumarol concentration then rises insidiously, as phenobarbital is slowly eliminated, and may go unnoticed for several weeks after discontinuing the barbiturate until, perhaps, a hemorrhagic crisis occurs.

STUDY PROBLEMS

(Answers to Study Problems are in Appendix II.)

1. Briefly comment on the accuracy of the following statements.
   a. Drug interactions are often detected when an interacting drug is initiated or withdrawn.
   b. Displacement of Drug A by Drug B occurs when the molar concentration of Drug B approaches that of the protein that binds Drug A.
   c. Displacement interactions are generally not *therapeutic drug interactions*.
   d. Of the various mechanisms of drug interaction, inhibition of metabolism is of primary therapeutic importance.
   e. Drug interactions are generally graded.
2. The graphs below show the concentration-time curves following the method of administration given. Sketch the expected plasma concentration-time profile of each drug (low clearance, large volume of distribution) if administered again during the coadministration of another drug that is at steady state. The parameter given is altered twofold. Each graph should clearly indicate the consequence of a change in CL, V, and $t_{1/2}$ (or a combination).
   a. fu increased, constant-rate i.v. infusion

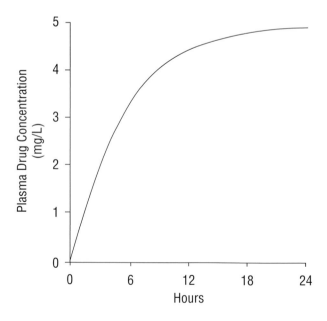

Fig. 17–11.

b. CL_{int} decreased, multiple i.v. doses

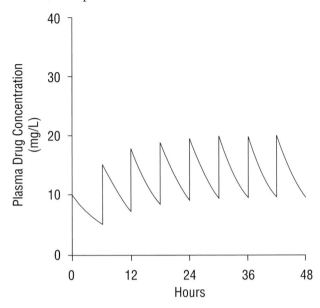

Fig. 17–12.

3. Chlordiazepoxide, a benzodiazepine, was administered to six healthy volunteers (45 mg, i.v. bolus) in crossover fashion alone or on the fifth day of a daily 400-mg dose of ketoconazole, an antifungal agent. For the purpose of this problem, the drug has one-compartment model characteristics. Mean values of $C(o)$ and $t_{1/2}$ for chlordiazepoxide are shown in Table 17–4.

Table 17-4.

	WITHOUT KETOCONAZOLE	WITH KETOCONAZOLE
$C(o)$ (mg/L)	2.0	2.0
$t_{1/2}$ (hr)	23.9	43.4

Adapted from data in Brown, M.W., Maldonado, A.L., Merdeith, C.G., and Speeg, K.V.: Effect of ketoconazole on hepatic oxidative drug metabolism. Clin. Pharmacol. Ther., *37*:290–297, 1985.

a. 1. Prepare a semilogarithmic plot of the mean concentration-time profiles of chlordiazepoxide in the presence and absence of ketoconazole. Label both axes and identify both curves.
   2. Complete the following table.

	Without Ketoconazole	With Ketoconazole
V (L)		
CL (L/hr)		

b. Given that chlordiazepoxide is eliminated by biotransformation in the liver, what physiologic mechanism(s) (Q_H, fu, fu_T, CL_{int}) is responsible for the interaction of ketoconazole with chlordiazepoxide? Justify any assumptions that you make.

4. The data in Table 17–5 show the time course of the concentration of theophylline during treatment with an oral 300-mg sustained-release dosage form every 12 hr. On days 6 and 7, mexiletine, an orally effective antiarrhythmic agent, is coadministered (200 mg every 8 hr starting at the time of blood sampling on day 6). The oral absorption of theophylline is virtually complete ($F = 1$) and C_b/C is approximately 1. Insufficient information was provided to conclude whether or not mexiletine altered the half-life of theophylline.

Table 17–5. Mean Trough Theophylline Concentrations in Plasma Sampled Before the Morning Dose (12 hr after 300-mg Evening Dose)[a]

DAY OF TREATMENT	1	2	3	4	5	6[b]	7[b]	8	9	10
Concentration (mg/L)	0	6.0	7.0	6.7	7.0	6.2	11.7	12.5	8.0	5.5

[a]Adapted from Hurwitz, A., Vacek, J.L., Botteron, G.W., Sztern, M.I., Hughes, E.M., and Jayaraj, A.: Mexiletine effects on theophylline disposition. Clin. Pharmacol. Ther., 50:299–307, 1991.
[b]Mexiletine coadministered for 5 doses (200 mg every 8 hr).

    a. Give an explanation for the effect of mexiletine on theophylline kinetics. The explanation should be based on a change in only *one* of the following parameters: fu, fu_T, CL_{int}, Q_H. Give the parameter involved and indicate the direction of its change.
    b. Briefly discuss the explanation in question "a" above in terms of one physiologic mechanism (e.g., enzyme induction, competition for active reabsorption in renal tubule, inhibition of biliary excretion) that could produce the interaction.
  5. Drug A is given by infusion at a rate of 25 mg/hr to maintain a constant plasma concentration. The data in Table 17–6 are obtained in a subject who is infused at this rate in the absence and presence of Drug B (assume that it is at steady state when present).

Table 17–6.

PLATEAU PLASMA CONCENTRATION OF DRUG B (mg/L)	DATA FOR DRUG A			
	PLATEAU PLASMA CONCENTRATION (mg/L)	URINARY EXCRETION RATE AT STEADY STATE (mg/hr)	FRACTION UNBOUND IN PLASMA	HALF-LIFE (hr)
0	10.0	15	0.1	12
20.0	6.7	4	0.3	8

Given this information and the observation that the creatinine clearance in this subject is 120 mL/min,
    a. Determine if there is evidence for Drug A being secreted and/or reabsorbed in the kidneys.
    b. Determine the mechanism(s) by which Drug B interacts with Drug A.
    c. Discuss the therapeutic implications of coadministering Drug A with Drug B.
  6. Table 17–7 contains pharmacokinetic values for an individual subject that typify what is known about the interaction between quinidine and digoxin.

Table 17–7.

	ORAL BIOAVAILABILITY	CLEARANCE (mL/min)	RENAL CLEARANCE (mL/min)	VOLUME OF DISTRIBUTION (L)	FRACTION UNBOUND
Digoxin alone	0.75	140	101	500	0.77
Digoxin plus quinidine[a]	0.75	72	51	240	0.79

[a]When the $C_{ss,av}$ of quinidine is 1–3 mg/L.

    a. Briefly comment on how quinidine affects the distribution of digoxin.
    b. Using the appropriate digoxin parameter values in Table 17–7, calculate the probable "loading" dose of digoxin needed when therapy with this drug is initiated in a patient who is undergoing antiarrhythmic therapy with quinidine. The therapeutic concentration range, 1 to 2 µg/L, remains the same for digoxin.
    c. Knowing that the half-lives of digoxin and quinidine are about 2 days and 8 hr, respectively, briefly discuss (in terms of the digoxin concentration) the therapeutic

consequence of administering quinidine to a patient who is receiving digoxin therapy. This is the more common situation in which the interaction is observed. Use the digoxin parameter values in Table 17–7 and consider the events upon both initiating and discontinuing quinidine coadministration.

d. Do you think quinidine would affect the dosage requirements for digoxin in a patient with severe renal function impairment? Briefly discuss.

7. Bergstrom *et al.* studied the pharmacokinetic interaction of the antidepressants fluoxetine and desipramine. Figure 17–13 and Table 17–8 summarize the observations following a single oral dose of desipramine (50 mg) alone and 3 hr after the eighth daily dose of fluoxetine (60 mg each). The concentration of fluoxetine during the time desipramine is quantified remains relatively constant (half-life of fluoxetine = 3 to 4 days after multiple doses). The value of *fe* for desipramine is about 0.03.

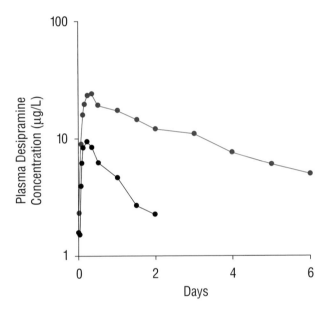

Fig. 17–13. Mean plasma concentration of desipramine after a 50-mg oral dose given alone (black) and after 8 daily doses (60 mg each) of fluoxetine (color). (Modified from Bergstrom, R.F., Peyton, A.L., and Lemberger, L.: Quantification and mechanism of the fluoxetine and tricyclic antidepressant interaction. Clin. Pharmacol. Ther. *51*:239–248, 1992.)

Table 17–8. Pharmacokinetics of Desipramine When Administered Orally in a Single 50-mg Dose Alone and After Eight Daily Doses of Fluoxetine[a]

PARAMETER	GIVEN ALONE (n = 6)	AFTER MULTIPLE DOSES OF 60 mg/day of FLUOXETINE (n = 5)
AUC (o–∞) (µg · hr/L)	284 ± 244	2110 ± 900
C_{max} (µg/L)	9.4 ± 5.4	23.9 ± 5.6
t_{max} (hr)	5.3 ± 1.6	6.8 ± 1.1
$t_{1/2}$ (hr)	16.1 ± 5.2	63.8 ± 19.3
CL/F (L/hr)	289 ± 168	27.1 ± 10.3
V/F (L/kg)	77.1 ± 39.8	29.7 ± 7.7

[a]Data are mean values ± SD.

a. Given that the blood/plasma concentration ratio of desipramine is close to 1.0, that the drug is metabolized only in the liver, and that the "well-stirred" model of hepatic elimination applies, calculate the value of $CL_{int} \cdot fu$ in the presence and absence of fluoxetine.

b. Suggest one mechanism (combination of mechanisms is not acceptable) for the pharmacokinetic interaction observed. Document how you arrived at your conclusion.

   c. Briefly explain why the factor by which half-life is altered is not the same as that of *CL/F*.

   d. What implications do the observations of these authors have for the concurrent administration of these two antidepressants? Briefly discuss.

8. Normal values for the pharmacokinetic parameters: clearance, fraction unbound, and fraction excreted unchanged are listed in Table 17–9 for Drugs A through G. Situations are presented that alter the kinetics of each of these drugs. On the right indicate whether the value of each parameter would be observed to increase (↑), decrease (↓), or show little or no change (↔). All drugs are administered orally and have volumes of distribution greater than 50 L.

9. Tolbutamide, an oral hypoglycemic agent, has the following pharmacokinetic parameters in a 70-kg adult: $F = 1.0$, $V = 9$ L, $CL = 1.1$ L/hr, $fe = 0.03$. Elimination is almost exclusively via oxidation to hydroxytolbutamide.

   a. Calculate the average plateau concentration and time to reach it when tolbutamide is administered in a regimen of 0.5 g orally twice daily.

Several drugs inhibit the metabolism of tolbutamide and cause excessive accumulation and hypoglycemic crises unless the maintenance dose of tolbutamide is reduced.

   b. Given the following information about a competitive inhibitor: $F = 1.0$, $V = 13$ L, $CL = 0.6$ L/hr, $fu = 0.03$, $K_I = 0.6$ mg/L, calculate the following:

     1. The expected new average plateau plasma concentration of tolbutamide after the addition of a dosage regimen of 1.0 g twice daily of the inhibitor to a patient previously stabilized on tolbutamide. The regimen of tolbutamide is continued unchanged.

     2. The time taken to reach this new plateau.

     3. A practical regimen of tolbutamide that maintains a similar average preinhibitor plateau concentration, when coadministered in the presence of the inhibitor. Tolbutamide is available as a scored 500-mg tablet.

Table 17-9.

DRUG	NORMAL VALUES CLEARANCE[a] (mL/min)	FRACTION[a] UNBOUND	FRACTION EXCRETED UNCHANGED	SITUATIONS	OBSERVATIONS CLEARANCE[a]	VOLUME OF DISTRIBUTION[a]	HALF-LIFE	FRACTION EXCRETED UNCHANGED	ORAL BIOAVAILABILITY
A	420	0.5	0.7	Simultaneous administration of a competitive inhibitor of renal secretion					
B (acid, renal clearance pH sensitive)	200	0.1	1.0	Urine pH increased by another drug					
C	1200	0.5	0.99	Simultaneous administration of a competitive inhibitor of metabolism of Drug C					
D	1200	0.05	0.01	Simultaneous administration of a drug that displaces Drug D from plasma proteins					
E	50	0.4	0.5	Simultaneous administration of a drug that displaces Drug E from tissue binding sites					
F	10	0.1	0.01	Simultaneous administration of a drug that displaces Drug F from plasma proteins					
G	1300	0.7	0.95	Simultaneous administration for several days of an inducer of enzymes that metabolize Drug G					

[a]Based on measurement of drug concentration in blood.

CONCENTRATION MONITORING

OBJECTIVES

The reader will be able to:

1. List the criteria for determining when monitoring of plasma drug concentrations and applying target concentration strategy are appropriate.

2. Describe how population information can be used to obtain initial estimates of an individual's pharmacokinetics.

3. Estimate the likely pharmacokinetic parameter values in an individual patient, based on both population and patient characteristics, for digoxin, gentamicin, phenobarbital, and theophylline.

4. Calculate the plasma drug concentration(s) expected at the time(s) of sampling, using estimated pharmacokinetic parameter values and dosing history of the patient.

5. Upon evaluation of a pharmacokinetic problem observed during chronic drug therapy, ascribe the problem to a change in bioavailability, compliance, clearance, volume of distribution, or a combination of these values.

6. Revise pharmacokinetic parameters from measured plasma concentration data acquired under either steady-state or nonsteady-state conditions.

7. Use the revised parameters (in objective 6) to calculate any modification in dosage required to ensure that the plasma concentration lies within the therapeutic window.

Drugs are administered to achieve a therapeutic objective. Once this objective is defined, a drug and its dosage regimen are chosen for the patient (Chap. 13). Drug therapy is subsequently managed as shown schematically in Fig. 18–1 together with steps required to initiate therapy. This management is usually accomplished by monitoring incidence and intensity of both therapeutic and toxic effects. Examples of this method of individualizing therapy are given in Table 18–1.

Although preferable, it is not always possible to use a direct measure of the desired effect as a therapeutic endpoint. Sometimes, signs of toxicity are used as a dosing guide. The dose of salicylates, for example, when used in the treatment of rheumatic diseases, is often increased until tinnitus or nausea and vomiting intervene. In moderate-to-severe asthmatic cases, theophylline too is frequently titrated to a toxic endpoint. Excessive dryness of the mouth is a common measure of the upper dosage of atropine when used as a spasmolytic agent.

The therapeutic effects of salicylates, theophylline, and atropine, although often subjective and vague, can be assessed and hence used in judging the success of therapy. This is not so readily accomplished for antiepileptic drugs; the therapeutic effect here is the non-occurrence of seizures. Seizures may be infrequent, and as a result, delays and difficulties

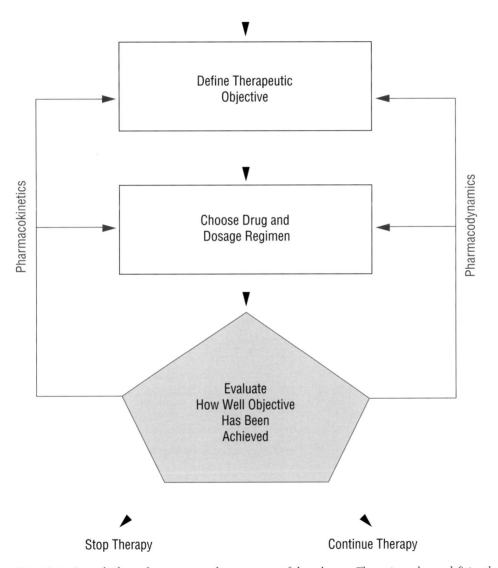

Fig. 18–1. General scheme for initiation and management of drug therapy. The major tasks are defining the therapeutic objective, choosing the drug and its dosage regimen, and evaluating how well the objective has been achieved. Monitoring response assists in accomplishing the last two tasks. Monitoring plasma drug concentration may also be helpful, especially if responses (therapeutic and toxic) are not well quantified. Both kinds of evaluation are accomplished through feedback (colored lines). The feedback occasionally requires redefinition of the therapeutic objective as well.

exist in assessing therapeutic success. Toxic effects that can be readily measured, e.g., nystagmus and ataxia, have therefore been used to assist in determining the upper limit of an epileptic patient's dosage requirement. A similar situation arises in the use of oral anticoagulants; the therapeutic objective is the prevention of thromboembolic complications. Again, the therapeutic objective cannot readily be assessed, and therefore an alternative, simple, and rapid laboratory test, prothrombin time, which measures the tendency of blood to clot, is substituted as the therapeutic objective. Likewise, for antihypercholesterolemic, hypoglycemic, and uricosuric agents, clinical laboratory tests are employed as alternative therapeutic endpoints. Clearly, to be useful, alternative tests must be graded and closely related to the true therapeutic effect.

The seriousness of the first toxic effect observed is a major determinant of whether it can or cannot be used as an endpoint. The titration of young adults with rheumatoid arthritis and on salicylate therapy to the occurrence of tinnitus is relatively safe, as tinnitus is an easily measured mild toxicity. However, tinnitus does not always occur before the advent of more serious toxicity, particularly in young children and patients with impaired hearing. Titrating dosage of digoxin and related glycosides to cardiac toxicity is always unsafe.

Table 18-1. Examples of Monitoring Drug Therapy by the Effects Produced or by Alternative Tests

DRUG	CONDITION	OBSERVATION SUGGESTING INCREASED DOSAGE	OBSERVATION SUGGESTING HOLDING OR DECREASING DOSAGE	SEVERE TOXIC SIGNS
Group I. Drugs Monitored by Clinical Signs and Symptoms				
Salicylates	Rheumatoid arthritis or rheumatic fever	Inadequate reduction of inflammation and pain	Tinnitus, nausea, vomiting	Metabolic acidosis
Furosemide	Edema associated with congestive cardiac failure, cirrhosis, renal disease	Excessive edema	Fluid and electrolyte imbalance associated with excessive dehydration	Severe hypotension, cardiac disturbances
Desipramine	Depression	Inadequate elevation of mood	Dry mouth, blurred vision, decreased effectiveness	Cardiac toxicity, orthostatic hypotension
Carbidopa/ levodopa	Parkinson's disease	Inadequate control of disease	Dyskinesias, blepharospasm	Involuntary movements, mental changes, and depression
Thiopental	Induction of anesthesia	Insufficient anesthesia	Anesthesia too deep	Respiratory failure
Group II. Drugs Monitored by Tests *in Vitro*				
Warfarin	Thromboembolic disease	Prothrombin time too short	Prothrombin time too long	Hemorrhage
Cyclosporine	Organ transplantation	Signs of tissue rejection	Decreased renal function	Severe depression of renal function
L-Thyroxine	Hypothyroidism	Decreased unbound triiodothyronine (T_3) and thyroxine (T_4) in plasma	Elevated T_3 and T_4	Hyperthyroidism
Pravastatin	Hypercholesterolemia	Elevated cholesterol	Asymptomatic elevation of transaminases and creatine phosphokinase	Marked persistent rise in transaminases, myopathies
Uricosurics	Gout	Elevated serum uric acid	Decreased serum uric acid	Gastrointestinal irritation

Monitoring of therapeutic responses and toxicity is best accomplished when integrated with kinetic concepts. Half-life determines the time course of accumulation and hence the development of responses. It is also a determinant of the time for a toxic response to resolve. Time is also a factor in the development of response to many drugs, even when the plasma concentration is constant. For example, the response to warfarin (Chap. 5, p. 63–64) is delayed because of the time required for the clotting factors to decline to values that produce an adequate and stable degree of anticoagulation. Tailoring dosage to an individual's needs clearly requires integration of kinetic principles.

Another approach more explicitly incorporating kinetic principles is the use of plasma concentrations. Such measurements serve as an intermediate to distinguish pharmacokinetic and pharmacodynamic domains.

At a minimum, the plasma concentration can serve as an additional piece of information to guide and assess drug therapy. The application of the plasma concentration measurements to therapy involves *target concentration strategy*. The basic idea is to apply a strategy to achieve and maintain a target concentration or a target range of concentrations for an individual patient.

TARGET CONCENTRATION STRATEGY

This strategy is useful as an adjunct in initiating and monitoring drug therapy when a number of criteria listed below are satisfied. Some of the criteria are absolute in nature, others are relative. Most of them, however, must be met for the strategy to be routinely effective.

The plasma concentration of a drug must correlate quantitatively with both the intensity and probability of therapeutic or toxic effects. A direct relationship between concentration and effect may be insufficient grounds for plasma concentration monitoring if the therapeutic effect itself is easily monitored, which is frequently the case. The strategy becomes particularly attractive when a therapeutic endpoint is difficult to quantify, as with the nonoccurrence of epileptic seizures. The strategy is most pertinent when the objective is to maintain a therapeutic effect by maintaining a concentration within a limited range (Chap. 5) and when the likelihood of toxicity can be predicted from the concentration.

Target concentration strategy is also indicated when there is a high probability of encountering a therapeutic failure, i.e., either a lack of effect or an occurrence of undue toxicity. A therapeutic failure is most likely to arise if the drug has a low therapeutic index and a great variability in its pharmacokinetics or if the patient is at particular risk because of genetic factors (Chap. 14), concurrent disease (Chap. 16), or multiple drug therapy (Chap. 17). A higher frequency of therapeutic failures is also anticipated when either noncompliance or erratic absorption is likely.

Examples of drugs for which target concentration strategy has been found to be appropriate, together with general information pertinent to their monitoring, are listed in Table 18–2.

For some drugs the strategy is applied only when a problem arises. The problem may be a lack of response at usual or even higher dosages as a result of one or more of the following conditions: noncompliance, poor bioavailability, unusually rapid elimination, or a pharmacodynamic resistance to the drug. Measurement of the plasma concentration permits distinction to be made among the causes of the problem. Similarly, the cause of a toxic or unusual response at customary or lower dosages may be ascertained.

Efficient use of the strategy requires prior knowledge of the pharmacokinetic parameters of the drug, the conditions in which these parameters and the target concentrations are likely to be altered, and if altered, the extent of the changes. The last two requirements are relative in that, by monitoring the concentration, adjustments in dosage can be made for altered pharmacokinetics.

A sensitive, accurate, and specific assay for the drug must be available. In addition, to be useful, the results should be available before the next therapeutic decision is to be made. The half-life is a useful index of this "turn-around" time because it is the time frame in which accumulation on multiple dosing and disappearance on discontinuing a drug occur.

THE TARGET CONCENTRATION

The target concentration initially chosen is the value or range of values with the greatest probability of therapeutic success (Table 5–2, p. 59), keeping in mind that the population value (or range) may be inappropriate for an individual. Higher concentrations may be appropriate when the condition is severe, and the converse when the condition is mild. If altered plasma protein binding is anticipated, such as in uremia, after surgery, or when displacing drugs are also administered, then the target total concentration should be adjusted to attain the same unbound concentration.

The principles for establishing a dosage regimen to achieve a desired concentration or to keep within concentration limits are presented in Chap. 7. Adjustment in the usual dosage regimen can often be anticipated based on the patient's age, weight, and clinical status, especially renal, hepatic, and cardiovascular functions (Chaps. 13 to 16). Yet, even after taking these factors into account, sufficient uncertainty often remains in the kinetics of the drug in the individual patient to warrant monitoring the plasma concentration. From such observations the patient's current pharmacokinetic parameters can be estimated, and a new dosage regimen can be designed to more closely achieve the target value(s).

Table 18-2 Information Pertinent to the Plasma Concentration Monitoring of Selected Drugs

DRUG	CONCURRENT DISEASE STATES	PLASMA PROTEIN BINDING	CONCURRENT DRUG THERAPY	ACTIVE METABOLITES	OTHER PERTINENT INFORMATION
Cyclosporine	Autoimmune diseases	Extensively bound to lipoproteins and blood cells	Phenobarbital, rifampin, erythromycin, ketoconazole	Some metabolites have activity	Renal toxicity is major concern
Digoxin	Renal disease, congestive cardiac failure, thyroid disease	—[a]	Diuretics	—	Distribution characteristics
Gentamicin	Renal disease	—	Some penicillins	—	Composed of three isomers
Nortriptyline	Alcoholic hepatic disease	Extensively bound to α_1-acid glycoprotein	Quinidine, fluoxetine, carbamazepine	10-Hydroxynor-tryptyline	Polymorphic hydroxylation
Phenytoin	Renal disease, chronic hepatic disease	Extensively bound to albumin	Valproic acid, carbamazepine, cimetidine	—	Saturable metabolism
Theophylline	Pneumonia, chronic obstructive pulmonary disease, congestive cardiac failure, hepatic cirrhosis, acute pulmonary edema	Moderately bound to albumin	Enoxacin, erythromycin, phenobarbital	—	Available in many dosage and salt forms

[a]Therapeutically unimportant.

Frequency of monitoring is a function of the presumed change in the factors that influence drug response. For example, the plasma concentration of phenobarbital in epileptic patients, whose state of health and drug therapy remains stable, may need to be monitored only a few times a year; more frequent monitoring may be indicated if the patient's health deteriorates or if therapy with other drugs is altered. Daily or even more frequent monitoring of plasma theophylline concentrations may be needed for optimal use of theophylline in the treatment of an asthmatic patient in an intensive care unit, especially if congestive cardiac failure, pneumonia, hepatic cirrhosis, and smoking are all present. These conditions alter theophylline clearance, which is likely to be quite variable and unpredictable in this situation.

PERTINENT INFORMATION NEEDED

Several kinds of information, given in Table 18–3 are needed to evaluate a measured plasma concentration efficiently. A history of drug administration, which includes doses and times of dosing is mandatory as are the times of sampling.

Specific patient population pharmacokinetic information for monitoring digoxin, gentamicin, phenobarbital, and theophylline concentrations is given in Table 18–4. These four drugs are used throughout the remainder of this chapter as examples of the application of the principles of plasma drug concentration monitoring.

EVALUATION PROCEDURE

Using the dosing history and the time(s) of sampling, judgment is needed on whether the measured value(s) is a good estimate of the maximum, average, or minimum concentration at steady state on a fixed regimen or of a nonsteady-state concentration(s) obtained either shortly after starting dosing or following an erratic schedule. Having established the conditions and an appropriate kinetic model, a generally recommended procedure to evaluate one or more concentrations is as follows:

1. Estimate the likely values of the pharmacokinetic parameters (F, CL, V, and hence $t_{1/2}$) in the patient based on population parameters, taking into account the patient's age, weight, renal function, concurrent diseases, drug therapy, dosage form, route of administration, and any other information about the patient known to affect the kinetics of the

Table 18–3. Data Collection

History of Drug Administration
      Drug, dose, dosage forms, routes of administration, times of administration, compliance, inpatient or outpatient
Time of Sampling (relative to previous dose)
Present and Previous (if any) Plasma Drug Concentrations
Clinical Status of Patient
      Weight, age, gender, condition being treated, smoking, ethnicity, concurrent disease states (especially cardiovascular, hepatic, and renal diseases)
Laboratory Data
      Renal function (serum creatinine, creatinine clearance)
      Hepatic function (prothrombin time, serum albumin, serum bilirubin)
      Protein binding (albumin, total plasma proteins)
Concurrent Drug Therapy
      Interacting drugs
      Assay interferences
Active Metabolites
Assay Method (reproducibility, sensitivity, and specificity)
Usual Pharmacokinetic Parameters Associated With Type of Patient in Question
      Bioavailability, absorption rate constant, volume of distribution, unbound fraction in plasma, total clearance, renal clearance

drug. A major intent here is to identify the subpopulation to which the patient belongs (Chap. 13).

2. Using the appropriate kinetic model and the parameter values above, estimate the plasma concentration(s) expected at the time(s) of sampling, taking into account the dosing history of the patient.

3. Compare the observed and expected concentrations. If they are in agreement, then one's confidence in knowing the parameters in the patient is increased. A clinical decision to modify the dosage in the patient depends on the concentration observed and on several other factors including, most importantly, the current response(s) of the patient.

4. If observed and expected concentrations are judged to be different, then one may wish to revise the pharmacokinetic parameter estimates. Here it is necessary to weigh how much confidence one has in the initial parameter estimates from previous population studies relative to that in the estimates obtained from the measured plasma concentration(s).

5. A recommendation for dosage adjustment or patient education (non-compliance) may be appropriate. In addition, comments to the clinician could aid in the interpretation of the drug concentration. Such comments include the need to adjust the therapeutic window when altered protein binding is expected and when a change in time of sampling is appropriate.

Table 18-4. Patient Population Pharmacokinetic Parameters of Digoxin, Gentamicin, Phenobarbital, and Theophylline[a]

PARAMETERS	DIGOXIN	GENTAMICIN	PHENOBARBITAL	THEOPHYLLINE[b]
Salt form factor	1.0	1.0	1.0 0.9 (Na salt)	0.85 hydrous aminophylline 0.8 anhydrous aminophylline (i.v. use)
Oral bioavailability	0.75 tablets 0.8 elixir 0.95 liquid-filled capsules	<0.01	1.0	1.0
Volume of distribution (L/kg)	[c]	0.22	0.55	0.5
Clearance (L/hr/kg)	—[d]	Cl_{cr}[e]	0.0037	0.04[f]
Half-life (hr)	44[g]	[h]	104	8.7[i]
Fraction excreted unchanged	0.7	>0.95	0.3	0.13
Therapeutic window (mg/L)	0.0008–0.002	peak >6, trough <2[j]	10–30	10–20
(μM)	0.001–0.0025	peak >11, trough <4[j]	43–130	55–110

[a]Adapted from data in Applied Pharmacokinetics, 3rd ed., Edited by W.E. Evans, J.J. Schentag, and W.J. Jusko. Spokane, Applied Therapeutics, 1992.
[b]Many controlled release dosage forms are available.
[c]V (L/kg) = 3.8 + 52 Cl_{cr}; Cl_{cr} in L/hr/kg for adults.
[d]In severe congestive cardiac failure patients, Cl(L/hr/kg) = 0.9 Cl_{cr} + 0.02; in mild-to-moderate conditions, Cl = Cl_{cr} + 0.048, where Cl_{cr} is in L/hr/kg.
[e]Approximately the same as patient's creatinine clearance.
[f]Multiply 0.04 by the factor below to adjust for smoking, age, disease, and concurrent drugs. Consider the factors to be multiplicative when more than one condition is present.

Smoking	1.6	Concurrent Drugs		Age (years)	
Diseases		Phenytoin	1.5	Child 1–4	2.4
Cirrhosis	0.5	Rifampin	1.8	Child 5–17	1.6
Cor pulmonale	0.7	Cimetidine	0.6		
Pulmonary edema	0.5	Erythromycin	0.7		
Congestive cardiac failure		Phenobarbital	1.3		
	0.4	Troleandomycin	0.5		

[g]$t_{1/2}$ = 0.693 V/Cl; V and Cl estimated from footnotes c and d.
[h]$t_{1/2}$ = 0.15/Cl_{cr}; Cl_{cr} in L/hr per kg.
[i]$t_{1/2}$ = 8.7/m; value of m is the factor determined in footnote f.
[j]Desired peak (30 min after the end of a 30-min infusion) and trough concentrations are indicated for an 8-hourly dose.

DOSING SCENARIOS

Chapters 6 and 7 contain the basic relationships needed for evaluating concentrations obtained during constant-rate and multiple-dose regimens. These relationships are now supplemented with equations, which are useful for four additional, frequently occurring scenarios. These are when one or more doses is missed; when a patient is on a four-times-a-day regimen in which the intervals are not equal, for example, 9 A.M., 1 P.M., 5 P.M., 9 P.M. (subsequently called a 9-1-5-9 regimen); when the drug is repeatedly infused over a period of time approaching its half-life; and when the doses vary and the dosing intervals are erratic. Emphasis here is on step 2 (evaluation procedure), particularly on determining the appropriate kinetic model for estimating concentration(s) at time(s) of sampling.

For each of the scenarios, absorption is assumed to be much more rapid than elimination; i.e., the intravenous (i.v.) bolus approximation applies. Absorption decreases fluctuation; it should be taken into account, when necessary, using the principles previously given in Chap. 7, Extravascular Dose. Unless otherwise noted, dosing and sampling times are subsequently based on the 24-hour clock.

Missed Dose

Although it would seem that missed doses would greatly complicate the evaluation of a measured concentration, it is not necessarily so. Figure 18–2 shows a fixed-dose, fixed-interval multiple-dose regimen in which one dose is missed. To account for the missed dose, one needs to subtract the concentration expected at the time of sampling, if only the missed dose had been given, from that expected if no dose was missed. This correction is based on the principle of additivity of concentrations from each dose at all times. In this example, a concentration is measured at time t_1 within a dosing interval. The concentration expected with no missed dose is

$$C_{ss}(t_1) = \frac{F \cdot S \cdot Dose}{V} \cdot \frac{e^{-kt_1}}{(1 - e^{-k\tau})} \qquad 1$$

The parameter S, salt form factor, is a coefficient correcting for the fractional content of drug. Its use is unnecessary if the dose and concentrations are expressed in molar units.

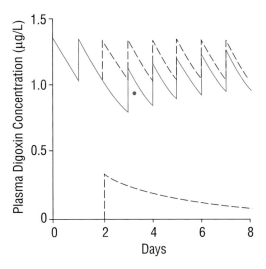

Fig. 18–2. A missed dose results in the lowering of the fluctuating concentrations from the steady-state values. The degree of this lowering is equivalent to the concentration remaining from the missed dose. The expected concentration at any time following the missed dose (colored line) can then be estimated by the difference between the value expected with no missed dose (---) and the concentration expected at that time had only the missed dose been given (bottom curve). The observed concentration on the day after the missed dose, 0.9 μg/L, is superimposed (●). The parameters used in the figure are those expected in the patient in the digoxin example case history (1 mg/L = 1.3 μM).

The concentration expected from giving only a single dose at the time of the missed dose is

$$C_{(missed\ dose)} = \frac{F \cdot S \cdot Dose}{V} \cdot e^{-kt_2} \qquad 2$$

where t_2 is the time since the missed dose. The concentration expected in the therapeutic setting is then

$$C = \frac{F \cdot S \cdot Dose}{V}\left[\frac{e^{-kt_1}}{(1 - e^{-k\tau})} - e^{-kt_2}\right] \qquad 3$$

If two doses were missed then

$$\frac{F \cdot S \cdot Dose}{V}\left[\frac{e^{-kt_1}}{(1 - e^{-k\tau})} \cdot e^{-kt_2} - e^{-kt_3}\right]$$

where t_3 is the time since the other dose was missed.

9-1-5-9 Regimen

In institutional settings many drugs are given in regimens similar to the one portrayed in Fig. 18–3. Such regimens have a 24-hour repetitive or regular cycle, even though the dosing intervals within the day are unequal. The expected concentration at any time during the day can be viewed simply as the sum of the steady-state concentrations resulting from each of the four daily doses. When given once daily, the first dose of the day is expected to yield a concentration, $C(t_1)$, at steady state, given by

$$C(t_1) = \frac{F \cdot S \cdot Dose}{V} \cdot \frac{e^{-kt_1}}{(1 - e^{-k\tau})} \qquad 4$$

Fig. 18–3. The plasma theophylline concentration varies extensively at steady-state (24-hour repeating pattern) with a "9-1-5-9" type of regimen in an average 6-year-old child. In this example the concentration, 2.1 mg/L, at the time of the morning dose (9:00 = "zero" time) would be ineffective (therapeutic window = 7 to 20 mg/L). An increase in the dose to overcome this low trough value, however, may cause toxicity, particularly during the evening hours after the dose at 21:00 (12 and 36 hr). The observed trough concentration of 6.3 mg/L (●) is superimposed. The parameter values used are those in the theophylline case history (1 mg/L = 5.5 μM).

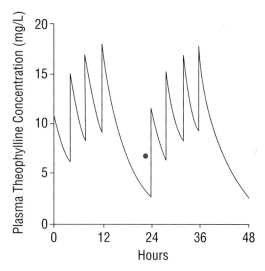

where t_1 is the time during the day between giving the dose and sampling the blood. The concentration resulting from giving only the second dose on a daily regimen is

$$C(t_2) = \frac{F \cdot S \cdot \text{Dose}}{V} \cdot \frac{e^{-kt_2}}{(1 - e^{-k\tau})} \qquad 5$$

where t_2 is the time between the administration of the second dose and the time of blood sampling, and so on. Thus, the concentration expected on such a regimen is

$$C = \frac{F \cdot S \cdot \text{Dose}}{V} \cdot \left[\frac{(e^{-kt_1} + e^{-kt_2} + e^{-kt_3} + e^{-kt_4})}{(1 - e^{-k\tau})} \right] \qquad 6$$

where τ is 24 hr, the dosing interval in each of the once daily regimens.

Intermittent Infusion Model

The aminoglycosides, e.g., gentamicin, are often administered every 6 to 8 hours by a constant-rate infusion of each dose over 30 to 60 min. This form of administration is neither a multiple-dose i.v. bolus regimen nor a constant-rate infusion, but rather an *intermittent infusion* regimen. When the infusion time approaches the half-life of a drug, a multiple-dose i.v. bolus model is no longer adequate for predicting concentrations and revising parameter values. The appropriate steady-state model, shown in Fig. 18–4 is

$$C = \underbrace{\frac{R_0 \cdot (1 - e^{-kt_{inf}})}{CL}}_{\text{I}} \cdot \underbrace{\frac{1}{(1 - e^{-k\tau})}}_{\text{II}} \cdot \underbrace{e^{-k(t - t_{inf})}}_{\text{III}} \qquad 7$$

where τ is the dosing interval; t_{inf} is the duration of the infusion; $R_o = S \cdot \text{Dose}/t_{inf}$; and t is the time in the last dosing interval between the start of the infusion and the withdrawal of the blood sample. Part I of the equation is the concentration expected just at the end of the infusion, at rate $S \cdot D/t_{inf}$. Part II is the accumulation factor for repeated administration to steady state (see Appendix I–E), and part III is the fraction remaining at postinfusion time, $t - t_{inf}$, after achieving the peak steady-state concentration, the product I · II.

Dose and Interval Unequal

The situation in which neither dose nor interval have any degree of regularity is frequently observed in therapeutic monitoring. In this situation, one can simply sum up drug that remains from previous doses with the realization that doses given more than four patient half-lives ago can be disregarded, since so little drug remains in the body from each of them. The plasma concentration expected after three doses, for example, is

$$C = \frac{F \cdot S}{V}\left(Dose_1 e^{-kt_1} + Dose_2 e^{-kt_2} + Dose_3 e^{-kt_3}\right) \qquad 8$$

where $Dose_1$, $Dose_2$, and $Dose_3$ represent the doses taken at times t_1, t_2, and t_3 before sampling.

Confidence in Estimates

To revise pharmacokinetic parameter values properly, one must consider several pieces of information. Information about compliance, bioavailability, times(s) of sampling (actual versus reported), assay reproducibility and specificity, and dosing history are of paramount importance. One must also weigh the relative confidence one has in the parameter values estimated from literature data, previous experience, and concentration data. Recall (Chap. 13) that literature parameter values are those estimated to apply to the subpopulation to which the patient belongs. Misassignment of the subpopulation and variability in the expected parameter values are, of course, concerns here.

Additional kinetic factors affect one's confidence in the use of a concentration value. Consider, e.g., the case of sampling while drug rises during a constant-rate i.v. infusion. A

Fig. 18–4. The plasma concentration of gentamicin, predicted during an 8-hour dosing interval at steady state and following the repeated 45-min constant rate infusion of the drug, shows similarities with repeated i.v. boluses, except for less fluctuation. When the input time (infusion duration, t_{inf}) is a significant part of the half-life (1.9 hr here), intermittent infusion can result in considerable error unless the *intermittent infusion model* is used to calculate expected concentrations within the interval. These calculations are based on the parameter values expected for the patient in the third case history. The two observed concentrations, 4.9 and 0.4 mg/L, are superimposed (●) (1 mg/L = 1.8 μM).

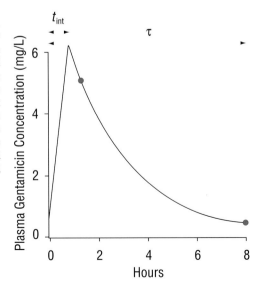

plasma concentration obtained during such an infusion is a function of rate of administration, clearance, and volume of distribution (Chap. 6).

$$C = \frac{R_O}{CL}(1 - e^{-(CL/V)t}) \qquad\qquad 9$$

Evaluation of a plasma concentration requires knowing whether clearance or volume of distribution is the more variable and appreciating on which of these two parameters the concentration is more dependent. The latter may be considered from the events depicted in Fig. 18–5 during the infusion of a drug in three separate situations. In Case A, the values of the clearance and volume parameters are those anticipated, the average values. In the other two situations, the half-life is three times greater than the average value, in Case B due to a threefold reduction in clearance and in Case C due to a threefold increase in volume of distribution.

With little drug having been eliminated, an early concentration is primarily a function of infusion rate and volume of distribution. Accordingly, there is little virtue in taking a sample before the usual half-life to estimate the dosage requirements needed to achieve therapeutic concentrations. A steady-state concentration depends only on the rate of administration and the value of clearance (Chap. 6). Accordingly, sampling at this time provides the most confidence in estimating dosing rate requirements.

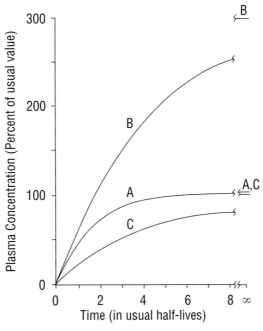

Fig. 18–5. Following a constant-rate infusion, monitoring the concentration at one usual half-life does little to distinguish between a patient with average values of clearance and volume of distribution, Case A, and one with a threefold reduction in clearance and an average volume of distribution, Case B. Distinguishing between these patients, without producing undue toxicity, is probably best done by monitoring at four usual half-lives. Although a threefold increase in volume of distribution, Case C, is readily detected at one usual half-life, this observation provides little information on the final plateau concentration to be achieved.

Sampling between the time of initiating the infusion and steady state often leads to inconclusive information. At two usual half-lives, the observation of the concentration expected, Case A, does not mean that CL and V have the expected values. They may both differ and fortuitously give the expected concentration. The lower-than-expected concentration at two usual half-lives, Case C, could be due to either an increased clearance or an increased volume, as shown. In contrast, the observation at this time of a concentration equal to or above the expected steady-state value, Case B, is a clear indication that clearance is less than usual. Indeed, the greater this difference, the lower is the probable value of clearance and the greater the need to reduce the rate of administration to avoid toxicity.

In the region of 2 to 6 usual half-lives, a major consideration in interpreting a single observation is whether clearance or volume of distribution is the more variable. For example, clearance (in units of L/hr/kg) of theophylline varies over an eightfold range or more, particularly if age and disease state are considered. The range of values for the volume of distribution (L/kg) is only about twofold. Thus, estimates of the clearance of theophylline can be made from nonsteady-state values obtained within this time span.

Although the preceding concepts regarding estimates of parameters were developed for administration by infusion, they generally apply to all forms and schedules of drug administration intended to produce a plateau concentration.

Revision of Parameter Values

Differences in observed and expected concentrations suggest a number of possibilities. For example, the patient's kinetics may be different than expected, he or she may have been noncompliant, the sampling times may not have been noted correctly, or an assay problem may have occurred.

The major decision is how much to rely on the measured concentration relative to information known about patients such as the one being treated. Such decisions are beyond the scope of this chapter but are very important in concentration monitoring. For the purpose of this chapter, the concentrations, dosing histories, sampling times, and assay procedures are considered to be accurate. The next step is then how to determine the pharmacokinetic parameters in the patient.

The model used for predicting the concentration(s) must be appropriate for determining the individual's parameter values. For example, if intravenously infused to steady state, the expected concentration is determined from $C_{ss} = R_0/CL$. Rearranging, clearance can be estimated from $CL = R_0/C_{ss}$. More complex models for nonsteady-state and multiple dosing situations, as detailed above, can often be similarly rearranged. Practice in doing so and special procedures for situations in which rearrangement is not possible are presented in the case histories below.

CASE HISTORIES

To demonstrate the principles of plasma drug concentration monitoring, the subsequent case histories are evaluated by the procedure suggested above. The population parameter estimates for the drugs utilize the information given in Table 18–4. Included are values for select subpopulations of patients. For gentamicin and digoxin, several parameter values depend on an estimate of renal function, e.g., creatinine clearance (Chap. 16). Parameter estimates of theophylline are obtained by multiplicative factors. For example, the clearance of theophylline in a 62-year-old, 65-kg female smoker (1.6) with congestive cardiac failure (0.4) and concurrently taking phenytoin (1.5) is calculated as follows:

$$0.04 \times (1.6 \times 0.4 \times 1.5) \times 65 = 2.5 \text{ L/hr}$$

where 0.04 L/hr/kg is the typical value for theophylline in the nonsmoking patient population. No correction for the age of this adult is included. One expects a decrease in clearance with age, especially in the elderly patient. However, current methods for estimating parameter values for theophylline do not include such an adjustment. It is important to note that rules developed here are intended to be examples and not to summarize all that is currently known about the drugs and the strategies employed for them. Certainly, as more information is obtained, new and more refined relationships will be forthcoming.

Case 1. *Digoxin*. Mrs. D.H., a 53-year-old, 82-kg patient with congestive cardiac failure for the past 3 years, was admitted on April 16 to the hospital at 16:00 because of a worsening of her congestive cardiac failure symptoms. Her admission history indicated that she had taken her digoxin tablet (0.25 mg) that morning at the usual time (8:00–9:00), but had failed to take a tablet on the previous day (April 15). A plasma sample (blood withdrawn at 17:00) was obtained to see if the symptoms were consistent with noncompliance. A plasma digoxin concentration of 0.9 μg/L and a serum creatinine of 0.9 mg/dL were reported.

Step 1. *Estimation of Expected Parameter Values*. From age, gender, weight, and serum creatinine, the creatinine clearance (Table 16–2, p. 258) is

$$CL_{cr} \text{ (mL/min)} = \frac{(140 - 53) \times 82}{85 \times 0.9} = 93 \text{ mL/min}$$
$$(5.6 \text{ L/hr or}$$
$$0.068 \text{ L/hr/kg})$$

Clearance of digoxin (Table 18–4) is then

$$CL \text{ (L/hr/kg)} = 0.9 \times 0.068 + 0.02$$
$$(0.0812 \text{ L/hr/kg}$$
$$\text{or } 6.66 \text{ L/hr})$$

and volume of distribution is

$$V\text{(L/kg)} = 3.8 + 52 \times 0.068 \ (7.34 \text{ L/kg or } 602 \text{ L})$$

Elimination rate constant and half-life are then

$$k = CL/V = 0.011 \text{ hr}^{-1}$$
$$t_{1/2} = 63 \text{ hr}$$

The values of S and F for digoxin tablets are 1.0 and 0.75, respectively.

Step 2. *Estimation of Expected Concentration at Time of Sampling*. The first question to be addressed is that of the appropriate kinetic model for evaluating this concentration. Presumably, the patient has been taking digoxin for 3 years. The dosing history indicates a single, recently missed dose. Thus, a steady-state model incorporating the missed dose is appropriate. Because the expected half-life is 63 hr and the dosing interval is 24 hr, the fluctuation in concentration should be minor and a constant-rate infusion model should apply. Alternatively, a steady-state, multiple-dose model could be employed. Using the constant-rate infusion model, the concentration expected, $C(t)$ (Fig. 18–2), is then $C_{ss} - C(t_1)$, where $C(t_1)$ is the concentration expected 32 hr after administration had only the missed dose been given.

$$C(t) = \underbrace{\frac{F \cdot S \cdot \text{Dose}}{CL \cdot \tau}}_{C_{ss}} - \underbrace{\frac{F \cdot S \cdot \text{Dose} \cdot e^{-kt_1}}{V}}_{C(t_1)}$$

Using a steady-state, multiple-dose model, the concentration expected is that 8 hr (t_2) into the 24-hour dosing interval (τ) minus $C(t_1)$, as defined above ($t_1 = 32$ hr).

$$C(t) = \frac{F \cdot S \cdot \text{Dose}}{V} \cdot \left[\frac{e^{-kt_2}}{1 - e^{-k\tau}} - e^{-kt_1} \right]$$

The values are 0.95 and 1.01 mg/L, a difference explained by the assumption of *average* steady-state concentration in the first model.

Step 3. *Comparison of Observed and Expected Concentrations.* The observed (0.9 µg/L) and expected (1.01 µg/L) values are virtually the same. Step 4, revision of parameter values, is unnecessary. Furthermore, the clinician now has some confidence that the patient is handling the drug as expected and that the concentration present may be inadequate to control her congestive cardiac failure. A decision must now be made on how much higher a concentration is needed, or if therapy should be augmented with other drugs or changed.

Case 2. Theophylline. J.T., a 6-year-old, 22-kg boy suffering from asthma and epilepsy, was taking a 100-mg aminophylline tablet ($S = 0.85$) four times a day at 8:00, 12:00, 16:00, and 20:00. Because of poor control of both his asthma and his seizures, a blood sample was obtained at 8:00, just before the next dose, for determination of theophylline and phenobarbital concentrations. The theophylline concentration was 6.3 mg/L.

Step 1. *Estimation of Expected Parameter Values.* To estimate the clearance of theophylline, the patient's age and concurrent drug therapy need to be considered. The clearance (Table 18–4) is then

$$CL = 0.04 \times 1.6 \times 1.3 \times 22 = 1.83 \text{ L/hr}$$

Note that the clearance per kilogram in the 6-year-old boy is adjusted by a factor of 1.6; younger children (1 to 4 years of age) are adjusted by a factor of 2.4 (Table 18–4). These numbers are close to the values expected for adjustment based on surface area (Chap. 15). The factor 1.3 is an adjustment for the concurrent administration of phenobarbital, which induces theophylline metabolism. Volume of distribution (0.5 L/kg times weight in kg) is 11 L. Elimination rate constant and half-life are then 0.17 hr^{-1} and 4.2 hr, respectively. Values of other pertinent parameters are $F = 1$, $S = 0.85$.

Step 2. *Estimation of Expected Concentration at Time of Sampling.* Using Eq. 6, the concentration at 8:00 is

$$C = \frac{0.85 \times 100}{11} \times \left[\frac{e^{-k \cdot 24} + e^{-k \cdot 20} + e^{-k \cdot 16} + e^{-k \cdot 12}}{(1 - e^{-k \cdot 24})} \right] = 2.1 \text{ mg/L}$$

A similar situation is depicted in Fig. 18–3.

Step 3. *Comparison of Observed and Expected Concentrations.* The observed concentration (6.3 mg/L) is three times greater than that expected (2.1 mg/L) on the assumption that the information on compliance, dosing schedule, sampling history, and assay is accurate.

Step 4. *Revision of Parameter Values.* Apparently, either volume or clearance, or both, needs revision. The questions are: Which one? and How much should it be revised? One approach would be to assume that the volume term is correct and change the value of k (or CL, since $k = CL/V$) in the equation above until the right side of the equation is equal to 6.3. The following values are determined:

k (hr^{-1})	RIGHT SIDE OF EQUATION (mg/L)
0.166	2.1
0.12	4.3
0.10	6.2
0.08	9.1

This procedure, called *iteration*, is used frequently in clinical pharmacokinetics. Note that the most likely value of k, to explain an observation of 6.3 mg/L, is about 0.10 hr^{-1}, a value not too different from that expected, 0.17 hr^{-1}.

A similar analysis could be carried out assuming that the value of clearance is that expected and the observation is a result of an unexpected volume of distribution. In this case,

$$C(mg/L) = \frac{0.85 \times 100}{V} \times \left[\frac{e^{-1.83 \times 24/V} + e^{-1.83 \times 20/V} + e^{-1.83 \times 16/V} + e^{-1.83 \times 12/V}}{(1 - e^{-1.83 \times 24/V})} \right]$$

By iteration, the following values are determined:

V (L)	RIGHT SIDE OF EQUATION (mg/L)
11	2.1
20	4.0
40	5.7
60	6.4

Note that a large increase in V is necessary to account for the observed concentration. Population data on theophylline show that clearance is much more variable (larger coefficient of variation) than volume of distribution. Accordingly, the prudent decision is to adjust clearance and not volume of distribution in this patient.

The procedure whereby the sensitivity of the observed measurement to changes in parameter values is assessed is called *sensitivity analysis*. It is accomplished by systematically substituting various values for each parameter, in turn, into the appropriate kinetic model. The concentration is insensitive to a parameter when large changes in the parameter produce small changes in concentration and the converse. We conclude from such an analysis, and from our general knowledge of the population pharmacokinetics of theophylline, that clearance ($k \cdot V$) in this patient is about 1.1 L/hr. The concentration is sensitive to clearance, as only a small change in its value (1.8 to 1.1 L/hr) produces a three-fold difference in observed and expected concentrations.

Step 5. *Recommendation for Adjustment of Dosage*. The maximum concentration expected after the dose at 20:00 is the trough value times $e^{+k \cdot 12}$, a value derived from the maximum having decayed by a factor of $e^{-k \cdot 12}$. In this case, the best estimate of the maximum concentration is 21 mg/L. The concentration range between a trough of 6.3 mg/L and a peak of 21.0 mg/L renders concentrations outside the recommended therapeutic window. A regimen of 6-hourly fixed doses may not be practical here. A more logical solution is to switch to a controlled-release dosage form. The patient's daily need is about 400 mg. A 200-mg dose with an appropriate controlled-release product, to be taken twice daily, is recommended here.

Case 3. *Gentamicin.* Mr. B.G., a 23-year-old, 58 kg patient with a gram-negative pneumonia, was being treated with gentamicin and ampicillin. Gentamicin had been given as an i.v. infusion (80 mg) over 45 min every 8 hr. Blood samples were obtained just before and 30 min after the end of the fourth infusion to prevent toxicity and to evaluate his therapy. The gentamicin concentrations reported were 0.4 and 4.9 mg/L. The serum creatinine in the patient was 1.2 mg/dL.

Step 1. *Estimation of Parameter Values.* The creatinine clearance in this patient, estimated from the patient's age, weight, gender, and serum creatinine (Table 16–2), is 79 mL/min (4.7 L/hr). The clearance of gentamicin is approximated by creatinine clearance (Table 18–4). The volume of distribution is 12.8 L (0.22 L/kg $\times$ 58 kg). The elimination rate constant and half-life are then 0.37 hr^{-1} and 1.9 hr, respectively.

Step 2. *Estimation of Expected Concentrations at Times of Sampling.* The samples are obtained under steady-state conditions (expected half-life = 1.9 hr), and the drug is constantly infused over a period of time, 45 min (0.75 hr), approaching the half-life. The intermittent infusion model (Eq. 7, F = 1) is appropriate. The concentration just before the next infusion is equivalent to the value at the end of the dosing interval (see Fig. 18–4). Thus, the concentrations 30 min after the end of the infusion (1.25 hr after starting the infusion) and at the end of the 8-hr interval can be calculated from

$$C = \frac{80}{4.7 \times 0.75} \frac{(1 - e^{-0.37 \times 0.75})}{(1 - e^{-0.37 \times 8})} \cdot e^{-0.37(t - 0.75)}$$

The expected concentrations are 4.8 and 0.4 mg/L, respectively (Fig. 18–4).

Step 3. *Comparison of Observed and Expected Concentrations.* Since the observed and expected values are virtually the same, the estimated parameter values are assumed to apply to this patient.

Case 4. *Phenobarbital.* Mrs. J.P., an 82-year-old, 55-kg patient with a seizure disorder, has been receiving 100 mg of phenobarbital at bedtime for years. She moved into a nursing home on February 17 after having a seizure on the 15th in her own apartment. On the morning of February 18, she had a blood sample taken, which showed a plasma phenobarbital concentration of 12 mg/L. Her physician increased her nightly dose to 200 mg (started on the 18th). On February 28 another blood sample was obtained; a concentration of 26 mg/L was then reported.

Step 1. *Estimation of Parameter Values.* Clearance and volume (from Table 18–4) are estimated to be 0.20 L/hr and 30 L, respectively. The resulting elimination rate constant and half-life values are 0.0067 hr^{-1} and 104 hr. F and S are equal to 1.0.

Step 2. *Estimation of Expected Concentrations at Times of Sampling.* It is uncertain whether the first concentration is a steady-state value, as the concentration obtained 10 days (240 hr) later is more than twice the first value, even when only 2.5 expected half-lives have elapsed. If the first had been a steady-state value, the concentration calculated for this time is

$$C(t_1) = \frac{F \cdot S \cdot Dose}{CL \cdot \tau} = \frac{100\ mg}{0.2\ L/hr \cdot 24\ hr} = 21\ mg/L$$

A steady-state constant-rate infusion model may be used because of the short dosing interval (1 day) relative to the half-life (4 days) and because the blood is sampled near the midpoint of the dosing interval. The second level can be calculated from a bolus plus constant-rate infusion model.

$$C(t_2) = C(t_1)\, e^{-kt} + \frac{F \cdot S \cdot \text{Dose}}{CL}(1 - e^{-kt})$$

$$= 21\, e^{-0.0067\,hr^{-1} \times 240\,hr} + \frac{200\ \text{mg/day} \times \dfrac{1\ \text{day}}{24\ \text{hr}}}{0.2\ \text{L/hr}}(1 - e^{-0.0067\,hr^{-1} \times 240\,hr})$$

$$= 38\ \text{mg/L}$$

Step 3. *Comparison of Observed and Expected Concentrations.* Clearly, the patient's observed values are well below the predicted ones. Revision of parameter values is in order.

Step 4. *Revision of Parameter Values.* As neither concentration is a steady-state value, non-steady-state methods must be used. Two approaches might be considered. First, the model above might be used.

If the value of V has only minor variability within the adult population, as is the case for phenobarbital, then the value of clearance can be calculated by iteration as in Case 2. The clearance value obtained is 0.3 L/hr.

Another approach comes from mass balance concepts. The net rate of change of drug in the body $(V \cdot dC/dt)$ is the difference between the rates in $(F \cdot S \cdot \text{Dose}/\tau)$ and out $(CL \cdot C)$, that is

$$V \cdot \frac{dC}{dt} = \frac{F \cdot S \cdot \text{Dose}}{\tau} - CL \cdot C$$

In conditions in which the concentration changes from one value, $C(t_1)$, to another $C(t_2)$, dC/dt can be approximated by $(C(t_2) - C(t_1))/(t_2 - t_1)$ and C by $(C(t_1) + C(t_2))/2$. The equation then becomes

$$V \cdot \frac{(C(t_2) - C(t_1))}{(t_2 - t_1)} = \frac{F \cdot S \cdot \text{Dose}}{\tau} + CL \cdot \frac{(C(t_1) + C(t_2))}{2}$$

On rearrangement,

$$CL = \frac{\dfrac{F \cdot S \cdot \text{Dose}}{\tau} - \dfrac{V \cdot (C(t_2) - C(t_1))}{(t_2 - t_1)}}{\dfrac{(C(t_1) + C(t_2))}{2}}$$

Substitution of the values for each symbol on the right side of the equation gives

$$CL = \frac{\dfrac{200}{24} - \dfrac{30 \times (26 - 12)}{(240 - 0)}}{\dfrac{(12 + 26)}{2}} = 0.35\ \text{L/hr}$$

a value close to the estimate from the first method. In both cases, an estimate of V had to be used. The second method is an approximation, with considerable error when $C(t_1)$ and $C(t_2)$ are close to each other $[(C(t_2) - C(t_1))/(t_2 - t_1)$ can then have a high error] or when $C(t_1)$ and $C(t_2)$ are far apart $[(C(t_1) + C(t_2))/2$ is then not a good estimate of the average value of C during the interval]. In general, the iterative method is preferred.

Other approaches are now available in computer programs that incorporate population mean and variability information in the parameter values and the characteristics of the kinetic model as well as the time(s) of sampling and dosing history.

Step 5. *Recommendation for Adjustment of Dosage.* If the daily dose of 200 mg is continued, a steady-state concentration of 28 mg/L is expected ($F \cdot S \cdot Dose/\tau \cdot CL$, $CL = 0.3$ L/hr). A daily dose of 100 mg then gives a corresponding value of 14 mg/L. Both values are within the therapeutic window. It seems appropriate to conclude that the patient has a higher (50%) clearance than expected, and that she had been compliant before admission to the nursing home. A decision now is needed on the proper dosage. Because she had a seizure on 100 mg/day, a daily dose between 150 and 200 mg seems appropriate.

Arguably, in all four of the preceding examples, dosage could have been adjusted solely by titrating to the effects observed. A point in favor of concentration measurement is that an assessment could be made as to why toxicity or a lack of effect occurred. These measurements also permitted facile and rapid estimation of the patient's dosage requirement, which otherwise might have required a considerable degree of readjustment from observing the effects alone. The fineness of the adjustment was also much greater with the plasma concentration data than it would have been without them.

STUDY PROBLEMS

(Answers to Study Problems are in Appendix II.)

1. List and briefly describe the criteria for performing drug concentration monitoring and applying target concentration strategy.
2. An 85-kg, 42-year-old female patient is receiving 120-mg doses of gentamicin in short-term, constant-rate infusions over 45 min every 8 hr. The patient has a serum creatinine of 1.2 mg/dL. Plasma samples were obtained just before and 45 min after the end of the fourth dose.
   a. Estimate the values of clearance, volume of distribution, and half-life expected in this patient.
   b. Estimate the gentamicin concentration in plasma expected at each of the two sampling times.
3. The plasma concentrations at the times of sampling in the patient in problem 2 were 2.5 and 7.2 mg/L, respectively.
   a. Using these concentrations, revise the estimates of clearance, volume of distribution, and half-life in this patient.
   b. Is it possible to adjust the dose (τ same) to keep the trough concentration below 2 mg/L and the peak above 6 mg/L?
4. Given the usual parameter values for theophylline (Table 18–4), provide a pharmacokinetic interpretation for each of the following theophylline concentrations, obtained in three different adult patients during an infusion of aminophylline at a constant rate of 0.8 mg/hr/kg. No theophylline was present in the body at the start of the infusion. In your interpretations include both a comparison of observed and expected plasma concentrations and an estimation of the values of clearance and half-life in each patient. Assume that the volume of distribution (liters/kg) is the same in all three patients and that they are nonsmoking, healthy adults, except for their asthmatic condition.

PATIENT	TIME OF SAMPLING (hours into infusion)	PLASMA THEOPHYLLINE CONCENTRATION (mg/L)
1	3	3.5
2	16	18
3	30	6

5. **Mr. V.J. is a 70-kg, 65-year-old asthmatic patient with congestive cardiac failure. He is started on aminophylline tablets orally and has a plasma theophylline concentration measured as noted in Table 18–5. He smokes 2 packs of cigarettes a day.**

Table 18–5. Dosing and Sampling History

DATE	TIME	TIME WHEN PLASMA SAMPLE IS OBTAINED (hr)	ORAL DOSE (mg)
June 1	18:00	24	400
	22:00	20	200
June 2	8:00	10	300
	12:00	6	300
	18:00	Plasma sample obtained C = 18 mg/L	

  a. Estimate the values of clearance, volume of distribution, and half-life expected for theophylline in this patient.
  b. Estimate the concentration expected at the time of sampling.
  c. Compare the observed and estimated concentrations.
  d. State which parameters you think need to be revised and by how much to account for any difference between observed and estimated concentrations.

6. **Mr. D.W., a 68-year-old, 74-kg, alcoholic, epileptic patient, has been taking phenobarbital (200 mg at bedtime) for 3 years. He has been free of seizures for at least 1 year. He was admitted to the hospital on January 10 with ataxia and general central nervous system depression, without alcohol on his breath. A plasma phenobarbital concentration of 56 mg/L was measured in a blood sample drawn at 11:00 of that day. The drug was discontinued (including no dose on January 10), and another blood sample was obtained on January 16 at 10:00 to determine if the patient was metabolizing the drug more slowly than expected, as the patient had signs of hepatic cirrhosis. The second concentration was 16 mg/L.**

  a. Evaluate the data in the sequential manner requested in problem 5.
  b. Given that clearance is much more variable than volume of distribution (Table 13–2), state the likely cause of the observations made and provide a recommendation for his future antiepileptic therapy with phenobarbital.

7. **Ms. K.D., a 70-kg, 68-year-old was admitted to the hospital at 13:30 on April 9 because of shortness of breath and wheezing. Congestive cardiac failure and asthma were confirmed by clinical symptoms. To treat the asthma, she was administered 300 mg of aminophylline intravenously at 14:00, and an infusion of 30 mg/hr was begun immediately. At 18:00 on April 10, a plasma sample was obtained. The theophylline concentration was reported to be 20 mg/L. On April 11, her physician switched her to oral therapy. The infusion was discontinued at 9:00, and the first oral dose (200 mg every 6 hr) was given at 13:00. Evaluate this case using the 5 steps recommended in the text.**

SELECTED TOPICS

DISTRIBUTION KINETICS

OBJECTIVES

The reader will be able to:

1. State why the one-compartment model is sometimes inadequate to describe kinetic events within the body.

2. Compare the sum of two exponentials with the compartment model for representing plasma concentration data showing distribution kinetics.

3. Estimate clearance and the half-life of the phase associated with the majority of elimination given plasma concentration-time data of a drug showing distribution kinetics.

4. Define and estimate the distribution parameters: initial dilution volume (V_1), volume during the terminal phase (V), and volume of distribution at steady state (V_{ss}).

5. Describe the impact of distribution kinetics on the interpretation of plasma concentration-time data following administration of a single dose.

6. Explain the influence of distribution kinetics and duration of administration on the time-courses of concentration in plasma and amount in tissue during and after stopping a constant-rate infusion.

7. Describe how distribution kinetics influences the fluctuations of plasma and tissue levels with time during a multiple-dose regimen.

8. Explain how distribution kinetics can influence the interpretation of plasma concentration-time data and terminal half-life when clearance is altered.

The first four sections cover most of the fundamentals of pharmacokinetics. Section Five now expands on selected topics; it begins with chapters on distribution kinetics and pharmacologic response. Subsequent chapters deal with metabolite kinetics, dose and time dependencies, turnover concepts and dialysis. These topics do not build on each other as extensively as do the previous topics. Notable exceptions to this statement are found in applications of distribution kinetic concepts in the chapters on pharmacologic response, turnover concepts, and dialysis.

Portraying the body as a single compartment is appropriate for establishing the fundamental principles of pharmacokinetics but is an inaccurate representation of events that follow drug administration. A basic assumption of the concept of a one-compartment representation of distribution is that equilibration of drug between tissues and blood occurs spontaneously. In reality, distribution takes time. The time required depends on tissue perfusion, permeability characteristics of tissue membranes for drug, and its partitioning between tissues and blood (Chap. 10). Ignoring distribution kinetics is reasonable so long as the error incurred is acceptable. This error becomes unacceptable when the one-compartment representation fails to adequately explain observations following drug administration; there is a danger of significant misinterpretation of the observations; and major discrepancies occur in the calculation of drug dosage. Such situations are most likely to arise when either substantial amounts are eliminated or response occurs before distribution equilibrium is achieved. This chapter deals with the pharmacokinetic consequence of distribution kinetics. The impact of distribution kinetics on pharmacologic response is dealt with in the next chapter, Pharmacologic Response.

EVIDENCE OF DISTRIBUTION KINETICS

Evidence of distribution kinetics is usually inferred from an early rapid decline in plasma (blood) concentration following an i.v. bolus dose; when little drug has been eliminated, and from the rapid onset and decline in the pharmacologic effect of some drugs during this early phase. Data in Fig. 19–1, which show the concentration of thiopental in various tissues after an i.v. bolus dose of this preoperative general anesthetic to a dog, provide direct evidence of distribution kinetics. Thiopental is a small, highly lipid-soluble drug for which distribution into essentially all tissues is perfusion rate-limited. The results seen with this drug are therefore typical of those observed with many other small lipophilic drugs.

Notice that thiopental in liver, a highly perfused organ, reaches distribution equilibrium with that in plasma by 5 min (the first observation), and thereafter, the decline in liver parallels that in plasma. The same holds true in other highly perfused tissues, including brain and kidneys.

Redistribution of thiopental from well-perfused tissues to less well-perfused tissues, such as muscle and fat, primarily accounts for the subsequent decline in plasma concentration over the next 3 hr; less than 20% of the dose is eliminated during this period. Due to a combination of poor perfusion and high partitioning, even by 3 hr distribution equilibrium in adipose tissue has not been established. Analysis of the situation indicates that this does not occur for several more hours, at which time the majority of thiopental remaining is in fat. Recall: The greater the partition of a drug into fat, or into any tissue, the longer is the time required to achieve distribution equilibrium (Chap. 10). However, only if the ap-

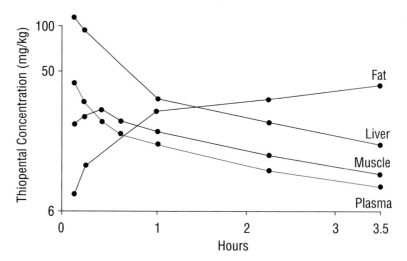

Fig. 19–1. Semilogarithmic plot of the concentration of thiopental in various tissues and plasma (colored line) following an i.v. bolus dose of 25 mg/kg to a dog. Note the early rise and fall of thiopental in the well-perfused tissues (e.g., liver) and in lean muscle tissue. After 3 hr much of the drug remaining in the body is in adipose tissue (1 mg/kg = 4.1 µmol/kg). (Redrawn from Brodie, B.B., Bernstein, E., and Mark, L.: The role of body fat in limiting the duration of action of thiopental. J. Pharmacol. Exp. Ther., *105*:421–426, 1952. © Williams & Wilkins (1952).)

parent volume of distribution of a tissue ($K_p \cdot V_T$) is a major fraction of the total volume of distribution does uptake into that tissue substantially affect events within plasma. With thiopental, which has an adipose-to-plasma partition coefficient of 10, fat (0.12 L/kg) constitutes approximately 40% of the total volume of distribution (2.3 L/kg). Accordingly, the plasma concentration of thiopental not only falls markedly, but distribution takes many hours. For other drugs, distribution may take even longer if partitioning into tissues is more extensive than for thiopental. In contrast, distribution is complete within 30 min after administration of theophylline (Fig. 3–1). Either theophylline does not enter poorly perfused tissues or if it does the partition coefficients are very low. It is impossible to distinguish between these two possibilities by measuring theophylline only in plasma, as events here may poorly reflect those that might occur elsewhere.

INTRAVENOUS BOLUS DOSE

Presentation of Data

Sum of Exponential Terms. The early rapid and subsequent slower decline in the plasma concentration of aspirin in an individual subject following a 650-mg i.v. bolus dose (Fig. 19–2) is typical of many drugs. Had no samples been taken during the first 10 min, the terminal linear decline of the plasma concentration when plotted on semilogarithmic graph paper would have been characterized by a monoexponential equation, and one-compartment disposition characteristics would have been applied to aspirin. Recall: The monoexponential equation is $C(0) \cdot e^{-kt}$, where k is the rate constant with an associated half-life, given by $0.693/k$, and $C(0)$ is the anticipated initial plasma drug concentration, given as the intercept on the plasma concentration axis when the line is extrapolated back to time zero. For aspirin k is 0.050 min^{-1}, the corresponding half-life is 14 min, and $C(0)$ is 33 mg/L. Going further, the volume of distribution [Dose/$C(0)$] is 20 L and clearance ($k \cdot V$) is 0.98 L/min.

Notice that the early plasma concentrations are higher than those anticipated by back extrapolation of the terminal slope and that the earlier the time, the greater is the difference. When the difference at each sample time is plotted on the same graph, all the difference values fall on another straight line, which can be characterized by a monoex-

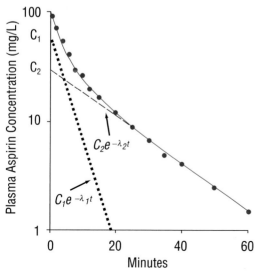

Fig. 19–2. When displayed semilogarithmically, the fall in the plasma concentration of aspirin is initially rapid but then slows after an i.v. bolus dose of 650 mg to a subject. The decline in concentration (——) can be characterized by the sum of two exponential terms: $C_1 e^{-\lambda_1 t}$ (●■●■) and $C_2 e^{-\lambda_2 t}$ (– – –) (1 mg/L = 5.5 μM). (Redrawn from Rowland, M., and Riegelman, S.: Pharmacokinetics of acetylsalicylic acid and salicylic acid after intravenous administration in man. J. Pharm. Sci., 57:1313–1319, 1968.)

ponential equation, $B(0)e^{-\alpha t}$, where α is the decay rate constant and $B(0)$ is the corresponding zero-time intercept. For aspirin, $\alpha = 0.23$ min^{-1}, $t_{1/2} = 3.0$ min, and $B(0) = 67$ mg/L.

Because all the plasma concentrations at the later times can be fitted by one equation, $C(0)e^{-kt}$ and because at the earlier times, all the difference values can be fitted by another equation, $B(0)e^{-\alpha t}$, it follows that the entire plasma drug concentration (C) versus time data can be fitted by the *sum* of these two exponential terms. That is

$$C = B(0)e^{-\alpha t} + C(0)e^{-kt} \qquad 1$$

For example, the biexponential equation $C = 67e^{-0.23t} + 33e^{-0.050t}$, where t is time in minutes, adequately describes the decline in the plasma aspirin concentration following a 650-mg bolus dose. Sometimes, when using this difference procedure, known commonly as the *method of residuals*, a sum of three and occasionally four exponential terms is required to adequately fit the observed concentration-time data. Since the principles in approaching such data are the same as those used to analyze and interpret events described by a biexponential equation, only the simpler case is considered further in this book.

To facilitate the discussion a more uniform set of symbols is needed. Rather than using the different symbols α and k, the general symbol λ is used to denote the exponential coefficient. Thus, Eq. 1 can be rewritten as

$$C = C_1 e^{-\lambda_1 t} + C_2 e^{-\lambda_2 t} \qquad 2$$

where the subscripts 1 and 2 refer to the first and second exponential terms respectively, and C_1 and C_2 refer to the corresponding zero-time intercepts, or coefficients. By convention, the exponential terms are arranged in decreasing order of λ. For example, in the case of aspirin $C_1 = 67$ mg/L, $\lambda_1 = 0.23$ min^{-1}, $C_2 = 33$ mg/L, and $\lambda_2 = 0.050$ min^{-1}.

With aspirin, two exponential terms and hence two phases are seen when plasma concentration-time data are displayed on a semilogarithmic plot. Commonly, the last phase is called the *terminal phase*. With aspirin and many other drugs it is a correct description. Sometimes, however, there is an additional, still slower phase, indicating that distribution equilibrium has not been achieved with all tissues. The terminal phase is often missed because the assay procedure employed is insufficiently sensitive to measure the drug concentration at these later times. This certainly was the case with aminoglycosides and some amine drugs before the advent of more sensitive assays. With increased potency of many new compounds, analytical sensitivity continues to be an occasional problem in drug development. In the subsequent discussion, the observed terminal phase is assumed to be correctly designated.

At time zero the anticipated plasma concentration is, by reference to Eq. 2, equal to the sum of the coefficients, $C_1 + C_2$. At that time the amount in the body is the dose. Hence, by definition, the volume into which drug appears to distribute initially, the *initial dilution volume*, V_1, is given by

$$V_1 = \frac{\text{Dose}}{(C_1 + C_2)} \qquad 3$$

For aspirin, the anticipated initial concentration is 100 ($= 67 + 33$) mg/L so that the initial dilution volume of aspirin is 6.5 L.

It is important to realize that the time for concentration to fall by one-half is only equal to a half-life during the terminal phase. Before then, the plasma concentration falls in half in a period of less than one terminal half-life but more than one initial half-life. This is clearly evident on comparing the fall in plasma aspirin concentration in the earlier moments with the decline of the first exponential term.

A Compartmental Model. Although for the majority of situations in pharmacokinetics the desired information can be obtained directly from modification of Eq. 2, it is sometimes conceptually helpful to represent disposition pictorially. Figure 19–3, a *two-compartment model*, is a common form of such a representation. Compartment 1, the initial dilution volume mentioned above, is also frequently called the central compartment because drug is administered into and distributed from it. As mentioned, the initial dilution volume of aspirin is 6.5 L; for many other drugs it is much larger. These values are clearly greater than the plasma volume, 3 L, and therefore this initial dilution volume must be composed of additional spaces into which drug distributes extremely rapidly. These spaces must be in well-perfused tissues, which probably include liver and kidneys, the major eliminating organs. Elimination is therefore usually depicted as occurring *directly* and *exclusively* from the central compartment. Drug distributes between this central compartment and a peripheral compartment, composed of tissues into which drug distributes more slowly.

Several points are worth mentioning here. First, the model is defined by the data. The number of compartments or pools required equals the number of exponential terms needed to describe the plasma concentration-time data. Thus, a three-compartment model is needed when the data are best fitted by a triexponential equation. Next, the model depicted in Fig. 19–3, or any other model for which drug elimination is portrayed as occurring exclusively from the central compartment, is not unique. Three two-compartment models can adequately describe a biexponential plasma concentration decay curve: the one depicted in Fig. 19–3, one with elimination occurring from both compartments, and one with loss occurring exclusively from the peripheral compartment. No distinction between these three possibilities can be made from plasma concentration-time data alone, and while the model depicted in Fig. 19–3 is the most favored one, based on such physiologic considerations as the initial dilution volume exceeding the plasma volume, elimination can sometimes occur in tissues of the peripheral compartment. Moreover, occasionally the liver (or kidneys) is not part of the central compartment. For example, the initial dilution volume of indocyanine green, a dye used as a dynamic test of hepatic function, is only 3 L, the plasma volume. The major peripheral tissue, in this instance the liver, is also the primary site of elimination via biliary excretion. A two-compartment model, with elimination occurring only from the peripheral compartment, therefore best describes the disposition kinetics of this dye. Last, drug distribution within a compartment is not homogenous. Although the concentrations of drug within and among such tissues usually vary enor-

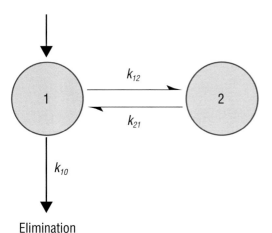

Fig. 19–3. A two-compartment model of the body. Drug is administered into and eliminated from compartment 1 and distributes between compartments 1 and 2. The rate constants for the processes are indicated.

mously, tissues are lumped together into a compartment because the times to achieve distribution equilibrium in each tissue are similar.

In Fig. 19–3 movement of drug between compartments can be characterized by transfer rate constants, where k_{12} denotes the rate constant associated with movement of drug from compartment 1 into compartment 2, and k_{21} is the rate constant associated with the reverse process. The rate constant k_{10} is associated with loss of drug from compartment 1 by metabolism and excretion. The unit of all three rate constants is reciprocal time.

Rate equations can be written for movement of amounts between the compartments and for drug elimination. Following an i.v. bolus dose these equations are

$$
\text{Rate of change} = \quad -k_{12} \cdot A_1 \quad - \quad k_{10} \cdot A_1 \quad + \quad k_{21} \cdot A_2
$$

Rate of change = $-k_{12} \cdot A_1$ − $k_{10} \cdot A_1$ + $k_{21} \cdot A_2$
of amount of
drug in
compartment 1 | Rate of movement from compartment 1 to compartment 2 | Rate of elimination | Rate of movement from compartment 2 to compartment 1

4

Rate of change = $k_{12} \cdot A_1$ − $k_{21} \cdot A_2$
of amount of
drug in
compartment 2 | Rate of movement from compartment 1 to compartment 2 | Rate of movement from compartment 2 to compartment 1

5

where A_1 and A_2 are the amounts of drug in compartments 1 and 2, respectively. Integration of these rate equations provides a biexponential equation, of the same form as Eq. 2, for the decline of drug from plasma, except that the coefficients and exponents are recast in terms of the parameters defining the compartmental model. Equivalent relationships between the biexponential and two-compartment models are listed in Table 19–1.

Table 19–1. Equivalent Relationships Between the Biexponential and Two-Compartment Models[a]

PARAMETER/VARIABLE	SUM OF EXPONENTIALS	TWO-COMPARTMENT MODEL
Plasma concentration (C)	$C_1 e^{-\lambda_1 t} + C_2 e^{-\lambda_2 t}$	$\left[\dfrac{\text{Dose}}{V_1} \cdot \dfrac{(k_{21} - \lambda_1)}{(\lambda_2 - \lambda_1)}\right] e^{-\lambda_1 t} + \left[\dfrac{\text{Dose}}{V_1} \cdot \dfrac{(k_{21} - \lambda_2)}{(\lambda_1 - \lambda_2)}\right] e^{-\lambda_2 t}$
	λ_1	$1/2[(k_{12} + k_{21} + k_{10}) + \sqrt{(k_{12} + k_{21} + k_{10})^2 - 4k_{21}k_{10}}]$
	λ_2	$1/2[(k_{12} + k_{21} + k_{10}) - \sqrt{(k_{12} + k_{21} + k_{10})^2 - 4k_{21}k_{10}}]$
	$\lambda_1 + \lambda_2$	$k_{12} + k_{21} + k_{10}$
	$\lambda_1 \cdot \lambda_2$	$k_{21} \cdot k_{10}$
Clearance (Cl)	$\text{Dose}/\left(\dfrac{C_1}{\lambda_1} + \dfrac{C_2}{\lambda_2}\right)$	$V_1 \cdot k_{10}$
Initial dilution volume (V_1)	$\text{Dose}/(C_1 + C_2)$	V_1
Volume of distribution (V) during terminal phase (V)	Cl/λ_2	$V_1 \cdot k_{10}/\lambda_2$
Volume of distribution at steady state (V_{ss})	$\dfrac{\text{Dose}\left[\dfrac{C_1}{\lambda_1^2} + \dfrac{C_2}{\lambda_2^2}\right]}{\left[\dfrac{C_1}{\lambda_1} + \dfrac{C_2}{\lambda_2}\right]^2}$	$V_1 \cdot (1 + k_{12}/k_{21})$

[a]Model in which drug is eliminated from the initial dilution volume only.

Although expressing data in terms of a compartmental model and associated parameters may appear to give greater insight into the data, caution should be exercised in doing so. Remember that the compartmental model chosen is often not unique, and one can rarely assign a physical or physiologic meaning to the value of any of the rate constants. Accordingly, much of the subsequent discussion is related to describing drug disposition by the sum of exponentials. However, pharmacokinetic observations are discussed in terms of the compartmental model when this procedure facilitates general understanding.

Pharmacokinetic Parameters

Clearance. Elimination occurs at all times. Just as plasma concentration is highest immediately following an intravenous bolus dose, so is rate of elimination $(CL \cdot C)$. Subsequently, both plasma concentration and corresponding rate of elimination fall rapidly. To calculate the amount eliminated in a small unit of time, dt, recall that

$$\text{Amount eliminated within interval } dt = \text{Clearance} \cdot C \cdot dt \qquad 6$$

where $C \cdot dt$ is the corresponding small area under the plasma concentration-time curve within the interval dt. The total amount eliminated, the dose administered, is the sum of all the small amounts eliminated from time zero to time infinity. Therefore,

$$\text{Dose} = \text{Clearance} \cdot AUC \qquad 7$$

where AUC is the *total* area under the plasma drug concentration-time curve. Accordingly, as with the simpler one-compartment model, clearance (CL) is most readily estimated by dividing Dose by AUC. The area may be determined from the trapezoidal rule (Appendix I–A) or, more conveniently, by realizing that the total area underlying each exponential term is the zero-time intercept divided by its corresponding exponential coefficient. Thus, the total area corresponding to Eq. 2 is given by

$$AUC = \underbrace{\frac{C_1}{\lambda_1}}_{\substack{\text{Area associated} \\ \text{with} \\ \text{initial term}}} + \underbrace{\frac{C_2}{\lambda_2}}_{\substack{\text{Area associated} \\ \text{with} \\ \text{last term}}} \qquad 8$$

When inserting the appropriate values for the aspirin example into Eq. 8, the value of AUC associated with the 650-mg dose is 951 mg-min/L, so that the total clearance of aspirin in the individual is 683 mL/min. Notice that clearance is considerably smaller than the value calculated assuming a one-compartment model, 985 mL/min. The latter is an overestimate of the true value, because more drug is eliminated during the attainment of distribution equilibrium than accounted for by the last term. If instead of the first phase a later phase is missed, the error in estimating clearance is large only if the missed area is a major fraction of the total area. Obviously, given the ease of estimating total area and provided that blood sampling times are adequate, the true value for clearance should always be calculated.

Volume of Distribution. One purpose of a volume term is to relate plasma concentration to amount in the body. The initial dilution volume fulfills this purpose initially. Subsequently, however, as drug distributes into the slowly equilibrating tissues, the plasma concentration declines more rapidly than does the amount in the body (A). Accordingly, as illustrated in Fig. 19–4 the effective volume of distribution (A/C) increases with time until distribution equilibrium between drug in plasma and all tissues is achieved; this occurs during the terminal phase. Only then does decline in all tissues parallel that in plasma and is proportionality between plasma concentration and amount in body achieved.

The volume of distribution during the terminal phase (V) can be calculated as follows. During this phase the concentration is given by $C_2 e^{-\lambda_2 t}$ (Fig. 19–2), and correspondingly,

$$\begin{matrix}\text{Amount of drug}\\ \text{in body during}\\ \text{terminal phase}\end{matrix} = V \cdot C = V \cdot C_2 e^{-\lambda_2 t} \qquad\qquad 9$$

Hence, extrapolating back to time zero, $V \cdot C_2$ must be the amount needed to give a plasma concentration of C_2, had drug spontaneously distributed into the volume, V. The amount, $V \cdot C_2$, remains to be calculated. When placed into the body, the amount, $V \cdot C_2$, is eventually matched by an equal amount eliminated. As the amount remaining to be eliminated is the product of clearance and area, and as C_2/λ_2 is the associated area, it follows that

$$\underset{\substack{\text{Amount in}\\ \text{body}}}{V \cdot C_2} = \underset{\substack{\text{Amount remaining}\\ \text{to be}\\ \text{eliminated}}}{CL \cdot \frac{C_2}{\lambda_2}} \qquad\qquad 10$$

or

$$\underset{\substack{\text{Volume of}\\ \text{distribution}}}{V} = \frac{CL}{\lambda_2} \qquad \frac{\text{Total clearance}}{\text{Terminal exponential coefficient}} \qquad\qquad 11$$

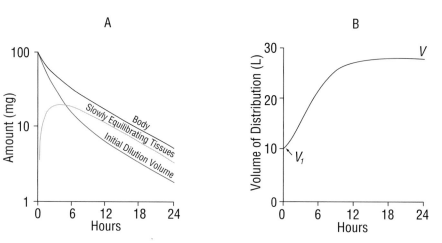

Fig. 19–4. Several events occur following a single i.v. bolus dose. *A*, Loss of drug from the initial dilution volume, of which plasma is a part, is due to both elimination from the body and distribution into the more slowly equilibrating tissues. The fall in amount of drug in the body is therefore initially less than the fall in the amount in the initial dilution volume. Only when distribution equilibrium has been achieved do the declines in the amounts in the initial dilution volume and in plasma parallel (same slope) that in the body. *A*, reflecting these events, the apparent volume of distribution (*A/C*), which just after giving the dose equals the initial dilution volume (V_1), increases with time approaching a limiting value (*V*), which occurs when distribution equilibrium is achieved.

Returning to the example of aspirin, $CL = 683$ mL/min and $\lambda_2 = 0.050$ min^{-1}, therefore its volume of distribution is 13.7 L. That is, if during the terminal phase the plasma concentration is 10 mg/L, then the amount in the body is 137 mg. Since 65 mg (10 mg/L $\times$ 6.5 L) are in the initial dilution volume, the remaining 71 mg must be in the tissues with which aspirin slowly equilibrates.

A comparison of Eq. 11 with the one that has been used in all previous chapters to define the volume of distribution $(V = CL/k)$ shows them to be the same, recognizing the equivalence of k and λ_2, the terminal exponential coefficient.

The ratio V_1/V gives an estimate of the degree of error in predicting the initial plasma concentration using a one-compartment model. For example, for aspirin, with values for V_1 and V of 6.5 and 13.7 L, respectively, the error in predicting initial concentrations from the plasma concentration-time data during the terminal phase can be relatively large. The error can be even larger when predicting conditions beyond the measured final phase if a still slower one exists. This last error is only of concern if there is an appreciable accumulation of drug in this phase during chronic administration, a point considered subsequently in this chapter.

Distribution Kinetics and Elimination

During the initial rapidly declining phase, more elimination occurs than would have been expected had distribution been spontaneous. Additional elimination is due to the particularly high concentrations of drug presented to organs of elimination during this period. For many drugs this increased elimination is small and, with respect to elimination, viewing the body as a single compartment is adequate. For other drugs, the additional elimination represents a major fraction of the administered dose, and approximating the kinetics with a one-compartment model is inappropriate. Area considerations are a basis for making this decision.

Recall from Eq. 9 that elimination associated with the concentrations defined by the terminal exponential term, $C_2 e^{-\lambda_2 t}$, gives an amount equal to $CL \cdot C_2/\lambda_2$. Expressing this amount as a fraction, f_2, of the administered dose and utilizing the relationship in Eq. 8 gives

$$\text{Fraction of elimination associated with last exponential term} = f_2 = \frac{C_2/\lambda_2}{AUC} \qquad\qquad 12$$

The remaining fraction, f_1, must therefore have been eliminated as a result of concentrations above those expected had spontaneous distribution occurred, i.e., those concentrations defined by $C_1 \cdot e^{-\lambda_1 t}$.

Applying Eq. 12 to the case of aspirin, elimination of 69% of the dose is associated with the terminal slope; the remaining 31% therefore must be associated with plasma concentrations above those expected had spontaneous distribution occurred. Although distribution kinetics cannot be ignored, the majority of aspirin elimination is clearly associated with events defined by the terminal phase, which has a half-life of 14 min. Based on the same reasoning, the terminal half-life is the elimination half-life for most drugs. There are some drugs, however, for which the calculated value of f_2 is low. Gentamicin is an example. Over 98% of an i.v. bolus dose is eliminated before distribution equilibrium within the body has been achieved. In this case, the reason lies in a permeability-limited distribution of gentamicin into certain tissues. Clearly, for gentamicin and similar drugs, the appropriate half-life (biexponential model) defining elimination after a bolus dose is $0.693/\lambda_1$.

A Mathematical Aid

For all but the mathematically inclined, analysis and prediction of plasma concentration-time data for a drug that displays multiexponential disposition characteristics are difficult. A useful mathematical aid to facilitate such analyses and predictions is to imagine that each exponential term arises from the independent administration of a different drug having one-compartment characteristics, and that the sum of their individual concentrations is the observed one. For example, imagine that a biexponential equation, $C_1 e^{-\lambda_1 t} + C_2 e^{-\lambda_2 t}$, arises from administration of two hypothetical drugs, Drug 1 and Drug 2; Drug 1 produces the curve $C_1 e^{-\lambda_1 t}$ and Drug 2 produces the curve $C_2 e^{-\lambda_2 t}$. Furthermore, assume that each hypothetical drug has the same clearance, CL. Therefore, because the two drugs have different rate constants, λ_1 and λ_2, they have different volumes of distribution, which are given by CL/λ_1 and CL/λ_2, respectively. To complete the analysis, the doses of the hypothetical drugs are needed. These are obtained from area considerations as follows. Since dose is the product of clearance and area, the respective doses are $CL \cdot (C_1/\lambda_1)$ and $CL \cdot (C_2/\lambda_2)$. Furthermore since $CL(C_1/\lambda_1 + C_2/\lambda_2)$ equals the total dose administered, it follows from Eq. 12 that $f_1 \cdot$ dose and $f_2 \cdot$ dose are the corresponding doses. Hence, the total observed concentration is given by

$$C = \frac{f_1 \cdot \text{Dose } e^{-\lambda_1 t}}{(CL/\lambda_1)} + \frac{f_2 \cdot \text{Dose } e^{-\lambda_2 t}}{(CL/\lambda_2)} \qquad \qquad 13$$

Although the above equation is a device that cannot, for example, predict events in slowly equilibrating tissues, it readily permits calculation of events in plasma under a variety of circumstances, as subsequently shown.

CONSTANT-RATE INFUSION

Figure 19–5 illustrates the anticipated effect of distribution kinetics on the plasma concentration upon stopping a constant-rate infusion at various times during approach to pla-

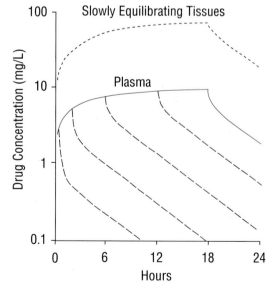

Fig. 19–5. Events in plasma (colored line) and in slowly equilibrating tissues (– – –) during and after stopping a constant-rate infusion. As concentration in the slowly equilibrating tissues rises during the infusion, the net tendency of drug to enter these tissues decreases. Consequently, on stopping the infusion, the distribution phase in plasma (– – –) appears shallower, the more prolonged the infusion. For simplicity, only the decline in tissue concentration when the infusion is stopped at plateau is shown. Eq. 20 describes the plasma concentration during an infusion. At the end of an infusion of duration τ, the concentration, $C(\tau)$, is therefore $C_{ss}[f_1(1 - e^{-\lambda_1 \tau}) + f_2(1 - e^{-\lambda_2 \tau})]$. Furthermore, on stopping the infusion, the plasma concentration is given by $C_{ss}[f_1(1 - e^{-\lambda_1 \tau}) \cdot e^{-\lambda_1 t_{post}} + f_2(1 - e^{-\lambda_2 \tau}) \cdot e^{-\lambda_2 t_{post}}]$, where t_{post} is the time after stopping the infusion. The last equation can be derived using the mathematical aid (Eq. 13), recognizing, for example, that $f_1 \cdot C_{ss}(1 - e^{-\lambda_1 \tau})$ is the concentration at the end of the infusion associated with the first phase, and $e^{-\lambda_1 t_{post}}$ is the corresponding fraction remaining at time t_{post}.

teau. At early times, a pronounced distribution phase is seen upon stopping an infusion, because distribution equilibrium has yet to be achieved between drug in blood and that in many tissues. With a more prolonged infusion, more drug enters the tissues. The tendency of drug to move from blood to tissues is then much reduced, and the distribution phase appears much shallower upon stopping the infusion. Even at plateau, however, some distribution may still be seen upon stopping the infusion. At plateau, the rates of drug entry into and out of the tissues are equal. Upon stopping the infusion, elimination of drug from plasma, along with a subsequent fall in plasma concentration, creates a gradient for return of drug from tissues. Initially, the rate of elimination from plasma exceeds the rate of efflux from tissues, and plasma concentration falls rapidly. Eventually, however, the rate of return from the tissues limits the rate of elimination from plasma. The body then acts, once again, as a single compartment; plasma concentration and amount in the tissues, and hence in the body as a whole, fall with a half-life equal to that seen during the terminal phase following an i.v. bolus dose.

The actual events seen after stopping an infusion at steady state depend largely on the kinetics of distribution. If distribution from tissues is slow relative to elimination from plasma, the plasma concentration falls substantially before the terminal phase is reached. Conversely, distribution may be so fast that, on stopping the infusion, drug in tissue and plasma stay in virtual equilibrium and only the terminal monoexponential decay is seen. The latter situation contrasts with events that would be seen following an i.v. bolus dose; a biexponential curve is invariably seen if blood is sampled early enough. As a guiding principle, a frank biphasic curve, on stopping an infusion at steady state, is seen when f_2 is small, i.e., when the majority of drug in plasma (and rapidly equilibrating tissues) is eliminated before distribution equilibrium is achieved.

Returning to events during infusion, two basic questions remain: What controls the plateau concentration? How long does it take to reach plateau?

Events at Plateau

Plateau Plasma Concentration. The plateau is reached when rate of drug elimination matches rate of infusion, R_0. The plasma concentration, C_{ss}, is therefore readily given by the familiar equation

$$C_{ss} = \frac{R_0}{\text{Clearance}} \qquad\qquad 14$$

Thus, as long as clearance is accurately determined, the rate of infusion needed to produce a given steady-state concentration can be calculated. Conversely, clearance can be determined from the concentration at steady state.

Volume of Distribution at Steady State. Although the volume of distribution, V, usefully relates amount in body to plasma concentration during the terminal phase, its value is influenced by elimination. As seen in Fig. 19–6, the faster a drug is eliminated, the greater is the ratio of drug in slowly equilibrating tissues to that in plasma during the terminal phase and, correspondingly, the larger is the apparent volume of distribution. A need, therefore, exists to define a volume term to reflect purely distribution. This volume term applies to steady state when drug is infused at a constant rate. This volume term, volume distribution at steady state, V_{ss}, is defined by

$$V_{ss} = \frac{\text{Amount in body at steady state}}{\text{Plasma concentration at steady state}} \qquad\qquad 15$$

Conceptualization of this volume may be helped by considering the two-compartment model depicted in Fig. 19–3. At steady state, the rates at which drug enters and leaves the slowly equilibrating tissues are exactly matched. It then follows from Eq. 5 that the amount in the slowly equilibrating compartment at steady state, $A_{ss,2}$ is given by

$$A_{ss,2} = \frac{k_{12}}{k_{21}} \cdot A_{ss,1} \qquad\qquad 16$$

The amount in the body at steady state, A_{ss}, is the sum of $A_{ss,1}$ and $A_{ss,2}$. Therefore,

$$A_{ss} = A_{ss,1} \left[1 + \frac{k_{12}}{k_{21}} \right] \qquad\qquad 17$$

Finally, as $A_{ss,1} = V_1 \cdot C_{ss}$ and $A_{ss} = V_{ss} \cdot C_{ss}$, it follows that

$$V_{ss} = V_1 \left[1 + \frac{k_{12}}{k_{21}} \right] \qquad\qquad 18$$

Volume of
distribution at
steady state

In practice, as amount in the body cannot be determined physically, V_{ss} is usually calculated from the disposition parameters (C_1, λ_1, C_2, and λ_2) following i.v. bolus adminis-

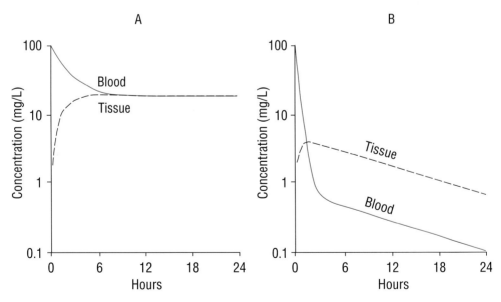

Fig. 19–6. Elimination influences volume of distribution during the terminal phase. To appreciate this statement, consider the distribution of a drug between blood (volume, V_B, 5 L) and a tissue (volume, V_T, 20 L). Furthermore, let $K_p = 1$, so that the concentrations in each compartment at equilibrium are equal if no elimination occurs (A). The volume of distribution at equilibrium is then 25 L. With elimination of drug, the concentration in the tissue (– – –) lags behind that in blood (———) during the terminal phase, thereby giving rise to a higher apparent value of K_p, $K_{p_{app}}$ (B). Consequently, the apparent volume of distribution ($V_B + K_{p_{app}} \cdot V_T$) is increased above that expected under true equilibrium conditions, $V_B + K_P \cdot V_T$.

tration (Table 19–1). The inter-relationships between V_{ss} and other pharmacokinetic parameters are best understood from the concept of mean residence time (Chap. 24, Turnover Concepts, and Appendix I–D).

The value of V_{ss} lies between the initial dilution volume, V_1, and the volume of distribution during the terminal phase, V. In general, the difference between the values of V_{ss} and V is small. Much depends on the disposition kinetics of the drug. The difference is larger, the greater the extent of elimination before distribution equilibrium is achieved. To appreciate this last point, consider three drugs, aspirin, salicylic acid, and gentamicin. The disposition kinetics, normalized to a 100-mg i.v. bolus dose for a 70-kg subject are aspirin, $C = 9.7\,e^{-13.8t} + 5.1\,e^{-3.0t}$; salicylic acid, $C = 10.2\,e^{-2.8t} + 8.7\,e^{-0.23t}$; gentamicin, $C = 7.1\,e^{-0.42t} + 0.05\,e^{-0.015t}$, where C is in mg/L and time in hours. Substitution of these parameter values into the respective equations listed in Table 19–1 yields: for aspirin, $V = 13.6$ L, $V_{ss} = 10.4$ L; for salicylic acid, $V = 10.5$ L, $V_{ss} = 10.2$ L; and for gentamicin, $V = 345$ L, $V_{ss} = 56$ L. Notice, for aspirin and salicylic acid, that the values of V_{ss} are very similar; they are both acids, predominantly bound to albumin, and accordingly have small volumes of distribution. The greater value of V relative to V_{ss} for aspirin rises because appreciable elimination ($CL = 41$ L/hr) occurs before distribution equilibrium is achieved; for salicylic acid, the difference between V and V_{ss} is small because of a lower clearance ($CL = 2.4$ L/hr). Finally, for gentamicin V is much larger than V_{ss}, because most of the administered drug is eliminated before distribution equilibrium is attained. In such circumstances, estimating V_{ss} is worthwhile if, for any reason, disposition kinetics were altered and one wished to assign the change to altered distribution or elimination, or to both.

Another view of distribution at steady state is to consider the ratio of amount in body (A_{ss}) to amount in the initial dilution volume ($A_{ss,1}$). The ratio is V_{ss}/V_1. For aspirin and salicylic acid, this ratio is approximately 2, indicating that these drugs are equally distributed between the initial dilution volume and the rest of the body. For gentamicin the ratio is 4, indicating that at steady state much more of this antibiotic resides outside, than inside, the initial dilution volume.

Finally, a connection needs to be made between V_{ss} and the volume of distribution used to consider the influence of plasma and tissue binding on distribution, e.g., $V = V_P + V_T \cdot fu/fu_T$ (Chap. 10). They are essentially the same. The term V_{ss} applies to a model in which no elimination occurs and distribution equilibrium (steady state) has been achieved (Fig. 10–7). In practice, elimination always occurs and confounds the estimation of a purely distributional volume term; V_{ss}, and not V (during the terminal phase) is the closest estimate of it.

Time to Reach Plateau

Recall that for practical purposes plateau is said to be reached when the concentration is 90% of C_{ss}. Because of distribution kinetics, the time to reach plateau differs between plasma and tissue.

Events in Plasma. The terminal half-life of the antihypertensive agent nicardipine is approximately 12 hr. Therefore, one would normally expect 50% of the plateau plasma concentration to be reached by 12 hr during a constant-rate infusion. Instead it takes only 1 hr (Fig. 19–7). Also, 90% of the plateau is reached by approximately 15 hr instead of the expected 40 hr ($3.3 \cdot t_{1/2}$).

This difference arises because nicardipine's disposition kinetics are biphasic, with substantial elimination occurring during the first phase, which has a half-life of approximately only 20 min. The result is a rapidly rising initial curve followed by a much slower approach to plateau.

The importance of not only the half-lives but also the relative rates of distribution and elimination on the approach of the plasma concentration to plateau can be appreciated by the events depicted in Fig. 19–8, for which the values of λ_1 and λ_2 are fixed and the fractional term associated with the terminal phase, f_2, is varied between 0.01 and 1. When $f_2 = 1$, drug distributes spontaneously relative to elimination; the body appears as a single compartment and, as expected, all the drug is eliminated during the terminal (and only) phase. In this case, it takes 1 terminal half-life ($0.693/\lambda_2$) and 3.3 such half-lives to reach 50% and 90% of the plateau, respectively. However, at lower values of f_2, more drug is correspondingly eliminated before distribution equilibrium is established. As a result, the time to achieve, e.g. 50% of the plateau occurs earlier until, when $f_2 = 0$; the time required

Fig. 19–7. By approximately 1 hr into a 48-hr, constant-rate i.v. infusion of nicardipine (0.5 mg/hr), the plasma concentration has risen to 50% of the plateau value (14 µg/L) despite a terminal half-life of 12 hr. This rapid approach to plateau is a result of events in plasma being primarily controlled by an initial phase, with a half-life of 20 min, during which time significant elimination occurs following a bolus dose. The data are the means of 37 patients with mild-to-moderate hypertension (1 mg/L = 2.1 µM). (Redrawn from Cook, E., Clifton, G.G., Bienvenu, G., Williams, R., Sambol, N., Mc-Mahon, G., Grandy, S., Lai, C.-M., Quon, C., Anderson, C.R., Turlapaty, P., and Wallin, J.D. Pharmacokinetics, pharmacodynamics and minimum effective clinical dose of intravenous nicardipine. Clin. Pharmacol. Ther., 47:706–718, 1990.)

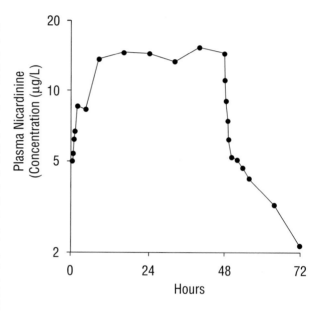

Fig. 19–8. Approach to plateau in plasma, during a constant-rate i.v. infusion, for a drug that displays biexponential disposition kinetics, is determined by the relative rates of distribution and elimination. In this example the two exponential coefficients λ_1 and λ_2 are kept constant (with $\lambda_1 = 10\lambda_2$), and the fractional elimination term associated with the terminal phase, f_2, is varied from 0.01 to 1. When drug distributes rapidly compared with elimination (f_2 approaches 1), the terminal half-life controls the time to approach plateau. When f_2 is very low, e.g., 0.01, implying elimination occurs much faster than distribution, the approach to plateau is determined primarily by λ_1. Included for reference is the expected curve when the drug exhibits one-compartment characteristics ($f_2 = 1$), in which case 50% and 90% of the plateau are reached by 1 and 3.3 terminal half-lives, respectively. Note that time is expressed in units of terminal half-life.

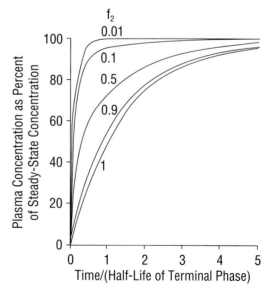

is the half-life of the first phase, $0.693/\lambda_1$. The body once again acts as a single compartment, but with a smaller volume of distribution, V_1. For most drugs f_2 exceeds 0.8, and so the terminal half-life primarily determines the time to reach plateau. For nicardipine, significant elimination occurs before distribution equilibrium is achieved and hence the observation in Fig. 19–7. For gentamicin, with f_2 close to 0, it is the half-life of the first phase, usually 2 to 4 hr, that primarily determines the time for this aminoglycoside to reach plateau in plasma.

Another view of events in plasma relates to the expanding volume of distribution on approach to distribution equilibrium (Fig. 19–4). A plateau is reached when the rates of infusion and elimination are equal. When distribution into the tissue is slow, the effective volume of distribution remains for some time close to the initial dilution volume, V_1, so that for a given rate of input the plasma concentration rises much faster than if distribution into tissue is rapid. Therefore, as rate of elimination $= CL \cdot C$, it follows that, for a given clearance value, the approach to plateau occurs earlier, the slower the distribution to tissues.

The plasma concentration at any time on approach to plateau can be calculated using concepts presented in Fig. 19–8. Remember for a drug with one-compartment characteristics the concentration at any time during an infusion is given by

$$C = \frac{R_0}{CL}(1 - e^{-kt})$$

For a drug that exhibits biexponential disposition characteristics, the corresponding equation is

$$C = \frac{f_1 R_0}{CL}(1 - e^{-\lambda_1 t}) + \frac{f_2 R_0}{CL}(1 - e^{-\lambda_2 t}) \qquad\qquad 19$$

or

$$C = C_{ss}[f_1(1 - e^{-\lambda_1 t}) + f_2(1 - e^{-\lambda_2 t})] \qquad\qquad 20$$

These relationships follow by imagining that total concentration is the sum derived from two hypothetical drugs, each with the same clearance value, infused at rates $f_1 \cdot R_0$ and $f_2 \cdot R_0$, respectively. Equations 19 and 20 emphasize the importance of f_2 (and hence C_1 and C_2) as well as λ_1 and λ_2 in determining the events in plasma following a constant-rate infusion. Equation 20 also permits ready calculation of the percent of plateau reached at any time. For example, if the half-lives associated with the first and terminal exponential terms are 1 and 12 hr, respectively, and $f_2 = 0.5$, then at 6 hr, the concentration is 64% of plateau. The converse, i.e., the time required to reach a certain percent of plateau, cannot be calculated directly, because there are two exponential terms containing the unknown, time. The time can be determined by iteration (Chap. 18), i.e., by substituting different times into Eq. 20 until the right answer is reached. In the example above, the time taken to reach 50% of plateau is 2.75 hr.

Events in Peripheral Tissue. As illustrated in Fig. 19–9 the time to achieve plateau in slowly equilibrating tissues is primarily determined by the terminal half-life, irrespective of the time required to achieve plateau in plasma. To appreciate this point, consider events in terms of the two-compartment model depicted in Fig. 19–3. When distribution occurs rapidly, drug in tissue for most of the time is virtually at equilibrium with drug in plasma. That is,

$$k_{21}A_2 \simeq k_{12}A_1$$

Rate of drug   Rate of drug   21
leaving tissue   entering tissue

and therefore

$$A_2 \simeq \frac{k_{12}}{k_{21}} \cdot A_1 \qquad\qquad 22$$

which shows that the amount in tissue parallels that in plasma. When, however, distribution is slow relative to elimination, the concentration in plasma approaches its plateau before much drug has entered the slowly equilibrating tissue. The situation is then analogous to a constant-rate input into a compartment from which loss occurs. Accumulation is determined by the elimination half-life, which in this case is associated with k_{21}, the exit rate constant from the slowly equilibrating tissue. In reality, the situation is somewhat more complex because of the reversible movement of drug between plasma and tissue. Nonetheless, under these circumstances, the constant for transfer out of the slowly equilibrating tissue is a major determinant of the terminal rate constant, λ_2.

Bolus Plus Infusion

Lidocaine is used to control ventricular arrhythmias in emergency settings. A bolus is given to rapidly achieve an effective concentration and is followed by a constant-rate infusion to maintain the concentration. Although the infusion eventually achieves the last objective, initially it cannot match the fall in plasma concentration associated with distribution into the tissues, potentially leading to a period of ineffective concentrations. The events are depicted schematically in Fig. 19–10. A larger bolus dose would overcome the problem but would also increase the likelihood of toxicity because of the initially higher concentrations. A common practical solution is to give supplementary bolus doses or an initially higher rate of infusion during this period of potential deficiency. A more elegant solution lies in giving a supplemental, exponentially declining infusion. The object of the supplemental

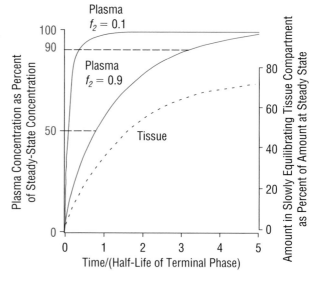

Fig. 19–9. Shown are events in plasma and slowly equilibrating tissue for two drugs that both display biexponential disposition kinetics. They have the same values for each of the exponential coefficients (λ_1 and λ_2) but differ in the contribution of each phase to elimination, signified by the value of f_2. For one drug $f_2 = 0.1$, for the other $f_2 = 0.9$. Despite differences seen in plasma, reproduced from Fig. 19–8, the approach to plateau in the slowly equilibrating tissue (. . .) during a constant-rate i.v. infusion is primarily controlled by the terminal half-life, which is the same for both drugs. Note that time is expressed in terminal half-lives. The horizontal dashed lines correspond to 50% and 90% of the plateau plasma concentration.

infusion is to match the net rate of movement into tissue. This rate is highest initially, when no drug is in tissue. However, as the tissue concentration rises toward plateau, the net movement into tissue progressively declines.

AN EXTRAVASCULAR DOSE

Often, absorption is slower than distribution, so approximating the body as a single compartment after an extravascular dose is reasonable. Occasionally, it is not, as illustrated with digoxin in Fig. 19–11. Following oral administration, digoxin is absorbed before much distribution has occurred, and consequently, the distribution phase is still evident beyond

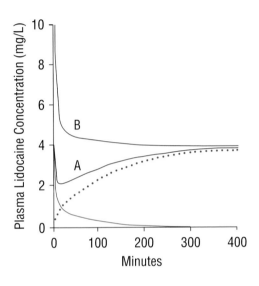

Fig. 19–10. Although a bolus ($V_1 \cdot C_d$) can be given to initially achieve a desired plasma lidocaine concentration of 4 mg/L, C_d, constant infusion at a rate required to maintain this value (rate = $CL \cdot C_d$) fails to do so in the early moments, owing to distribution kinetics. Note that the observed plasma concentration (————, A) is the sum of that associated with the bolus (colored solid line) (Eq. 2) and that associated with the constant-rate infusion (colored dotted line) (Eq. 20). A larger bolus dose can be given to prevent the concentration falling below 4 mg/L, but the resulting high initial plasma concentrations (————, B) may increase the chance of toxicity (1 mg/L = 4.3 μM).

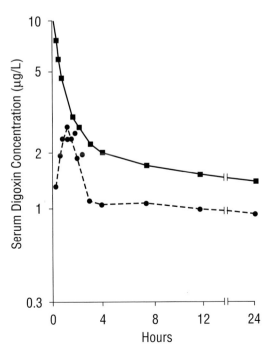

Fig. 19–11. Depicted is a semilogarithmic plot of the mean concentration of digoxin following 0.5 mg administered orally (two 0.25-mg tablets, ●) and i.v. (■) to four volunteers. Because absorption is much faster than distribution, a biphasic curve is still seen after attainment of the peak concentration following the oral dose (1 mg/L = 1.3 μM). (Taken from Huffman, D.H. and Azarnoff, J.: Absorption of orally given digoxin preparations. JAMA, 222:957–960, 1972. Copyright 1972, American Medical Association.)

the peak concentration. In this situation the peak concentration and the time of its occurrence depend on the kinetics of both absorption and distribution and minimally on elimination. The implication of these events to drug therapy and monitoring depends on whether the site of action resides in a rapidly or a slowly equilibrating tissue. Digoxin distributes slowly into the heart, the target organ. Accordingly, it is inappropriate to relate plasma concentration to effect until distribution equilibrium is achieved, 6 hr is a conservative estimate for this drug in most patients. Before then, response increases due to a rising cardiac concentration, even when plasma concentration is declining, making any interpretation of the plasma concentration extremely difficult (Chap. 20 p. 358). In contrast to digoxin, many drugs equilibrate rapidly with such highly perfused tissues as heart and brain; then plasma concentration correlates positively with response at all but the earliest times.

As with the simple one-compartment model, bioavailability is given by $F = CL \cdot AUC/$ Dose, and relative bioavailability is estimated by comparison of AUC values following different formulations or routes of administration, correcting for dose.

MULTIPLE DOSING

The impact of distribution kinetics on events during multiple dosing is illustrated by the data in Fig. 19–12, obtained following an 8-hourly i.m. regimen of gentamicin administered

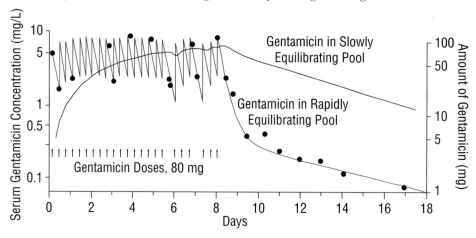

Fig. 19–12. Depicted are semilogarithmic plots of the levels of gentamicin in the body occurring during and after i.m. administration, 80 mg, almost every 8 hr (times indicated by arrows) to a patient for just over 8 days. The biphasic decline in serum concentration (●) when administration was stopped was fitted by a model that assumes that gentamicin distributes between a slowly equilibrating compartment and a rapidly equilibrating compartment from which elimination, entirely by renal excretion, occurs (see Fig. 19–3). The lines are the predicted concentrations (colored line, left-hand ordinate), the amount in the rapidly equilibrating compartment (colored line, right-hand ordinate), a value obtained by multiplying the serum concentration by the estimated initial dilution volume, and the predicted amount in the slowly equilibrating compartment (black line, right-hand ordinate). Little accumulation and large fluctuations of drug occur in plasma and the rest of the rapidly equilibrating pool. In contrast, the gentamicin slowly, but extensively, accumulates in the slowly equilibrating pool during drug administration, with little fluctuation within a dosing interval; disappearance of drug from the slowly equilibrating tissues is also slow on stopping gentamicin. During administration, the concentration in plasma after the Nth dose can be calculated from the formula

$$C = \frac{D_M}{V_1} \left\{ f_1 \left[\frac{1 - e^{N\lambda_1\tau}}{1 - e^{-\lambda_1\tau}} \right] e^{\lambda_1 t} + f_2 \left[\frac{1 - e^{N\lambda_2\tau}}{1 - e^{-\lambda_2\tau}} \right] e^{-\lambda_2\tau} \right\}$$

where D_M is the maintenance dose given every τ, t is the time since the last dose, and V_1 is the initial dilution volume. This equation can be derived using the multiple-dosing equation (Appendix I–D), assuming instantaneous absorption, and the mathematical aid (p. 322) (1 mg/L = 1.8 µM). (Adapted from Schentag, J.J., and Jusko, W.J.: Renal clearance and tissue accumulation of gentamicin. Clin. Pharmacol. Ther., 22:364–370, 1977. Reproduced with permission of C.V. Mosby.)

to a patient for the treatment of a serious infection for 8 days. Seen are large fluctuations in concentration resulting from this regimen and a long terminal half-life on stopping therapy. In common with other aminoglycosides, gentamicin is polar, and while it distributes rapidly into the extracellular water space, approximate volume of 15 L, it enters cells very slowly. Accordingly, although gentamicin has a long terminal half-life, 87 hr in this patient, the majority of a dose is eliminated by 8 hours, associated with the 4-hr half-life of the first phase in the patient. Indeed, as a reasonable approximation, the terminal phase can be ignored with respect to events in plasma, as was done previously when considering gentamicin dosing (Chap. 18, Concentration Monitoring). The reasonableness of this approximation is borne out by the observed rapid establishment of a plateau in plasma and by the continuance of large fluctuations in concentration, a result expected for a drug with a half-life of 4 hr when it is given every 8 hr. Associated with this regimen, however, is a slow but continual accumulation of drug in the slowly equilibrating tissues, where it takes approximately 12 days (3.3 terminal half-lives) to reach plateau. However, at plateau, accumulation is so extensive that more gentamicin exists in these tissues than, on average, in the rapidly equilibrating pool. Furthermore, little fluctuation of drug occurs in the slowly equilibrating pool, because of slow distribution.

Accumulation, both time-course and extent thereof, are clearly dependent on site of measurement. For gentamicin little accumulation occurs in plasma, and a plateau is reached soon after initiating therapy. In contrast, extensive accumulation occurs in the slowly equilibrating tissues, where it takes much longer to attain plateau. In Chap. 7, based on consideration of the minimum amount of drug after the first dose and at plateau (p. 87), a proposed index of accumulation was $1/(1 - e^{-k\tau})$. As a reasonable approximation, this index can also be employed here using the appropriate exponential coefficient. For example, in plasma ($\lambda_1 = 0.17\,\text{hr}^{-1}$; $t_{1/2} = 4\,\text{hr}$) with $\tau = 8\,\text{hr}$, the accumulation index for gentamicin is only 1.35, whereas in the slowly equilibrating pool ($\lambda_2 = 0.008\,\text{hr}^{-1}$), it is as much as 16.

The events on stopping gentamicin administration are predictable. The plasma concentration falls rapidly for the first 2 days, with a half-life controlled by the first phase. Eventually, however, elimination of drug from plasma is rate-limited by return from the slowly equilibrating tissues. Except for the high degree of fluctuation, the events seen in plasma with gentamicin are those expected following a constant-rate infusion for any drug with a low value of f_2 (Fig. 19–9).

Significant clinical implications arise from the distribution kinetics of gentamicin. Most organisms against which gentamicin is used reside in the rapidly equilibrating extracellular space, and so frequent administration is needed to maintain an adequate antimicrobial concentration. Unfortunately, ototoxicity and nephrotoxicity, associated with the accumulation of drug at slowly equilibrating sites within the ears and kidneys, can eventually occur. Accumulation cannot be avoided if an effective plasma concentration is to be maintained. To minimize the problem, a prudent practice is to limit the total duration of gentamicin administration whenever possible. Monitoring the plasma concentration also may help. Of the measures in plasma, the trough value is the most sensitive indicator of the rising concentration in the slowly equilibrating tissues, although as illustrated in Fig. 19–11, even this measurement is not that sensitive. Nonetheless, monitoring of trough concentrations is of value, particularly if the concentration continues to rise, indicating a greater-than-expected rise in the slowly equilibrating pool with a corresponding increase in the potential for toxicity.

A comment needs to be made about the application of volume terms to multiple dosing when distribution kinetics prevails. The purpose of a volume term is to relate plasma concentration to amount in the body. To appreciate the issues involved, consider the events at steady state. Following a constant-rate infusion, V_{ss} is the appropriate volume term to relate plasma concentration to amount in the body. With multiple dosing a true steady

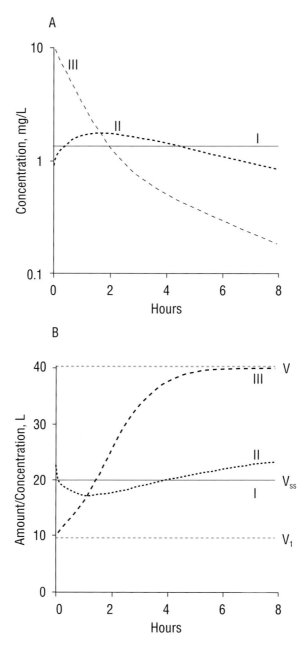

Fig. 19–13. The utility of the volume terms V and V_{ss} for calculating amount in the body from plasma concentration within a dosing interval at steady state, during a multiple-dose regimen, depends on the degree of departure from the true steady state. Shown are the logarithm of the plasma concentration (A) and the ratio of amount in body to plasma concentration (B) within a dosing interval at steady state for three situations (I, II, III). Also shown in B are the values for V, V_{ss} and V_1. In Case I, a constant-rate infusion, V_{ss} applies throughout the equivalent of an 8-hr dosing interval at steady state. In Case II, input is first-order and sufficiently slow that the fluctuation in plasma concentration is small. Here the use of V_{ss} to calculate amount in body is still reasonable. In Case III, bolus dose administration, the deviation from steady state is now too large to render V_{ss} of use. Distribution equilibrium is virtually achieved, however, toward the end of the dosing interval. Then, V can be used to calculate the amount in the body. At earlier times, the volume needed to estimate amount in the body is changing rapidly. Calculations have been made using the following parameter values: Disposition kinetics (single 100-mg i.v. bolus dose); C(mg/L) $= 9\ e^{-1.386t} + 1\ e^{-0.231t}$ (t in hours). Input kinetics: Case I, constant rate of infusion of 12.5 mg/hr; Case II, input half-life of 4 hr, $F = 1$; Cases II and III, 100-mg doses, 8-hr dosing interval.

state does not apply throughout a dosing interval; the plasma concentration fluctuates around a steady-state value, creating a concentration gradient between plasma and tissues. However, as illustrated in Fig. 19–13, as long as the fluctuation in plasma concentration is small, the condition is sufficiently close to the true steady state that V_{ss} can still be applied to estimate amount in the body. This condition exists when input into the body is slow, relative to disposition kinetics, or when the dosing interval is short relative to the time to achieve distribution equilibrium. As one moves away from this condition, either with use of more rapid input (extreme being an i.v. bolus) or by widening the dosing interval, the deviation from the true steady state increases so that V_{ss} has less application. Indeed, if the dosing interval is long enough so that distribution equilibrium is achieved, then V becomes the appropriate volume term to use but, clearly, only during the terminal phase. The problem is exaggerated when distribution equilibrium is not achieved within the dosing interval, as is the case with gentamicin (Fig. 19–12). Then the ratio of amount in body to plasma concentration is continually changing, and neither volume term, V or V_{ss}, is very useful. Frequently, however, distribution is sufficiently rapid to allow one-compartment disposition characteristics to apply on multiple dosing at steady state. Then, V and V_{ss} are almost equal, and either can be used to gain a reasonable estimate of amount in the body.

ALTERED CLEARANCE

When discussing the use of gentamicin in patients with renal insufficiency (Chap. 18, p. 306), the terminal phase is ignored in adjusting dosing regimens to achieve therapeutic concentrations. The reasonableness of this approach is illustrated in Fig. 19–14. Only the initial half-life is altered among patients with varying degrees of renal insufficiency; the terminal half-life is virtually unaffected. The observation may be rationalized in the following manner. When renal function is unimpaired, gentamicin in the rapidly equilibrating pool is mostly eliminated before distribution equilibrium is either achieved after administration of a bolus dose (Fig. 19–15) or re-established on stopping administration after chronic dosing (Fig. 19–14). Under these circumstances elimination may be viewed as

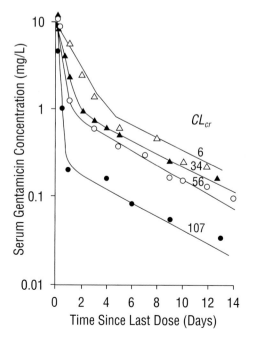

Fig. 19–14. Semilogarithmic plots of the decline in the serum concentration of gentamicin in four patients with different degrees of renal function, as assessed by creatinine clearance, CL_{cr}, after stopping gentamicin administration. Notice that renal function impairment primarily affects the half-life of the first phase and the depth of the decline in concentration before the terminal phase is reached (1 mg/L = 1.8 μM). (Redrawn from Schentag, J.J., Jusko, W.J., Plaut, M.E., Cumbo, T.J., Vance, J.W., and Abrutyn, E.: Tissue persistence of gentamicin in man. JAMA, 238:327–329, 1977. Copyright 1977, American Medical Association.)

occurring from volume V_1 with a clearance, CL. Hence the rate constant for decline in the rapidly equilibrating pool (including plasma) approaches CL/V_1, with a corresponding half-life of $0.693 \cdot V_1/CL$. Reduction in clearance is then reflected by an almost proportional increase in half-life of the first phase. In contrast, during the terminal phase, loss of drug from plasma (and the rapidly equilibrating pool) is controlled by return from the slowly equilibrating tissues and not by its clearance from plasma. Accordingly, the terminal half-life is unchanged. However, with a reduction in clearance, distribution equilibrium takes somewhat longer to be established and, because less drug is eliminated by then, the concentration of gentamicin in plasma is higher compared with that in a patient with unimpaired renal function (Figs. 19–14 and 19–15). Ultimately, if renal function is sufficiently low, the terminal half-life is sensitive to renal function. Then the first phase primarily reflects distribution, as shown in Fig. 19–15. To appreciate the last point, consider administration of a bolus dose of drug to a patient with no renal function. Drug in plasma would still decline initially with a half-life determined solely by distribution. Between this extreme and unimpaired renal function is a range over which the terminal half-life changes noticeably with renal function. For gentamicin, calculation shows this to occur when renal function is less than 7% of normal. Then, albeit slowly for gentamicin, distribution is achieved before much drug is eliminated, the condition that normally prevails for most drugs. Now, to return to a point made previously about V and V_{ss}. As renal function diminishes, so does the value of V. This is a result of less drug being eliminated before distribution equilibrium is achieved. In contrast, the value of V_{ss} remains unchanged.

With gentamicin, concern exists for excessive accumulation in the slowly equilibrating tissues during chronic dosing, particularly in patients with renal insufficiency. However, provided that dosing rate has been adjusted to compensate for diminished renal function, the risk of toxicity in patients with renal insufficiency should be no greater than in those with unimpaired renal function. This conclusion is based on consideration of events at plateau. The amount in the slowly equilibrating tissues at steady state is the difference between the amount in the body ($V_{ss} \cdot C_{ss}$) and that in the rapidly equilibrating pool ($V_1 \cdot C_{ss}$). That is,

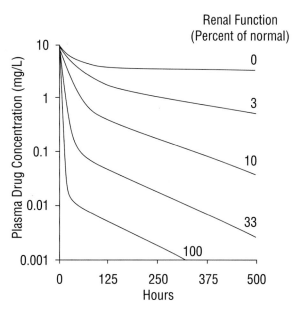

Fig. 19–15. Semilogarithmic plots of the simulated decline in the plasma concentration after i.v. bolus administration of a drug, with disposition characteristics similar to gentamicin, for different degrees of renal function from 0 to 100% of normal. Notice that renal function primarily affects the half-life of the first phase and the depth of decline in concentration before the terminal phase is reached, until renal function is very low. When renal function is very low, the initial decline is determined primarily by distribution, and the impairment is reflected by changes in the terminal half-life.

$$\text{Amount of drug in slowly equilibrating tissues at steady state} = (V_{ss} - V_1) \cdot C_{ss} \qquad 23$$

From this last relationship it is seen that, provided dosing rate is adjusted to maintain a given steady-state plasma concentration, the amount in the slowly equilibrating tissues is unaltered, as both V_1 and V_{ss} are purely distribution terms that, at least for gentamicin, are unaltered by renal insufficiency.

Changes in Concentration and Half-life

A concluding comment is needed here about changes in plasma concentration and half-life. Consider the following three questions. What is the time needed for the plasma concentration to fall by one-half following an i.v. bolus dose? How long does it take to reach 50% of plateau following a constant rate infusion? What is the dosing interval needed to ensure that the maximum and minimum plasma concentrations at plateau differ twofold following a fixed-dose multiple i.v. bolus regimen? When disposition kinetics is characterized by a one-compartment model, the answers to all three questions are simple and the same: the (elimination) half-life. It should be apparent, however, from what has been discussed in this chapter, that the answers cannot be directly inferred from the terminal half-life when distribution kinetics is evident. Then, terminal half-life, or indeed any half-life, ceases to have simple application. The answers no longer lie just in the half-life value of an exponential term but rather in all the parameters that define the entire pharmacokinetic model (e.g., C_1, λ_1, C_2, λ_2). Knowing these parameters, the time to achieve any concentration can be calculated during and following drug administration.

STUDY PROBLEMS

(Answers to Study Problems are in Appendix II.)

1. Define the following terms: initial dilution volume, volume of distribution during terminal phase, and volume of distribution at steady state.
2. Comment on the following statements.
   a. All drugs are expected to exhibit distribution kinetics.
   b. For most drugs it is reasonable to represent the disposition kinetics by a compartmental model, with elimination occurring exclusively from the central compartment.
   c. Following an i.v. bolus dose of drug, essentially all drug is eliminated from the body by 5 terminal plasma half-lives.
3. Aspirin possesses analgesic, anti-inflammatory, and antiplatelet activity. To characterize the disposition kinetics of this drug, Rowland and Riegelman intravenously administered a 650-mg bolus dose of aspirin, as its N-methylglucamine salt, to subjects. Table 19–2 lists the plasma concentration-time data obtained in one representative subject.

Table 19–2.[a]

TIME (min)	1	2	4	8	12	15	20	30	45	60	70
Plasma Aspirin Concentration (mg/L)[b]	98	82	58	33	22	17	12	7.5	3.7	1.8	1.2

[a]Adapted from data in Rowland, M., and Riegelman, S.: Pharmacokinetics of acetylsalicylic acid and salicylic acid after intravenous administration in man. J. Pharm. Sci., *57*:1313–1319, 1968.
[b]One mg/L = 5.6 μM.

   a. Prepare a semilogarithmic plot of these data. Using the method of residuals, estimate the values of the parameters of the biexponential equation that fit these data (C_1, λ_1, C_2, λ_2) and the initial and terminal half-lives.

   b. From the parameter values in "a", calculate CL, V_1, and V.
   c. From the biexponential equation, predict the plasma concentrations at 10, 50, and 75 min after the bolus dose.
   d. Had another 650-mg bolus dose of aspirin been administered 30 min after the first, what would the plasma concentration be 30 min later?
4. Hamilton et al. (reference in Table 19–3) assessed the effect of acetylator phenotype on the disposition kinetics of amrinone, a positive inotropic agent with vasodilatory properties. The acetylator status was determined for the subjects with isoniazid. Each subject then received a 75-mg bolus dose intravenously (infused over 10 min). Table 19–3 lists the plasma concentration-time data in one slow and one fast acetylator. The drug is metabolized (probably in the liver) and is excreted unchanged. Both subjects weighed the same, and the doses were given instantaneously.

Table 19–3.[a]

| | PLASMA AMRINONE CONCENTRATION (mg/L)[b] | |
TIME (hr)	SLOW ACETYLATOR	FAST ACETYLATOR
0.16	1.30	1.20
0.25	1.03	0.93
0.33	0.89	0.76
0.5	0.72	0.54
0.67	0.64	0.42
1	0.59	0.31
2	0.52	0.19
3	0.47	0.13
4	0.42	N.D.[c]
8	0.27	N.D.[c]
12	0.17	N.D.[c]
15	0.12	N.D.[c]

[a]Problem adapted from data in Hamilton, R.A., Kowalsky, S.F., Wright, E.M., Cernak, P., Benziger, D.P., Stroshane, R.M., and Edelson, J.: Effect of acetylator phenotype on amrinone pharmacokinetics. Clin. Pharmacol. Ther., 40:615–619, 1986.
[b]One mg/L = 5.3 μM.
[c]N.D. Below detection limit of assay.

   a. Prepare semilogarithmic plots of both sets of data and, using the method of residuals, determine the values of the parameters of the biexponential equations that fit each set of data: C_1, λ_1, C_2, and λ_2.
   b. From the values in "a", calculate CL, V_1, and V. Which of these parameters show(s) major differences between the slow and fast acetylator phenotypes?
   c. Is the assumption that the liver and kidneys are part of the initial dilution volume reasonable?
   d. Had data only been available from 1 hr onward, so that only the terminal phase is evident, what values for V and CL would be calculated? Compare these values for the slow and fast acetylators with those obtained in part "b."
   e. What fraction of the dose eliminated is associated with the terminal exponential term for each subject?
   f. Is it reasonable to conclude, for both subjects, that the terminal half-life will principally determine the time to reach plateau in plasma following a constant-rate infusion?
5. In Fig. 21–9 (Metabolite Kinetics, p. 380) the plasma concentrations of the benzodiazepine halazepam are shown during and following an oral dosage regimen of 40 mg of the drug every 8 hr for 14 days.
   a. Why is the plasma concentration of halazepam fluctuating markedly even at steady state?
   b. Can the terminal half-life of halazepam be determined during administration of the dosage regimen?

6. A moderately polar drug is eliminated entirely by renal excretion. Following a 50-mg i.v. bolus dose to a 68-kg healthy subject, the plasma drug concentration was observed to decline biexponentially: C (mg/L) $= 2.71e^{-0.19t} + 0.034e^{-0.0095t}$, where t is in hours. The fraction of the drug in plasma unbound is 0.37 and is independent of drug concentration over the range seen in plasma.

   a. Given that elimination occurs only from the initial dilution volume (central compartment), calculate the following pharmacokinetic parameters: V_1, CL, V (V_{ss}, optional).

   b. Comment on the mechanism of renal excretion of the drug and the appropriateness of the assumption that elimination occurs only from the central compartment.

   c. Optional: comment on the discrepancy between V and V_{ss}.

   d. Calculate the fractions of the dose eliminated that are associated with each exponential term, and comment on the question, "What is the half-life of the drug?"

   e. The drug is given by a constant-rate infusion.

      1. Using an iterative procedure, calculate how long it takes for the plasma concentration to reach 50% and 90% of the steady-state value. Comment on the statement, "It takes 1 half-life to reach 50% of plateau and 3.3 half-lives to reach plateau."

      2. Comment on why a pronounced biexponential curve is seen in the decline of plasma concentration postinfusion after steady state has been reached.

      3. Would you expect to have detected a biexponential curve on stopping the infusion at steady state had the disposition kinetics of the drug following a 50-mg bolus dose been defined by the equation $C(t) = 0.56e^{-0.19t} + 0.14e^{-0.0095t}$. That is, the same exponential coefficients, but different coefficients compared with the i.v. bolus dose.

7. The fractions of drug normally excreted unchanged after i.v. administration of both the neuromuscular blocking agents d-tubocurarine and pancuronium are similar at approximately 0.65. Yet, as seen in Fig. 19–16, the effect of compromised renal function on the disposition kinetics of these drugs is different. For pancuronium the terminal half-life is prolonged, whereas for d-tubocurarine the terminal half-life is unchanged. Briefly discuss the reason for the difference in the effect of renal dysfunction on these two drugs.

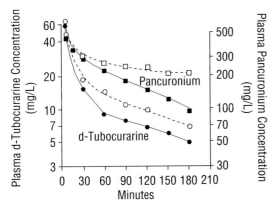

Fig. 19–16. The disposition kinetics of d-tubocurarine ($\bigcirc$, $\bullet$) and pancuronium ($\square$, $\blacksquare$) for patients with both normal (colored lines) and impaired renal function (– – –). (Redrawn from Miller, R.D.: Pharmacokinetics of muscle relaxants and their antagonists. In Pharmacokinetics of Anesthesia. Edited by C. Pry-Roberts and C.C. Hug. Oxford, Blackwell Scientific Publications Limited, 1984, p. 255.)

8. In Table 19–4 are listed the disposition kinetic parameters of three i.v. anesthetic drugs, alfentanil, fentanyl, and sufentanil. Notice each required the sum of three exponential terms to adequately describe the kinetics after single i.v. bolus doses.

Table 19-4. Disposition Kinetic Parameters of Three Intravenous Anesthetic Drugs[a]

DRUG PARAMETERS	ALFENTANIL	FENTANYL	SUFENTANIL
C_1'[b]	0.830	0.90	0.84
$\lambda_1 (min^{-1})$	1.03	0.67	0.48
C_2'	0.120	0.080	0.15
$\lambda_2 (min^{-1})$	0.052	0.037	0.030
C_3'	0.050	0.020	0.010
$\lambda_3 (min^{-1})$	0.0062	0.0015	0.0012
Terminal half-life (min)	111	462	577

[a]Abstracted from Hughes, M.A., Glass, P.S.A., and Jacobs, J.R. Context-sensitive half-time in multicompartment pharmacokinetic models for intravenous anesthetic drugs. Anesthesiology, 76:334–341, 1992.
[b]$C_1' = C_1/(C_1 + C_2 + C_3); C_2' = C_2/(C_1 + C_2 + C_3); C_3' = 1 - C_1' - C_2'$

One of the critical factors in the use of these drugs is the time taken for the plasma concentration to fall on stopping administration. Generally, the shorter the time, the quicker the patient recovers, a desirable characteristic.

The equations below describe the plasma concentration at the end of an infusion of duration τ, $C(\tau)$, and the fraction of that concentration at time t_{post} after stopping the infusion.

$$C(\tau) = C_{ss} \cdot [f_1(1 - e^{-\lambda_1\tau}) + f_2(1 - e^{-\lambda_1\tau}) + f_3(1 - e^{-\lambda_3\tau})]$$

$$\text{Fraction of } C(\tau) \text{ at } t_{post} = [f_1 (1 - e^{-\lambda_1\tau}) e^{-\lambda_1 t_{post}} + f_2(1 - e^{-\lambda_2\tau}) e^{-\lambda_2 t_{post}} + f_3(1 - e^{-\lambda_3\tau}) e^{-\lambda_3 t_{post}}]/C(\tau)$$

where

$$f_1 = \frac{\dfrac{C_1'}{\lambda_1}}{\left(\dfrac{C_1'}{\lambda_1} + \dfrac{C_2'}{\lambda_2} + \dfrac{C_3'}{\lambda_3}\right)}, \quad f_2 = \frac{\dfrac{C_2'}{\lambda_2}}{\left(\dfrac{C_1'}{\lambda_1} + \dfrac{C_2'}{\lambda_2} + \dfrac{C_3'}{\lambda_3}\right)} \quad \text{and } f_3 = 1 - f_1 - f_2$$

C_1', C_2' and C_3' are defined in footnote b of Table 19.5. These equations are expansions of those given in the legend to Fig. 19–5, which apply when the disposition kinetics are described by a biexponential equation.

a. Calculate the values of f_1, f_2, and hence f_3 for alfentanil, fentanyl and sufentanil.

b. Calculate the fraction of the final concentration for each drug at the following times after stopping an infusion of 1-hr duration ($\tau = 60$ min).

Alfentanil	$t_{post} = 24.5$ min
Fentanyl	$t_{post} = 15.6$ min
Sufentanil	$t_{post} = 14.8$ min

c. Given that the patient awakens when the plasma concentration falls by 50% after stopping the 1-hr infusion, by reference to your answer to "b", comment on the utility of the terminal half-life (Table 19–4) in predicting duration of action of the three i.v. anesthetic drugs.

d. Would the ranking be any different if the plasma concentration had to fall by 50% after stopping an infusion at steady state before the patient awakens? (Hint: In answering this question you need to determine, by iteration, the value of t_{post} in each of the above equations that gives a fraction of the steady-state concentration of 0.5).

e. Comment on the impact of the duration of infusion when attempting to rank the duration of action of these three drugs on stopping administration.

9. The disposition kinetics of salicylic acid following a 500-mg bolus dose is characterized by the equation $C(\text{mg/L}) = 37\ e^{-0.17t} + 57\ e^{-0.0027t}$, where t is in min.

a. Using the appropriate equation in Table 19–1, calculate the V_{ss} for this drug.

b. The data can also be described by a two-compartment model. Using the appropriate equivalent relationships, calculate the values V_1 and the microscopic rate constants k_{12}, k_{21}, and k_{10}. (Hint: Use the equivalent relationship for C_1 to calculate k_{21}, and that for $\lambda_1 \lambda_2$ to calculate k_{10}.)

c. Confirm that the value of V_{ss}, calculated from V_1 and the microscopic rate constants, agrees with your answer to "a."

d. Utilizing the appropriate values for the microscopic rate constants, calculate the expected parameter values of the biexponential equation for salicylic acid when the clearance of this drug is reduced by 50%. All distributional parameters remain unchanged.

PHARMACOLOGIC RESPONSE

OBJECTIVES

The reader will be able to:

1. Describe, with examples, the relationship generally expected between a graded response and concentration at the site of action.

2. Show graphically how one can readily detect when response is delayed compared to plasma drug concentration after a single dose, and give at least two explanations for the delay.

3. Describe the parameters of the model that often characterize the relationship between response and plasma concentration.

4. Explain why duration of response is often proportional to the logarithm of an intravenously administered dose, and when it is, calculate both the minimum effective dose and the effective half-life.

5. Describe the influence of distribution kinetics on the relationship between duration of response and logarithm of the dose following single i.v. boluses.

6. Show graphically how duration and intensity of response change on repetitive dosing when each dose is given just as the response and concentration fall to predetermined levels for drugs showing one- or two-compartment distribution characteristics.

7. Show why response of reversibly acting drugs declines linearly with time when response is proportional to the logarithm of the concentration and concentration declines exponentially.

The basic principles surrounding the establishment of an appropriate dosage regimen are presented in Chap. 5. These principles rest heavily on there being a functional relationship, albeit sometimes complex, between concentration of drug at site(s) of action and response produced. Some evidence supporting this view is presented in Chap. 5, together with short commentaries on such additional considerations as delays in drug response, role of active metabolites, and tolerance. In this chapter some of these aspects are considered in greater depth and the temporal relationship between dose (or concentration) and response is explored. The chapter begins with an examination of the concentration–response relationship and concludes with a discussion of hysteresis in a plot of response versus concentration.

CONCENTRATION AND RESPONSE

Because sites of action lie mostly outside the vasculature, delays often exist between placement of drug into blood and response produced. Such delays can obscure underlying relationships between concentration and response. One potential solution is to measure concentration at the site of action. Although this may be possible in an isolated organ system, it is rarely a practical solution in humans. Apart from ethical and technical issues that arise, many responses observed *in vivo* represent an integration of multiple effects at numerous sites. Another approach is to develop a model that incorporates the time-course of drug movement between plasma and site of action, thereby predicting "effector site" concentrations that can then be related to response. Yet another approach is to relate plasma concentration to response under steady-state conditions, which obviates consideration of distribution kinetics. Whatever the approach adopted, the resulting concentration–response relationships for most drugs have features in common. Response increases with concentration at low concentrations and tends to approach a maximum at high values. Recall from Chap. 5 that this was observed for the bronchodilating effect of terbutaline. Such an effect is also seen for the anesthetic ketamine, as illustrated in Fig. 20–1. R($-$)-ketamine and S($+$)-ketamine are optical isomers which, as the racemate, constitute the commercially available intravenous (i.v.) anesthetic agent, ketamine. Although both compounds have an anesthetic effect, they clearly differ from each other. Not only is the maximum effect (E_{max}) with R($-$)-ketamine less than that with S($+$)-ketamine, but the plasma concentration required to produce 50% of E_{max}, referred to as the EC_{50} value, is also greater (1.8 mg/L versus 0.7 mg/L). Moreover, the response curve for R($-$)-ketamine appears shallower than that for S($+$)-ketamine. Although the reason for the differences are unclear, these observations stress the importance that stereochemistry can have in drug response.

General Equation

A general equation to describe the types of observations seen in Figs. 5–1 and 20–1 is

$$\text{Intensity of Effect} = \frac{E_{max} \cdot C^{\gamma}}{EC_{50}^{\gamma} + C^{\gamma}} \qquad 1$$

where E_{max} and EC_{50} are as defined above and γ is the *shape factor* that accommodates the shape of the curve. The intensity of response is usually a change in a measurement from its basal value expressed as either an absolute difference, or a percent change. Examples are an increase in blood pressure and a decrease in percent of neuromuscular blockade.

Although empirical, Eq. 1 has found wide application. Certainly, it has the right properties. Fig. 20–2A shows the influence of γ on the shape of the concentration–response relationship. The larger the value of γ, the greater is the change in response with concen-

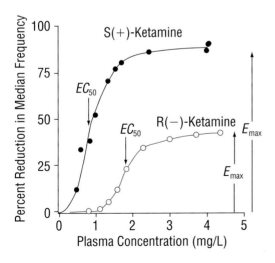

Fig. 20–1. Changes in the electroencephalographic median frequency were followed to quantify the anesthetic effect of R($-$)-ketamine and S($+$)-ketamine in a subject who received an infusion of these two optical isomers on separate occasions. Shown is the percent reduction in the median frequencies *versus* plasma concentration. Although characteristic S-shaped, or sigmoidal, curves are seen with both compounds, they differ in both maximum effect achieved, E_{max}, and concentration needed to produce 50% of E_{max}, the EC_{50}. These relationships may be considered direct ones as no significant time delay was found between response and concentration (1 mg/L = 4.2 μM). (Redrawn from Schuttler, J., Stoeckel, H., Schweilden, H., and Lauvan, P.M.: Hypnotic drugs. *In* Quantitation, modeling and control in anaesthesia. Edited by H. Stoeckel. Stuttgart, George Thieme Verlag, 1985, pp. 196–210.)

tration around the EC_{50} value. For example, if $\gamma = 1$ then, by appropriate substitution into Eq. 1, the concentrations corresponding to 20% and 80% of maximal response are 0.25 and 4 times EC_{50}, respectively, a 16-fold range. Whereas, if $\gamma = 2$, the corresponding concentrations are 0.5 and 2 times EC_{50}, only a fourfold range. Using the percent decrease in heart rate during a standard exercise as a measure of response to propranolol, the average value of γ is close to 1 (Fig. 20–3). Generally, the value of γ lies between 1 and 3. Occa-

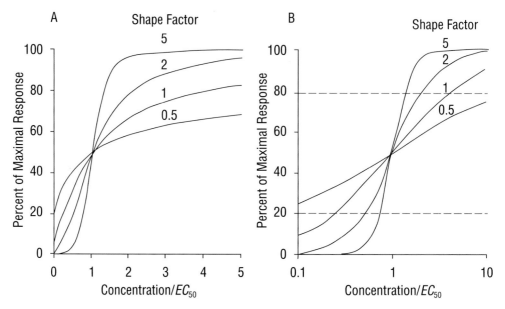

Fig. 20–2. Linear (*A*) and semilogarithmic (*B*) concentration-response plots, predicted according to Eq. 1, for three hypothetical drugs that have the same EC_{50} value but different values of the shape factor, γ. At low concentrations the effect increases almost linearly with concentration (*A*), when $\gamma = 1$, approaching a maximal value at high concentrations. The greater the value of γ, the steeper is the change in response around the EC_{50} value. Between 20 and 80% of maximal effect (colored dashed lines), the response appears to be proportional to the logarithm of the concentration (*B*) for all values of γ. Concentrations are expressed relative to EC_{50}.

Fig. 20–3. Response, measured by the percent decrease in exercise-induced tachycardia, to propranolol increases with the unbound concentration of the drug in plasma. The data points represent measurements after single and multiple (daily) oral doses of two 80-mg tablets of propranolol (●) or a 160-mg sustained-release capsule (○) in an individual subject. The colored line is the fit of Eq. 1 to the data. The response appears to follow the E_{max} model with a γ of 1, an E_{max} of 40%, and an EC_{50} of 5.3 μg/L. (Redrawn from Lalonde, R.L., Straka, R.J., Pieper, J.A., Bottorff, M.B., and Mirvis, D.M.: Propranolol pharmacodynamic modeling using unbound and total concentrations in healthy volunteers. J. Pharmacokinet. Biopharm., *15*:569–582, 1987.)

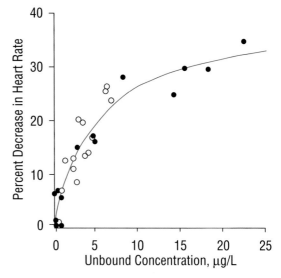

sionally, it is much greater, in which case the effect appears almost as an all-or-none response, because the range of concentrations associated with minimal and maximal responses becomes so narrow.

Patients differ widely in their values of EC_{50} and γ for a given drug. Part of the variability in EC_{50} may be due to differences in plasma protein binding, as response depends on unbound drug at the site of action. Even when based on unbound concentration, as is the case in Fig. 20–3, the EC_{50} value may still vary, indicating differences in sensitivity to the drug among patients. Variability may also exist in E_{max} so that the maximal response produced in one individual differs from that in another.

A common form of representing concentration–response data is a plot of the intensity of response against the *logarithm* of concentration. Figure 20–2B shows this transformation of the curves in Fig. 20–2A. This transformation is popular because it expands the initial part of the curve, where response is changing markedly with a small change in concentration, and contracts the latter part, where a large change in concentration produces only a slight change in response. It also shows that between approximately 20% and 80% of maximum, response appears to be proportional to the logarithm of concentration. This relationship occurs with propranolol within the range of unbound concentrations of 1 and 10 µg/L, as shown in Fig. 20–4 after transformation of the data in Fig. 20–3. The greatest response that may be produced *in vivo* for some drugs is less than the maximum. For example, the entire cardiovascular system may deteriorate, and the patient may die long before the heart rate approaches its maximum value. Other toxicities of the drug or metabolite(s) may further limit the maximally tolerated concentration *in vivo*.

All the preceding examples are graded responses. Eq. 1 has also been found to describe concentration-response curves involving a quantal response in which the response is expressed as the incidence or probability of occurrence. In such cases, the EC_{50} refers to the concentration that produces a 50% probability of response, and γ determines the shape of the cumulative probability-concentration curve. Figure 20–5 shows not only the application of Eq. 1 to describe probability data arising from a study with the opioid analgesic alfentanil but also that the concentration needed to produce an effect may vary with the specific application. Assessed was the frequency of patients who received alfentanil to supplement

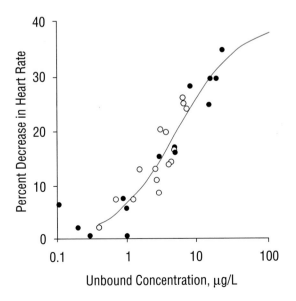

Fig. 20–4. The response data in Fig. 20–3 are replotted versus the logarithm of the unbound plasma concentration, a common representation of the concentration–response relationship. The colored line is the same as that in Fig. 20–3, namely, the best fit of Eq. 1 to the data. Note that the response does not become appreciable until a concentration of about 0.5 µg/L is present and that a limiting response is apparent above about 15 µg/L. ($\bullet$ = two 80-mg tablets of propranolol; $\circ$ = one 160-mg sustained-release capsule.)

nitrous oxide anesthesia and who did not exhibit a series of clinical endpoints indicative of less than optimal anesthetic control during surgery. In Fig. 20–5 the mean percent probability of attaining satisfactory control is plotted against the mean arterial alfentanil concentration for groups of patients undergoing breast, lower abdominal, or upper abdominal surgery. In common with other opioids, the concentration-response curve is very steep in all three groups. In addition, the mean EC_{50} values for the three surgical procedures were in the order, upper abdominal > lower abdominal > breast, and all were greater than the EC_{50} value required for satisfactory spontaneous ventilation at the end of surgery. Collectively, these data indicate that different operative conditions require different drug concentrations. They also show that alfentanil administration must be finely adjusted to the individual's need in order to maintain adequate anesthetic control, yet, by minimizing respiratory problems, permit rapid recovery after surgery.

Time Effects

So far, the examples considered are ones in which response is sustained as long as concentration at the site of action is maintained. Although this is frequently the case, occasionally it is not. *Tolerance* can develop, whereby the response is diminished with time for a given concentration (Chap. 5). The time course of tolerance can vary from minutes to weeks. The mechanism for tolerance also varies. It may involve depletion of either an endogenous transmitter or the receptors to which drug must bind to initiate a response. Tolerance may also be caused by a homeostatic mechanism whereby, through feedback control, the measurement returns toward the predrug value.

An example of tolerance is that associated with the repeated administration of nicotine (Fig. 20–6). When nicotine is readministered within 1 hr, the drug accumulates extensively, but the peak cardioaccelerating response appears to diminish. If the doses are separated by 3.5 hr, accumulation is less, but the peak response is now increased. These results indicate a rapid development of tolerance to the cardioaccelerating effect of nicotine; the mechanism of the tolerance is unknown.

When acute tolerance exists, the *rate* at which the concentration is changing may be as important as the concentration itself. The effect of nifedipine on hemodynamics illustrates this last statement. Nifedipine, a calcium channel blocking agent, both increases heart rate (tachycardia) and lowers diastolic blood pressure when given to patients as a rapidly disintegrating capsule. Fig. 20–7 shows the changes in heart rate and blood pressure, together with the plasma concentrations of nifedipine, following two schedules of i.v. administration to a group of normotensive subjects. When a regimen is employed that promptly attains

Fig. 20–5. Mean arterial concentration–response relationships obtained for alfentanil, an opioid analgesic, during the intraoperative period in each of three surgical groups of patients during nitrous oxide anesthesia. The lines are those predicted from Eq. 1, using mean EC_{50} and γ values determined by averaging the estimates of individual patients. The respective mean values of EC_{50} and γ for the three surgical procedures are: breast (0.27 mg/L, 21), lower abdomen (0.31 mg/L; 21), and upper abdomen (0.31 mg/L, 21) (0.41 mg/L, 11). The horizontal lines at 50% are the standard deviations of the respective EC_{50} values (1 mg/L = 2.0 μM). (Redrawn from Ausems, M.E., Hug, C.C., Stanski, D.R., and Burm, A.G.L.: Plasma concentrations of alfentanil required to supplement nitrous oxide anesthesia for general surgery. Anesthesiology, 65:362–373. 1986. Reproduced by permission of J.B. Lippincott.)

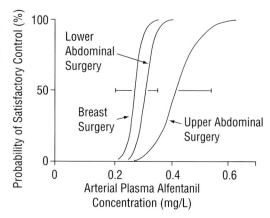

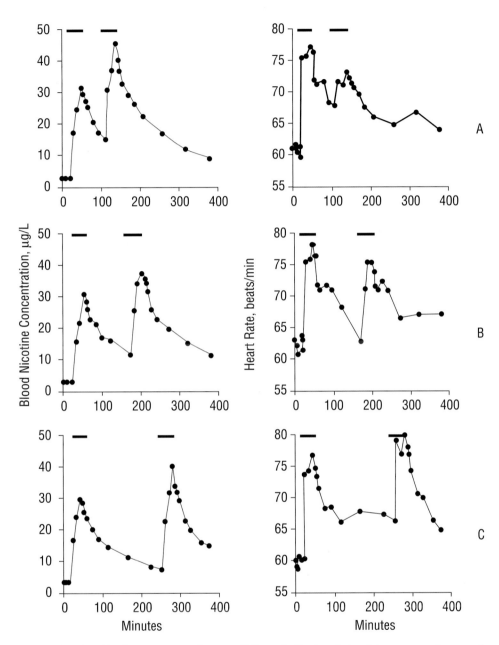

Fig. 20–6. Mean blood concentration of nicotine (left panels, line in color) and the corresponding mean heart rate (right panels) in eight subjects after two 30-min i.v. infusions of 25 µg/min/kg separated by 1 hr (*A*), 2 hr (*B*), and 3.5 hr (*C*). The short bars at the top of each graph indicate the periods during which nicotine was infused. The longer the separation between the doses, the smaller is the increase in the plasma concentration, but the greater the maximum response following the second dose. The effect on heart rate is clearly diminished when the doses quickly follow each other, a phenomenon called *tolerance*. (Adapted and redrawn from Porchet, H.C., Benowitz, N.L., and Sheiner, L.B.: Pharmacodynamic model of tolerance: Application to nicotine. J. Pharmacol. Exp. Ther., *244*:231–236, 1988. The American Society for Pharmacology and Experimental Therapeutics.)

and then maintains a constant plasma concentration (regimen I), a sustained increase in heart rate but no fall in diastolic blood pressure is observed. In contrast, a fall in diastolic blood pressure but no tachycardia occurs when a constant-rate infusion is employed alone, despite a comparable steady-state concentration of nifedipine. Nifepidine's primary action is arteriolar vasodilation. This causes a reduction in peripheral resistance and blood pressure, followed by an increase in cardiac output and heart rate through activation of the baroreceptor reflex. Apparently, if drug input is slow enough, the adaptive control system has sufficient time to respond and so maintain the basal heart rate. Further evidence supporting this hypothesis is the increase in heart rate produced when a small supplementary bolus dose is administered at the end of the constant-rate-alone schedule, which momentarily raises the plasma nifedipine concentration above an already high steady-state concentration. The failure to observe a lowering of blood pressure with the constant-rate-alone regimen is at variance with the consistent lowering achieved in patients. These results

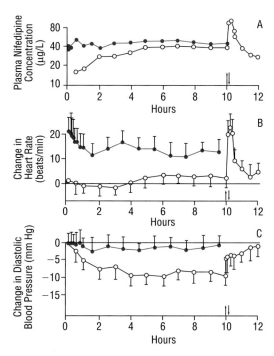

Fig. 20–7. The rate of change of plasma concentration can be a major determinant of response, as demonstrated here with the hemodynamic effects produced by nifedipine. Each of six subjects received nifedipine in distinct regimens on two different occasions. Regimen I—by means of a computer-controlled infusion pump, the rate was adjusted to immediately attain and then maintain a relatively constant plasma concentration for 9.5 hr. Regimen II—a constant-rate infusion of 1.3 mg/hr for 10 hr at which time the infusion rate was increased 10-fold, to 13 mg/hr for 10 min (the period denoted by ⇅). A, the plasma concentration (colored line) in one subject associated with regimens I (●) and II (○). B and C, the corresponding mean group changes in heart rate and diastolic blood pressure, respectively. The slow approach to plateau associated with regimen II caused a fall in diastolic blood pressure but no tachycardia, whereas with regimen I, the converse was obtained. Further supporting the importance of rate considerations is the sharp rise in concentration and heart rate when the infusion rate was increased sharply and momentarily at the end of regimen I, before which the plasma concentrations produced by the two regimens were comparable. The mechanism for this regimen-dependent difference produced by nifedipine is still not fully understood but may be associated with the time needed for the baroreceptor reflex to respond to a change in arteriolar vasodilation produced by nifedipine (1 mg/L = 2.9 µM). (From Kleinbloesem, C.H., van Brummelen, D., Danhof, M., Faber, H., Urquhart, J., and Breimer, D.D.: Rate of increase in the plasma concentration of nifedipine as a major determinant of its hemodynamic effects in humans. Clin. Pharmacol. Ther., *41*:20–30, 1987. Reproduced with permission of C.V. Mosby.)

underline the need to complement baseline studies in healthy subjects with studies in patients. Nonetheless, the observations described in Fig. 20–7 may have a practical application. The primary use of nifedipine is to lower blood pressure; tachycardia is an undesirable side effect. The data suggest that the latter effect can be reduced by slowing absorption.

Another time effect that complicates the concentration–response relationship is that of irreversible binding to the active site. A notable example is the inhibition of acetylcholinesterase by diisopropylfluoridate, an organophosphate inhibitor. This compound binds covalently to the enzyme. Return of acetylcholinesterase activity is, in large part, dependent on synthesis of new enzyme. This compound shows "hit and run" action, i.e., the plasma concentration literally vanishes, while the activity persists. Clearly, the concentration–response relationship expressed by Eq. 1 does not apply here.

RAPID DISTRIBUTION

The onset, duration, intensity, and time course of response are related to drug disposition. First consider drugs with one-compartment characteristics. For these drugs, distribution to the site of action is so rapid relative to other kinetic events that, effectively, a constant proportionality, always exists between unbound drug in plasma and at the site of action.

Onset, Duration, and Intensity

Given the many complexities determining the temporal pattern of response, concepts that have universal application do not exist. The subsequent discussion is restricted to drugs that act reversibly and directly at the site of action to produce a response as described by Eq. 1. Furthermore, metabolites are considered to be either inactive or not to reach a sufficiently high concentration to contribute to response.

Before proceeding, it is important to realize that the amount of drug involved in producing a response is usually only a minute fraction of the total amount in the body. Consequently, drug so involved has no effect on its own pharmacokinetics. An exception is a drug, like propranolol, that reduces both cardiac output and hepatic blood flow and has a high hepatic extraction ratio.

Onset of Effect. An effect occurs when the concentration at the site of action reaches a critical value. The time of onset of effect is governed by many factors: release rate of drug from its dosage form, route of administration, distribution to target site, and other time delays, as discussed previously in this chapter and elsewhere in the book. Additional factors affecting time of onset are dose and the concentration–response relationship.

Increasing the dose shortens the onset of effect by shortening the time required to achieve the critical concentration at the site of action. For the same dose, the time of onset of effect is also shortened in an individual with a low EC_{50} value, because less time is needed to reach the concentration producing the effect.

Duration. An effect lasts as long as the minimum effective concentration at the site of action is exceeded. The duration of effect is, therefore, a function of both dose and rate of drug removal from the site of action. Removal can result from either elimination or redistribution from the site to more slowly equilibrating tissues, a situation subsequently discussed under Slow Distribution. When a drug distributes rapidly to all tissues, including the site of action, and response immediately reflects the concentration of drug at the site of action, the relationship between duration and kinetics is readily conceived following single bolus doses and following doses repeated every time the response falls to a minimum value.

Single Bolus Dose. Consider a drug that distributes into a volume V, is eliminated by first-order kinetics, and is characterized by rate constant k. After a bolus dose, the plasma concentration falls exponentially, i.e.,

$$C = \frac{\text{Dose}}{V} \cdot e^{-kt}$$ 2

Eventually, a time is reached, the duration of effect (t_d), when the plasma concentration falls to a value (C_{min}), below which the response is less than that minimally desired (Fig. 20–8). The relationship between C_{min} and t_d is given by appropriately substituting into the preceding equation; thus,

$$C_{min} = \frac{\text{Dose}}{V} \cdot e^{-k \cdot t_d}$$ 3

Upon rearrangement and taking logarithms, an expression for t_d is obtained,

$$t_d = \frac{1}{k} \left[\ln \text{Dose} - \ln \left(C_{min} \cdot V \right) \right]$$ 4

where $C_{min} \cdot V$ is the minimum amount needed in the body, A_{min}. According to Eq. 4 a plot of duration of effect against ln dose should yield a straight line with a slope of $1/k$ and an intercept, at zero duration of effect, of ln A_{min} (Fig. 20–8, inset). For example, the duration of effect of many local anesthetics is proportional to the logarithm of the injected dose. The muscle relaxant effect of succinylcholine conforms to this last equation. Figure

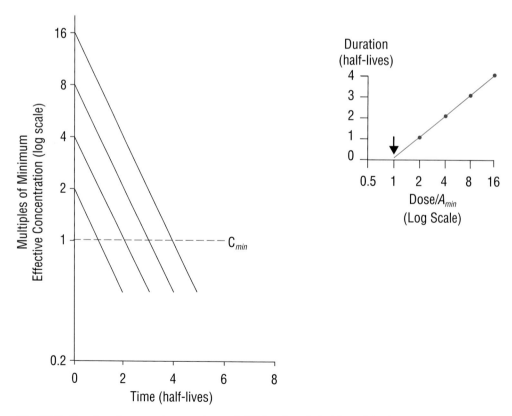

Fig. 20–8. Duration of response increases by one half-life with each doubling of the dose as determined by the increase in time required for the concentration to decline to C_{min} (graph on left). Duration is also proportional to the logarithm of dose (graph on right).

20–9 shows the times to 10 (T_{10}), 50 (T_{50}), and 90% (T_{90}) recovery of muscle twitch (a measure of neuromuscular block after stimulation of a nerve) following i.v. injections of 0.5-, 1-, 2-, and 4-mg/kg bolus doses of succinylcholine. As expected, the slope, $1/k$, is independent of the endpoint chosen, which only influences the value of A_{min}. The value of k, estimated from the slope, is 0.2 min^{-1}; the half-life is 3.5 min.

To further appreciate the last equation, consider the following statement: "Duration of effect increases by one half-life with each doubling of dose." This must be true. To prove that it is, let a given dose D_O produce a duration of effect, t_d. When $2 \cdot D_O$ is given, the amount in the body falls by one-half in one half-life, that is, to D_O; the duration of effect beyond one half-life must be t_d. The total duration of effect produced by the larger dose is, therefore, $t_{1/2} + t_d$. The increase in the duration of effect is, therefore, one half-life. For example, as 0.5 mg/kg of succinylcholine results in a T_{10} of approximately 4.5 min, the duration of effect following 1 mg/kg is 8 min (Fig. 20–9). The increase in the time to recover, 3.5 min, is the half-life of succinylcholine at the site of action. By inspecting each of the T_{10}, T_{50}, and T_{90} curves in Fig. 20–9, it is apparent that the same t_d is obtained on doubling the dose.

Multiple Bolus Doses. Extending the duration of effect by increasing the dose rapidly results in a condition of diminishing returns, especially for a drug with a short half-life and a narrow therapeutic index. For example, when duration of effect is extended by two half-lives, the quadrupled dose required may produce too great an initial response or may substantially increase the chance of toxicity. Multiple smaller doses are then called for.

Instead of fixing the dose and dosing interval, a safer approach is to give the same dose each time the effect reaches a predetermined value, e.g., just when the effect wears off (Fig. 20–10). With this approach, an increase in duration and, if the response is graded, an increase in intensity is expected with the second dose. The reason is readily apparent. Immediately after giving the second dose, the amount in the body is not the dose, but Dose + A_{min}. How much intensity or duration of effect increases, therefore, depends on the relative magnitude of dose and A_{min}. If A_{min} is small relative to dose, very little remains from the first dose when the second one is given, and little increase in response, or duration of effect, is expected. In contrast, large increases in both response and duration are expected when the response from the first dose wears off before much drug is lost.

No further increase in intensity or duration of effect is anticipated with third or subsequent doses, because the amount in the body always returns to the same value, A_{min}, before the next dose is given. Stated differently, from the second dose onward, during each dosing interval, the amount lost equals the dose given.

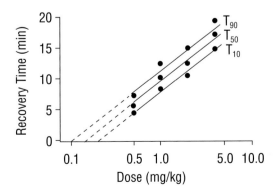

Fig. 20–9. The time to recover from succinylcholine paralysis is proportional to the logarithm of the dose injected. T_{90}, T_{50}, and T_{10} indicate 90, 50, and 10% recovery of muscle twitch (a measure of the degree of return of muscular function). (Redrawn from the figure by Levy, G.: Kinetics of pharmacologic activity of succinylcholine in man. J. Pharm. Sci., 56:1687–1688, 1967. The original data are from Walts, L.F., and Dillon, J.B.: Clinical studies of succinylcholine chloride. Anesthesiology, 28:372–376, 1967.)

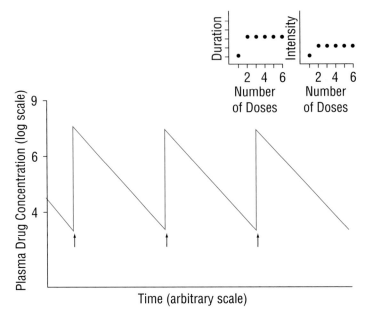

Fig. 20–10. Both the duration and the intensity of a graded response increase with the second, but not with subsequent bolus doses when each dose is given, indicated by an arrow, at the time the effect (or concentration) reaches a predetermined level.

Concentration, Intensity, and Time

An effect subsides when concentration at the site of action falls. How the intensity of response varies with time therefore depends, as does the duration of effect, on dose and rate of removal from the site of action. It also depends on the region of the concentration-response curve covered during the decline. Here, discussion is limited to the situation in which the concentration–response relationship is maintained at all times and drug distributes in a single compartment from which it is eliminated by first-order kinetics.

Intravenous Bolus Dose. To appreciate the relationships among dose, intensity of response, and time, consider the events, depicted in Fig. 20–11, that follow the i.v. administration of a 10-mg bolus dose of a drug with a half-life of 1 hr. A plot of intensity of response against logarithm of the plasma concentration is shown in the inset.

A complete description of the entire time-course of response can be gained by substituting the equation defining the relationship between concentration and time into Eq. 1. However, for didactic purposes it is convenient to divide the plot into three regions. In *region 1*, up to 20% maximal response, intensity of response is directly proportional to the plasma concentration; in *region 2*, covering 20 to 80% of maximal response, intensity is proportional to the logarithm of concentration; and in *region 3*, response slowly approaches the maximal value despite large changes in concentration. As the initial concentration lies in region 3, despite a rapid fall in concentration in the first hour, intensity of response remains almost constant and maximal. Only after 2 hr, when concentration falls below 3 units and response falls below 80% of the maximal value, does response begin to decline more rapidly. Then, for the next 2.5 hr, on passing through region 2, response declines at an almost constant rate of 22% hr. The reason for this constant decline in response, while the plasma concentration declines exponentially, is apparent from the inset of Fig. 20–11, because in region 2

$$\text{Intensity} = m \cdot \ln C + b \qquad\qquad 5$$

where m and b are the slope and intercept of the relationship.

Substituting $C(o) \cdot e^{-kt}$ for C in Eq. 5, where $C(o)$ is the concentration upon entering region 2 from region 3, and collecting terms therefore yields:

$$\text{Intensity} = (m \cdot \ln C(o) + b) - m \cdot k \cdot t \qquad\qquad 6$$

Letting $I(o)$ be the intensity of response when the concentration is $C(o)$ gives

$$\text{Intensity} = I(o) - m \cdot k \cdot t \qquad\qquad 7$$

Thus, *the intensity of effect falls linearly with time* in region 2. Note that the rate of decline, $m \cdot k$, depends on both slope of the intensity-ln concentration curve and half-life of the drug. In this instance, for example, $m = 31$ (in region 2 the intensity of response changes by 31% of the maximal response for a 1-ln change in C), and as $k = 0.7 \ \text{hr}^{-1}$, a constant rate of 22%/hr in the decline of activity is anticipated.

Beyond 5 hr, when the concentration has fallen below 0.3 unit and entered region 1, the fall in response parallels that of drug. In theory, the half-life can be determined from intensity of response-time data in this region; here, half-life is the time for intensity to fall by one-half. In practice, being close to a variable baseline, measurements in this region are often too imprecise to permit accurate assessment of the half-life. The foregoing equations

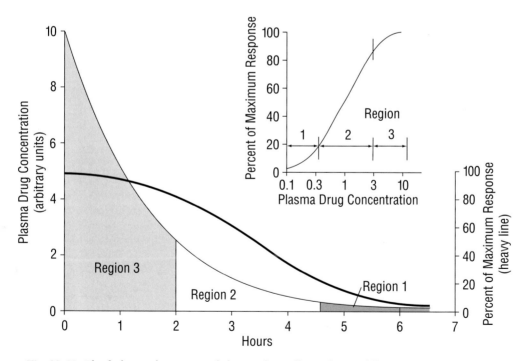

Fig. 20–11. The decline in the intensity of pharmacologic effect with time, following a single large dose, has three parts corresponding to the regions of the concentration-response curve (inset). Initially, in region 3, the response remains almost maximal despite a 75% fall in the concentration. Thereafter, as long as the concentration is within region 2, intensity of response declines approximately linearly with time. Only when concentration falls into region 1 does decline in response parallel that of drug in the body. The concentration–response relationship is defined by Eq. 1, with $EC_{50} = 1$ and $\gamma = 1$.

are expressed in terms of concentration. The corresponding equations using dose admin-istered and amount in body are obtained by multiplying each respective concentration term by volume of distribution. The numerical value of b also changes.

The concepts developed above are now illustrated with degree of muscle paralysis pro-duced by succinylcholine. Changes in degree of muscle paralysis with time, following a 0.5 mg/kg bolus dose of succinylcholine to a patient, are shown in Fig. 20–12. The 1-min delay before onset of effect is probably accounted for by the time required for blood to circulate from injection site to muscle and, in part, by the time for succinylcholine to diffuse into the neuromuscular junction. Once at the site, however, full response ensues promptly; the time between onset and total paralysis is less than 1 min. Total paralysis is then maintained for a full 2 min despite the continual rapid inactivation of this agent. Subsequently, the effect subsides. As predicted, between 20% and 80% of maximal response, the effect de-clines at a constant rate: in this instance, 22%/min. At higher doses, the duration of effect is longer (Fig. 20–13), but once 80% of maximal response is reached, the amount in the body should be the same and the subsequent rate of decline (slope) in intensity should be constant. This is indeed so. Knowing both the rate of decline $(m \cdot k)$ and k (from the duration-log dose plot, Fig. 20–9), the value for m, the slope of the intensity of the response-log (amount in body) curve, can be calculated; for succinylcholine, $m = 109$. It is the short half-life (3.5 min) and the steep response-dose curve that make succinylcholine such a useful agent clinically. Changes in muscle paralysis can be produced within a few minutes of changing an infusion rate, which allows fine and continuous control of response. Also, once the infusion is stopped, the patient promptly recovers.

Other Modes of Administration. Concentration–intensity–time relationships after a single i.v. bolus dose are expected to be different from those seen following other modes

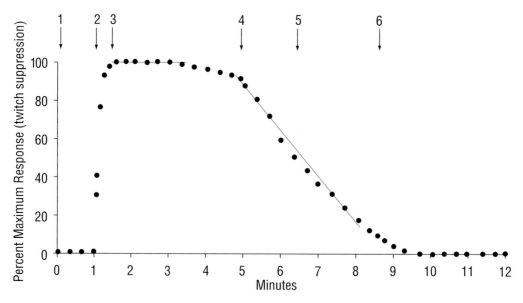

Fig. 20–12. Changes in the degree of muscle paralysis (assessed as the suppression of a twitch produced in response to ulnar nerve stimulation) following an i.v. bolus dose of 0.5 mg/kg succinylcholine to a subject. 1, Time of injection; 2, onset of twitch suppression; 3, complete twitch suppression; 4, 5, and 6, recovery of twitch to 10% (T_{10}), 50% (T_{50}), and 90% (T_{90}) of the maximum twitch height. The straight lines cover the regions of maximum response (horizontal colored line) and where the response declines (between 4 and 6) essentially linearly with time (declining colored line). (Modified from Walts, L.F., and Dillon, J.B.: Clinical studies on succinylcholine chloride. Anesthesiology, 28:372–376, 1967.)

of administration. A recurring question for drugs of short half-life is whether they are best administered as multiple-dose regimens or as constant-rate infusions. There is no general answer, but it is likely that the outcome may be different, even for the same total daily dose. Such a difference is illustrated in Fig. 20–14 with the diuretic furosemide (half-life is about 90 min). The same 40-mg dose is administered as a single i.v. bolus and following an 8-hr constant rate of infusion (4 mg/hr) after a loading bolus of 8 mg. The naturetic effect is clearly greater after the infusion as is the diuretic effect (5.8 vs. 4.6 L of urine in 8 hr). Clearly, concentration–response–time relationships can be more complex following

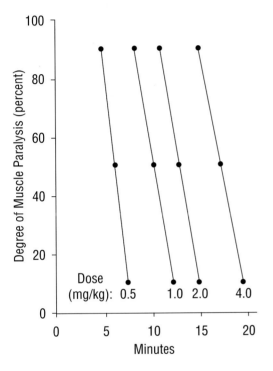

Fig. 20–13. Irrespective of the dose of succinylcholine administered, once 90% of maximal paralysis is reached, the rate of decline in muscle paralysis is constant at 22%/min. (Redrawn from the figure by Levy, G.: Kinetics of pharmacologic activity of succinylcholine in man. J. Pharm. Sci., 56:1687–1688, 1967. The original data are from Walts, F., and Dillon, J.B.: Clinical studies on succinylcholine chloride. Anesthesiology, 28:372–376, 1967.)

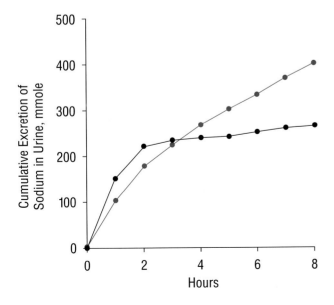

Fig. 20–14. Mean cumulative urinary excretion of sodium during an 8-hr period after a single 40-mg bolus dose (black line) and after the same amount given as an 8-mg bolus loading dose followed by an 8-hr infusion of 4 mg/hr of furosemide (colored line) in eight male volunteers. Although the same amount was given, the rate of delivery of furosemide is clearly a determinant of its cumulative naturetic effect. (Redrawn from van Meyel, J.J.M., Smits, P., Russel, F.G.M., Gerlag, P.G.G., Tan, Y., and Gribnau, F.W.J.: Diuretic efficiency of furosemide during continuous administration versus bolus injection in healthy volunteers. Clin. Pharmacol. Ther., 51:440–444, 1992.)

multiple-dose regimens and single extravascular doses than those seen following single i.v. bolus doses.

SLOW DISTRIBUTION

The onset, duration, and intensity relationships are now considered for those drugs that slowly distribute into tissues. A two-compartment model (Chap. 19) is emphasized.

Onset, Duration, and Intensity

The impact of distribution kinetics on duration and intensity of effect depends on two factors: speed of equilibration of drug at site of action and size of the dose.

Single Bolus Dose. Consider first the situation in which the site of action is in a rapidly equilibrating, and hence well-perfused, tissue. The peak effect is seen almost immediately after an i.v. bolus dose, and thereafter the effect is directly related to the plasma concentration. Typical plasma concentration-time curves observed after various bolus doses are shown in Fig. 20–15A; the curves only become linear on this semilogarithmic plot when distribution equilibrium is achieved in all tissues. If dose is small (here less than 10 units), plasma concentration falls to the minimum effective value, and response wears off, during the distribution phase. In that case, on increasing dose, duration of effect increases disproportionally with the logarithm of dose (Fig. 20–15B). It takes disproportionally longer to reach the minimum effective concentration due to a slowing in the decline of plasma concentration with time. Only when the effect wears off well into the terminal phase is duration of effect proportional to the logarithm of dose.

Supporting these expectations are the times of recovery to 10% (T_{10}), 50% (T_{50}), and 90% (T_{90}) of normal muscle twitch after i.v. injection of bolus doses (between 4 to 16 mg per m^2) of the neuromuscular blocking agent d-tubocurarine (Fig. 20–16A). The plasma concentration-time profile displays pronounced distribution kinetics; it takes an hour before the plasma concentration reaches the terminal exponential phase (Fig. 20–16B). Relative

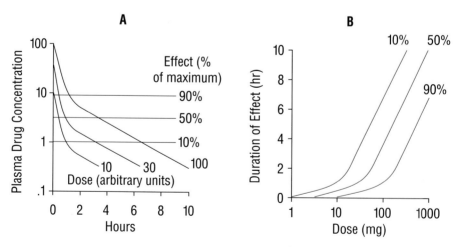

Fig. 20–15. Duration of effect increases linearly with the logarithm of dose only when the effect wears off well into the terminal phase of a drug for which the site of action is in a rapidly equilibrating tissue. When the effect wears off during the distribution phase, because either the dose is small or substantial response still exists at the predetermined end point, duration of effect increases disproportionally for small increases in dose. Shown are semilogarithmic plots of simulated plasma concentration-time profiles for different i.v. bolus doses of a drug that displays pronounced multiexponential disposition kinetics (A), and the corresponding duration of response-versus-log dose plots for predetermined endpoints corresponding to different degrees of maximal response (B).

to this time frame, drug equilibrates quite rapidly between plasma and neuromuscular junction, the site of action. The recovery time increases proportionally with the logarithm of the dose when the duration of effect is well in excess of 1 hr. This condition is met only at the highest doses of d-tubocurarine and when a small response, T_{90}, is chosen as the endpoint. At lower doses and when a greater response, T_{10}, is chosen, the duration of effect is seen to increase disproportionally with the logarithm of dose.

Multiple Dosing. Fig. 20–17 illustrates the expected results when the same size dose is administered each time response falls to a predetermined value, or when the response has just worn off. The second dose produces a higher concentration in plasma and all tissues of the body and a correspondingly more intense response than that achieved after the first dose. Also, since the tendency for drug to return from the tissues is also increased, the duration of effect is greater than after the first dose. Up to this point the result is the same as expected for a drug displaying one-compartment characteristics (Fig. 20–9), but differences do emerge on administering the third and successive doses. On repeating administration and as drug in the slowly equilibrating tissues rises, the tendency to distribute out from blood and other rapidly equilibrating tissues diminishes. Accordingly, the duration of effect becomes progressively longer until, within a dosing interval, the amount eliminated from the body equals the dose administered. Only then are the concentrations of drug in any tissue the same at the beginning and end of the dosing interval. In contrast to duration,

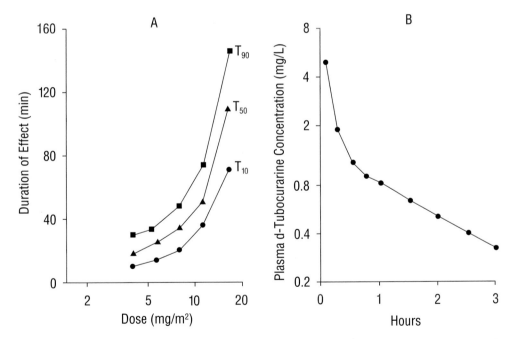

Fig. 20–16. A, Relationship between the median duration of response and size of the bolus dose (log scale) of d-tubocurarine given i.v. to a group of subjects. T_{90}, T_{50}, and T_{10} indicate 90, 50, and 10% recovery of muscle twitch (a measure of the degree of return of muscle function). B, Semilogarithmic plot of estimated mean plasma d-tubocurarine concentration-time profile following a 0.5-mg/kg i.v. bolus dose of drug to a group of 10 subjects. (A: Redrawn from the figure by Gibaldi, M., Levy, G., and Hayton, W.: Kinetics of elimination and neuromuscular blocking effect of d-tubocurarine in man. Anesthesiology, 36:213–218, 1972. The original data from Walts, L.F., and Dillon, J.B.: Duration of action of d-tubocurarine and gallamine. Anesthesiology, 29:498–504, 1968. Reproduced with permission of J.B. Lippincott. B: Redrawn from the data of Sheiner, L.B., Stanski, D.R., Vozeh, S., Miller, R.D., and Harm, J.: Simultaneous modeling of pharmacokinetics and pharmacodynamics: Application to d-tubocurarine. Clin. Pharmacol. Ther., 25:358–371, 1979. Reproduced with permission of C.V. Mosby.)

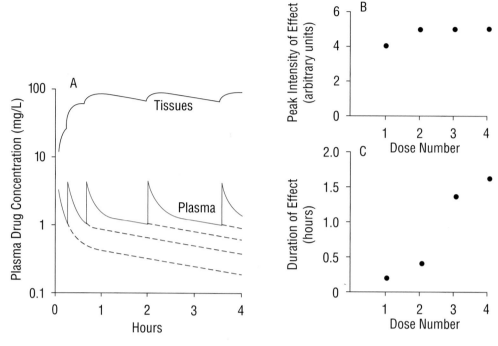

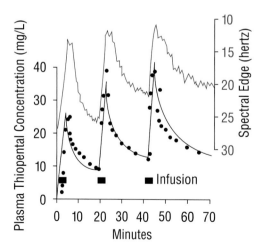

Fig. 20–17. *A,* When the same dose size is administered repeatedly each time the response wears off and the response is directly related to the plasma concentration, the duration of response (time above a predetermined value following each successive dose) increases for a drug showing distribution kinetics. The increase in duration is explained by accrual of drug in tissues. This reduces the tendency for net movement from plasma into tissue and slows the decline of plasma concentration on repetitive dosing (colored line). Also shown is the plasma concentration expected had the successive doses not been given (–––). *B,* Note that the peak intensity of response is expected to increase only with the second dose *C.* This is in contrast to duration of effect. Notice how duration increases dramatically when the time the response wears off moves into the terminal phase of the concentration-time curve (graph A).

Fig. 20–18. Both plasma concentration of thiopental (●) and spectral edge (jagged colored line), an electroencephalographic measure of anesthetic effect, were monitored in a subject who received three successive short-term i.v. infusions of thiopental. The tendency for concentration to fall in plasma and in rapidly equilibrating tissues such as the brain diminishes, and response is prolonged, on the second and third doses, associated with the rise of drug concentration in slowly equilibrating tissues. To minimize the increase in maximal effect, above that produced with the first dose (8.4 mg/kg), the sizes of the two successive doses were reduced (to 5.7 mg/kg). The solid line close to the plasma concentration values is the predicted concentration after fitting a biexponential disposition model to the plasma concentration-time data. Because thiopental produces a diminution in the spectral edge, the spectral edge scale is inverted for clarity (1 mg/L = 4.1 μM). (Redrawn from Hudson, R.J., Stanski, D.R., Saidman, L.J., and Meathe, E.: A model for studying depth of anesthesia and acute tolerance to thiopental. Anesthesiology, 59:301–308, 1985. Reproduced with permission of J.B. Lippincott.)

intensity of response does not increase beyond the second dose, because the concentration at the site of action just before the next dose is always the same.

The events shown in Fig. 20–18 with thiopental are illustrative of dosing to a minimum effect. Following repetitive i.v. dosing, the plasma concentration declines more slowly and the effect lasts longer after the second and third doses, even though these doses were smaller than the first to prevent too great a response. The data with thiopental also indicate that the brain is a rapidly equilibrating site, with a minimal delay in response. In addition, these data do not support a common suggestion that tolerance to the hypnotic effect of thiopental occurs acutely. If tolerance had occurred, the sensitivity to thiopental would have decreased; it would have been expressed as a higher EC_{50} value. No such increase in EC_{50} value with time is observed, however.

Major differences between rapidly and slowly equilibrating sites of action are apparent on administering a drug on a fixed-dose, fixed-interval regimen, as illustrated in Fig. 20–19. When drug at the effector site equilibrates rapidly, response follows the plasma concentration with minimal delay. When, however, equilibration is slow, it may take several doses before the maximal response is seen, even though the plasma concentration is at virtual steady state. In addition, upon stopping administration, response wears off slowly and may remain noticeably long after the plasma concentration falls below detection. In the absence of such insight, there may be a temptation to mistakenly classify the drug as one with hit-and-run characteristics.

Along similar lines, binding of drug at the site of action can conceivably be so tight that its removal, and subsequent decline in effect, is slower than the overall decline of drug in the body. An example is that of methotrexate, an anticancer drug that binds avidly to the site of action, namely, tetrahydrofolate reductase. Under such conditions, plasma concentration correlates poorly with the temporal pattern of drug effect. Clearly, a failure to detect drug in plasma does not mean it is absent from the site of action.

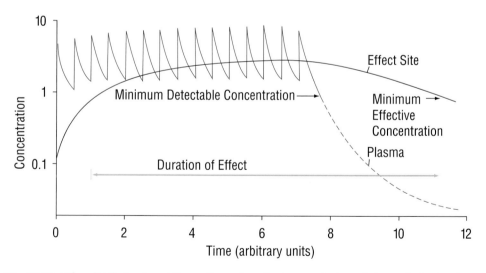

Fig. 20–19. When distribution to and from a tissue where the drug acts is slow relative to elimination, drug in the tissue accumulates slowly on multiple dosing. This delays the onset of effect, even when the drug is given i.v. After discontinuing drug administration, the plasma concentration may quickly fall below the detectable limit, but the concentration at the site of action may persist for some time. The dashed line represents the time course of the plasma concentration below the detection limit. (Modified from Gibaldi, M., Levy, G., and Weintraub, H.: Drug distribution and pharmacologic effects. Clin. Pharmacol. Ther., *12*:734–742, 1971. Reproduced with permission of C.V. Mosby.)

Concentration, Intensity, and Time

Time Delays. Drug response often lags behind plasma concentration. A striking example of such a delay is the rise in left ventricular ejection time index, a measure taken from an electrocardiogram, while the plasma concentration falls during the first 4 hr after an i.v. bolus dose of digoxin (Fig. 20–20). Certainly, these data do not mean that less drug is needed to produce a greater response. Rather, distribution of digoxin into cardiac tissue is slow. Therefore, to use plasma concentration as a guide to digoxin therapy, one should wait until distribution equilibrium with cardiac tissue is reached, which is about 6 hr after a dose of digoxin. On relating response to concentration before 6 hr, an absurd relationship is observed (Fig. 20–21). The response is nil when the concentration is highest and the converse. Were the response to be followed with time, it would eventually (days) decline toward zero, as approximated by the dashed line in Fig. 20–21.

Following an i.v. infusion or an extravascular dose, plasma drug concentration rises and falls. This may lead to *hysteresis* in the concentration–response relationship, a useful diagnostic of the temporal features of drug response. An example of such a curve is shown

Fig. 20–20. The prolongation in the left ventricular ejection time index (○), a measure of effect, increases as the plasma digoxin concentration (colored line) declines for 4 hr after i.v. administration of a 1-mg dose of digoxin. Average data from six normal subjects (1 mg/L = 1.3 μM). (Redrawn from data of Shapiro, W., Narahara, K., and Taubert, K.: Relationship of plasma digitoxin and digoxin to cardiac response following intravenous digitalization in man. Circulation, *42*:1065–1072, 1970. Reproduced by permission of the American Heart Association, Inc.)

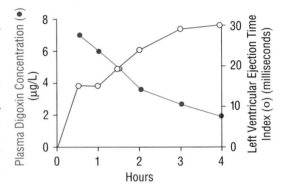

Fig. 20–21. When the response data in Fig. 20–20 are related to the plasma concentration of digoxin, the response is seen to be highest at the lowest concentration and the converse (colored line). The extrapolation to the right is toward earlier times where the concentration is high. At some time, probably many days later as the half-life is about 44 hr, response should return to zero (dashed line on left).

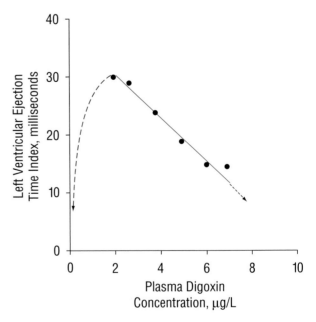

in Fig. 20–22 following the i.v. infusion of alfentanil, an opioid analgesic. Shown in Fig. 20–22A are the plasma concentrations and the reduction of spectral edge, an electroencephalographic measure of response, in a subject during and after a 5-min infusion of the drug. Although there is a suggestion of a time lag between plasma concentration and response from this graph, the delay is much more apparent when response is plotted directly against the corresponding plasma concentration (Fig. 20–22B), yielding a characteristic hysteresis loop. Initially, during the infusion, effect lags behind the rise of alfentanil in plasma. Subsequently, while the plasma concentration falls rapidly, there is little change in effect. Only after 10 min does response follow the fall in plasma concentration. Notice that the chronologic sequence of the paired concentration-response observations moves in a counterclockwise direction. With alfentanil, as with many other drugs, this counterclockwise hysteresis is most likely caused by delayed distribution to the site of action. Other explanations for delayed response include the formation of an active metabolite, which takes time to reach an adequate concentration (see Chap. 21, Metabolite Kinetics); the situation in which the observed response is an indirect measure of the true effect (see Chap. 23, Turnover Concepts); and the condition in which the concentration of an endogenous material is reduced, but only when the concentration falls below a critical value does a reaction that produces the observed response become rate-limiting.

Many drugs are lipophilic and equilibrate rapidly across well-perfused tissues, e.g., heart and brain, which are often target organs. For these tissues, because the period of obser-

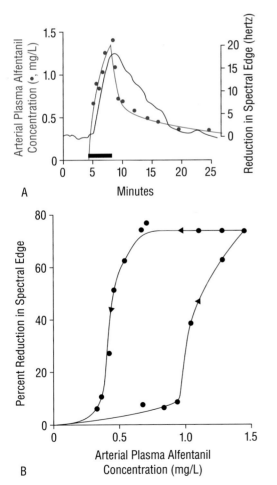

Fig. 20–22. *A,* Time-course of the reduction in the spectral edge (an electroencephalographic measure of effect on the central nervous system) and the arterial plasma alfentanil concentration (●) in a subject during and following a 1.5 mg/min infusion of alfentanil for 5 min (solid bar). *B,* Percent reduction of spectral edge versus arterial plasma alfentanil concentration, demonstrating a counterclockwise hysteresis loop probably caused by delayed distribution of drug into the brain. The arrows indicate the time sequence of the observations (1 mg/L = 2.0 µM). (From Scott, J.C., Pongania, K.V., and Stanski, D.R.: EEG-quantitation of narcotic effect: The comparative pharmacodynamics of fentanyl and alfentanil. Anesthesiology, 62:234–241, 1986. Reproduced by permission of J.B. Lippincott.)

vation in clinical practice is often hours if not days, any time delay in effect is likely to be minimal and drug in plasma can be correlated directly with effect. This was the case in the study from which the propranolol data in Fig. 20–4 were obtained. Propranolol was given orally in single and multiple doses, and measurements were made over several hours, particularly after the peak plasma concentration had been reached. The statements above apply even if distribution throughout the body has not been achieved; all that is required is that distribution equilibrium between plasma and target organ be reached.

Emergency admissions and surgical procedures are special settings during which responses are frequently measured in minutes rather than hours. Here, delays in response after drug administration are almost always noticed. Even though plasma concentration monitoring is unlikely to be employed in these circumstances, it is still important to delineate the determinants of the time-course of response to improve general understanding and to optimize treatment procedures and drug use.

Effect Compartment. A delay in achieving a response, as shown by hysteresis, can be modeled as a delay in reaching an *effect compartment* or in triggering a number of events

Fig. 20–23. The mean pain index difference (corrected for placebo response) in a dental model of analgesic pain relief as a function of the unbound plasma concentration of naproxen, following an oral 500-mg dose. *A*, Pain relief clearly shows hysteresis, in that different responses are apparent at the same unbound plasma concentration. *B*, When an effect compartment is used, the counterclockwise hysteresis is removed. The response can now be related to the effect site concentration at all times. The time of sampling from 1 to 8 hr is noted next to each point in both graphs. (Drawn from data kindly provided by Syntex, U.S.A. Inc.)

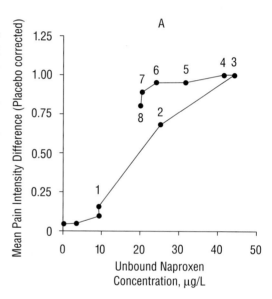

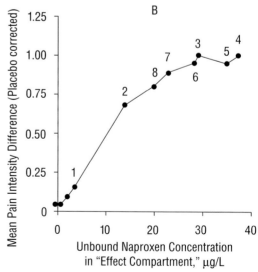

that have a time constant associated with the delay. To this end a pharmacodynamic model with an effect compartment linked to the plasma concentration has been used. The relationship between response and concentration in the effect compartment can then be modeled as in Eq. 1. This procedure has been applied to naproxen, an analgesic, antipyretic, and anti-inflammatory agent.

Figure 20–23A shows hysteresis in the mean pain index in a dental pain model as a function of time after a single 500-mg oral dose of naproxen. When an effect compartment is added, the relationship between response and concentration in the effect compartment

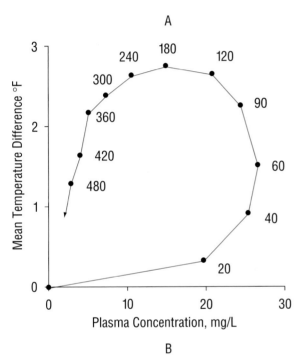

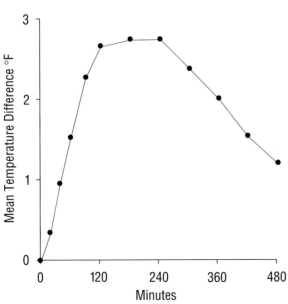

Fig. 20–24. The mean temperature difference (observation minus baseline in degrees Fahrenheit, 1.8°F = 1.0°C) after a 6-mg/kg dose of ibuprofen in 36 children from 6 months through 11 years of age. *A*, Relationship between the temperature difference and plasma ibuprofen concentration. Note the large degree of hysteresis present. The time of sampling is indicated next to each point. *B*, Temperature difference as a function of time. (Redrawn from Kelley, M.T., Walson, P.D., Edge, J.H., Cox, S., and Mortensen, M.E.: Pharmacokinetics and pharmacodynamics of ibuprofen isomers and acetaminophen in febrile children. Clin. Pharmacol. Ther., 52:181–189, 1992.)

now shows no dependence on time (Fig. 20–23B). This relationship may now be modeled by Eq. 1.

Interpretation of Hysteresis Curves. Response is an all-embracing term applied to a wide variety of measurements. The response may be direct or indirect. It may be an observation that integrates past effects, as in the case of the naturetic effect of furosemide (Fig. 20–14). Two more examples follow, which show that one must be careful in interpreting concentration-response curves.

In the first example, ibuprofen, an analgesic and antipyretic agent, is administered as a racemate to 36 children with rectal temperatures, reported in degrees Fahrenheit between 102 and 104.9°F (38.8 and 40.5°C, 6 months through 3 years) and between 101 and 103.9°F (38.3 and 40°C, 4 through 11 years). The mean fall in temperature is noted in Fig. 20–24A relative to the concentration of drug. The relationship implies that the drug has little effect at early times when the concentration is high and maximal effect when the concentration has dropped to 15 mg/L. Actually, the effect of the drug is greatest at early times and has partially worn off by the time the temperature is minimal (Fig. 20–24B). Temperature is an integrated response that measures the cumulative effect of the drug. Using specific heat to relate temperature change, dT/dt, to net heat transfer, then

$$\frac{\text{Specific}}{\text{heat}} \cdot \frac{dT}{dt} = \frac{\text{Rate of heat}}{\text{production}} - \frac{\text{Rate of}}{\text{heat loss}}$$

Even if heat production is instantly reduced, time is required for body temperature to fully reflect the reduction. This phenomenon is further discussed in Chap. 23, Turnover Concepts, for the anticoagulant response to warfarin.

The hysteresis in Fig. 20–24A is therefore not readily interpretable. Clearly, if the data were to be collapsed by the use of an effect compartment, the results would be nonsense. This is particularly so if a correlation between response and effect site concentration were then to be attempted.

The second example is that of the effect produced following i.v. administration of erythropoietin, an antianemic agent given to patients with end-stage renal disease. Figure 20–25

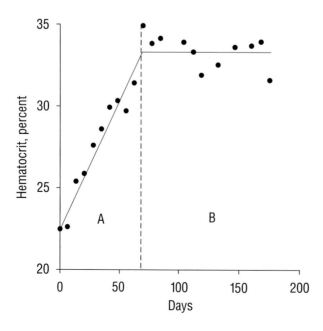

Fig. 20–25. The hematocrit in a uremic patient undergoing dialysis and receiving erythropoietin after dialysis three times a week increases for 70 days and then levels off. *A*, The drug increases erythrocyte production rate; hematocrit increases because the newly produced erythrocytes do not die at this early stage. *B*, Erythropoietin continues to stimulate production of erythrocytes. However, after reaching one lifespan, 70 days, erythrocytes die at the current production rate, and a new steady state is reached. (Redrawn from Uehlinger, D.E., Gotch, F.A., and Sheiner, L.B.: A pharmacodynamic model of erythropoietin therapy for uremic anemia. Clin. Pharmacol. Ther., *51*:76–89, 1992.)

shows the results from a patient who received 4000 units of erythropoietin three times a week. The hematocrit rises for about 70 days and then levels off. One might be tempted to conclude that the effect of the drug takes time to develop. In fact, the drug increases the rate of production of red blood cells throughout the entire course of its administration. The observation is the accumulation of newly formed cells until they have reached their lifetime potential and begin to die. The rates of production and death of the cells subsequently come into a new steady state; the hematocrit now fully reflects the increased production of cells induced by the drug.

STUDY PROBLEMS

(Answers to Study Problems are in Appendix II.)

1. Indicate whether the following statements are true (T) or false (F).
   a. For a drug showing first-order disposition kinetics and producing a graded response, the duration of effect increases linearly with dose.
   b. A hysteresis loop in a response versus plasma drug concentration curve is not expected to be observed after i.v. administration of a bolus dose.
   c. For a graded response, the EC_{50} is the plasma drug concentration at steady state that produces 50% of the maximum response.
   d. For responses less than 20% of the maximum, the response is directly proportional to drug concentration only when γ of Eq. 1 equals one.
   e. One should wait for distribution equilibrium between drug in plasma and that at the site of action to be established before attempting to use plasma monitoring as a guide to therapy.
2. The concentration–response relationship for a drug that produces a graded response is characterized by an EC_{50} of 10 mg/L and a γ of 2.5. To be effective, the response to the drug must be kept between 20% and 80% of the maximal value. Calculate the range of concentrations that are needed to achieve this objective. Drug at the site of action equilibrates rapidly with drug in plasma.
3. The data in Table 20–1 were obtained in humans with AF-DX116, a cardioselective muscarinic agent. In parallel with measurement of heart rate, blood samples were drawn and centrifuged for measurement of the plasma concentration of the drug.

Table 20–1. Increase in Heart Rate and Plasma Concentration Following a Single 40-mg Oral Dose of AF-DX116[a]

INCREASE IN HEART RATE (beats/min)	PLASMA CONCENTRATION OF AF-DX116 (moles/L)
0	0
0.70[b]	1.00×10^{-8}
1.73	3.08×10^{-8}
4.08	7.97×10^{-8}
6.05	8.32×10^{-8}
6.8	9.89×10^{-8}
7.65	1.52×10^{-7}
8.4	1.98×10^{-7}
11.6	2.06×10^{-7}
15.8	3.17×10^{-7}
17.8	3.17×10^{-7}
21.1	4.69×10^{-7}
24.7	1.71×10^{-6}
29.1[b]	1.00×10^{-5}
30[b]	1.00×10^{-4}

[a]Adapted from Schute, B., Volz-Zang, C., Mutschler, E. Horne, C., Palm, D., Wellstein, A., and Pitschner, H.F.: AF-DX 116, a cardioselective muscarinic antagonist in humans: Pharmacodynamic and pharmacokinetic properties. Clin. Pharmacol. Ther., 50:372–378, 1991.
[b]Points added for didactic exercise.

a. Prepare a plot of the increase in heart rate versus logarithm of plasma drug concentration.

b. Estimate the approximate values for E_{max}, EC_{50}, and γ using the model

$$E = \frac{E_{max} \cdot C^\gamma}{EC_{50}^\gamma + C^\gamma}$$

4. An experimental anesthetic agent, CI-581, produces coma in human subjects. Table 20–2 shows the mean duration of coma as a function of the i.v. dose of CI-581 administered (Domino, E.F., Chodoff, P., and Corssen, G.: Pharmacologic effects of CI-581, a new dissociative anesthetic, in man. Clin. Pharmacol. Ther., 6:279–291, 1965).

Table 20-2.

Dose (mg/kg)	0.5	1.0	1.5	2.0
Duration of coma (min)	1.7	5.8	9.0	10.0

Several subjects, immediately after the initial coma had ended following the 1.0-mg/kg dose, received a second 1.0-mg/kg dose. The duration of coma associated with this second dose was 8.0 min. Assuming a one compartment model,

a. Determine the minimum dose of CI-581 required to produce coma.

b. Is the increase in duration of coma seen with the second dose consistent with the information obtained following the single dose?

5. A compound is given as an i.v. bolus to a patient requiring a minimum plasma concentration of 40 mg/L for a therapeutic effect. Given that Dose = 1000 mg; k = 0.10 hr^{-1}; V = 8 L, and assuming a one-compartment model,

a. Calculate how long the clinical effect lasts with this dose.

b. Calculate how long the clinical effect lasts following a 2000-mg dose.

c. Determine the duration of effect following a 1000-mg dose, if k = 0.05 hr^{-1} and the change in the k is a result of (1) a twofold decrease in clearance; and (2) a doubling of the volume of distribution by increased nonspecific tissue binding.

d. Does doubling the dose of a drug yield the same change in duration of clinical effect as doubling the half-life?

6. Galeazzi et al. measured the plasma and saliva concentrations of procainamide, an antiarrhythmic agent, as well as the prolongation of the QT interval, an electrocardiographic measure of drug response. The mean data are given in Table 20–3. In these studies, four volunteers received 500 mg of procainamide hydrochloride by constant-rate i.v. infusion over 30 min. Each saliva sample was obtained during a period of 2 to 4 min spanning the time of venous blood collection. The plasma and saliva concentrations listed are means of the concentrations of each individual calculated, by model fitting, to have occurred at the time of the electrocardiographic recording.

a. Plot response versus plasma procainamide concentration. Is there evidence of hysteresis in the relationship and, if so, is it clockwise or counterclockwise?

b. Plot response versus saliva procainamide concentration. Is the observation similar to that in "a"? Briefly discuss.

c. Is hysteresis observed in a plot of saliva versus plasma procainamide concentrations? Compare the plot to those in parts "a" and "b."

d. Response versus concentration plots that show hysteresis are sometimes modeled with an "effect compartment." Briefly explain why this approach may be useful.

Table 20-3. Mean Plasma and Saliva Concentrations and Prolongation of QT Interval After Infusion of 500 mg Procainamide Hydrochloride Over 30 min in Each of Four Volunteers[a]

TIME (Minutes After Start of Infusion)	PLASMA CONCENTRATION (mg/L)	SALIVA CONCENTRATION (mg/L)	PROLONGATION OF QT INTERVAL (Milliseconds)
0	0	0	0
8	2.3	1.9	3.7
12	3.0	3.5	15.7
23	4.2	6.7	17.6
33	4.1	8.7	20.3
44	2.37	7.0	16.9
52	1.88	5.6	16.0
70	1.54	4.1	12.3
97	1.35	3.4	12.9
127	1.20	3.0	11.3
157	1.06	2.6	11.2
194	0.92	2.2	7.2
257	0.74	1.73	8.3
370	0.50	1.04	0.3

[a]Adapted from Galeazzi, R.L., Benet, L.Z., and Sheiner, L.B.: Relationship between the pharmacokinetics and pharmacodynamics of procainamide. Clin. Pharmacol. Ther., 20:278–289, 1976.

7. Table 20–4 lists the duration of effect achieved with the neuromuscular blocking agent pancuronium following the administration of a 0.02 mg/kg i.v. dose each time the response returned to 10% of maximal effect. Assume that drug at the site of action rapidly equilibrates with drug in plasma.

Table 20-4. Neuromuscular Blocking Effect of Successive Doses[a] of Pancuronium

DOSE NUMBER	1	2	3	4
Duration of Effect (min)[b]	14	20	36	>54

Abstracted from summary in Gibaldi, M., Levy, G., and Weintraub, H. Clin. Pharmacol. Ther., 12:734–742, 1971. Original data from Norman, J., Katz, R.C., and Seed, R.F.: The neuromuscular blocking action of pancuronium in man during anesthesia. Br. J. Anaesth., 42:702–710, 1970.
[a]0.02 mg/kg i.v.
[b]Time to recover 90% of normal function.

    a. Suggest why the duration of effect progressively increases each time a dose is administered.

    b. Will the duration of effect continue to increase if drug administration continues to be administered in the same manner?

8. McDevitt, D.G., and Shand, D.G.: (Plasma concentrations and the time-course of beta blockade due to propranolol. Clin. Pharmacol. Ther., 18:708–715, 1975) observed a linear relationship between effect (percent reduction in exercise tachycardia) and the logarithm of plasma concentration of propranolol. The slope of the line was 11.5%. Table 20–5 lists the effect with time after i.v. administration of 20 mg propranolol.

Table 20-5.

TIME (hr)	0.25	1	2	4	6
Percent reduction in exercise tachycardia	28	25.5	22	15	8

    a. Estimate the apparent half-life of propranolol in plasma.

    b. Calculate how long the reduction in exercise tachycardia is expected to remain above 15% (1) after a 40-mg i.v. dose and (2) after a 60-mg i.v. dose.

9. Predict the general tendencies (clockwise, counterclockwise or no hysteresis) for the observed relationship between response and plasma drug concentration after a single oral dose of a drug as a consequence of each of the following conditions.

   a. Slow distribution to site of action.

   b. Rapid development of tolerance to the drug.

   c. Drug given in controlled-release dosage form. Activity resides solely with drug, which equilibrates rapidly between plasma and site of action.

METABOLITE KINETICS

The reason for our interest and concern with metabolites can be summed up in four words: action, toxicity, inhibition, and displacement. All too often metabolites are thought of as weakly active or inactive waste products. For many this is so, but as seen in Table 21–1 for many others it is not. Sometimes the agent administered is an inert prodrug, which depends on metabolism for activation. Examples are enalapril, which is hydrolyzed to enalaprilat, an active angiotensin-converting enzyme (ACE) inhibitor, and prazepam, which is metabolized to the active benzodiazepine desmethyldiazepam. Some metabolites have pharmacologic properties in common with the parent drug and augment its effect. Some metabolites have a different pharmacologic profile and may even be the cause of toxicity. Other metabolites are inactive but may, by acting as inhibitors, prolong or enhance the response to a drug. Still others may affect the disposition of a drug by competing for plasma and tissue binding sites. It is not sufficient, however, to know that a metabolite possesses the potential for any or all of these properties. Unless a sufficient concentration exists at the site of action, the presence of a metabolite is of little therapeutic concern.

This chapter examines the factors that influence the kinetics of metabolites in the body and the consequences that ensue. The pathways involved and the sites of metabolism are discussed in Chap. 11, Elimination. For purposes of clarity, it is assumed that the body acts as a single compartment for both drug and metabolites, that all kinetic processes are first-order, and that no change in plasma protein binding occurs, unless stated otherwise. The situation in which metabolism is saturable is discussed in Chap. 22, Dose and Time Dependencies.

Information about a metabolite is usually obtained following drug administration. Although this information is arguably the most relevant to drug therapy, situations do arise that require independent information on the pharmacokinetics and activity of the metabolite. Then the metabolite must be administered separately.

SINGLE DOSE OF DRUG

Rate-Limiting Step

To appreciate the factors influencing the amount of metabolite in the body, $A(m)$, with time following a single i.v. dose of drug, consider the scheme:

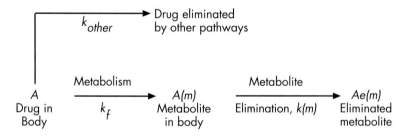

Table 21-1. Representative Therapeutically Important Metabolites

COMPOUND ADMINISTERED	METABOLITE	COMPOUND ADMINISTERED	METABOLITE
Acetylsalicylic acid	Salicylic acid	Isosorbide dinitrate	Isosobide 5-mononitrate
Amiodarone	Desethylamiodarone	Lidocaine	Desethyllidocaine
Amitriptyline	Nortriptyline	Meperidine	Normeperidine
Carbamazepine	Carbamazepine-10,11-epoxide	Morphine	Morphine-6-glucuronide
		Pentoxifylline	5-hydroxypentoxifylline
Cefotaxime	Desacetylcefotaxime	Prazepam	Desmethyldiazepam
Chlordiazepoxide	Desmethylchlordiazepoxide	Prednisone	Prednisolone
Chlorpromazine	7-hydroxychlorpromazine	Primidone	Phenobarbital
Codeine	Morphine	Procainamide	N-Acetylprocainamide
Diazepam	Desmethyldiazepam	Propranolol	4-Hydroxypropranolol
Diltiazem	Desacetyldiltiazem	Quinidine	3-Hydroxyquinidine
Enalapril	Enalaprilat	Sulindac	Sulindac sulfide
Encainide	O-desmethylencainide	Verapamil	Norverapamil
Fluoxetine	Norfluoxetine	Zidovudine	Zidovudine triphosphate
Imipramine	Desipramine		

in which drug is converted to a metabolite that, in turn, are eliminated. The two steps are characterized by the respective first-order rate constants k_f and $k(m)$. The overall elimination rate constant of drug (R) is the sum of k_f and k_{other}, the rate constant for other routes of drug elimination. Also, at any time

$$\text{Rate of change of amount of metabolite in body} = \underset{\text{Rate of formation}}{k_f \cdot A} - \underset{\text{Rate of elimination}}{k(m) \cdot A(m)} \qquad 1$$

Strictly speaking $k_f \cdot A$ refers to rate of entry of metabolite into the systemic circulation. It may not be its rate of formation. Sometimes, a metabolite formed within an organ is further metabolized while there, so that only a fraction of the formed metabolite is released from the organ into the bloodstream. This is referred to as *sequential metabolism* during passage through an organ. A metabolite formed within the liver may also be excreted into the feces via the bile. For simplicity, in the subsequent discussion, only the case in which all of the metabolite formed reaches the systemic circulation is considered.

In the scheme above, either step can be rate-limiting; the rate-limiting step has the smaller rate constant. Figure 21–1, two semilogarithmic plots of the amounts of drug and metabolite in the body against time following a single dose of drug, shows the consequence of a rate limitation in each step.

A rate limitation in drug disposition, the most common situation, has a number of consequences. First, the half-life of drug is longer than that of the metabolite. Second, there is always more drug than metabolite in the body. Last, *metabolite elimination is formation rate-limited*; i.e., metabolite is cleared so rapidly that during its decline phase whatever is formed is almost immediately eliminated. Approximately, therefore

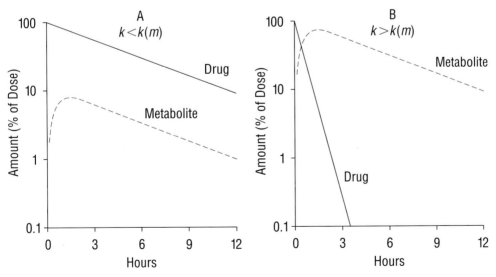

Fig. 21–1. Consequences of a rate limitation shown in semilogarithmic plots of drug and metabolite. *A*, When the elimination rate constant of the drug is smaller than that of metabolite, metabolite (colored dashed line) declines in parallel with the drug. *B*, Conversely, when the elimination rate constant of metabolite is smaller than that of drug, metabolite (colored dashed line) declines more slowly than drug. In the former case (*A*), decline of metabolite is governed by elimination of drug and, in the latter case (*B*), by its own elimination. The graphs are simulated using k_f, k_{other}, and $k(m)$ values of 0.2, 0, and 2 hr^{-1}, respectively, in the former case, and 2, 0, and 0.2 hr^{-1}, respectively in the latter.

$$k(m) \cdot A(m) \quad \approx \quad k_f \cdot A$$

Elimination rate   Formation rate   2
of metabolite   of metabolite

and on rearranging,

$$\text{Amount of metabolite in body} \approx \left(\frac{k_f}{k(m)} \right) \cdot \text{Amount of drug in body} \qquad 3$$

In this case, the metabolite declines with the same half-life as the drug.

A metabolite accrues substantially in the body only when its elimination is the slower step. That is, the half-life of metabolite is longer than that of the drug. When this occurs, drug is mostly eliminated by the time the metabolite peak is reached; decline of metabolite is then controlled by its elimination half-life.

In Eqs. 1 to 3, $k(m)$ refers to the rate constant for metabolite elimination. Just how many pathways are involved in metabolite elimination is not important. What is important is to know whether the drug or metabolite elimination is the rate-limiting step. In any sequence, substances formed beyond the rate-limiting step decline with the half-life of this slowest step. To emphasize this point consider the following scheme:

in which A refers to the drug, C through I refer to metabolites, J is the excreted metabolite I, and the number above each arrow is the value of the respective rate constant in hr^{-1}.

Q. What is the rate-limiting step in the entire sequence?
A. Elimination of metabolite G, $t_{1/2} = 0.693/0.05 = 13.9$ hr.

Q. What are the half-lives for decay of A, D, E, H, and I from the body following administration of drug?
A. Disposition of A rate limits decline of D and E, $t_{1/2} = 0.693/(0.03 + 0.2 + 0.3) = 1.31$ hr for A, D, and E. Elimination of G rate-limits terminal decline of H and I, $t_{1/2} = 13.9$ hr.

Occasionally, the half-lives of drug and metabolite are comparable, and then neither step is rate-limiting. However, metabolite declines more slowly than anticipated from its half-life alone because some drug remains to sustain the level of metabolite for much of its elimination.

Plasma Concentration

The preceding discussion, helpful in realizing the importance of rate-limiting steps, deals with amounts of drug and metabolite in the body. However, plasma concentrations are measured and are of greater interest. Furthermore, in most cases, a metabolite has not been cleared for human use by regulatory authorities to permit determination of its volume of distribution and, therefore, its amount in the body. However, much can be gained from clearance concepts, as illustrated with several examples.

The first example concerns methylprednisolone. Owing to low solubility, formulation of an i.v. preparation is difficult. Yet, clinical situations, e.g., treatment of shock, sometimes demand rapid input of this steroid. One solution has been to administer the water-soluble hemisuccinate ester which is rapidly hydrolyzed to methylprednisolone by esterases within the body. Shown in Fig. 21–2 are the plasma concentrations of both the hemisuccinate and methylprednisolone following an i.v. bolus dose of the ester. It is readily apparent that the hemisuccinate is so rapidly hydrolyzed to steroid that elimination of methylprednisolone is not rate-limited by its formation. These data also permit the conclusion to be drawn that the clearance of methylprednisolone (metabolite), $CL(m)$, is much lower than that of its hemisuccinate. The argument is as follows:

At any time,

$$\text{Rate of change of amount of metabolite in body} = \underbrace{CL_f \cdot C}_{\substack{\text{Rate of}\\\text{metabolite}\\\text{formation}}} - \underbrace{CL(m) \cdot C(m)}_{\substack{\text{Rate of}\\\text{metabolite}\\\text{elimination}}} \qquad 4$$

where CL_f is the clearance associated with the hydrolysis of the hemisuccinate ester to methylprednisolone, sometimes referred to as the *formation clearance*. $CL(m)$ is the total clearance of this metabolite, and C and $C(m)$ are the respective plasma concentrations of drug and metabolite.

Integrating the foregoing equation gives the amount of metabolite in the body at any time. As no methylprednisolone is present in the body initially or at infinity, it follows, upon integrating Eq. 4 between these time limits, that

$$\frac{AUC(m)}{AUC} = \frac{CL_f}{CL(m)} \qquad 5$$

where $AUC(m)$ and AUC are the total areas under the metabolite and drug concentration-

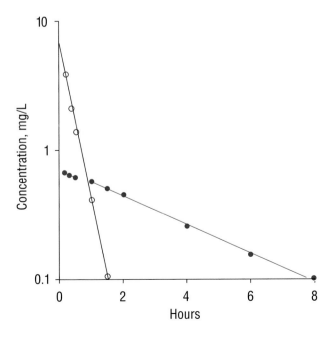

Concentration, mg/L

Hours

Fig. 21–2. Displayed semilogarithmically are the plasma concentrations of methylprednisolone (●) and its water-soluble hemisuccinate ester (○) following an i.v. bolus injection of 80 mg of the ester; values of 11 subjects. The decline of methylprednisolone ($t_{1/2}$ = 2.7 hr) is rate-limited by its disposition, not by the disposition of its hemisuccinate ester ($t_{1/2}$ = 0.25 hr). The clearance of methylprednisolone is lower than that of its hemisuccinate, a conclusion drawn from the observation (seen on a corresponding linear plot) that the AUC of methylprednisolone is the larger of the two. (Redrawn from Derendorf, H., Mollmann, H., Rohdeward, P., Rehder, J., and Schmidt, E.W.: Kinetics of methylprednisolone and its hemisuccinate ester. Clin. Pharmacol. Ther., 37:502–507, 1985.)

time profiles, respectively. Substituting $fm \cdot CL$ for CL_f, where fm is the fraction of an i.v. dose of drug converted to systemically available metabolite, the following relationship is obtained:

$$\frac{AUC(m)}{AUC} = fm \cdot \frac{\text{Clearance of drug}}{\text{Clearance of metabolite}} \qquad\qquad 6$$

Returning to Fig. 21–2, the data suggest that the area for methylprednisolone ($AUC(m)$) is greater than that for the administered ester (AUC). Calculation confirms this; the respective areas are 3.9 and 2.1 mg-hr/L. Accordingly, since the value of fm cannot exceed unity, the clearance of methylprednisolone must be less than that of its ester. If the ratio of areas had been less than 1, then, unless the value of fm is known, the relative total clearance values cannot be assessed. Because no knowledge of the amount of drug in the body is necessary to arrive at the above conclusion, this area method of interpreting metabolite data can be extremely useful, especially in cases of drug poisoning in which the amounts ingested and absorbed are frequently unknown.

The second example deals with propranolol. Based on the data in Fig. 21–3, obtained after giving propranolol intravenously, the drug has the following characteristics: total clearance, 1.1 L/min; volume of distribution, 380 L; and elimination half-life, 4 hr. Other data suggest that almost the entire dose is metabolized in the liver. Metabolites of propranolol include one or more glucuronides and naphthoxylactic acid, which was measured specifically in this study. What can be learned from the data displayed semilogarithmically in Figure 21–3?

From considerations of areas of drug and metabolite, one must conclude that the clearance of naphthoxylactic acid is much lower than that of propranolol. However, the parallel decay of metabolite and drug indicates that elimination of this metabolite is rate-limited by its formation. Hence, the elimination half-life of this more polar metabolite must be shorter, and the amount in the body always lower, than that of the parent drug (see Fig. 21–1A).

The only explanation consistent with these observations is that volume of distribution of metabolite, $V(m)$, must be smaller than that of parent drug by a factor even greater than

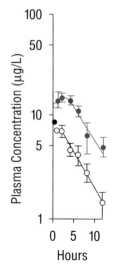

Fig. 21–3. Semilogarithmic plot of the plasma concentrations of propranolol (○) and of one of its metabolites, naphthoxylactic acid (●, color), (mean ± SEM) after a single i.v. dose of 3.7 mg propranolol to three subjects. Note that the elevated metabolite concentration declines in parallel with parent drug because of a lower total clearance and a smaller volume of distribution of naphthoxylactic acid compared with propranolol. For a strict comparison, the naphthoxylactic acid should be expressed in propranolol equivalents, but the difference in their molecular weights (260 and 284, respectively) is small (1 mg/L of propranolol = 3.9 µM). (Redrawn from Walle, T., Conradi, E.C., Walle, K., Fagan, T.C., and Gaffney, T.E.: Naphthoxylactic acid after single and long-term doses of propranolol. Clin. Pharmacol. Ther., 26:548–554, 1979. Reproduced with permission of C.V. Mosby.)

the ratio of clearance values. This conclusion follows from a comparison of the elimination rate constants for metabolite and drug:

$$\frac{k(m)}{k} = \frac{CL(m)/CL}{V(m)/V} \qquad\qquad 7$$

For $k(m)/k$ to be greater than 1, the ratio $V(m)/V$ must be smaller than $CL(m)/CL$. Confirming this conclusion is a concentration of metabolite much higher than that of the parent drug (Fig. 21–3), despite a much lower amount of metabolite in the body when elimination of metabolite is formation rate-limited (Fig. 21–1A). The findings with propranolol are quite commonly encountered, particularly with basic drugs that are converted to acidic metabolites. The volumes of distribution of these basic drugs are often in excess of 100 L, whereas those of their acidic metabolites are closer to 10 to 20 L. These metabolites not only are more polar and tend to bind less to tissue constituents than the parent drug but also are bound more strongly to albumin, thereby further restricting their distribution.

Kinetically, giving an i.v. bolus of drug and measuring the plasma metabolite concentration is similar to giving an oral dose of drug and measuring its plasma concentration. In both situations, the appearance and disappearance of a species (metabolite in one case, drug in the other) are monitored after placing a bolus dose in the preceding compartment, thus

Metabolism

$$A \xrightarrow[\text{Metabolism}]{k_f} A(m) \xrightarrow{k(m)} \text{Elimination of metabolite}$$

Drug in body Metabolite in body

Absorption

$$Aa \xrightarrow[\text{Absorption}]{k_a} A \xrightarrow{k} \text{Elimination of drug}$$

Drug at absorption site Drug in body

Recall from Chap. 4 (Extravascular Dose) that the peak plasma concentration of a drug given extravascularly reflects the balance between rates of drug absorption and elimination. Correspondingly, the 1.5 to 2 hr required for naphthoxylactic acid to reach a peak in Fig. 21–3 reflects the balance between rates of formation and elimination of this metabolite.

The last example concerns tolbutamide, an effective oral hypoglycemic agent. This drug is extensively metabolized to hydroxytolbutamide, which, although active, is therapeutically unimportant. As seen in Fig. 21–4, the concentrations of hydroxytolbutamide are so low that they never augment the effect of tolbutamide. One possible explanation for the low concentration of metabolite is that little is formed. However, in the case of tolbutamide, based on urinary recovery, almost all the drug is converted to hydroxytolbutamide. That is, fm is close to 1. Accordingly, the 20-fold ratio of drug and metabolite areas reflects a corresponding ratio in total clearance values, with that of hydroxytolbutamide being the much higher of the two.

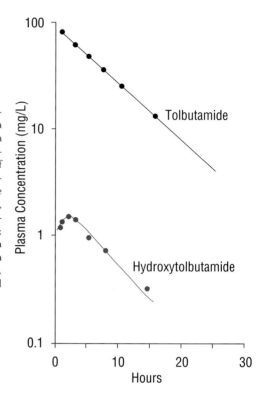

Fig. 21–4. A subject receives a 1-g i.v. bolus of tolbutamide. The concentration of tolbutamide in plasma falls with a half-life of 4 h. Although oxidation to hydroxytolbutamide is almost obligatory for tolbutamide elimination, the plasma concentration of this metabolite is always very low, owing to its extremely high clearance. As a consequence, since the volumes of distribution are similar (0.15–0.30 L/kg), oxidation of tolbutamide rate limits hydroxytolbutamide elimination. (Tolbutamide: 1 mg/L = 3.7 μM; Hydroxytolbutamide: 1 mg/L = 3.5 μM.) (Redrawn from Matin, S.B., and Rowland, M.: Determination of tolbutamide and metabolites in biological fluids. Anal. Letters, 6:865–876, 1973, by courtesy of Marcel Dekker, Inc.)

Impact of Hepatic Extraction

Ingesting drugs that are cleared by the liver is like taking a mixture of drug and metabolite. The reason, as mentioned in Chap. 2, is that all ingested drug must pass through the liver before entering the general circulation. The composition of the mixture leaving the liver depends on the hepatic extraction ratio of the drug. When the extraction ratio is high, metabolism during absorption is extensive, and the situation comes close to that of administering just metabolite. Table 21–2 lists some drugs undergoing extensive first-pass hepatic elimination and forming active metabolites. For them, caution must be taken against attempting to relate plasma drug concentration alone to effect following oral administration.

To appreciate the impact of first passage of drug through the liver on the plasma concentration of metabolite, consider the data in Fig. 21–5, obtained following oral adminis-

Table 21–2.   Representative Drugs Undergoing Extensive First-Pass Hepatic Extraction and Their Active Metabolites

DRUG	ACTIVE METABOLITE[a]	DRUG	ACTIVE METABOLITE[a]
Alprenolol	4-Hydroxyalprenolol	Imipramine	Desipramine
Amitriptyline	Nortriptyline	Isosorbide dinitrate	Isosorbide 5-mononitrate
Buspirone	1-Pyrimidinylpiperazine	Meperidine	Normeperidine
Codeine	Morphine	Metoprolol	α-Hydroxymetoprolol
Desipramine	10-Hyroxydesipramine	Morphine	Morphine-6-glucoronide
Dextropropoxyphene	Norpropoxyphene	Naloxone	6-β-Hydroxynaloxone
Dihydroergotamine	8′-Hydroxydihydroergotamine	Pentoxifylline	5-Hydroxypentoxifylline
Diltiazem	Desacetyldiltiazem	Propranolol	4-Hydroxypropranolol
Doxepin	Desmethyldoxepin	Quinidine	3(S)-Hydroxyquinidine
Encainide	O-Desmethylencainide	Verapamil	Norverapamil

[a]For some drugs more than one active metabolite is formed.

tration of propranolol. Compared to the situation following an i.v. dose (see Fig. 21–3), the naphthoxylactic acid-to-propranolol concentration ratio is much higher, and the metabolite concentration peaks as early as the parent drug. These observations are understood by examining the following scheme:

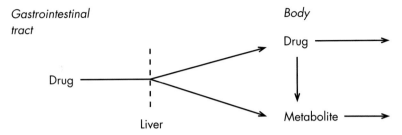

As anticipated from its high hepatic clearance and confirmed by comparing *AUC* values after oral and i.v. administration with correction for differences in dose, only 21% of an oral dose of propranolol filters past the liver; the majority enters the body directly as metabolites. The small fraction of propranolol absorbed systemically is then handled like an i.v. dose of the drug. Thus, the observed concentration of each metabolite is the sum of the amounts derived from the two sources (Fig. 21–6).

The therapeutic implications of the preceding discussion depend on the activities of drug and metabolite. A shorter onset and a more intense response may occur when giving a compound orally, rather than intravenously, if the compound is a prodrug, is rapidly absorbed, and undergoes extensive first-pass conversion to an active metabolite. In this case, a low bioavailability of prodrug does not mean a poor therapeutic effect following oral administration. On the other hand, if only the administered compound is active, a larger oral than parenteral dose is required to achieve an equivalent therapeutic response. The situation with propranolol appears to lie somewhere between these two extremes. Following a single oral dose, the pharmacologic effect is maximal at the peak propranolol concentration, but for a given plasma concentration of propranolol, the response seen after an oral dose is greater than that observed following an i.v. dose. The explanation appears to be the presence of a significant concentration of one or more pharmacologically active

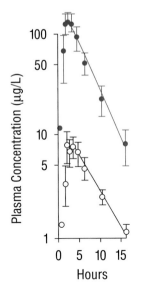

Fig. 21–5. Semilogarithmic plot of the plasma concentrations of propranolol (○) and naphthoxylactic acid (●, color), (mean ± SEM) after a single 20-mg oral dose of propranolol to five subjects. As a consequence of extensive hepatic metabolism, only a small fraction of the dose is absorbed intact. The remainder appears as metabolites, such as naphthoxylactic acid, which reach a peak value at the same time as propranolol, 1.5 to 2-hr after drug administration. For a strict comparison, the naphthoxylactic acid should be expressed in propranolol equivalents, but the difference in their molecular weights (260 and 284 g/mole, respectively) is small (1 mg/L of propranolol = 3.9 μM). (Redrawn from Walle, T., Conradi, E.C., Walle, K., Fagan, T.C., and Gaffney, T.E.: Naphthoxylactic acid after single and long-term doses of propranolol. Clin. Pharmacol. Ther., 26:548–554, 1979. Reproduced with permission of C.V. Mosby.)

metabolites, formed on the first pass through the liver. Certainly, one identified metabolite, 4-hydroxypropranolol, is as active as propranolol.

In Chap. 9 (Table 9–2), examples of drugs stated to be partially metabolized within the gastrointestinal tract are given. For some, evidence favoring this site of metabolism is the failure to detect a metabolite when drug is given parenterally, yet significant concentrations of this metabolite are measured after oral drug administration. Were metabolism to occur primarily within the liver, then the fraction of the dose converted to the metabolite should be independent of the route of drug administration. Thus, given that ingested drug entirely traverses the gastrointestinal wall and that hepatic metabolism is the only route of elimination, drug, whether given orally or parenterally, is equally and fully available to the liver for metabolism. The oral bioavailability of the drug may be low if its hepatic extraction ratio is high, but the fraction of dose converted to a metabolite must be independent of the route of drug administration. The data in Fig. 21–7 support this last point. Morphine is highly and almost exclusively cleared by the liver. Using *AUC* as a measure of the amount of material entering the body, the oral bioavailability of morphine is low (21%), but the amount of the active metabolite, morphine-6-glucuronide, formed is the same, when comparing results after oral and i.v. drug administration. Likewise, the equality of areas of naphthoxylactic acid following oral and i.v. administration of propranolol (Figs. 21–3 and 21–5) appropriately correcting for differences in dose administered, supports the formation of this metabolite, primarily if not totally, in the liver. The finding does not support formation in the gastrointestinal tract.

CONSTANT-RATE DRUG INFUSION

In Chap. 6, the kinetics of a constant-rate i.v. infusion was examined. Recall that infusion rate and clearance determine the plateau concentration and that half-life alone determines the time to approach plateau. These observations can be extended to metabolite. The essential features can be understood by considering the constant-rate infusion of drug, the scheme on p. 368 for metabolite formation and elimination, and the events depicted in Fig. 21–8.

Fig. 21–6. Following an oral dose of drug, the observed plasma concentration of metabolite (——) is the sum of metabolite from two sources: that formed during the absorption of drug (· · ·) and that formed from absorbed drug (– – –). Note, on this semilogarithmic plot, the decline of metabolite formed during absorption is determined by the elimination half-life of the metabolite, whereas decay of metabolite formed from the absorbed drug is determined by the half-life of the drug, the rate-limiting step here. If the hepatic extraction ratio of the drug is high, then most of the dose is converted to metabolite during the absorption of drug, and the decline phase appears biphasic. In this simulation, drug and metabolite have half-lives of 3.5 and 1.1 hr, respectively, and 90% is converted to metabolite during drug absorption.

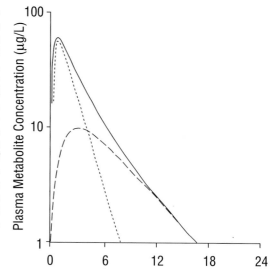

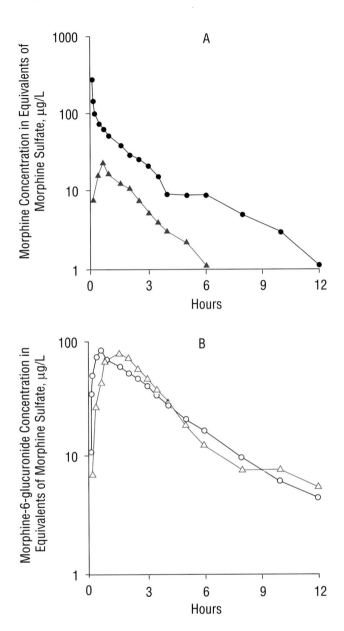

Fig. 21–7. Subjects received morphine sulfate orally (11.7 mg, colored lines) and intravenously (5 mg, black lines) on separate occasions. Plasma concentrations of drug (▲, oral; ●, i.v.) (*A*) and an active metabolite, morphine-6-glucuronide (△, oral; ○, i.v.) (*B*) were measured. Average data in 10 subjects are shown; concentrations of drug (*A*) and metabolite (*B*) are normalized to a 10-mg dose morphine sulfate. The data following oral administration are colored. As a consequence of extensive first-pass hepatic metabolism, the oral bioavailability of morphine is low ($F = 0.20$). Even so, the same amount of metabolite enters the circulation, as judged by the equality of $AUC(m)$ associated with the metabolite following the two routes of morphine administration (1 mg/L morphine sulfate = 3.5 μM). (Data from Osbourne R., Joel, S., Trew, D., and Slevin, M.: Morphine and metabolite behavior after different routes of morphine administration. Demonstration of the importance of the active metabolite morphine-6-glucuronide. Clin. Pharmacol. Ther., *47*:12–19, 1990.)

The Plateau

At any time during drug infusion,

$$\text{Rate of change of metabolite in body} = \underbrace{k_f \cdot A}_{\substack{\text{Rate of} \\ \text{metabolite} \\ \text{formation}}} - \underbrace{k(m) \cdot A(m)}_{\substack{\text{Rate of} \\ \text{metabolite} \\ \text{elimination}}}$$

8

or, expressing the equation in terms of plasma concentrations

$$\text{Rate of change of metabolite in body} = CL_f \cdot C - CL(m) \cdot C(m) \qquad 9$$

When steady state is reached for both drug and metabolite, the rates of infusion and drug elimination are equal and so are the rates of metabolite formation and elimination. Equations 8 and 9 then simplify to

$$\text{Amount of metabolite in body at steady state} = \frac{k_f}{k(m)} \cdot A_{ss} \qquad 10$$

and

$$\text{Concentration of metabolite in plasma at steady state} = \frac{CL_f}{CL(m)} \cdot C_{ss} \qquad 11$$

As fm is the fraction of an i.v. dose of a drug converted to metabolite, the term $fm \cdot R_o$ must be equal to the rate of metabolite formation at the plateau, namely $k_f \cdot A_{ss}$ or $CL_f \cdot C_{ss}$. So

$$\text{Amount of metabolite at steady state} = \frac{fm \cdot R_o}{k(m)} \qquad 12$$

and

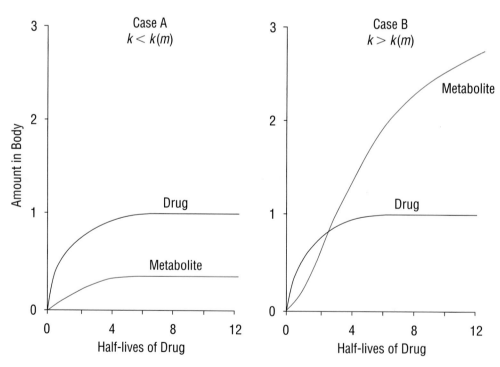

Fig. 21–8. Two situations following constant-rate drug infusion are depicted. In case A, the more usual situation, the metabolite half-life is shorter than that of the drug. Throughout most of drug accumulation, metabolite elimination is formation rate-limited; therefore, the approach to the metabolite plateau is determined by the half-life of the drug. In the less common situation, case B, the half-life of drug is less than that of metabolite. Drug is at steady state well before metabolite. Approach of the metabolite to plateau is now determined by its half-life.

$$\text{Concentration of metabolite at steady state} = \frac{fm \cdot R_o}{CL(m)} \qquad 13$$

Suppose, for example, that a drug is infused at 5 mg/hr, fm is 0.5, $k(m)$ is 0.1 hr^{-1}, and $CL(m)$ is 1.0 L/hr. Then,

$$\text{Amount of metabolite at plateau} = \frac{0.5 \times 5 \text{ mg/hr}}{0.1 \text{ hr}^{-1}} = 25 \text{ mg}$$

$$\text{Plasma concentration of metabolite at plateau} = \frac{0.5 \times 5 \text{ mg/hr}}{1.0 \text{ L/hr}} = 2.5 \text{ mg/L}$$

Time to Plateau

Bolus Plus Infusion. The time required for a metabolite to reach plateau depends on whether or not a bolus of drug is given at the start of the constant-rate drug infusion. If a bolus is given and the infusion maintains that amount of drug in the body, then the approach of the metabolite toward plateau depends only on its half-life. This point becomes apparent when one realizes that at constant drug concentration, metabolite is formed at a constant rate, $fm \cdot R_o$. As this is analogous to giving a constant-rate infusion of metabolite, it follows (from Chap. 6) that the approach to plateau is governed *solely* by the metabolite's half-life. Thus, 50% and 90% of the plateau are reached in 1 and 3.3 metabolite half-lives, respectively. Hence, metabolites with short half-lives reach plateau quickly.

Infusion Alone. If no bolus is given, the situation is more complicated. The time for a metabolite to reach plateau can be governed primarily by either the drug's or metabolite's half-life, *whichever is the longer*. To appreciate this point, consider two situations, both shown in Fig. 21–8. In the more prevalent situation, Case A, the drug has the longer half-life. As expected, the amount of drug in the body reaches plateau in approximately 3.3 drug half-lives. The amount of metabolite and hence the rate of metabolite elimination also rises. However, because elimination of the metabolite is a much faster process than that of the drug, the rate of metabolite elimination soon becomes limited by and approximately equal to its rate of formation. Metabolite is then at virtual steady state with respect to, and cannot rise any faster than, drug. This follows, since under this condition (Eq. 3)

$$\text{Amount of metabolite} \approx \left(\frac{k}{k(m)}\right) \cdot \text{Amount of drug}$$

i.e., the amount of metabolite proportionally reflects the amount of drug. Therefore, the metabolite reaches plateau within approximately 4 drug half-lives.

In Case B, the drug is eliminated faster than metabolite. Now drug reaches steady state before the level of the metabolite has barely risen. From then on, the rate of metabolite formation is constant, and as observed previously, when an appropriate bolus of drug is given, accumulation of metabolite to plateau is controlled by its half-life. Examples of Cases A and B are the oxidation of tolbutamide to hydroxytolbutamide and the hydrolysis of methylprednisolone hemisuccinate to methylprednisolone, respectively.

Postinfusion

As should now be anticipated, on stopping an infusion, the decline of metabolite is governed by the longer half-life, i.e., drug or metabolite. For example, on stopping a tolbutamide infusion, hydroxytolbutamide would decline by one-half each tolbutamide half-life, whereas methylprednisolone's decline would be determined by its half-life after stopping an infusion of its hemisuccinate ester.

MULTIPLE-DOSE DRUG REGIMEN

The concepts that apply to metabolite following administration of drug as a single dose or a constant-rate infusion can readily be applied to the most common situation of a multiple-dose oral drug regimen. As with infusion of drug, accumulation of metabolite to plateau depends as much on its half-life as on that of the parent drug. For example (Fig. 21–9), accumulation of N-desalkylhalazepam, a metabolite of the benzodiazepine, halazepam, lags behind parent compound during drug administration and falls more slowly after administration is stopped. Both observations occur because this metabolite has a longer half-life than that of the drug. In addition, the plateau concentration of N-desalkylhalazepam is higher than that of halazepam, signifying that the metabolite has the lower clearance. Fluctuations in the plasma concentrations of both drug and metabolite are the only noticeable differences expected between an infusion and a multiple-dose regimen. The degree of fluctuation depends on the dosing frequency and half-lives of drug absorption, drug elimination, and metabolite elimination.

PREDICTION FROM SINGLE-DOSE DATA

The concentration of metabolite during an oral multiple-dose drug regimen can readily be calculated from the plasma metabolite concentration-time profile after a single oral dose of drug. The approach is analogous to that taken for drug alone (Chap. 7, p. 87). The metabolite concentration at any time into the drug regimen is obtained by adding the

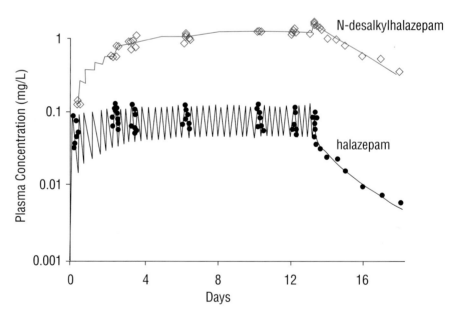

Fig. 21–9. Because it has the longer half-life, the metabolite N-desalkylhalazepam (◇ , color) both accumulates more extensively and falls more slowly than its parent drug, halazepam (●), during and after stopping the ingestion of 10 mg halazepam every 8 hr for 13 consecutive days. The metabolite also has a lower clearance, indicated by its higher plateau concentration, and undergoes less fluctuation compared with parent drug. (Halazepam: 1 mg/L = 2.8 μM; desalkylhalazepam: 1 mg/L = 3.7 μM). (Redrawn from Chung, M., Hilbert, J.M., Gural, R.P., Radwanski, E., Symchowicz, S., and Zampaglione, N.: Multiple-dose halazepam kinetics. Clin. Pharmacol. Ther., 35:838–842, 1984. Reproduced with permission of C.V. Mosby.)

metabolite concentrations expected from each of the previous doses; there is no need to know any pharmacokinetic parameter of either drug or metabolite. For example, if four oral doses of drug are given at 0, 12, 24, and 36 hr, then the concentration of metabolite at 48 hr is equal to the sum of the metabolite concentrations at 48, 36, 24, and 12 hr after a single dose of drug. The average concentration of metabolite at plateau can also be readily calculated from AUC considerations. The area under the metabolite concentration-time curve after a single dose of drug, $AUC(m)_{single}$, is given by

$$AUC(m)_{single} = \frac{F_m \cdot Dose}{CL(m)} \qquad\qquad 14$$

where F_m is the fraction of the administered dose of drug that enters the general circulation as metabolite. At plateau, metabolite formed is lost within a dosing interval, τ, so that the average metabolite concentration, $C(m)_{ss,av}$, is

$$C(m)_{ss,av} = \frac{F_m \cdot Dose}{\tau \cdot CL(m)} \qquad\qquad 15$$

Substituting Eq. 14 into Eq. 15 gives

$$C(m)_{ss,av} = \frac{AUC(m)_{single}}{\tau} \qquad\qquad 16$$

For example, if the $AUC(m)_{single}$ is 120 mg-hr/L after a 100-mg dose of drug, then the expected plateau metabolite concentration is 10 mg/L when this dose is given every 12 hr. Obviously, if the observed average plateau metabolite concentration differs from that expected, then either F_m, clearance of metabolite, or both, have been altered during chronic drug administration.

VARIABILITY

As with parent drug, the pharmacokinetics of a metabolite varies widely in the patient population. With additional variability in clearance of metabolite formation, this often means that interpatient variability in metabolite concentration can be even greater than that seen with parent drug. Sources of variability in metabolite kinetics are the same as those affecting parent drug and include genetics, age, disease, and interacting drugs. Differences exist among patients in both clearance and volume of distribution of metabolite and as with a drug itself, preferably all parameters should be related to the unbound species.

Concern about metabolites is greatest when they contribute significantly to therapeutic response or toxicity. Frequently, the concentration of metabolite is too low to produce an effect, because only a small fraction of drug is converted to a particular metabolite and the clearance of the metabolite is high. Situations can arise, however, in which metabolites reach concentrations high enough to be of concern. This occurs particularly in patients with renal insufficiency, because many metabolites are relatively polar and are primarily excreted unchanged. For example, the elimination of morphine-6-glucuronide, an active metabolite of morphine is reduced in patients with renal dysfunction.

Prediction of the total activity of drug and dosage adjustment needed in patients with renal insufficiency is therefore more complex than usual. There are ways of treating such situations. The most useful is by the steady-state approach. To illustrate the use of this approach, consider the scheme in Fig. 21–10, which shows the input and disposition of a drug and its active metabolite. Table 21–3 lists average values for several pharmacokinetic parameters of this drug and its active metabolite in the typical patient with unimpaired renal function. In this example both drug and active metabolite are equipotent and equitoxic in terms of plasma concentration (with each activity additive). The average rate of drug administration is 100 mg/hr.

At steady state, the plasma drug concentration may be calculated from average rate of absorption and total clearance,

$$C_{ss,av} = \frac{0.8 \times 100 \text{ mg/hr}}{30 \text{ L/hr}} = 2.7 \text{ mg/L}$$

The rate of formation of the active metabolite is 0.3 times the rate of input of the drug; therefore,

$$C(m)_{ss,av} = \frac{0.3 \times 0.8 \times 100 \text{ mg/hr}}{10 \text{ L/hr}} = 2.4 \text{ mg/L}.$$

In an anuric patient, total clearance is extrarenal clearance. For this drug, extrarenal clearance is 15 L/hr; for metabolite, it is 1.5 L/hr. Therefore, the predicted steady-state concentration of drug in the anuric patient, $C(d)_{ss,av}$, is

$$C(d)_{ss,av} = \frac{0.8 \times 100 \text{ mg/hr}}{15 \text{ L/hr}} = 5.3 \text{ mg/L}$$

Because 0.6 of the total elimination, $[CL_f/(CL - CL_R)$ or 9 L/hr/(30–15) L/hr$]$ goes to the active metabolite in the anuric patient, the steady-state concentration of metabolite, $C(m,d)_{ss,av}$, is

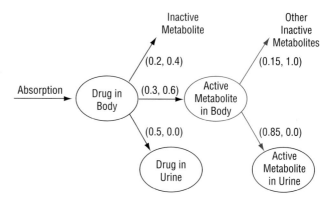

Fig. 21–10. Model for absorption and disposition of a hypothetical drug and disposition of its active metabolite (color). The first number in parentheses refers to the fraction of drug or metabolite that is normally eliminated by the pathway shown with an arrow. The second number refers to the same fraction when there is no renal function.

Table 21–3. Average Pharmacokinetic Parameters of a Drug and Its Active Metabolite

PARAMETER	DRUG	ACTIVE METABOLITE
Total clearance	30 L/hr	10 L/hr[a]
Renal clearance	15 L/hr	8.5 L/hr
Fraction excreted unchanged	0.5	0.85[a]
Oral Bioavailability	0.8	0.3[b]

[a]Obtained following administration of metabolite.
[b]Fraction of drug converted to active metabolite.

$$C(m,d)_{ss,av} = \frac{0.6 \times 0.8 \times 100 \text{ mg/hr}}{1.5 \text{ L/hr}} = 32 \text{ mg/L}$$

Note that the average drug concentration is twice as great in the anuric patient, while the active metabolite concentration is increased 13 times. With drug and active metabolite equipotent and additive in their activities, the rate of administration in the anuric patient should be $(2.7 + 2.4)/(5.3 + 32)$ or 0.14 that of normal. Thus, the anuric patient would require only 14 mg/hr. This example illustrates clearly that although a metabolite may make a minor contribution to the total activity in patients with normal renal function, in an anuric patient, it may be primarily responsible for activity.

ADDITIONAL CONSIDERATIONS

Four other aspects of metabolite kinetics warrant consideration. One is response, another is interconversion between metabolite and drug, and the other two are the use of metabolite data to quantify metabolite clearance and to identify possible causes of a change in pharmacokinetics.

Response

When all activity or toxicity resides with a particular metabolite, relating response to metabolite concentration is relatively straightforward. The problem is more difficult when both drug and metabolite contribute to activity or toxicity. Occasionally, it may be possible to relate the response to a linear combination of the plasma concentrations of drug and metabolite as was done in the last section. More often, however, the relationship between response and concentration is more complicated, and no simple relationship exists. For example, if the response produced by the drug alone approaches the maximum, E_{max}, the response changes little with increases in the concentration of a metabolite that acts as a competitive agonist. Although there are mathematical approaches to this problem, based for example on modification of Eq. 1 in Chap. 20 (Pharmacologic Response) they are unlikely to be used clinically. Nonetheless, measurement of an active metabolite concentration can help to explain an observation and account for variability in drug response. Accordingly, such measurements can serve as useful semiquantitative guides to therapy.

Interconversion

Among the list of therapeutically important metabolites in Table 21–1 are some that are enzymatically converted back to the administered drug substance; they include prednisolone, the metabolite of prednisone, and sulindac sulfide, the metabolite of sulindac. Both drugs are prescribed as anti-inflammatory agents, but in each case the activity resides with the metabolite. These and other examples of drug-metabolite pairs that undergo interconversion are listed in Table 21–4.

Figure 21–11 illustrates some common features of interconversion. Shown are the plasma concentrations of prednisolone and prednisone after administration of each steroid on separate occasions. Notice, irrespective of which is administered, both steroids are present in plasma. Also, the ratio of prednisolone to prednisone rapidly reaches a fixed value of 10:1, after which time the steroids decline in parallel on a semilogarithmic plot. How quickly the equilibrium is established and where the ratio lies depend not only on the kinetics of interconversion but also on the irreversible loss of each species from the body, as can be visualized in the scheme below.

$$\boxed{\text{Drug}} \rightleftarrows \boxed{\text{Metabolite}}$$
$$\downarrow \qquad\qquad\qquad \downarrow$$

Table 21–4. Representative Drugs That Undergo Metabolic Interconversion

DRUG	METABOLITE[a]	COMPOUND THAT PREDOMINATES AT EQUILIBRIUM IN PLASMA	COMMENT
Canrenone[b]	Canrenoate	Canrenone	Canrenoate is inactive
Clofibric acid[c]	Glucuronide	Clofibric acid	In renal impairment glucuronide elimination is reduced; this causes reduced apparent clearance of clofibric acid
Cortisol	Cortisone	Cortisol	Cortisone is inactive
Dapsone	Monoacetyldapsone	Dapsone	Acetylation shows genetic polymorphism; metabolite is less active
Haloperidol	Reduced haloperidol	Haloperidol	Haloperidol is reduced by a carbonyl reductase; the reduced form is oxidized by CPY2D6
Lovastatin[d]	Open-acid	Open-acid	The liver is the target organ
			Lovastatin, given orally, is extensively converted to metabolites during first pass through the liver
Methylprednisolone	Methylprednisone	Methylprednisolone	Methylprednisone is inactive
Prednisone[e]	Prednisolone	Prednisolone—[f]	Prednisone is inactive
Sulindac	Sulindac sulfide		Sulindac (a sulfoxide) is inactive, and therefore acts as prodrug for sulindac sulfide
Vitamin K	Vitamin K-epoxide	Vitamin K	Epoxide is inactive; oral anticoagulants work by blocking reduction of epoxide back to vitamin K, which is needed for blood clotting

[a]Definition of drug and metabolite somewhat arbitrary; the term drug tends to be reserved for administered compound.
[b]Canrenone, an active aldosterone antagonist, is the major metabolite of spironolactone.
[c]Clofibric acid is administered orally as the inactive ethyl ester, which is rapidly hydrolyzed during absorption.
[d]Lovastatin, a lactone, is hydrolyzed to the ring-opened acid.
[e]Commercially available as a drug substance.
[f]Situation complicated by enterohepatic cycling of sulindac and sulindac sulfide.

Fig. 21–11. Once equilibrium is established, the concentrations of prednisone (in color) and prednisolone (in black) in plasma are independent of which compound is administered. Data are obtained after a single oral dose of 50 mg prednisone (■—■) and an i.v. dose of prednisolone (●··●), as prednisolone succinate (40 mg), to a subject on separate occasions. Prednisolone succinate, not shown, is hydrolyzed very rapidly to prednisolone (1 mg/L prednisone = 2.8 μM). (Redrawn from Rose, J.Q., Yurchak, A.M., Jusko, W.J., and Powell, D.: Bioavailability and disposition of prednisolone tablets. Biopharm. Drug Disp., 1:247–258, 1980. Reprinted by permission of John Wiley & Sons, Ltd.)

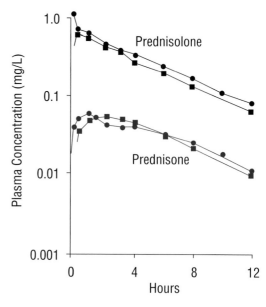

Each pathway is characterized by an associated clearance, and each species may differ in its volume of distribution. The terminal half-life of the interconverted pair is a hybrid of all these parameters. This scheme resembles the two-compartment distribution model discussed in Chap. 19 (Fig. 19–3), except the two compartments now represent drug and metabolite. The difference between the two models is that with interconversion loss can also occur from the "peripheral" (metabolite) compartment. Indeed, if no such loss occurs then, viewed from drug in plasma, the metabolite is effectively a component of drug distribution since, under these circumstances, no drug is irreversibly lost via this pathway.

The therapeutic importance of interconversion varies with the drug and the circumstance. For example, interconversion between sulindac and its sulfide helps to moderate and sustain the concentration of active sulfide. In contrast, interconversion between the antileprotic drug dapsone and its less active metabolite monoacetyldapsone has no therapeutic relevance; the equilibrium is always strongly toward dapsone, which is primarily eliminated via pathways other than N-acetylation. Normally, interconversion between clofibric acid (derived from the rapid hydrolysis of the administered ethyl ester, clofibrate) and its inactive glucuronide is not of concern; the glucuronide is excreted so rapidly that glucuronidation can be regarded as a pathway of irreversible loss of clofibric acid. Consequently, as only 6% of clofibric acid is usually excreted unchanged and all the activity resides with clofibric acid, no change in its pharmacokinetics is anticipated in patients with renal insufficiency. However, as shown in Fig. 21–12, the unbound clearance of clofibric acid is markedly reduced, and its half-life is prolonged, as renal function decreases. The explanation lies in reduced clearance of the glucuronide, which then accumulates and is hydrolyzed back to the parent acid; effectively, a major route of elimination of clofibric acid is increasingly blocked. To what extent the observation with clofibric acid applies to other drugs that depend heavily on glucuronidation for elimination is not known. Clofibric acid glucuronide is an ester; many other drugs form more stable ether glucuronides.

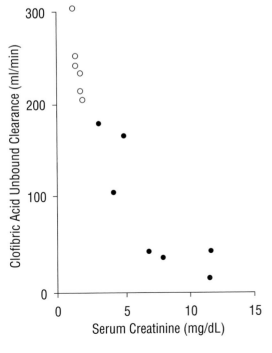

Fig. 21–12. Unbound clearance in patients with unimpaired (○) and compromised (●) renal function is shown. Although little clofibric acid is excreted unchanged ($fe(t) = 0.06$ to 0.1) when renal function is normal, the unbound clearance of clofibric acid decreases markedly with an increase in serum creatinine, an inverse measure of renal function. The apparent dependence of clofibric acid's unbound clearance on a patient's renal function is explained by its interconversion to a polar glucuronide, for which loss from the body depends on renal function (1 mg/L = 4.7 μM). (Redrawn from Gugler, P., Kurten, J.W., Jensen, C.J., Klehr, U., and Hartlapp, J.: Clofibrate disposition in renal failure and acute and chronic liver disease. Euro. J. Clin. Pharmacol., *15*:341–347, 1979.)

Estimation of Metabolite Formation

From Plasma Metabolite Concentration. The amount of administered dose of drug converted to systemically available metabolite can be calculated if metabolite clearance, $CL(m)$ is known, since this amount equals the amount of metabolite eliminated, $CL(m) \cdot AUC(m)$. To gain an estimate of $CL(m)$, the metabolite needs to be given intravenously. In the general case, the ratio $CL(m) \cdot AUC(m)$/Dose gives the fraction of administered drug available systemtically as metabolite. This ratio may be low, e.g., if a drug is given orally and it has a low bioavailability due to incomplete dissolution. An estimate of the importance of a particular metabolic pathway to the elimination of a drug can be made in the special case in which metabolite data are available following i.v. administration of both drug and metabolite on separate occasions. Such data for isosorbide-5-mononitrate are listed in Table 21–5. Isosorbide-5-mononitrate is one of the active metabolites of isosorbide dinitrate, an antianginal drug. The amount of metabolite formed following a 5-mg i.v. dose of parent drug $[CL(m) \cdot AUC(m)]$ is 8.3 L/hr $\times$ 0.37 mg-hr/L, i.e., 3.07-mg or 3.8-mg drug equivalents after correcting for differences in molecular weight (dinitrate, 236 g/mole: 5-mononitrate, 191 g/mole). Clearly, with 3.8 mg of a 5-mg dose converted to this metabolite, the formation of the 5-mononitrate is a major route of elimination of isosorbide dinitrate.

From Metabolite Excretion. Many metabolites are polar and eliminated almost exclusively by renal excretion. The elimination (excretion) of these metabolites in the terminal phase is frequently formation rate-limited, either because they have a much higher clearance, smaller volume of distribution, or both, compared with parent drug. Recall, when formation is rate-limiting, as a reasonable approximation during the terminal phase,

$$\frac{\text{Rate of metabolite excretion}}{\text{Rate of metabolite formation}} \simeq CL_f \cdot C \qquad 17$$

Thus, by measuring the rates of excretion of metabolite and the corresponding plasma drug concentration, clearance associated with formation of metabolite may be estimated. Note that when Eq. 17 applies, the fall in metabolite excretion rate is determined by, and can be used to estimate, the half-life of the drug. Equation 17 is most accurate under steady state conditions.

Detection of Changes in Pharmacokinetics

Comparison of drug and metabolite areas is helpful in identifying the organ of drug metabolism (i.e., gastrointestinal tract, liver) when drug is administered by different routes

Table 21–5. Mean Pharmacokinetic Data for Isosorbide-5-Mononitrate After Intravenous Administration of 5 mg of Isosorbide-5-Mononitrate and Isosorbide Dinitrate[a] on Separate Occasions

	ISOSORBIDE-5-MONONITRATE PARAMETERS	
	AFTER ISOSORBIDE 5-MONONITRATE	AFTER ISOSORBIDE DINITRATE[b]
AUC (mg-hr/L)	0.60	0.37
Cl (L/hr)	8.3	—
Half-life (hr)	4.2	4.3

[a]Data from Straehl, P., Galeazzi, R.L., and Soliva, M.: Isosorbide 5-mononitrate and isosorbide-2-mononitrate kinetics after intravenous and oral dosing. Clin. Pharmacol. Ther., 36:485–492, 1984.
[b]Data from Straehl, P., and Galeazzi, R.L.: Isosorbide dinitrate bioavailability, kinetics, and metabolism. Clin. Pharmacol. Ther., 38:140–149, 1985.

(p. 376). Area analysis can also be used to examine possible causes of a change in the pharmacokinetics of a drug or metabolite. Suppose, for example, that when given orally the plasma concentration of a drug of low clearance is reduced on Occasion B compared to the value on Occasion A. Possible explanations are: reduced oral bioavailability, increased clearance, or both. Examination of drug data alone might give a clue, but the situation is helped considerably by simultaneous use of metabolite data.

The following example is that of a single dose of drug. An analogous analysis can be extended to steady-state conditions. Following a single dose, the area ratios for drug are

$$\text{Occasion A:} \quad F_A \cdot \text{Dose} = CL_A \cdot AUC_A \tag{18}$$

$$\text{Occasion B:} \quad F_B \cdot \text{Dose} = CL_B \cdot AUC_B \tag{19}$$

and for metabolite the corresponding equations are

$$\text{Occasion A:} \quad fm_A \cdot F_A \cdot \text{Dose} = CL(m)_A \cdot AUC(m)_A \tag{20}$$

$$\text{Occasion B:} \quad fm_B \cdot F_B \cdot \text{Dose} = CL(m)_B \cdot AUC(m)_B \tag{21}$$

When the same dose is given on both occasions,

$$\frac{AUC_B}{AUC_A} = \frac{F_B}{F_A} \cdot \frac{CL_A}{CL_B} \tag{22}$$

$$\frac{AUC(m)_B}{AUC(m)_A} = \frac{F_B fm_B \cdot CL(m)_A}{F_A fm_A \cdot CL(m)_B} \tag{23}$$

and since $fm \cdot CL = CL_f$, then

$$\left[\frac{AUC(m)}{AUC}\right]_A = \frac{CL_{f,A}}{CL(m)_A} \tag{24}$$

$$\left[\frac{AUC(m)}{AUC}\right]_B = \frac{CL_{f,B}}{CL(m)_B} \tag{25}$$

Now consider the various possibilities.

Possibility 1. Reduced bioavailability that is due to incomplete dissolution of drug $(F_B < F_A)$. If this is so, as clearance of neither drug nor metabolite is altered, it follows from Eqs. 22 and 23 that

Expectation:

$$\frac{AUC_B}{AUC_A} = \frac{AUC(m)_B}{AUC(m)_A}$$

That is, the ratios of areas of drug and metabolite should be equal and less than 1. Of course, the reason could also be due to the patient's failing to take the dose as instructed, a compliance problem.

Possibility 2. Increased clearance of drug $(CL_B > CL_A)$. If this is the reason for the decreased drug concentration, then the expected outcome for the metabolite depends on the mechanism responsible for the increase in drug clearance namely, decreased binding of drug, enzyme induction, or increased renal clearance and also depends on the extraction ratios of drug and metabolite. Given a low extraction ratio, the expectation is the following:

a. *Decreased binding (fu ↑).*

If this occurs, CL_f is increased but fm is unaltered, because, clearances by all pathways of drug elimination are equally affected. As neither bioavailability nor metabolite clearance is altered,

Expectation:

$$\frac{AUC(m)_A}{AUC(m)_B} = 1$$

$$\left[\frac{AUC(m)}{AUC}\right]_B > \left[\frac{AUC(m)}{AUC}\right]_A$$

b. *Enzyme Induction.*

If this occurs, CL_f may or may not change depending on which metabolic pathway is induced. Remember, there is often more than one enzyme responsible for drug metabolism, and all are not equally susceptible to induction by a given inducing agent.

b1. *Formation of metabolite induced.*

Since CL_f is increased, it follows that

Expectation:

$$\left[\frac{AUC(m)}{AUC}\right]_B > \left[\frac{AUC(m)}{AUC}\right]_A$$

Whether the metabolite area ratio changes depends on whether or not the metabolite is the only pathway of drug elimination. If it is, then, since $fm = 1$ and cannot increase further, no change in the metabolite area ratio is expected. Otherwise,

Expectation:

$$\frac{AUC(m)_B}{AUC(m)_A} > 1$$

b2. *Another metabolic pathway induced.*

Since CL_f is not changed but fm is decreased (as CL is increased), it follows that

Expectation:

$$\left[\frac{AUC(m)_B}{AUC(m)_A}\right] > 1$$

$$\left[\frac{AUC(m)}{AUC}\right]_B = \left[\frac{AUC(m)}{AUC}\right]_A$$

c. *Increased renal clearance (CL_R ↑).*

The outcome in terms of the metabolite is the same as that predicted for case b2, because CL_f is unaltered and fm is decreased.

Expectation:

$$\left[\frac{AUC(m)_B}{AUC(m)_A}\right] < 1$$

$$\left[\frac{AUC(m)}{AUC}\right]_B = \left[\frac{AUC(m)}{AUC}\right]_A$$

From the above analyses it is apparent that metabolite data may help to narrow the number of likely reasons for reduced plasma concentrations of a drug. Giving drug intravenously would have resolved the issue, but it is not always possible or practical to do so. Measurement of protein binding and of drug in urine would certainly have helped distinguish between the various possibilities. Of course, it is possible that both bioavailability and clearance of both drug and metabolite had changed. Such changes complicate the interpretation. Notwithstanding such complications, it is often possible to make reasonable conclusions as to the likely cause of a change in drug pharmacokinetics from combined drug and metabolite data.

STUDY PROBLEMS

(Answers to Study Problems are in Appendix II.)

1. Elson et al. (Elson, J., Strong, J.M., Lee, W.-K., and Atkinson, A.J.: Antiarrhythmic potency of N-acetylprocainamide. Clin. Pharmacol. Ther., *17*:134–140, 1975) determined the ratio of plasma concentrations of active metabolite, N-acetylprocainamide (see Table 21–1), and procainamide in patients on long-term procainamide therapy. Figure 21–13 is a histogram of the results of 33 patients; there is considerable variation. Given, as is likely, that these values are reasonable estimates of the ratio at plateau, comment on which pharmacokinetic parameters of drug and metabolite contribute to the observed variability in the ratio.

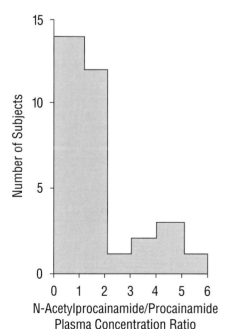

Fig. 21–13.

2. Which (if any) of the explanations offered below are consistent with the following statement? An increase in the ratio of $AUC(m)/AUC$ suggests that any of the following could have happened.
   a. Induction of the metabolite formation pathway.
   b. Reduction of the volume of distribution of the metabolite.
   c. Increase in dose of drug absorbed.
   d. Reduction in clearance of an alternative pathway of elimination of drug.
3. Carbamazepine-10,11-epoxide is an active and substantive metabolite of the antiepileptic drug carbamazepine. Listed in Table 21–6 are the mean steady-state plasma concentrations of carbamazepine and the ratio of the mean steady-state plasma concentrations of carbamazepine-10,11-epoxide and carbamazepine following increasing daily doses of carbamazepine. Given that carbamazepine is well absorbed, and that the clearance of the epoxide, to the diol, does not change with the dose of carbamazepine, what pharmacokinetic parameters of drug and epoxide metabolite have changed to explain the data in Table 21–6?

Table 21–6.   Mean Steady-state Carbamazepine and Metabolite Plasma Concentration Data Following Increasing Daily Doses of Carbamazepine[a]

Daily dose (mg)	100	200	400	800	1200
Carbamazepine concentration (mg/L)	2.6	4.3	5.7	7.3	9.0
Carbamazepine - 10,11-expoxide to Carbamazepine Ratio	0.1	0.15	0.17	0.20	0.21

[a]Abstracted from Kudriakova, T.B., Sirota, L.A., Rozova, G.I. and Gorkov, V.A.: Carbamazepine metabolism in man: Induction and pharmacogenetic aspects. Br. J. Clin. Pharmacol., 33:611–614, 1992. One mg/L carbamazepine = 4.23 µM.

4. Eichelbaum et al. (Eichelbaum, M., Tomson, T., Tybring, G., and Bertilsson, L.: Autoinduction and steady-state pharmacokinetics of carbamazepine and its major metabolites. Clin. Pharmacokinet., 10:80–90, 1985) found that the terminal half-lives of carbamazepine and its trans-diol metabolite were equal, approximately 30 hr, following oral administration of carbamazepine. Do the data suggest the possibility of a rate-limiting step in the process, and if so, where does it lie?
5. Glycine conjugation, with the formation of salicyluric acid, is one of the major pathways for the elimination of salicylic acid in humans. Salicylic acid is cleared slowly from the body, whereas salicyluric acid is cleared so rapidly and completely into urine that the plasma concentration of this metabolite is very low. Discuss why measuring salicyluric acid in the urine could be successfully used to assess its rate of formation.
6. As discussed in this chapter (p. 386), isosorbide dinitrate is extensively metabolized to the 2- and 5-mononitrates. Table 21–7 lists the mean pharmacokinetic data for isosorbide-2-mononitrate following independent i.v. administration of 5 mg of isosorbide dinitrate and the 2-mononitrate to a panel of volunteers. (Molecular weights: dinitrate, 236 g/mole; 2-mononitrate, 191 g/mole.)

Table 21–7.   Mean Pharmacokinetic Data for Isosorbide-2-Mononitrate

ISOSORBIDE-2-MONONITRATE PARAMETERS	AFTER i.v. ISOSORBIDE 2-MONONITRATE[a]	AFTER i.v. ISOSORBIDE DINITRATE[b]
AUC (mg-hr/L)	0.22	0.044
Cl (L/hr)	23.0	—
Half-life (hr)	1.93	1.82

[a]Data from Straehl, P., Galeazzi, R.L., and Soliva, M.: Isosorbide 5-mononitrate and isosorbide-2-mononitrate kinetics after intravenous and oral dosing. Clin. Pharmacol. Ther., 36:485–492, 1984.
[b]Data from Straehl, P., and Galeazzi, R.L.: Isosorbide dinitrate bioavailability, kinetics and metabolism. Clin. Pharmacol. Ther., 38:140–149, 1985.

    a. Calculate the fraction of isosorbide dinitrate metabolized to the 2-mononitrate.

    b. What assumptions have you made in your calculation?

    c. By reference to the corresponding data for the 5-mononitrate provided in this chapter (p. 386), what percentage of i.v.-administered isosorbide dinitrate is eliminated by de-nitration?

7. Dollery et al. (Dollery C.T., Davies, D.S., and Conolly, M.E.: Differences in the metabolism of drugs depending upon their routes of administration. Ann. N.Y. Acad. Sci., *179*:108–114, 1971) examined the influence of route of administration on the metabolic profile of isoproterenol. This beta-adrenergic-stimulating drug is methylated to O-methylisoproterenol; both drug and metabolite form sulfate conjugates. Table 21–8 lists the urinary recovery of all four compounds following administration of tritiated isoproterenol intravenously, orally, and by inhalation to volunteers. Only parent compound has a cardiostimulating effect.

Table 21–8. Percent Urinary Recovery Following Administration of Isoproterenol

	RECOVERY (% of Dose)			
ROUTE	ISOPROTERENOL	ISOPROTERENOL CONJUGATE	O-METHYL ISOPROTERENOL	O-METHYL ISOPROTERENOL CONJUGATE
i.v.	62.2	0	13.0	24.8
Oral	6.3	62.0	5.6	1.3
Inhalation	2.0	89.3	0.9	4.7

    a. On a dose basis, isoproterenol is much less active in increasing heart rate given orally than intravenously, which is due to a pronounced oral first-pass metabolic loss, principally by sulfate conjugation. Comment on the likely primary site for conjugation of isoproterenol administered orally.

    b. Do the data support any evidence for O-methylation occurring presystemically following oral administration?

    c. Given the relative similarity of the excretory profiles following the oral and inhaled routes, comment on the likely fate of much of the inhaled drug.

8. Osborne et al. (Osborne, R., Joel, S., Trew, D., and Slevin, M.: Morphine and metabolite behavior after different routes of morphine administration: Demonstration of the importance of the active metabolite morphine-6-glucuronide. Clin. Pharmacol. Ther., *47*:12–19, 1990) studied the pharmacokinetics of the analgesic morphine and its two glucuronide metabolites, the active morphine-6-glucuronide, and the inactive morphine-3-glucuronide. Table 21–9 lists mean ($\pm$ SD) AUC and C_{max} data obtained following administration of morphine sulfate as an i.v. bolus (5 mg), oral tablet (11.7 mg), and sublingual tablet (11.7 mg) to 10 healthy volunteers. Molecular weight of morphine is 285.3 g/mole; morphine sulfate, 669 g/mole, contains 85.3% morphine base.

Table 21–9. Mean ($\pm$SD) AUC and C_{max} Data[a] for Morphine and Its Glucuronides Following Administration of Morphine by Different Routes

		ROUTE		
SPECIES		i.v. BOLUS	ORAL	SUBLINGUAL
Morphine	AUC (nmol·hr/L)	229 $\pm$ 37	43 $\pm$ 13	48 $\pm$ 10
	C_{max} (nmol/L)	273 $\pm$ 65	21 $\pm$ 7.7	19 $\pm$ 4.5
Morphine-6-	AUC (nmol·hr/L)	313 $\pm$ 87	371 $\pm$ 159	298 $\pm$ 159
glucuronide	C_{max} (nmol/L)	80 $\pm$ 15	84 $\pm$ 26	74 $\pm$ 19
Morphine-3-	AUC (nmol·hr/L)	1765 $\pm$ 300	2180 $\pm$ 808	1664 $\pm$ 485
glucuronide	C_{max} (nmol/L)	407 $\pm$ 100	440 $\pm$ 125	386 $\pm$ 81

[a]All data are normalized to a 10-mg dose of morphine.

a. Calculate the bioavailability of morphine following oral administration.
b. Given that the blood-to-plasma concentration ratio of morphine is 0.55 and that 8% of an i.v. dose is excreted unchanged in urine, do the i.v. data for morphine itself suggest that its low oral bioavailability is due to a substantial first-pass hepatic loss?
c. Do the data for both glucuronides support the concept that the liver is the primary site of formation of these metabolites?
d. One reason for the use of sublingual tablets, in general, is to increase the systemic bioavailability of a drug that exhibits a high first-pass hepatic loss, as blood perfusing the buccal cavity drains directly into the superior vena cava. Do the data in Table 21–9 support this rationale for morphine?
e. Comment briefly as to what extent the estimation of oral bioavailability of morphine may be used to guide any difference in dosage requirements of morphine given orally and intravenously.
f. Suggest why the C_{max} for morphine-3-glucuronide is greater than that of morphine, after i.v. morphine administration.
g. Independently, Osbourne et al. (Osbourne, R., Thompson, P., Joel, S., Trew, D., Patel, N., and Slevin, M.A.: The analgesic activity of morphine-6-glucuronide. Br. J. Clin. Pharmacol., 34:130–138, 1992) studied the pharmacokinetics of morphine-6-glucuronide after i.v. administration of this glucuronide to cancer patients. Given that the clearance found, 5.8 L/hr, applies to the volunteers who participated in the study that generated the data in Table 21–9, calculate the fraction of orally administered morphine converted to the 6-glucuronide.

9. Shown in Fig. 21–14 are semilogarithmic plots of the mean (±SD) plasma concentrations of propranolol (○) and its active metabolite, 4-hydroxypropranolol (●), after oral administration of propranolol (80 mg) to six healthy subjects. Discuss why the plasma concentration of 4-hydroxypropranolol peaks earlier and initially declines more rapidly than that of propranolol.

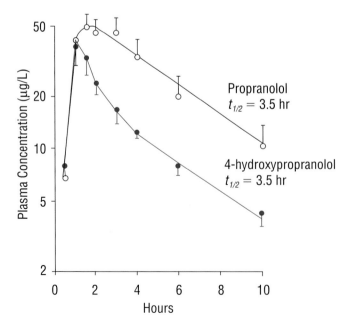

Fig. 21–14.

10. Listed in Table 21–10 are the plasma concentrations of a drug and one of its metabolites following oral administration of 1 g of drug to a subject. The drug is fully bioavailable when given orally, absorption is rapid relative to its elimination, and the volumes of distribution of drug and metabolite are equal. The molecular weight of the drug is 308 g/mole, that of the metabolite is 326 g/mole.

   a. Calculate the fraction of drug converted to metabolite, the formation clearance of metabolite, and the disposition kinetics of the metabolite.

   b. The recommended dosage regimen of the drug is 1 g orally, to be taken every 8 hr. The pharmacokinetics of both drug and metabolite do not change with time on chronic dosing. Calculate:

   1. The average plasma concentrations of drug and metabolite at plateau.
   2. The plasma concentration-time profiles of drug and metabolite within a dosing interval at plateau.
   3. The times required to reach their respective plateaus.

Table 21-10.

Time (hr)	0	0.5	1	1.5	2	3	4	6	8	12
Drug (mg/L)	0	25	32	30	32	16	9	4	1.2	—
Metabolite (mg/L)	0	10	22	31	44	42	32	25	16	8.5

11. Predict the general tendencies (clockwise, counterclockwise, or no hysteresis) for the observed relationship between response and plasma drug concentration after a single oral dose of a drug as a consequence of each of the following conditions. See problem 9 of Chap. 20 (p. 366) for complementary information on conditions producing hysteresis.

   a. Activity resides solely with a metabolite. Low-clearance drug with metabolite elimination rate-limiting the decline of the metabolite concentration in terminal phase.

   b. Activity resides solely with a metabolite. High first-pass metabolism of drug with drug elimination rate-limiting the decline of metabolite concentration in terminal phase.

DOSE AND TIME DEPENDENCIES

OBJECTIVES

The reader will be able to:

1. List at least 10 sources of dose (or time) dependence in drug absorption, distribution, and elimination.

2. Recognize dose- (or time-) dependent kinetics from either plasma or urine data showing such behavior.

3. Graphically depict the kinetic behavior of a drug when the situation and the cause of a dose (or time) dependence are given.

4. On analyzing data in which a dose (or time) dependence occurs, identify which pharmacokinetic parameters are affected, and assign probable causes to the observation.

5. Demonstrate the kinetic consequences at steady state of a change in the rate of input, Vm or Km, of a drug showing saturable Michaelis-Menten metabolism.

6. Define saturable first-pass metabolism, describe how it can occur, and discuss its kinetic consequences.

An epileptic patient who has not responded to phenytoin after 2 weeks on 300 mg/day is observed to have a plasma concentration of 4 mg/L. Twenty days after the daily dose has been increased to 500 mg, the patient develops signs of toxicity, nystagmus, and ataxia; the plasma concentration of phenytoin is now 36 mg/L. Why should only a 67% increase in daily dose give rise to a ninefold increase in plasma concentration? The answer lies in the dose-dependent kinetic behavior of this drug.

Normally, plasma (or blood) concentration, unbound concentration, and amount of drug and its metabolites excreted in urine at any given time all increase in direct proportion to dose, when drug is administered in either a single dose or in multiple doses. Therefore, on correcting such observations for the dose administered, the values should superimpose at all times. This is referred to as the *principle of superposition*. When superposition occurs, the pharmacokinetics of a drug is said to be *dose-independent*, or *linear*.

There are many reasons why the principle of superposition may not hold. Among them are the administration of a drug by different routes, in different dosage forms, or by different methods (bolus or infusion). These are examples of dependencies on dosage form and route of administration. They are not the subject of this chapter. Other reasons for lack of superposition include changes in pharmacokinetic parameters themselves with size of dose administered or dosing rate, when all other factors are held constant. The pharmacokinetics of such drugs are said to be *dose-dependent*. When there is a lack of superposition on administering a drug on separate occasions or a lack of predictability following repeated or continuous dosing, based on single-dose data, the drug is said to show *time-dependent kinetics*. Such behaviors are sources of variability in drug response. Although relatively uncommon, they occur frequently enough in drug therapy to warrant special consideration. In drug overdose, they are more the rule than the exception.

This chapter deals with identification and consequences of dose-dependent and time-dependent kinetics. The major intent is to establish a general awareness of this topic.

EVIDENCE

Five pharmacokinetic parameters (F, ka, V, CL_R, and CL_H) basically define and summarize the time-course of a drug in the body. Usually, none of these parameters systematically changes with dose in the same individual. But in *dose-dependent kinetics*, any one or a combination of these parameters appears to change with administration of different doses. The parameters change during continuous or repeated administration when kinetics show *time dependence*.

Both dose-dependent and time-dependent kinetic behaviors defy easy quantitative description and prediction. The first step in evaluating this behavior is to identify its occurrence. Subsequent steps involve determining the parameters affected and the likely mechanism(s) of the nonlinearity. There are many potential causes of dose and time dependencies. Table 22–1 lists examples of representative causes together with the pharmacokinetic parameters affected. Let us now consider examples of drugs for which there is evidence of nonlinear behavior in absorption or disposition. For many of these examples, therapeutic implications and means of accommodating or circumventing the problems are given.

ABSORPTION

Dose or time dependencies in drug absorption may be reflected by a change in either bioavailability or rate-time profile of absorption. These dependencies most often arise from three sources following oral administration. First are solubility and dissolution limitations in the release of drug from a dosage form in the gastrointestinal tract. Second is saturability

Table 22–1. Representative Causes of Dose- (or Time-) Dependent Kinetics and Selected Drug Examples

	EXAMPLE	PARAMETER AFFECTED[a]	
I. *Gastrointestinal Absorption*			
A. Saturable transport in gut wall	Amoxycillin	F	↓
B. Drug comparatively insoluble	Griseofulvin	F	↓
C. Saturable gut wall or hepatic metabolism on first pass	Nicardipine	F	↑
II. *Distribution*			
A. Saturable plasma protein binding	Naproxen	V, fu	↑
B. Saturable tissue binding		V, fu_T	↓; ↑
III. *Renal Excretion*			
A. Active secretion (saturable)	Penicillin G	CL_R	↓
B. Active reabsorption (saturable)	Ascorbic acid	CL_R	↑
C. Decrease in urine pH	Salicylic acid	CL_R	↓
D. Saturable plasma protein binding	Disopyramide	CL_R	↑
E. Nephrotoxicity[b]	Aminoglycosides	CL_R	↓
F. Increase in urine flow[b]	Theophylline	CL_R	↑
IV. *Hepatic Metabolism*			
A. Capacity-limited kinetics, cofactor limitation, etc.	Phenytoin	CL_H	↓
B. Enzyme induction[b]	Carbamazepine	CL_H	↑
C. Hepatotoxicity[b]	Acetaminophen	CL_H	↓
D. Saturable plasma protein binding	Prednisolone	CL_H	↑
E. Decreased hepatic blood flow	Propranolol	CL_H	↓
F. Inhibition by metabolite[b]	Lidocaine	CL_H	↓

[a]Direction of change: ↑ increase, ↓ decrease on increasing dose.
[b]Time-dependent as well as dose-dependent.

in a transport mechanism for passage across the gastrointestinal membranes. Last is saturability in metabolism during a drug's first pass through the gut wall and the liver.

Solubility

Dissolution can be the cause of dose dependency in bioavailability for drugs with low aqueous solubility, when given orally in relatively large doses. With a fixed transit time through the gastrointestinal tract, the amount of drug absorbed is unlikely to increase in proportion to the dose administered. An example is griseofulvin (Fig. 22–1). For this sparingly soluble drug (solubility is 10 mg/L), bioavailability decreases as the dose is increased from 250 to 500 mg.

Saturable Active Transport

For a few drugs, absorption from the gastrointestinal tract occurs by a capacity-limited transport mechanism. An example is that of amoxycillin, a polar β-lactam antibiotic. This drug is absorbed by a peptide transport mechanism in the small intestine. This conclusion is supported by the observation that bioavailability decreases with increased dose, but the peak time changes little (Fig. 22–2). The decrease in bioavailability is explained by the capacity-limited nature of the transport process. The lack of a major change in the peak time is a consequence of the limited region in the small intestine from which absorption can occur. The dose size does not influence the time between ingestion and movement past the site of transport.

Saturable First-Pass Metabolism

Nicardipine, a dihydropyridine calcium-channel blocker, exhibits dose dependence in its oral bioavailability (Table 22–2) because of saturability in its metabolism on first pass

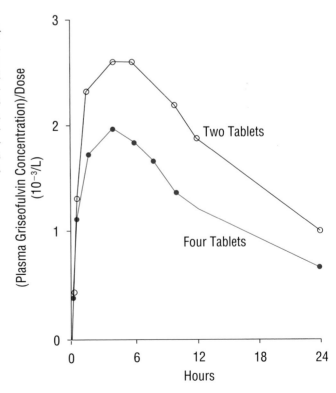

Fig. 22–1. Plasma concentration, normalized to dose, as a function of time following the oral administration of two tablets (upper curve ○) and four tablets (lower colored curve, ●) of ultramicronized griseofulvin (125 mg/tablet) (1 mg/L = 2.8 μM). (Adapted from data in Barrett, W.E., and Bianchine, J.R.: The bioavailability of ultramicronized griseofulvin (GRIS-PEG®) tablets in man. Curr. Ther. Res., *18*:501–509, 1975.)

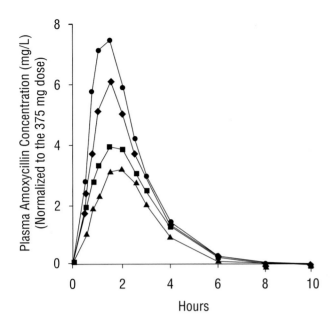

Fig. 22–2. Mean amoxycillin plasma concentrations after single oral doses of 375 (●), 750 (♦), 1500 (■), and 3000 (▲) mg. The concentrations are normalized to those expected for a 375-mg dose ($C = C$ (observed) × 375/ Dose(mg)). Note the decrease in the C_{max} and AUC values, and the similarity in t_{max} on increasing the dose. The observations are explained by oral bioavailability decreasing with dose with little or no change in peak time. (1 mg/L = 2.7 µM). (Data from Sjovall, J., Gunnar, A., and Westerlund, D.: Dose-dependent absorption of amoxycillin and bacampicillin. Clin. Pharmacol. Ther., 38:241–250, 1985. Interpretation from Reigner, B.G., Couet, W.R., Guedes, J.-P., Fourtillan, J.-B., and Tozer, T.N.: Saturable rate of cefatrizine absorption after oral administration to humans. J. Pharmacokinet. Biopharm., 18:17–34, 1990.)

Table 22–2. Saturable First-Pass Metabolism of Nicardipine Observed at Steady State Following Oral Doses of 10 to 40 mg Every 8 hr[a]

DOSE (mg)	BIOAVAILABILITY (%)
10	19(4)[b]
20	22(5)
30	28(5)
40	38(6)

[a]Data from Wagner, J.G., Ling, T.L. Mroszczak, E.J., Freedman D., Wu, A., Huang, B., Massey, I.J., and Roe, R.R.: Single intravenous dose and steady-state oral dose pharmacokinetics of nicardipine in healthy subjects. Biopharm. Drug. Dispos., 8:133–148, 1987.
[b]Mean and SE of data from 6 subjects.

through the liver. The data in the table were acquired during an 8-hr dosing interval at steady state (3 days into regimen). An i.v. radiolabeled tracer dose (0.885 mg) was given concurrently with the 30-mg dose to determine oral bioavailability.

Saturable first-pass metabolism occurs for a number of orally administered drugs that are highly extracted by the liver or intestinal tissues. Additional examples are listed in Table 22–3. For several of these drugs, dose dependence in oral bioavailability is observed without an apparent change in elimination half-life. This behavior can be understood by realizing that the concentration of drug reaching the liver during absorption can be much higher than that after absorption is over. Consider, for example, the following conditions: Distribution is instantaneous; all drug reaches the liver intact; input of drug from the gastrointestinal tract is first-order with a *ka* of 0.05 min-1 (14-min half-life); oral bioavailability at low doses is 0.1; volume of distribution is 250 L; total hepatic blood flow, Q_H, is 1.35 mL/min; and absorption is faster than elimination.

Table 22–3. Examples of Drugs Showing Saturable First-Pass Metabolism in the Liver or Gut Wall After Oral Administration of Therapeutic Doses

Alprenolol	Methoxysalen	Propranolol
5-Fluorouracil	Nicardipine	Salicylamide
Hydralazine	Propoxyphene	Verapamil

The initial rate of input into the portal vein, $ka \cdot$ Dose, is also the initial rate of entry of drug into the liver, $Q_H \cdot C_{initial}$. Consequently, after a 100-mg dose,

$$C_{initial} = \frac{ka \cdot \text{Dose}}{Q_H} = 3.7 \text{ mg/L} \qquad\qquad 1$$

The concentration in the blood entering the liver after absorption is finished would have a maximum value of

$$C_{max} = \frac{F \cdot \text{Dose}}{V} = 0.04 \text{ mg/L} \qquad\qquad 2$$

The actual value of C_{max} should be less because some drug is eliminated during the absorption phase. As can be seen, the contribution of absorbed drug to the concentration entering the liver during first pass is much greater than that recycled from the rest of the body. Indeed, the ratio of $C_{initial}$ to C_{max} is

$$\frac{C_{initial}}{C_{max}} = \frac{ka \cdot V}{F \cdot Q_H} = 92 \qquad\qquad 3$$

Thus, the larger the value of ka or V or the smaller the value of F at low (nonsaturating) doses, the greater is the ratio $C_{initial}/C_{max}$ and the more likely there is to be a separation in the degree of saturation of metabolism during absorption and elimination phases. All the drugs listed in Table 22–3 show saturable first-pass metabolism and have pharmacokinetic parameters that favor a high value of $C_{initial}/C_{max}$.

SATURABILITY OF PLASMA PROTEIN AND TISSUE BINDING

A limited number of binding sites exist on plasma proteins. Recall from Table 10–4 that the plasma concentration of albumin is usually 43 g/L or 600 μM (molecular weight = 67,000 g/mole). At one binding site per albumin molecule, there is then a limiting concentration of 600 μM for the bound drug. For α_1-acid glycoprotein, the limitation occurs at about 15 μM, a much lower concentration. The sites to which drugs bind in the tissues may be similarly limited. Consequently, the volume of distribution depends on drug concentration, a *concentration-dependent* behavior. Changes in binding tend to become appreciable when more than 20% of the available sites are occupied. This number, corresponding to 120 μM for one binding site on albumin, is arbitrary but useful for predicting the likelihood of concentration-dependent binding. For a drug with a molecular weight of 250, 120 μM corresponds to a concentration of 30 mg/L.

For drugs that show saturable binding to plasma proteins, the volume of distribution is expected to increase with plasma concentration, except when the volume of distribution is small (less than 0.2 L/kg, see Chap. 10, Distribution). Conversely, for drugs that show saturability in binding to tissues, the volume of distribution decreases as plasma concentration is increased. Because of the potential dependence on the fraction unbound in plasma and the dependence of half-life on both clearance and volume of distribution, dose dependence in distribution may be difficult to identify and quantify, unless plasma protein binding is measured. Consider the example of naproxen.

The *AUC* of naproxen following single doses fails to increase linearly with dose when doses above those maximally recommended (500 mg) are given (Fig. 22–3). Without any other information, this nonlinear observation might be explained by either a decrease in bioavailability or an increase in clearance, in that

$$AUC = \frac{F}{CL} \cdot Dose \qquad\qquad 4$$

The increase in clearance may be due to induction of metabolism or saturable binding to plasma proteins. As naproxen is a drug of low clearance (Dose/AUC calculated from data in Fig. 22–3A varies from 0.3 to 1.3 L/hr), the peak concentrations observed at doses of 1 to 4 g (Fig. 22–3B) provide information to distinguish between these possibilities. If one approximates a concentration of 110 mg/L when most of a 1000-mg dose is in the body, a value of V/F of approximately 9 L can be estimated. This small volume suggests strong binding to plasma proteins. The maximum concentrations obtained are in the region where nonlinear binding is expected for naproxen, a weak acid that binds to albumin. With a molecular weight of 230 g/mole, 100 and 200 mg/L correspond to concentrations of 430 and 870 μM, values approximating that (600 μM) of serum albumin. This is the condition in which *fu* is expected to increase with higher doses. Thus, with minimal information, a probable source of nonlinearity, saturable binding to plasma albumin, can be deduced.

The therapeutic consequence of decreased binding to plasma proteins at higher daily doses of a drug of low extraction ratio differs dramatically from that of drug-induced increased enzyme activity (autoinduction). When binding decreases (*fu* increases), the steady-state total plasma concentration is not increased much on doubling the rate of administration. The steady-state unbound concentration, however, doubles as a consequence of no change in unbound clearance. The intensities of toxic and therapeutic responses are expected to increase accordingly. In contrast, an increase in enzyme activity would affect both unbound and total concentrations proportionally. Thus, if autoinduction occurs, only a minor increase in response would be expected at higher rates of administration.

The expected change in the time-course of a drug in plasma when plasma protein binding exhibits nonlinear behavior is complex. Changes occur in both volume of distribution (Chap. 10) and clearance (Chap. 11). The magnitude of the changes depends on both the volume of distribution and the extraction ratio of the drug. Furthermore, because volume

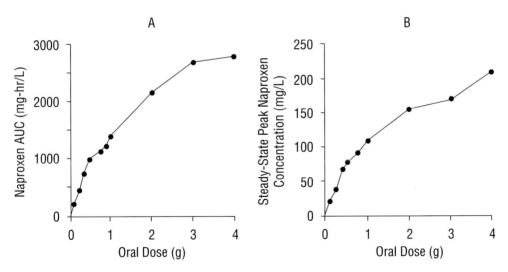

Fig. 22–3. The *AUC* of naproxen increases with the size of a single oral dose but not in direct proportion; the *AUC* appears to approach a limiting value (A). Nonlinearity is also observed in the peak concentration (B). These observations are consistent with either a decrease in *F* or an increase in *CL* with decreasing dose. As explained in the text, saturable binding to plasma albumin is most probably responsible (1 mg/L = 4.3 μM). (Modified from Runkel, R., Chaplin, M.D., Sevelius, H., Ortega, E., and Segre, E.: Pharmacokinetics of naproxen overdoses. Clin. Pharmacol. Ther., 20:269–277, 1976).

of distribution changes with amount in body, the decline of the plasma concentration does not reflect, in direct proportion, the disappearance of drug from the body. The slope of the semilogarithmic decline in the concentration-time curve is then not a good measure of the fractional rate of elimination. The qualitative effect of saturable binding to plasma proteins for a drug with a small volume of distribution is demonstrated by the decreasing slope of the unbound cefonicid concentration with time on a semilogarithmic plot (Fig. 22–4) after a single 30-mg/kg i.v. dose. The difference between the decline of the total and unbound concentrations (Fig. 22–4A) is explained by the decrease in the fraction unbound with time (Fig. 22–4B). The apparent one-compartmental nature of the total concentration decline is explained by virtually all drug in the body being bound to albumin.

The *ACE* inhibitor trandolaprilat, formed following oral administration of trandolapril, shows nonlinear plasma and tissue protein binding, as do other agents in this pharmacologic class. Evidence of nonlinearity in trandolaprilat kinetics is provided in Fig. 22–5. Both *AUC* (Fig. 22–5A) and plasma concentration (Fig. 22–5B), particularly during the terminal phase, fail to increase in direct proportion to the oral dose of trandolapril, over the eightfold range (0.5 to 4.0 mg) studied. Also, contrary to the expectation of linear kinetics, dosing daily, which is relatively frequent compared to the long terminal half-life, does not lead to extensive accumulation (Fig. 22–5C). Thus, when a 2-mg dose of trandolapril is administered orally for 10 days, the accumulation ratio of trandolaprilat ($AUC_{ss}/AUC_{(\tau,1)}$, Eq. 25, Chap. 7) is only 1.49. Direct evidence of concentration-dependent plasma protein binding of trandolaprilat is shown in Fig. 22–5D and Table 10–4. It should be noted that the range of concentrations, 0.5 to 5 µg/L, over which the fraction unbound changes threefold, covers most of the plasma trandiloprilat concentrations obtained following the oral doses of trandolapril (Fig. 22–5B, C).

The observations above can be rationalized as follows. The extremely low plasma concentration at which saturable binding occurs suggests a binding protein of much lower concentration than albumin or α_1-acid glycoprotein (see Table 10–4). The body of evidence

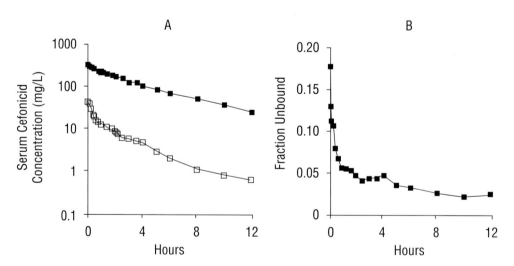

Fig. 22–4. *A*, Mean total (■) and unbound (□) plasma cefonicid concentrations with time in six volunteers after a single i.v. dose of 30 mg/kg given over 5 min. Note the much more rapid decline of the unbound concentration during the first 2 hr. *B*, The difference between the declines of the two curves in *A* is explained by a rapid decrease in the fraction unbound with time. As a consequence of the limited capacity of serum albumin to bind cefonicid, the high total concentrations at early times tend to approach the capacity for binding (1 mg/L = 1.84 µM). (Redrawn from Dudley, M.N., Shyu, W.-C., Nightingale, C.H., and Quintiliani, R.: Effect of saturable serum protein binding on the pharmacokinetics of unbound cefonicid in humans. Antimicrob. Agents Chemother.,

points to *ACE* itself being responsible. This high-affinity, low-capacity enzyme resides in both plasma and the endothelial linings of the vasculature, the latter site being interpreted as tissue binding when viewed from plasma data. Trandolaprilat, a relatively polar molecule, is restricted in its distribution mainly to extracellular spaces and is cleared systemically, mostly by renal excretion. Renal excretion is primarily via glomerular filtration, so that renal clearance shows concentration dependence associated with saturable protein binding. At high concentrations of trandolaprilat, which saturate *ACE*, renal clearance is high and elimination rapid. As the plasma concentration falls, the fraction bound to plasma and tissue *ACE* increases, thereby diminishing the unbound pool and lowering renal clearance. The net effect is a much slower elimination of material from the body. Thus, the biphasic decline of plasma trandolaprilat, seen in the semilogarithmic plots (Fig. 22–5B) is due to concentration-dependent protein binding and not distribution kinetics. Notice, that had only one dose of drug been administered, one could not have readily distinguished between concentration-dependent binding and distribution kinetics as the cause of the apparent biexponential decline of the plasma data. Finally, the lack of appreciable accumulation on multiple dosing arises because after each dose, most of the systematically available trandolaprilat is eliminated before reaching the terminal phase. Thus, nonlinear binding to the active site, *ACE*, appears to explain virtually all of trandolaprilat's odd kinetic behavior.

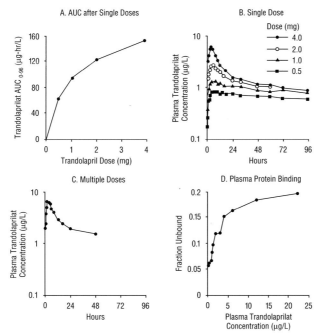

Fig. 22–5. Trandolaprilat, the active metabolite of trandolapril, exhibits nonlinear kinetic behavior. *A*, The *AUC* (0 to 96 hr) of the metabolite does not increase in direct proportion to the dose of trandolapril over the dose range of 0.5 to 4 mg. *B*, A semilogarithmic plot of mean plasma trandolaprilat concentrations after oral doses of 0.5, 1.0, 2.0, and 4.0 mg shows nonlinearity in that the curves are not equally spaced by a factor of 2 in the vertical direction for each of the successive doses. The lack of proportionality with dose is particularly evident at later times. *C*, Administration of 2.0 mg of trandolapril daily for 10 days fails to produce the degree of accumulation of trandolaprilat, as viewed from the concentration-time profile within a dosing interval at steady state (24 hr) that is predicted based on the long terminal decline in plasma concentration observed following a single 2.0-mg dose (see *B*). *D*, Binding of trandolaprilat to plasma proteins shows nonlinearity in that the fraction unbound increased with increasing concentration. (1 mg/L = 2.4 μM). (Data in *A* and *B* from Lenfant, B., Mouren, M., Bryce, T., De Lauture, D., and Strauch, G.: Trandolapril: Pharmacokinetics of single oral doses in male healthy volunteers, J. Cardiovasc. Pharmacol., in press, 1994; Data in *C* from Arnor, P., Wade, A., Engfelt, P., Mouren M., Stepniewski, J.P., Sultan, E., Bryce, T., and Lenfant, B: Pharmacokinetics and pharmacodynamics of trandolapril after repeated administration. J. Cardiovasc. Pharmacol., in press, 1994; Data in *D* from B. Lenfant, personal communication.)

CONCENTRATION-DEPENDENT RENAL EXCRETION

Renal clearance can vary with plasma concentration. Both filtration and reabsorption are usually passive processes, the rates of which are directly related to plasma concentration. In contrast, active secretion and active reabsorption are saturable processes with maximum capacities. This is shown in Fig. 22–6, for active secretion. The rate of tubular secretion increases in direct proportion to the plasma concentration until the transport approaches an upper limit often called the *TM* value. Consequently, clearance by secretion decreases as plasma concentration increases. This is observed for the antimicrobial agent dicloxacillin (Fig. 22–7). On increasing the dose from 1 to 2 g, the renal clearance, assessed by Ae_∞/AUC, is reduced. Extrarenal clearance is unaffected. With an *fu* of 0.04, the unbound renal clearance is about 2600 mL/min following the 1-g dose. This value greatly exceeds the usual glomerular filtration rate of 120 mL/min, indicating that this drug is extensively secreted into the tubular lumen (see Chap. 11, Elimination). At these doses, secretion shows concentration dependence and, as a consequence, the *AUC* increases disproportionately with dose. The body exposure to the drug and the half-life are disproportionately increased, considerations for the therapeutic use of large doses.

Secretion never occurs alone; filtration is always a component, and passive reabsorption may or may not be. Figure 22–6 also demonstrates how the rate of excretion of a drug that undergoes filtration and secretion, such as penicillin, always increases with plasma concentration. Even though the rate of secretion approaches an upper limit the rate of filtration continues to increase directly with unbound plasma concentration.

Fig. 22–6. The rate of renal secretion has a limiting value, the maximum transport rate (T_M), whereas the rate of filtration increases in direct proportion to the plasma concentration of a drug. Consequently, the rate of excretion of a drug that is both filtered and secreted, but not reabsorbed, increases with its plasma concentration. The increase, however, is not in direct proportion. Drug is either not bound in plasma or *fu* remains constant throughout the range of plasma concentrations.

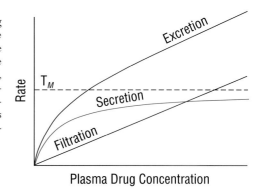

Fig. 22–7. Renal clearance of dicloxacillin, as measured by Ae_∞/AUC, is decreased following a 2-g i.v. dose relative to that observed after a 1-g i.v. dose. The extrarenal clearance is not affected by dose. Saturable secretion of drug into the renal tubule explains the decrease in renal clearance. Mean ± SD (bars) (1 mg/L = 2.1 μM). (Data from Naufa, E.H., and Mattie, H.: Dicloxacillin and cloxacillin: Pharmacokinetics in healthy and hemodialysis subjects. Clin. Pharmacol. Ther., *20*:98–108, 1976.)

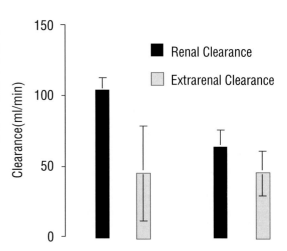

Renal clearance is the rate of drug excretion divided by its plasma concentration. A drug that is only filtered, and is not bound in plasma, has the same renal clearance at all concentrations, as shown schematically in curve A of Fig. 22–8. Curve B depicts the events that occur for a drug that is actively secreted. In the region of plasma concentrations well below those required to approach saturation, renal clearance is highest and is relatively insensitive to changes in drug concentration. The therapeutic concentrations of most actively secreted drugs lie within this region. At higher plasma concentrations, renal clearance decreases; the lower limiting value is that contributed by both filtration and passive reabsorption.

The renal clearances of ascorbic acid, disopyramide, and the protein superoxide dismutase all increase with increasing concentrations, but for different reasons. Ascorbic acid (vitamin C) is normally conserved in the body by active reabsorption from the renal tubule. When the plasma concentration is excessive, the capacity of the reabsorption mechanism is exceeded, and the vitamin appears in large amounts in the urine (Fig. 22–9). The consequence of nonlinear excretion following oral administration of vitamin C is illustrated by the data in Table 22–4. Although statistically significant, note that the plasma concentration does not increase much even when megadoses are given. Another nonlinear mechanism also contributes to this observation. The bioavailability of the vitamin decreases with increasing dose (not shown) because it is absorbed in the intestine by a saturable process. The combined effect of saturable gastrointestinal absorption and renal tubular reabsorption is that only a relatively small change in the steady-state plasma concentration occurs, even when the daily oral dose is increased greatly.

Rather than saturable reabsorption, nonlinear binding to α_1-acid glycoprotein causes renal clearance (based on total concentration) of disopyramide to be greater at earlier times after a 1.5-mg/kg i.v. dose (Fig. 22–10A). Unbound renal clearance, on the other hand, shows no evidence of nonlinearity (Fig. 22–10B). The greater total clearance coincides with a higher total concentration and a lower binding ($fu\uparrow$) at earlier times.

The nonlinearity in renal clearance of the experimental protein drug superoxide dismutase is related to renal metabolism (Fig. 22–11). This protein, protective against cell injury that is due to oxygen-derived free radicals or superoxides, is filtered and then partially

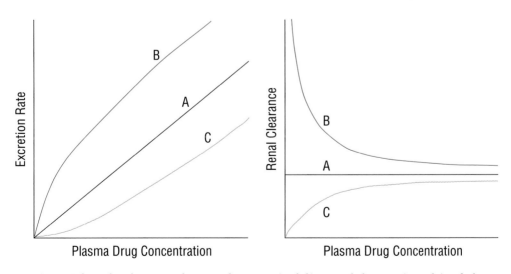

Fig. 22–8. Relationships between either rate of excretion (on left) or renal clearance (on right) and plasma concentration depend on whether the drug undergoes filtration only (curve A), filtration and secretion (curve B), or filtration and active reabsorption (curve C). The drug is either not bound to plasma proteins, or *fu* does not change in the concentration range shown.

metabolized in the renal tubular cells. At higher plasma concentrations, metabolism of the filtered drug becomes saturable with a resultant increase in renal clearance, an observation commonly reported for other proteins of comparable size. Note that the apparent upper limit of renal clearance (40 mL/min/70 kg) is less than the glomerular filtration rate, a probable consequence of filtration of this protein being incomplete because of its large molecular size (M.W. = 32,000 g/mole). Although no specific cut-off in molecular weight can be given, filtration of proteins above 30,000 g/mole falls off rapidly with increasing molecular size. Above 70,000 g/mole, only a small fraction is filtered except in glomerular disease (See Chap. 11, Elimination, p. 178).

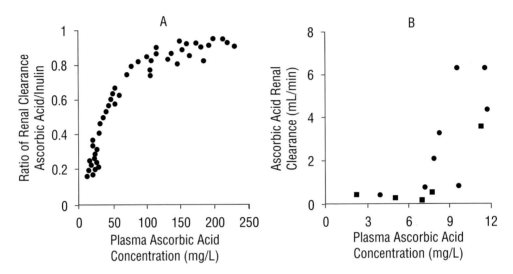

Fig. 22–9. *A,* The renal clearance of ascorbic acid relative to that of inulin increases dramatically at plasma concentrations well above the values of 4 to 15 mg/L typical for normal dietary conditions. The increase occurs at higher ascorbic acid plasma concentrations because the rate of filtration exceeds the capacity of the facilitated transport mechanism to reabsorb the vitamin from the tubular lumen. At high concentrations, the renal clearance of ascorbic acid approaches that of inulin, a compound that is only filtered. The high concentrations were produced following i.v. injections of 1500 to 6000 mg of ascorbic acid (1 mg/L = 5.7 μM). (Adapted from Ralli, E.P., Friedman, G.J., and Rubin, S.H.: The mechanism of the excretion of vitamin C by the human kidney. J. Clin. Invest., *17*:765–770, 1940.) *B,* In the plasma concentration range resulting from daily oral doses of 30 to 180 mg, renal clearance of ascorbic acid ranges from negligible to 4 to 8 mL/min (3 to 6% of the expected inulin clearance) in 22- to 45-year-old male subjects while on diets essentially free of vitamin C. Each symbol (●, ■) crepresents a group of subjects studied in one experiment with different intakes of ascorbic acid per day. (Adapted from Kallner, A., Hartmann, D., and Hornig, D.: Steady-state turnover and body pool of ascorbic acid in man. Am. J. Clin. Nutr., *32*:530–539, 1979.)

Table 22–4. Steady-State Trough Plasma Ascorbic Acid Concentrations in Healthy Adults Taking Various Doses of the Vitamin Twice Daily for 3 to 4 Weeks[a]

GROUP	PLASMA ASCORBIC ACID CONCENTRATION[b] (mg/L)
1. No supplementary dose, 6 subjects. Daily dietary intake of 50–75 mg expected.	9 ± 0.6[c]
2. 1 to 3 g/day, 11 subjects.	15.4 ± 1.6[d]
3. 8 to 12 g/day, 6 subjects.	19.5 ± 2.0[d]

[a]Adapted from Yew, M.-L.S.: Megadose vitamin C supplementation and ascorbic acid and dehydroascorbic acid levels in plasma and lymphocytes. Nutr. Rep. Intern., 30:597–601, 1984.
[b]Blood sampled in the morning before the next dose.
[c]Mean ± standard error of the mean.
[d]Significantly different from group 1.

Renal clearance may also show concentration dependence when the drug (1) produces changes in pH and its tubular reabsorption is pH-dependent, e.g., salicylate; (2) is a diuretic and renal passive clearance is flow-dependent, e.g., theophylline; or (3) causes nephrotoxicity, e.g., an aminoglycoside. The mechanisms of the last two drugs are also time-dependent. Theophylline produces diuresis soon after its administration, but this effect, and consequently its renal clearance, decrease with time. The nephrotoxic effect of

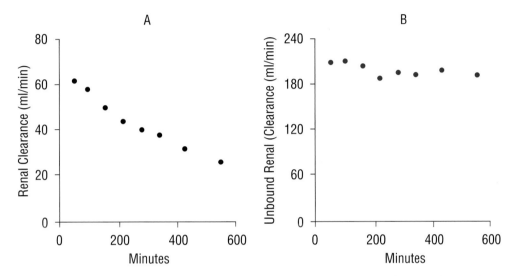

Fig. 22–10. *A*, The renal clearance of disopyramide in an individual subject shows changes with time after a single 1.5-mg/kg i.v. dose. *B*, Unbound renal clearance, on the other hand, does not appear to change over the corresponding time period. The initial plasma concentrations were in the range of 2 to 4 mg/L. These total concentrations are expected to produce nonlinear binding to α_1-acid glycoprotein, the protein to which this drug primarily binds in plasma (see Chap. 10, Distribution) (1 mg/L = 2.9 μM). (Modified from Giacomini, K.M., Swezey, S.E., Turner-Tamiyasu, K., and Blaschke, T.F.: The effect of saturable binding to plasma proteins on the pharmacokinetic properties of disopyramide. J. Pharmacokinet. Biopharm., *10*:1–14, 1982.)

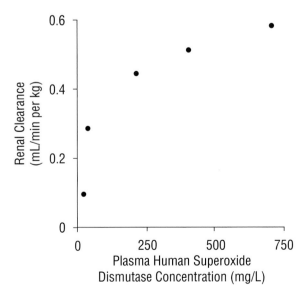

Fig. 22–11. Mean renal clearance of recombinant human superoxide dismutase increases at higher plasma concentrations after an i.v. dose of 45 mg/kg in eight subjects. The experimental drug is filtered in the glomerulus and partially metabolized by tubular cells. At higher plasma concentrations, the rate of filtration exceeds the ability of the tubular cells to absorb and metabolize the drug (1 mg/L = 0.031 μM). (Modified from Tsao, C., Greene, P., Odlind, B., and Brater, D.C.: Pharmacokinetics of recombinant human superoxide dismutase in healthy volunteers. Clin. Pharmacol. Ther., *50*:713–720, 1991.)

aminoglycosides, on the other hand, develops with dose and duration of exposure to the drug.

CAPACITY-LIMITED METABOLISM

Perhaps the most dramatic dose-dependent kinetic mechanism is that of *capacity-limited metabolism,* a characteristic typical of enzymatic reactions. Recall from Chap. 11 (Eq. 11) that

$$\text{Rate of metabolism} = \frac{Vm \cdot Cu}{Km + Cu} \qquad\qquad 5$$

for a drug showing saturable Michaelis-Menten kinetics. Also, recall that in this case

$$\text{Unbound metabolic clearance} = \frac{Vm}{Km + Cu} \qquad\qquad 6$$

The social and therapeutic consequences of Michaelis-Menten kinetics are now explored with two examples, alcohol and phenytoin.

Alcohol

At doses usually consumed, the metabolism of alcohol is capacity-limited. Although metabolized by both alcohol dehydrogenase and cytochrome P450-2E1, the elimination kinetics of alcohol has been approximated by a Michaelis-Menten model of a single enzyme. This simplified kinetic model is subsequently presented.

The maximum rate of metabolism, Vm, and the Michaelis constant, Km, are approximately 10 g/hr and 100 mg/L, respectively. The pharmacologic effects of alcohol, which does not bind to plasma proteins, become apparent when the plasma concentration is about 200 mg/L, concentrations above 5000 mg/L are potentially lethal. Thus, the concentration range in which alcohol exerts its pharmacologic effects is well above its Km.

Table 22–5 shows the calculated rate of metabolism and clearance of alcohol as a function of the concentration at the metabolic site. Note that rate of metabolism of alcohol is essentially constant, zero-order, and close to Vm throughout the range of concentrations associated with activity. Accordingly, clearance decreases at high concentrations. At low concentrations, the intrinsic clearance (Vm/Km) approaches 100 L/hr or 1.6 L/min, a value

Table 22-5. Calculated Rate of Metabolism and Clearance of Alcohol as a Function of the Concentration at the Metabolic Site

CONCENTRATION AT SITE (mg/L)	RATE OF METABOLISM[a] (g/hr)	CLEARANCE[b] (L/hr)
7000	9.9	1.4
5000	9.8	2.0
3000	9.7	3.2
1000	9.1	9.1
500	8.3	17
200	6.7	33
100	5.0	50
50	3.3	67
10	0.91	91

[a]Rate of metabolism = $Vm \cdot Cu/(Km + Cu)$; Vm = 10 g/hr, Km = 100 mg/L.
[b]Clearance = $Vm/(Km + Cu)$.

in excess of hepatic blood flow. Thus, at very low concentrations, the extraction ratio is sufficiently high so that the rate of metabolism is partially limited by hepatic perfusion. Under these conditions oral bioavailability is expected to be reduced.

The consequences of zero-order elimination can be dramatic. The usual-size drink, 45 mL, of 40% v/v whiskey contains about 18 mL, or 14 g, of alcohol. Drinking this quantity of alcohol each hour exceeds the eliminating capacity of the body. Consequently, alcohol accumulates until ultimately either coma or death intervenes.

Alcohol distributes evenly throughout total body water; its volume of distribution is therefore 42 L. Accordingly, approximately 200 g of alcohol are needed in the body to achieve a concentration, about 5000 mg/L, that can produce coma or, occasionally, death. But, since the rate of ingestion, 14 g/hr, exceeds the rate of metabolism, 10 g/hr, by only 4 g/hr, this rate of drinking must be maintained for at least 2 days (a total of 48 drinks) to accumulate 200 g of alcohol. This degree of accrual can occur within 5 hr (20 drinks) when four drinks are consumed every hour, because this rate of ingestion, 56 g/hr, exceeds the maximum metabolic capacity by 46 g/hr.

If the rate of ingestion is reduced to one-half drink (or 7 g/hr), then, with respect to the effect of alcohol, one can drink with virtual impunity as now shown. By definition, of steady state, rate of elimination matches rate of administration (or input), R_o.

$$R_o = \frac{Vm \cdot Cu_{ss}}{Km + Cu_{ss}} \qquad 7$$

or on rearrangement

$$Cu_{ss} = \frac{Km \cdot R_o}{Vm - R_o} \qquad 8$$

Using the previously given values for Km and Vm and an R_o value of 7 g/hr, the plateau concentration of alcohol is 230 mg/L, which produced only a marginal effect.

Reflect on the calculations above. Chronically imbibing one-half a drink of whiskey per hour produces little or no effect, but taking one drink per hour becomes lethal. There can be no standard dosage regimen to maintain the effects of alcohol. Maintenance of effect requires titration of dosage to the effect itself.

The consequence of capacity-limited metabolism on the time-course of a drug in the body when input rate is changed is also demonstrated with alcohol. When alcohol is administered 10 min after ingesting water, light cream, or a glucose solution (80 g/240 mL), the plasma concentration-time profiles differ profoundly (Fig. 22–12). Compared to water, administration of light cream and 33% glucose, foods that delay gastric emptying, lower both AUC and peak concentration and increase time to reach the peak. These observations can be explained by the nearly zero-order metabolism of alcohol. To emphasize the point, assume that both elimination and input are strictly zero-order, as shown in Fig. 22–13. Decreasing the input rate, for a given total dose administered, lowers AUC and peak concentration as well as increases the peak time. Clearly, oral bioavailability in the presence of zero-order elimination and variable input rates cannot be assessed by conventional area ratio methods.

Phenytoin

Therapeutic problems encountered with capacity-limited metabolism are classically exemplified by phenytoin. Typical Vm and Km values of this drug are 500 mg/day and 0.4 mg/L, although the values vary widely. The value of Km is usually expressed in terms of

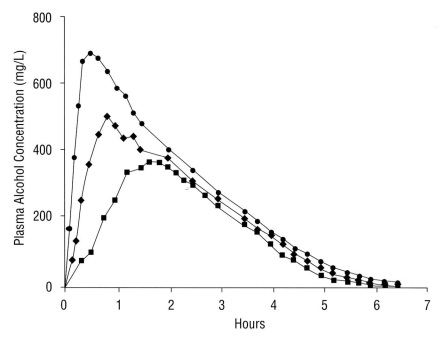

Fig. 22–12. A decrease in the absorption rate of alcohol, produced by slowing gastric emptying, causes peak concentrations and *AUC* to decrease and time to reach the peak to increase. The effect differs from that expected of first-order kinetics by the observed decrease in *AUC*. This observation is explained by a constant rate of elimination at almost all concentrations, as illustrated schematically in Fig. 22–13. Alcohol, 45 mL of 95% ethanol in 105 mL of orange juice, was administered 10 min after 240 mL of tap water (●); 240 mL of light cream (◆); or 240 mL of a 33% glucose solution (■) (1 mg/L = 22.0 μM). (Redrawn from data of Sedman, A.J., Wilkinson, P.K., Sakmar, E., Weidler, D.J., and Wagner, J.G.: Food effects on absorption and metabolism of alcohol. Reprinted by permission, from Journal of Studies on Alcohol, Vol. 37, pp. 1197–1214, 1976. Copyright by Journal of Studies on Alcohol, Inc., Rutgers Center of Alcohol Studies, New Brunswick, NJ 08903.)

Fig. 22–13. As a consequence of zero-order elimination, the plasma concentrations at the end of a 50-g dose of a drug by bolus injection (A) and constant-rate infusions of 1- (B), 2- (C), and 3- (D) hr durations are quite different from those expected with first-order kinetics. The amount in the body at the end of each infusion is the difference between dose and amount lost during the infusion period. Consequently, the concentration at the end of each of the infusions is the same as that expected at that time following the i.v. bolus dose. Note that the slower the input rate, the smaller is *AUC* and the lower is peak concentration. The time to peak is, of course, increased. Furthermore, if the dose had been infused over a 5-hr period, i.e., at 10 g/hr, output would have matched input and there would have been no *AUC* in this hypothetical example.

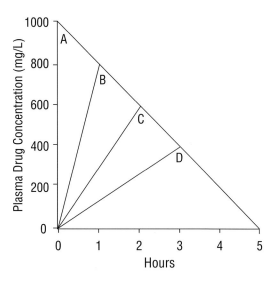

total, rather than unbound, concentration. Since fu is typically 0.1, the apparent Km for total concentration, Km', is equal to 4 mg/L.

Plateau. Perhaps the most striking consequence of the kinetics of this drug is the relationship observed between steady-state plasma concentration and rate of administration, as shown in Fig. 22–14. A greatly disproportionate increase in concentration is observed in, and above, the therapeutic concentration range, 10 to 20 mg/L. As a result, the difference between the daily dose giving ineffective therapeutic concentrations, less than 10 mg/L, and that producing potentially toxic concentrations, above 20 mg/L, is narrow.

The observed increase in concentration can be explained by rearrangement of Eq. 8.

$$\frac{Cu_{ss}}{Km} = \frac{C_{ss}}{Km'} = \frac{R_o}{Vm - R_o} \qquad 9$$

The consequences of Michaelis-Menten metabolism result when either the desired steady-state unbound concentration is above Km (Km' for total concentration) or the rate of administration required to achieve these concentrations approaches Vm.

Because of its kinetics, only small changes in phenytoin input caused, for example, by a change in salt form (acid and sodium salt are used) or in bioavailability can produce relatively large changes in the steady-state concentration. To illustrate this point, consider a male patient with Km' and Vm values of 3 mg/L and 425 mg/day, respectively, and who has an average steady-state concentration of 12 mg/L when taking 200 mg orally every 12 hr. On switching from his current dosage form (bioavailability = 0.85) to one with a bioavailability of 0.95, it is seen, by setting $R_o = F \cdot D/\tau$ in Eq. 9, that the average steady-state concentration is expected to increase to 25 mg/L. Thus, a minor change in bioavailability (0.85 to 0.95) causes a major change (12 to 25) in the steady-state concentration when the dosing rate approaches the Vm value.

Time to Plateau. Because of capacity-limited metabolism, the time to reach steady state varies with the rate of administration. Figure 22–15 shows the approach to plateau during each of four dosing rates, which increase by small increments from 300 to 425 mg/day, in a patient with typical Vm and Km' values. Note that the time to reach 90% of plateau increases progressively with the rate of administration. These disproportionate changes in the steady-state concentration and the time required to reach them are major problems in optimally dosing phenytoin and interpreting its concentrations. Even though

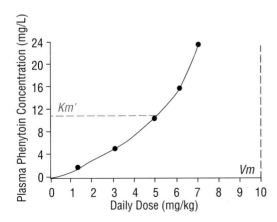

Fig. 22–14. The steady-state plasma phenytoin concentration increases disproportionately with rate of administration (given twice daily) of phenytoin, a drug that is virtually eliminated by a single metabolic pathway, that exhibits typical Michaelis-Menten enzyme kinetics. The estimated Vm, the maximum rate of metabolism, and Km', the total plasma concentration at which the rate is half of the maximum (colored line), are shown. All the data were obtained in the same individual whose Km' and Vm values are considerably higher than the typical ones of 4 mg/L and 7 mg/kg/day. (1 mg/L = 4.0 µM.) (Adapted from Martin, E., Tozer, T.N., Sheiner, L.B., and Riegelman, S.: The clinical pharmacokinetics of phenytoin. J. Pharmacokinet. Biopharm., 5:579–596, 1977. Reproduced with permission of Plenum Publishing Corp.)

the approach to plateau is usually somewhat quicker on reducing doses than on increasing them, it can still take a long time, as shown in Fig. 22–16.

Because clearance, and hence half-life, are functions of the plasma concentration, the meanings of these parameters are lost when capacity-limited metabolism occurs. For this reason, these parameters should not be used for predicting or summarizing the kinetics of drugs showing this kind of behavior. The parameters of choice are those of the appropriate nonlinear model (*Km* and *Vm* for Michaelis-Menten kinetics and *V*).

Alterations in Metabolism. Another therapeutically important facet of the kinetics of phenytoin is altered metabolism brought about by other drugs and disease states. Either *Km'* or *Vm* can be altered, but the effect on plasma concentration is different. From Eq. 9 it can be seen that the phenytoin concentration at steady state is directly proportional to *Km'*. Thus, a condition such as competitive inhibition of metabolism, which affects the *Km'* value, produces corresponding changes in the steady-state phenytoin concentration.

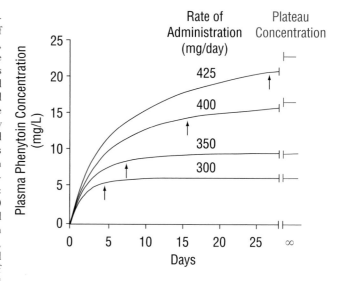

Fig. 22–15. Following administration (i.v. infusion is simulated) of phenytoin at constant rates of 300, 350, 400, and 425 mg/day, the plasma concentration approaches steady-state values of 6, 9.3, 16, and 22.7 mg/L, respectively (colored lines). Not only are the steady-state concentrations disproportionately increased, but so is the time required to approach the plateau. The arrows indicate the time required to reach 90% of the plateau value. The following parameter values were used: *Km'*, 4 mg/L; *Vm*, 500 mg/day; *V*, 50 L (1 mg/L = 4.0 µM). (Reproduced by permission of publisher. Redrawn from Winter, M.E., and Tozer, T.N., Phenytoin, Chap. 25, in Applied Pharmacokinetics: Principles of Therapeutic Drug Monitoring, 3rd edition, edited by W.E. Evans, J.J. Schentag, and W.J. Jusko, published by Applied Therapeutics, Inc., Spokane, Washington, 1992.)

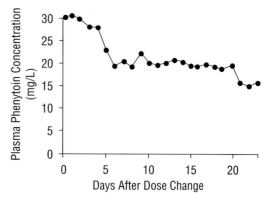

Fig. 22–16. On decreasing the daily dose from 250 to 200 mg/day, the plasma phenytoin concentration (obtained daily just before the morning dose) declines slowly toward a new steady state. Note that a 20% reduction in the daily dose leads to a 50% decrease in the concentration at steady state (the concentration stabilized after Day 23) (1 mg/L = 4.0 µM). (Redrawn from Theodore, W.H., Qu, Z.-P., Tsay, J.-Y., Pitlick, W., and Porter, R.J.: Phenytoin: The pseudosteady-state phenomenon. Clin. Pharmacol. Ther., 35:822–825, 1984. Reproduced with permission of C.V. Mosby.)

For example, when cimetidine inhibits phenytoin metabolism, thereby increasing Km' from 4 to 6 mg/L, the steady-state unbound and total phenytoin concentrations are expected to increase by 50% as well.

In contrast, either an increase in Vm, brought about by enzyme induction, or a decrease in Vm, caused by the presence of hepatic cirrhosis, is expected to produce disproportionate change in the steady-state phenytoin concentration. This is seen by taking the ratio of the two different concentrations, $Cu_{ss,1}$ and $Cu_{ss,2}$ (Eq. 9), that result from the unaltered, Vm_1, and altered, Vm_2, values, respectively.

$$\frac{Cu_{ss,2}}{Cu_{ss,1}} = \frac{Vm_1 - R_o}{Vm_2 - R_o} \qquad\qquad 10$$

For example, when R_o = 300 mg/day, Vm_1 = 500 mg/day, and Vm_2 = 400 mg/day, the unbound concentration at steady state is doubled, $Cu_{ss,2}/Cu_{ss,1}$ = 2. If Vm_2 is 600 mg/day, the ratio is 0.67. Thus, a 20% decrease in Vm doubles the steady-state concentration; whereas a 20% increase in Vm reduces the steady-state concentration by 33%. Note that a Vm of 300 mg/day results in a concentration approaching infinity, and that with a Vm below 300 mg/day, steady state can never be achieved. The input rate would then always exceed Vm, and Eqs. 5 to 10 would not be applicable.

Alcohol and phenytoin represent extreme cases in that almost all the elimination of each drug occurs by a single saturable pathway. More commonly, a drug is metabolized by several pathways, and only one or two of them approaches saturation. Then, saturation has less effect on total clearance. The extent of the effect depends on fm, the fraction of drug eliminated by the saturable pathway at low drug concentrations. Only if fm is 0.5, or greater, under nonsaturating conditions is total clearance materially affected by saturation of the pathway. Examples of drugs in this category include propranolol, theophylline, and salicylic acid.

TIME-DEPENDENT DISPOSITION

The study of changes in response to drug administration or kinetics with time of day, month, or year is an area called *chronopharmacology*. The pharmacokinetic component is *time-dependent kinetics* or *chronopharmacokinetics*. Carbamazepine shows time dependence in its disposition (Chap. 23, p. 430). The decrease in its peak concentration on repetitive oral administration indicates that either oral bioavailability decreases or clearance increases with time. The latter has been shown to explain the observation caused by carbamazepine inducing its own metabolism. This *autoinduction* is also dose- and concentration-dependent, a property common to many time-dependent processes.

Autoinduction has a number of therapeutic consequences. It affects the time to achieve steady state and limits one's ability to use information from a single dose to predict kinetics after repeated doses or continuous administration. Furthermore, it may be associated with the induction of metabolism (same enzymatic pathway) of coadministered drugs, producing a drug interaction.

Although enzyme induction is perhaps the most common cause of time-dependent kinetics, there are many other reasons for this behavior. For example, diurnal variations in renal function, urine pH, α_1-acid glycoprotein concentration, gastrointestinal physiology (food and drink), and cardiac output all occur. Chronic effects of a drug on its own renal and hepatic elimination have also been seen, as previously mentioned.

Aminoglycosides can produce renal toxicity with chronic administration. Because these antibiotics are primarily eliminated by renal excretion, a diminishing renal function with time may cause greater drug accumulation and therefore more toxicity. There is clearly a need to monitor therapy and to limit the duration of therapy, especially in patients who already have compromised renal function.

An example of diurnal changes in drug absorption and disposition is shown in Fig. 22–17. Median data are shown (because of skewed distribution of values) for eight subjects who received an oral 80-mg dose of verapamil at various times during the day. Note that administration in the evening produces a lower peak drug concentration and, as such, may produce less effect than does administration in the morning.

Food is a major cause of diurnal variations. Gastric emptying is slowed or delayed by food (see Fig. 9–7), often resulting in a decrease in the peak concentration and an increase in the time of its occurrence following a single dose.

NONLINEAR METABOLITE FORMATION OR ELIMINATION

Nonlinear formation or elimination of a metabolite is of therapeutic interest when it accounts for some or all of either the therapeutic response, or toxicity, or both. The consequences of such nonlinearities depend on the cause and the site of occurrence. At the end of Chap. 21, the ratio of AUC values for metabolite and drug was explored as a means of evaluating changes in drug metabolism from one occasion to another. The ratios can also be used to assess sources of dose dependence.

Table 22–6 lists kinetic changes expected for a drug that forms two sequential metabolites following a single i.v. dose. Using the principles given in Chap. 21, the consequences of capacity-limited metabolism at each of the sites in the metabolic scheme can be assessed. For a compound with nonlinear metabolism, AUC increases with respect to the dose administered; the AUC of the product of the nonlinear pathway decreases with respect to the AUC of its precursor. If the site of nonlinearity involves the first of three consecutive steps, the ratio of areas of the last two products remains constant, though both areas may be decreased with respect to the dose given.

Fig. 22–17. Median plasma verapamil concentration-time profiles for eight subjects, each given a single 80-mg tablet of drug at the following times: 4:00 A.M. (▲); 8:00 A.M. (○); noon (□); 4:00 P.M. (△); 8:00 P.M. (●), and midnight (■). Food was withheld 2 hr before to 2 hr after drug administration, as food is known to affect verapamil absorption. To minimize a delay in esophageal transit, subjects took the tablets while standing and remained so for 15 min. The kinetics of the drug appears to change with the time of administration during the day. Factors other than food and posture may be responsible, e.g., changes in hepatic blood flow (verapamil has a high hepatic extraction ratio), enzyme activity, or protein binding (1 mg/L = 2.2 μM). (From Hla, K.K., Latham, A.N., and Henry, J.A.: Influence of time of administration on verapamil pharmacokinetics. Clin. Pharmacol. Ther., 51:366–370, 1992.)

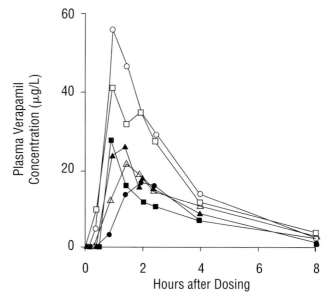

The general tendencies for changes in steady-state concentrations following chronic dosing are the same as those for *AUC* after a single dose. Here, however, the compound (drug or metabolite) with capacity-limited metabolism may not reach steady state if it is formed at a rate that exceeds its Vm.

Dose-dependence is expected in the degree of autoinduction for drugs that undergo this behavior. Such is observed with carbamazepine. As shown in Fig. 22–18A, the steady-state concentration of carbamazepine fails to increase in direct proportion to daily dose ($C_{ss,av}/(D/\tau)$ decreases). Furthermore, the ratio of the steady-state concentrations of the metabolite carbamazepine-10,11-epoxide and carbamazepine increase with dose (Fig. 22–18B). These results demonstrate nonlinearity in the formation of the metabolite. The directions of the changes suggest that formation clearance of the epoxide is increased.

RECOGNITION OF NONLINEARITIES

Nonlinearities are often apparent in graphic and tabular presentations of data. The interpretation of such kinetic behavior often requires a methodical analysis of the information. This analysis may be accomplished using the following steps:

1. Compare the observation to that expected for linear kinetics.
2. Identify the kinetic parameter(s) that appear(s) to be altered and the direction of the change.
3. Determine the primary pharmacokinetic parameter(s) CL_H, CL_R, V, ka, and F that appear to be affected. Also evaluate if fu is altered.
4. Consider the mechanism(s) consistent with the changes observed.

Urinary Recovery

Nonlinearities are often first identified from recovery of drug and metabolites in urine. This is the case for salicylic acid, as shown in Table 22–7.

Analysis

Step 1. Dose dependence in salicylic acid is apparent from changes in the fraction of a single oral dose recovered as unchanged drug and as the metabolites, salicyluric acid and glucuronide conjugates. With linear kinetics, the fraction of each compound recovered remains the same regardless of dose.

Table 22–6.   Consequences of Capacity-Limited Processes in the Sequential Metabolism of a Drug Given in a Single Dose

MODEL	$\dfrac{AUC}{DOSE}$	$\dfrac{AUC(m_1)}{AUC}$	$\dfrac{AUC(m_2)}{AUC(m_1)}$
1. $D \rightarrow M_1 \rightarrow M_2 \rightarrow$ $\qquad\downarrow$	$\leftrightarrow^a$	$\leftrightarrow$	$\leftrightarrow$
2. $D \Rightarrow^b M_1 \rightarrow M_2 \rightarrow$ $\qquad\downarrow$	$\uparrow^c$	$\downarrow$	$\leftrightarrow$
3. $D \rightarrow M_1 \Rightarrow M_2 \rightarrow$ $\qquad\downarrow$	$\leftrightarrow$	$\uparrow$	$\downarrow$
4. $D \rightarrow M_1 \rightarrow M_2 \Rightarrow$ $\qquad\downarrow$	$\leftrightarrow$	$\leftrightarrow$	$\uparrow$
5. $D \rightarrow M_1 \rightarrow M_2 \rightarrow$ $\qquad\Downarrow$	$\uparrow^c$	$\leftrightarrow$	$\rightarrow$

$^a\leftrightarrow$, little or no change; $\uparrow$, increase; $\downarrow$, decrease on increasing the dose.
$^b\Rightarrow$, capacity-limited metabolism of Michaelis-Menten type.
^{c}The affected pathway is the major route of elimination at nonsaturating doses. Otherwise, little change is expected.

Fig. 22–18. *A*, The steady-state concentration of carbamazepine fails to increase in direct proportion to the daily dose, evidence of nonlinear kinetics. *B*, The ratio of the concentrations of the metabolite, carbamazepine-10,11-epoxide, and carbamazepine increase with dosing rate. These observations indicate that either the clearance of formation increases or the clearance of elimination of the epoxide decreases at higher dosing rates. The former, a consequence of dose-dependent autoinduction of metabolite formation, is the explanation. Each point in both graphs is the mean of data from 77 patients. (Carbamazepine: 1 mg/L = 4.2 μM; carbamazepine 10,11-epoxide: 1 mg/L = 4.0 μM.) (Adapted from Kudriakova, T.B., Sirotsa L.A., Rozova, G.I., and Gorkov, V.A.: Autoinduction and steady-state pharmacokinetics of carbamazepine and its major metabolites. Br. J. Clin. Pharmacol., *33*:611–615, 1992.)

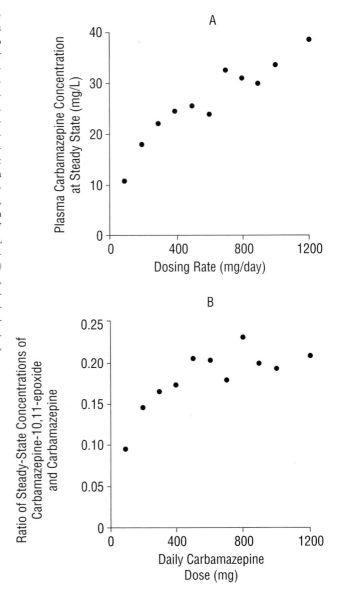

Table 22-7.   Urinary Recovery of Salicylic Acid and its Metabolites as a Percent of a Single Oral Dose[a]

DOSE (mg)	SALICYLIC ACID	SALICYLURIC ACID	SALICYL PHENOLIC AND ACYL GLUCURONIDES
192	3	83	17
767	5	70	24
1533	17	59	24
3000	14	50	30

[a]Dose and recovery expressed in equivalents of salicylic acid. (Adapted from Levy, G.: Pharmacokinetics of salicylate elimination in man. J. Pharm. Sci., *54*:959–967, 1965.)

Steps 2 to 4. The increased percent recovered as unchanged drug on increasing dose could be explained by an increased bioavailability, an increased renal clearance, or a capacity limitation in its metabolism. This is seen from the relationships $Ae_\infty/Dose = fe \cdot F$ and $fe = CL_R/(CL_R + CL_{NR})$. Without further information, these possibilities cannot be distinguished. The decreased recovery of the major metabolite, salicyluric acid, and the nearly complete total recovery (as drug and metabolites) at all of the doses suggest that increased bioavailability may not be the explanation (see Chap. 21). Increased bioavailability would increase metabolite recovery as well, which was not the case.

Concentration-Time Profile

Figure 22–19 is a semilogarithmic plot of plasma salicylic acid concentration with time after a single 3-g oral dose.

Analysis

Step 1. The slope of the decline is greater at low than at high concentrations. When linear kinetics operates, there is either no change in slope or a greater slope at early times while distribution is occurring (Chap. 19, Distribution Kinetics).

Step 2. The half-life shortens as time passes or as concentration declines.

Step 3. It appears that either CL increases or V decreases with time or with falling concentration.

Step 4. From the dose and maximum concentration (around 200 mg/L) and the conclusion based on urinary data (and independent i.v. data) that salicylic acid is totally absorbed after oral administration, the volume of distribution is estimated to be about 15 L. Being so small, V is unlikely to decrease much with either time or decreasing concentration. An increase in CL with time or at lower concentrations would occur if elimination of salicylic acid is capacity-limited. The data in Table 22–7 indicate that salicylic acid is extensively

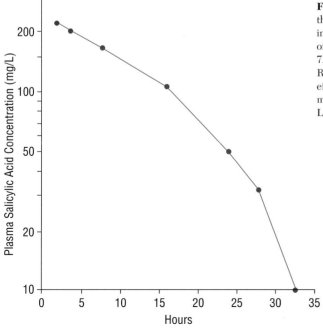

Fig. 22–19. Semilogarithmic plot of the plasma concentration of salicylic acid in a subject following a single oral dose of 3 g of sodium salicylate (1 mg/L = 7.2 μM). (Adapted from data in Salassa, R.M., Bollman, J.L., and Dry, T.J.: The effect of para-aminobenzoic acid on the metabolism and excretion of salicylate. J. Lab. Clin. Med., 33:1393–1401, 1948.)

converted to several metabolites. However, the pronounced increase in fraction excreted as unchanged salicylic acid with increasing dose (Table 22–7) implies that saturability of a major metabolic pathway is likely at the 3-g dose level.

Protein Binding Data

The incorporation of binding data further clarifies the nature of nonlinearities present, as shown in Fig. 22–20.

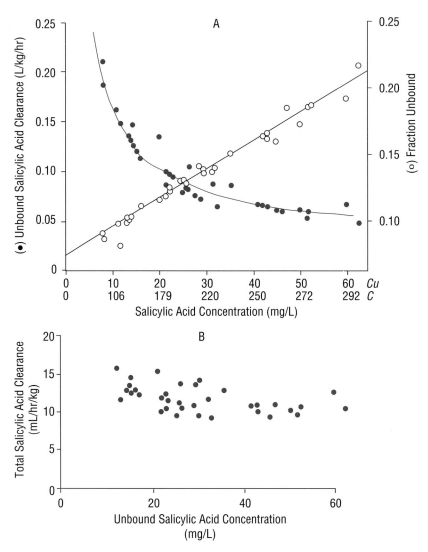

Fig. 22–20. *A,* The clearance of unbound drug (●, colored line), determined under steady-state conditions, and the fraction unbound in plasma (○) vary inversely with each other as the salicylic acid concentration is increased. The corresponding total plasma concentrations are superimposed on the linear scale of the unbound drug concentration (1 mg/L = 7.2 µM). (Redrawn from Furst, D.E., Tozer, T.N., and Melmon, K.L.: Salicylate clearance: The result of protein binding and metabolism. Clin. Pharmacol. Ther., 26:380–389, 1979. Reproduced with permission of C.V. Mosby.) *B,* The total clearance of salicylic acid, determined under steady-state conditions, remains essentially constant within the range of therapeutic concentrations; a fortuitous consequence of the essentially equivalent and opposing effects of saturable plasma protein binding and saturable metabolism (1 mg/L = 7.2 µM).

Analysis

Step 1. As observed in Fig. 22–20A, *fu* increases with increasing concentration in the antirheumatic therapeutic range, 100 to 300 mg/L, indicating nonlinearity of salicylic acid binding to plasma proteins. Nonlinearity in *CLu* is also uncovered. As shown in Fig. 22–20B, salicylic acid has a low clearance even at low concentrations. As such, *CLu* should remain constant if elimination processes are unaffected by the concentration (dose) of salicylic acid.

Steps 2–3. The parameters affected are identified in this case, *fu* and *CLu*.

Step 4. The mechanisms involved appear to be saturable binding to plasma proteins and some form of capacity-limited elimination. From the additional information in Table 22–7 and Fig. 22–19, the capacity limitation must lie with metabolism.

Interestingly, total clearance is relatively constant throughout the therapeutic range of salicylic acid (*Cu* between 10 and 60 mg/L). This is a consequence of the opposing tendencies of the two forms of nonlinearity. Clearance decreases with concentration because of capacity-limited metabolism. Saturable binding, on the other hand, tends to increase clearance at higher concentrations, $CL = fu \cdot CLu$. The decrease in unbound clearance, the consequence of saturability in two major metabolic pathways of salicylic acid (formation of salicyluric acid and salicyl phenolic glucuronide) leads to a disproportionate increase in unbound concentration with increasing dosing rate (Fig. 22–21). Further information on the specific nonlinear metabolic pathways requires isolating the metabolic pathways. This has been accomplished by comparing the rates of urinary excretion of each metabolite to the amount of salicylic acid in the body, a procedure analogous to the determination of renal clearance. The method is applicable if the rate of excretion of metabolite equals its rate of formation, as is the case for salicylic acid after a single dose and for all drugs under steady-state conditions.

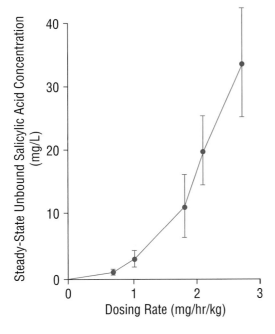

Fig. 22–21. The steady-state unbound concentration of salicylic acid in plasma (mean ± SD) increases disproportionately with the dosing rate of aspirin. Aspirin is completely converted to the measured metabolite, salicylic acid. The disproportionate increase reflects the saturability of two of salicylic acid's major pathways of elimination, formation of salicyl phenolic glucuronide and salicyluric acid (1 mg/L = 7.2 µM). (Redrawn from Tozer, T.N., Tang-Liu, D.D.-S., and Riegelman, S.: Linear vs. nonlinear kinetics. In Topics in Pharmaceutical Sciences. Edited by D. Breimer and P. Speiser. New York, Elsevier, 1981, pp. 3–17.)

THERAPEUTIC CONSEQUENCES

The therapeutic consequences of dose-dependent kinetics are perhaps best considered under steady-state conditions. Here, dose dependence in rate-time profile of absorption is of little or no consequence unless bioavailability (extent) is also altered. Alterations in bioavailability are important in that unbound concentration and amount in the body at steady state may change disproportionately on changing dose. Conditions that cause dose dependence in bioavailability may also produce increased variability in this parameter at the same dose. For example, consider two drugs, a dissolution rate-limited one, such as griseofulvin, and one that is highly extracted on passing across the gastrointestinal membranes or through the liver, such as alprenolol. Changes in gastric emptying and in other physiologic factors can produce large variations in the bioavailability of these drugs. The effect of rapid gastric emptying may be a decrease in bioavailability of griseofulvin because of less time for mixing and dissolution but an increase in bioavailability of alprenolol because of saturability in intestinal and hepatic metabolism.

Clinically, the most dramatic source of dose dependence is capacity-limited metabolism. Only small changes in bioavailability may produce large changes in the steady-state concentration. Under these conditions, careful titration of an individual patient's dosage requirement is needed, especially if the drug has a narrow therapeutic index. Moreover, this source of dose-dependence also produces large interpatient variability in steady-state concentration, as observed for phenytoin in Fig. 1–5.

Time-dependent kinetics is perhaps best typified by autoinduction. Another cause is decreased renal function on continued administration of a nephrotoxic drug. If the drug is primarily renally eliminated, the therapeutic consequence of the latter cause is clear and opposite to that of autoinduction.

In general, if two drugs are equivalent in all respects except for one showing either a dose- or time-dependent kinetic behavior, then the one showing linear kinetics is the drug of choice.

STUDY PROBLEMS

(Answers to Study Problems are in Appendix II.)

1. Circle the number(s) of the one or more *correct* answers to each of the following multiple-choice questions. Briefly discuss those answers that may be ambiguous (situations in which the statement may be true or false).
   a. Capacity-limited metabolism of a drug is associated with:
      1. A less than proportional increase in the steady-state plasma concentration on increasing the total daily dose.
      2. An apparent half-life that is longer at low than at high concentrations.
      3. A decrease in the rate of metabolism as the amount of drug in the body is increased.
      4. All of the above.
      5. None of the above.
   b. A mean steady-state plasma concentration obtained after 30 doses that is much higher than that predicted from the value of clearance obtained after a single dose suggests that:
      1. Induction has occurred.
      2. The volume of distribution has decreased.
      3. A metabolite may be acting as an inhibitor of drug elimination.
      4. None of the above.

c. The following steady-state plasma drug concentrations have been observed in a subject following various constant daily oral dosages:

DOSING RATE (mg/day)	STEADY-STATE PLASMA CONCENTRATION (mg/L)
500	45
1000	56
1500	62

These data are consistent with and may be explained by:
1. Decreased bioavailability
2. Increased clearance
3. Decreased plasma protein binding
4. Increased volume of distribution
on increasing the dosing rate.

d. The total cumulative amounts of drug collected in the urine within 48 hours (essentially Ae_∞) following various single oral doses of a drug, administered on separate occasions, are shown below.

DOSE (mg)	AMOUNT EXCRETED UNCHANGED IN 48 HR (mg)
50	1.1
100	2.8
200	9.0

These data are consistent with and may be explained by:
1. Saturable active transport in the wall of the gastrointestinal tract
2. Saturable first-pass metabolism
3. Saturable active renal tubular secretion
4. Saturable active renal tubular reabsorption

2. Define *saturable first-pass hepatic metabolism*, and describe how this dose-dependent kinetic behavior can be seen after oral administration without observing it after an equivalent i.v. bolus dose.

3. The steady-state plasma concentration of phenylbutazone relative to the dose administered decreased when given orally at anti-inflammatory doses of 200 to 400 mg/day (Fig. 22–22). The drug is primarily bound to albumin.
   a. Draw a line on both graphs of Fig. 22–22 (bottom of p. 420) showing the relationships expected when kinetics are linear.
   b. Suggest an explanation for the observations, given the additional information that only negligible amounts of phenylbutazone appear in urine and feces at all doses examined.

4. For *each* of the tables on the top of p. 420, indicate *all* of the possibilities in the following list that might explain the dose-dependent kinetics observed for each drug.

List of Explanations

   I. Saturable hepatic metabolism
  II. Saturable renal tubular reabsorption
 III. Saturable renal active secretion
  IV. Saturable plasma protein binding with extraction ratio approaching one in organs of elimination
   V. Saturable plasma protein binding with extraction ratio approaching zero in organs of elimination
  VI. Saturable metabolism during first pass of drug through the intestines or the liver
 VII. Saturable gastrointestinal transport

a.
Table 22-8.

Single oral dose (mg)	300	600	900
Area under blood concentration-time curve (mg·hr/L)	3	10	19

b.
Table 22-9.

Rate of i.v. infusion (mg/hr)	5	10	15
Steady-state plasma concentration (mg/L)	2	6.5	14

c.
Table 22-10.   One-Compartment Drug

Single i.v. dose (mg)	50	100	200	400
Initial blood concentration (mg/L)	1.1	2.0	4.3	8.7
Area under blood concentration-time curve (mg·hr/L)	20	55	160	410

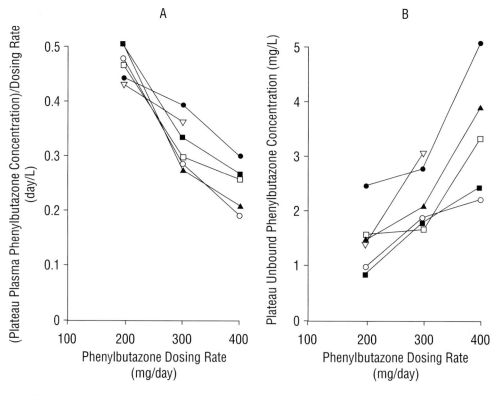

Fig. 22–22. Conditions at plateau for phenylbutazone. Events were monitored in patients receiving increasing daily doses (200 to 400 mg); each dose was maintained for a minimum of 3 weeks. Displayed are the total plasma concentration, normalized to the daily dose administered (A), and the unbound concentration (B) at plateau. Each symbol corresponds to data from one patient (1 mg/L = 3.2 µM). (Redrawn from Higham, C., Aarons, L.J., Holt, P.J.L., Lynch, M., and Rowland, M.: A chronic dose-ranging study of the pharmacokinetics of phenylbutazone in rheumatoid arthritic patients. Br. J. Clin. Pharmacol., 12:123–129, 1981. Reproduced with permission of Blackwell Scientific Publications.)

5. The relationship between glucose urinary excretion rate and its plasma concentration in a healthy individual is displayed in Table 22–11. Prepare a graph of glucose renal clearance in milliliters per minute as a function of its plasma concentration, and briefly explain the observation.

Table 22–11.　Glucose Excretion Rate at Various Plasma Glucose Concentrations

Excretion rate (mg/min)	5	66	151	256	400	520	631
Plasma glucose concentration (g/L)	2.00	3.01	3.98	5.03	6.05	7.08	7.99

6. The data in Table 22–12 were observed for disopyramide (M.W. = 339.5 g/mole) in two different subjects, each receiving various rates of i.v. infusion. Approximately 55% of disopyramide, a basic drug that binds to α_1-acid glycoprotein, is normally excreted unchanged in urine. The remainder is metabolized.

　　Based on the information above, give two possible explanations for the dose-dependence of disopyramide clearance.

Table 22–12.

SUBJECT	INFUSION RATE (mg/min)	STEADY-STATE CONCENTRATION (mg/L)
J.J.	0.039	0.70
	0.077	1.15
	0.154	2.01
	0.309	2.48
B.H.	0.08	0.82
	0.16	1.30
	0.32	2.30
	0.64	2.90
	1.05	4.09
	1.94	5.56

7. Table 22–13 is intended to summarize the direction of change expected in the disposition parameters and in total and unbound steady-state blood concentrations of a drug, relative to the rate of i.v. administration, when there is a dose dependency in absorption, distribution, or elimination. Complete the table by indicating ↑ for increase, ↓ for decrease, or ↔ for little or no change.

Table 22–13.　Disposition Kinetics and Total and Unbound Steady-State Blood Drug Concentrations as a Function of Dose-Dependency in Each of Several Sources Following Oral and i.v. Administrations

SOURCE OF DOSE DEPENDENCY	DIRECTION OF CHANGE[a] WITH INCREASED TOTAL DAILY DOSE	VOLUME OF[b] DISTRIBUTION	CLEARANCE	HALF-LIFE	$\left[\dfrac{\text{CONCENTRATION}}{\text{RATE OF ADMINISTRATION}}\right]$[c] TOTAL	UNBOUND
Oral Administration						
Bioavailability	↓	↔				
Absorption rate constant	↓	↔				
Intravenous Administration						
Fraction unbound in blood						
Low extraction ratio drug	↑	↑				
High extraction ratio drug	↑	↑				
Fraction unbound in tissue	↑		↔			
Metabolic clearance	↑		↑			
Renal clearance	↓		↓			

[a]Only one example of each direction of change is shown.
[b]The volume of distribution is at least ten times the blood volume.
[c]The average steady-state total and unbound blood drug concentrations relative to the rate of administration.

8. Four mechanisms that produce dose-dependent kinetics together with supplemental information obtained under linear conditions, are listed below. Graphically show, on the plots requested, the kinetic consequences of each of these mechanisms. Draw a *solid line* for the observation expected when the kinetics are linear and a *dashed line* for the situation in which dose-dependent behavior occurs. General tendencies, rather than specific functionalities, are sought.

Plot Requested

a. Saturable first-pass metabolism (oral administration of a single dose)
$\dfrac{Dose}{AUC}$ vs. Dose

b. Saturable reabsorption in the renal tubule ($F = 0.9$; $fe = 0.5$; drug given as single oral dose)
$\dfrac{Ae_{\infty}}{AUC}$ vs. Dose

c. Capacity-limited metabolism ($fe = 0.01$, drug infused intravenously at a constant rate)
C_{ss} vs. Infusion rate

d. Saturable binding to plasma proteins (single oral dose)
Cu vs. C

9. The data in Fig. 22–7 for dicloxacillin were presented without associated plasma protein binding information (not provided in the article). The renal clearance of the drug, as assessed from Ae_{∞}/AUC, decreased on increasing the dose from 1 to 2 g. Dicloxacillin, a weak acid with a molecular weight of 470 g/mole, is extensively bound to albumin ($fu = 0.04$ at 10 mg/L) and produces a peak concentration of about 60 mg/L after oral administration of 2 g. Could saturable binding to a plasma protein explain the decrease in Ae_{∞}/AUC with the larger dose?

10. Table 22–14 lists plasma heparin activity determined by the amount of hexadimethrine bromide required to neutralize heparin activity using thrombin-induced coagulation as an endpoint.

Table 22-14. Heparin Activity in Plasma After Single i.v. Injections of 25 and 75 Units/kg of Heparin on Separate Occasions in a Healthy Subject[a]

		HEPARIN ACTIVITY	
TIME (min)	DOSE (Units/kg)	25	75
10		0.313[b]	—
15		—	0.872
20		0.238	—
30		0.175	—
40		0.106	—
45		—	0.592
60		0.06[c]	0.420
90		—	0.249
120		—	0.228
150		—	0.161
180		—	0.083

[a]Modified from Bjornsson, T.D., Wolfram, K.M., and Kitchell, B.B.: Heparin kinetics determined by three assay methods. Clin. Pharmacol. Ther., *31*:104–113, 1982.
[b]Activity in units/mL.
[c]Point added for didactic purposes.

a. Plot both sets of activity-time data on the same semilogarithmic graph.

b. Do the data suggest dose-dependent kinetic behavior? If so, which pharmacokinetic parameters appear to be affected?

c. Could the kinetic behavior be explained by capacity-limited elimination of the Michaelis-Menten type? Briefly discuss.

d. Heparin is a natural heterogeneous mucopolysaccharide consisting of polymeric units of different chain length and chemical composition with molecular weights ranging from 3,000 to 40,000 g/mole. Could the nonlinear kinetic behavior be explained by the simultaneous assay of multiple components? Briefly discuss.

11. Using the data in Table 12–8 (problem 5 of Chap. 12 Study Problems) together with information in Fig. 22–23, answer the following questions.

    a. Briefly explain why the apparent *AUC* of (+)-methylphenidate is about 10 to 20 times higher than that for the (−)-isomer (Fig. 22–23A) following a 30-mg oral dose of racemate. Is your explanation consistent with the similar half-lives of the two isomers?

    b. Is your explanation in "a" consistent with the observed lack of a difference in the *AUC* values of the ritalinic acid metabolites of the respective isomers?

    c. The ritalinic acid metabolites appear to decline with the same half-life as the (+) and (−) isomers of methylphenidate after the 30-mg dose. How would you account for this observation?

    d. Explain why the plasma concentration of (−)-ritalinic acid appears to be about 20% higher in the first 2 hr than (+)-ritalinic acid.

    e. In Fig. 22–23B, the *AUC* of (+)-methylphenidate increases disproportionally with dose of racemate over the range 10 to 40 mg. How do you explain this apparent nonlinearity?

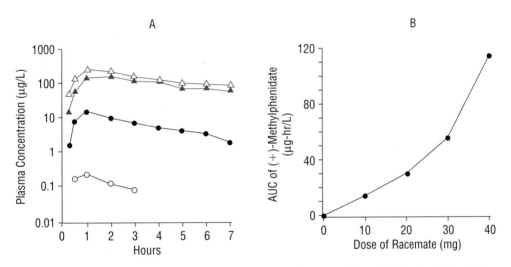

Fig. 22–23. *A,* The plasma concentrations of (+)-methylphenidate (●), (−)-methylphenidate (○) and their respective metabolites (in color), (+)-ritalinic acid (▲), and (−)-ritalinic acid (△) after the oral administration of 30 mg of racemic methylphenidate hydrochloride to a volunteer. *B,* The relationship between the *AUC* of (+)-methylphenidate and dose following oral administration of 10, 20, 30, and 40 mg of the racemate to the same volunteer. (Methylphenidate: 1 mg/L = 4.3 μM; ritalinic acid: 1 mg/L = 4.1 μM.) (Adapted from Aoyama, T., Kotaki, H., Sasaki, T., Sawada, Y., Honda, Y., and Iga, T.: Nonlinear kinetics of threo-methylphenidate enantiomers in a patient with narcolepsy and in healthy volunteers. Eur. J. Clin. Pharmacol., *44*:79–84, 1993.)

TURNOVER CONCEPTS

OBJECTIVES

The reader will be able to:

1. Define turnover and turnover rate and the following parameters: turnover time, fractional turnover rate, and mean residence time.

2. Determine turnover parameters and turnover rate of a one-compartment, first-order system when input or elimination is completely blocked.

3. Know the limitations of a single time-point determination in the interpretation of kinetic events when the turnover of a system is altered.

4. Determine turnover rate and mean residence time of a tracer or drug in a multicompartmental system in which elimination occurs only from the central sampling compartment, when data after a single bolus dose are provided.

5. Quantify the relationship between turnover rate of an endogenous substance and the plasma concentration of an inhibitor of its production, given appropriate data.

6. Estimate creatinine clearance from two serum creatinine concentrations obtained under non-steady-state conditions.

CONCEPT OF TURNOVER

Many drugs act by affecting the concentration of a normal (endogenous) constituent of the body. Examples are oral anticoagulants, which lower plasma concentrations of certain clotting factors by inhibiting their synthesis, and uricosuric agents, which lower the plasma concentration of uric acid by increasing its renal clearance. Some endogenous compounds are also used to assess various body functions. Thus, creatinine is commonly used to assess renal function, and bilirubin is used to assess hepatic function. Accordingly, to be able to relate sensibly the pharmacokinetics of a drug to its pharmacologic effect when an endogenous compound is involved or to interpret the concentration of an endogenous compound to assess body function, the kinetics of the endogenous compound must be understood.

The amounts of many body constituents remain fairly constant with time. This does not mean, however, that they are in a static state. Indeed, they are often being replaced or synthesized at a rapid rate; they are said to be "turning over." The concept of *turnover* can be applied to plasma proteins, enzymes, hormones, electrolytes, water, and in fact to virtually every substance in the body. The term *turnover*, however, does not indicate how rapidly the renewal process occurs. It only indicates the nature of the process.

Turnover implies that a substance is at steady state. Thus, the rate of renewal equals the rate of elimination. This rate, the *turnover rate*, does not fully convey the speed of the process. To do that, the turnover rate must be related to the amount of substance present, frequently called the *pool size*. The ratio of the turnover rate, R_t, to the pool size, A_{ss}, is called the *fractional turnover rate, k_t,* that is,

$$k_t = \frac{R_t}{A_{ss}}$$

1

A second useful parameter for measuring turnover is *turnover time, t_t*. It is the time required to renew the amount in the pool. Complete renewal actually requires an infinite period of time, because newly entering substance continuously mixes with that already in the pool. Turnover time can be readily defined, however, by the time required to bring into the pool the amount that is in it, therefore,

$$t_t = \frac{A_{ss}}{R_t}$$

2

Consequently, the relationship between turnover time and fractional turnover rate is

$$t_t = \frac{1}{k_t}$$

3

The input may be either synthetic or involve a transfer of substance into the pool from elsewhere, or both. A good example is total body water, which is both imbibed and synthesized by catabolism of foodstuffs.

Figure 23–1 schematically shows the turnover of water in the body. Using the data in the figure and Eqs. 1 to 3, the following average turnover values for water are obtained:

Turnover rate = 2.5 L (or kg)/day

Fractional turnover rate = 0.06 day^{-1}

Turnover time = 17 days

Although the turnover rate (2.5 kg/day) is a large value, the actual turnover of body water is quite slow as reflected by the fractional turnover rate (6%/day) or turnover time (17 days). Clearly, these two parameters characterize turnover better than turnover rate alone.

The output may involve several pathways. For body water, urinary and fecal excretion, perspiration, and respiration are the major routes of loss. In a hot, dry desert climate, the last two pathways, especially perspiration, may increase dramatically. Intake must then be increased to compensate for increased loss. The pool size remains essentially constant, although turnover rate may be increased to 21 L/day under these extreme conditions. In this situation, fractional turnover rate and turnover time of water become 0.5 day^{-1} and 2

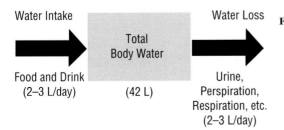

Fig. 23–1.   The turnover of total body water.

days, respectively. The pool size of many body constituents is kept constant by feedback control mechanisms that maintain homeostasis.

In contrast to these substances, the pool size, rather than fractional turnover rate or turnover time, of many other constituents changes when the turnover rate is altered. This results in a change in the concentration of the substance. Selected examples of these situations in which turnover is altered are listed in Table 23–1. These include induction of cytochrome P450 isozymes by phenobarbital, changes in plasma creatinine in acute renal impairment, and changes in plasma concentration of clotting factors on administration of oral anticoagulants.

Turnover concepts have a wide range of applications. Before considering particular applications, the similarity between turnover concepts and those that apply to constant-rate infusion should be noted. Consider, for example, Eq. 1. The analogous equation following constant rate infusion is $k = R_0/A_{ss}$. Thus, fractional turnover rate, k_t, is synonymous with elimination rate constant for a one-compartment model. Also, pool size is synonymous with amount in body at steady state. A major distinction between the two concepts exists with respect to the initial condition. In turnover, the initial condition is one of steady state. With constant rate infusion, it is not; initially, no drug is in the body. Notwithstanding this and other differences, such as feedback control, many of the concepts of constant rate input have application in turnover.

TURNOVER UNDER BLOCKING CONDITIONS

The turnover parameters of a system may be obtained if two of the following three are measured: turnover rate, amount in the pool, and fractional turnover rate. None can be obtained from measurement of steady-state plasma concentration alone. The turnover rate can be measured in some circumstances, e.g., the daily renal excretion of creatinine, but

Table 23–1. Selected Examples of Altered Turnover

| | | TURNOVER MEASURES | | | |
OBSERVATION	CAUSE	TURNOVER RATE (R_t)	FRACTIONAL TURNOVER RATE (k_t)	TURNOVER TIME (MRT)	EXAMPLE
I. Change in Pool Size					
Increased pool size (or concentration)	Increased synthesis or input	↑[a]	N/C[b]	N/C	Induction of a cytochrome P450 isozyme by phenobarbital
	Decreased ability to eliminate	N/C	↓[c]	↑	Plasma creatinine in acute renal function impairment
Decreased pool size (or concentration)	Decreased synthesis or input	↓	N/C	N/C	Decrease in concentration of certain clotting factors after oral anticoagulants
	Increased ability to eliminate	N/C	↑	↓	Decreased renal tubular reabsorption of serum uric acid by a uricosuric agent
II. Little or No Change in Pool Size					
Increased output (or elimination)	Increased input	↑	↑	↓	Increased water consumption in hot weather
Decreased output (or elimination)	Decreased input	↓	↓	↑	Sodium in urine on a low-salt diet

[a]↑ = increase.
[b]N/C = little or no change.
[c]↓ = decrease.

again, other parameters remain unknown. Except through the use of tracer amounts of isotopically labeled substances, which can be measured independently, fractional turnover rate can be measured only by perturbing steady state.

To appreciate the consequences of altering fractional turnover rate, consider the events in Fig. 23–2 (upper graph) in which elimination is immediately and completely blocked and input is unaltered. The rate at which the substance accumulates depends on its normal turnover. The time required for a doubling of the amount initially present, A_{ss}, is the turnover time, by definition. Similarly, if concentration is measured, turnover time is that required for the concentration to double the steady-state value. This last statement assumes that the system acts as a single compartment within the time frame of the measurements. To determine turnover rate, the steady-state amount in the body must be known or the converse.

The consequences of immediately and completely blocking input under conditions in which elimination is first-order, and unaffected, and the body acts as if it were a single compartment are depicted in Fig. 23–2 (lower graph). The situation is equivalent to stopping a constant-rate intravenous (i.v.) infusion of drug at steady state. Recall (Chap. 7) that the amount in the body (or plasma concentration) then falls exponentially by one half each half-life. Recall also that the fractional rate of elimination is the elimination rate constant k, and as $t_t = 1/k_t$, it follows that:

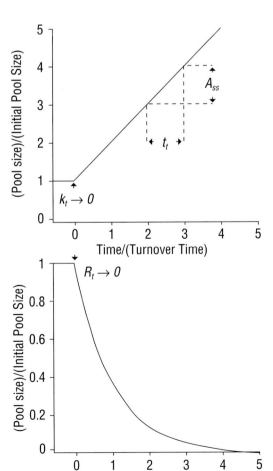

Fig. 23–2. *Upper graph*, The pool size increases linearly with time when (at arrow) elimination is completely blocked and input rate remains unchanged. The slope is the original turnover rate, A_{ss}/t_t. *Lower graph*, The pool size decreases with time when (at arrow) input is completely blocked. The decline is exponential when first-order elimination and one-compartment distribution pertain. The rate constant for the decline (slope of semilogarithmic plot) is the fractional turnover rate. In both graphs, pool size is expressed relative to the original value, and time is related to the original turnover time.

$$t_t = \frac{1}{k_t} = \frac{1}{0.693/t_{1/2}} = 1.44 \cdot t_{1/2} \qquad\qquad 4$$

or

$$t_{1/2} = 0.693 \cdot t_t \qquad\qquad 5$$

To illustrate the consequence of blocking synthesis, consider the effect of the oral anticoagulant warfarin on prothrombin complex activity. Prothrombin complex activity reflects the activity of the four vitamin K_1-dependent clotting factors whose syntheses are inhibited by warfarin. On administering of a blocking dose of warfarin, this complex declines monoexponentially with a half-life of 15 hr, as shown in Fig. 23–3. Hence, its turnover time is 21.6 hr. The consequence of blocking degradation is different as illustrated with creatinine. Creatinine is totally excreted unchanged. Accordingly, as shown in Fig. 23–4, serum creatinine is expected to rise linearly, not exponentially, with time in a patient with acute oliguria, due to virtually no residual renal function. Notice that the actual rate of rise (dC/dt) is about 3.5 mg/dL/day (0.31 mM/day), from which the turnover of creatinine can be calculated as follows:

Equation 6 expresses the interrelationships between turnover time, rate of rise of plasma creatinine on blocking its elimination, and other parameters.

$$t_t = \frac{A_{ss}}{R_t} = \frac{V \cdot C_{ss}}{V \cdot dC/dt} = \frac{C_{ss}}{dC/dt} \qquad\qquad 6$$

Clearly, to define the normal turnover of creatinine, both its volume of distribution (V) and normal plasma concentration (C_{ss}) are needed. Although neither value is known for the patient, the usual values, which do not vary widely among normal healthy individuals, are likely to apply. The volume of distribution of creatinine is 42 L/70 kg, because it

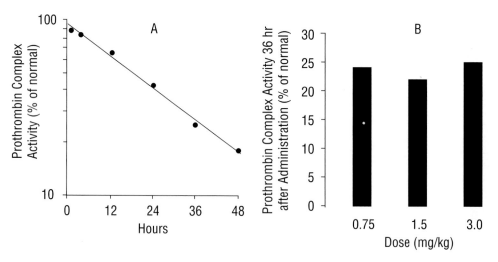

Fig. 23–3. *A*, A blocking dose of warfarin, 1.5 mg/kg orally as the sodium salt, caused the prothrombin complex activity to decline exponentially over the first 48 hr after administration to a subject. *B*, As expected, higher (oral and i.v.) doses of warfarin produced no further change in the rate of decline of the complex activity, as determined by the activity remaining at 36 hr. (Redrawn from Nagashima, R., O'Reilly, R.A., and Levy, G.: Kinetics of pharmacologic effect in man: The anticoagulant action of warfarin. Clin. Pharmacol. Ther., *10*:22–35, 1969.)

distributes into total body water and is unbound within the body. A typical plasma concentration is 0.9 mg/dL (0.08 mM). Hence, the turnover rate of creatinine, R_t, is 1500 mg/day, and the turnover time is 6 hr [0.9 mg/dL/((3.5 mg/dL/day) · (1 day/24 hr))].

ESTABLISHMENT OF A NEW STEADY STATE

Instead of the two extreme cases of complete blockade considered above, input or elimination is usually only partially affected. Quantitation of such a situation is difficult. When either the input rate or fractional turnover rate is immediately shifted to a new constant value, it takes time for the pool size to reach a new steady state and therefore to reflect the shift in turnover, as illustrated below.

Turnover Rate Altered to a New Constant Value

Changes in pool size with time on increasing or decreasing input (turnover rate) by a factor of four are shown, respectively, by the solid lines in Fig. 23–5. The new steady states reflect changes in turnover rate. Notice that, as the elimination half-life is unaltered, the time to reach the new steady state is the same. This is seen by the time required to reach one-half the way to the new steady state. Indeed, this statement is true irrespective of the extent of change in turnover rate, as shown in the upper graph of Fig. 23–5. Had the turnover time been 1 hour, then it would have taken 42 min (0.693 · t_t) to reach this point; if it had been 1 week, then it would have taken about 5 days. This lack of change in the time to go from one steady state to another distinguishes altered turnover rate from altered fractional turnover rate.

One common example of altered turnover rate is enzyme induction, whereby a compound (the inducer) increases the synthesis rate of a drug-metabolizing enzyme. The result is an increase in the pool size of the enzyme, which in turn is normally reflected by a proportional increase in the Vm, and hence intrinsic clearance, of a substrate. The half-lives of drug metabolizing enzymes vary from hours to days so that the full effect of induction may not be seen for some time after an inducing agent is administered. Occasion-

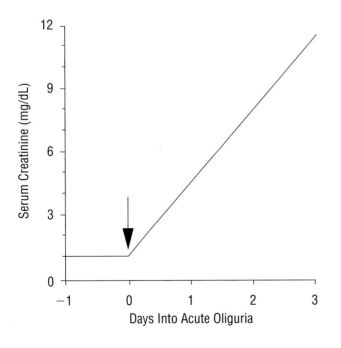

Fig. 23–4. Acute renal failure causes the serum concentration of creatinine to rise at a constant rate of 3.5 mg/dL/day (1 mg/L = 8.8 μM).

Fig. 23–5. *Upper graph.* Pool size increases to a value four times the original when (at arrow) turnover rate (solid line) increases by four. A fourfold decrease in fractional turnover rate (stippled line) gives the same end result; however, it takes four times as long to reach the new steady-state (in color). *Lower graph.* Pool size decreases to a value one-fourth of the original when (at arrow) turnover rate decreases (solid line) by a factor of four. A fourfold increase in fractional turnover rate (stippled line) again produces the same new steady state (in color); however, the new value is approached four times more rapidly.

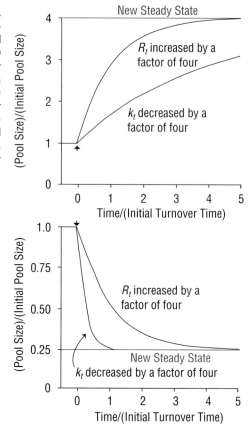

Fig. 23–6. Carbamazepine undergoes autoinduction as evidenced by the declining plasma concentration (●), assessed on days 7, 8, 15, 16, 22, and 23 of an oral multiple-dose regimen of 6 mg/kg taken by a subject once daily in the morning for 22 consecutive days. Predictions based on single-dose pharmacokinetic data, obtained previously in the subject and based on the assumption that no induction occurs, are shown by the *stippled line.* Predictions assuming an autoinduction model for carbamazepine, in which the turnover time of the affected enzyme is approximately 5 days, are indicated by the *solid colored line* (1 mg/L = 4.2 µM) (Copyright 1976 by the American Pharmaceutical Association, *Clinical Pharmacokinetics: Concepts and Applications,* Second Edition. Reprinted with permission of the American Pharmaceutical Association.)

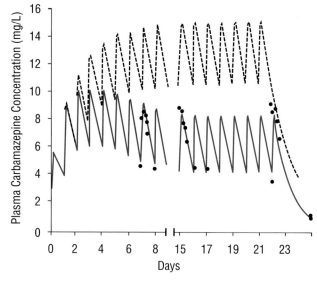

ally, a drug induces its own metabolizing enzymes, *autoinduction*, as illustrated with carbamazepine (Fig. 23–6). As can be seen, it takes approximately 3 weeks to achieve the full effect of autoinduction of this antiepileptic drug, indicating that the turnover time of the affected enzyme is about 5 days. Interpretation of the exact drug concentration–time relationship is complicated by the graded nature of the induction process, as the degree of induction changes continuously with drug concentration.

Fractional Turnover Rate Altered to a New Constant Value

The consequences of changing elimination rate constant (fractional turnover rate) are quite different from changing input (turnover) rate. The difference is shown by the stippled lines in Fig. 23–5. It can be seen that a fourfold decrease in the elimination rate constant quadruples pool size, but it takes four times as long to reach the same new steady state as it did after quadrupling turnover rate. A fourfold increase in elimination rate constant, on the other hand, reduces pool size by a factor of four, and the new steady state is reached much more quickly than by the former mechanism.

The principle is illustrated by creatinine. If renal function drops immediately to a value that is 50, 33, 25, or 20% of normal, the plasma creatinine concentration rises to a new steady state that is 2, 3, 4, or 5 times the normal value, respectively, as shown in the lower

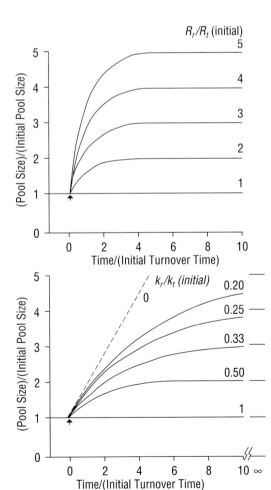

Fig. 23–7. *Upper graph,* The pool size is increased from one to five times its original value when (at arrow) the turnover increases by the factor R_t/R_t *(initial)*. The time (half-life, turnover time) to approach each new steady state is the same. *Lower graph,* The approach to the new steady state is prolonged when (at arrow) the fractional turnover rate decreases by the factor k_t/k_t *(initial)*. When the value of k_t approaches zero (stippled line), steady state is never achieved. The prolonged approach to the new steady state for the other conditions can be expressed by the time (half-life) required to reach the pool size half-way between the initial and final values.

graph of Fig. 23–7. The new steady-state concentration is directly proportional to the turnover time. The turnover time and the half-life of creatinine elimination at various degrees of renal function are shown in Table 23–2.

The time required for a plasma creatinine concentration to reflect a change in renal function can be greatly prolonged with severe renal function impairment. Interpretation of a plasma creatinine value in a clinical situation is therefore dependent on the acuteness of the change in renal function and on the degree to which renal function is impaired. Furthermore, in bedridden or only partially ambulatory patients with severe renal dysfunction, the muscle mass is typically decreased, leading to a reduced production rate of creatinine and a rise of only about 1 to 3 mg/dL (0.09 to 0.27 mM)/day in plasma creatinine between hemodialysis treatments (used to remove accumulated polar substances, see Chap. 24, Dialysis).

Distinction between decreased turnover rate and increased fractional turnover rate is similar with the analysis above, but here pool size decreases, as shown in Fig. 23–8. The time required to approach the new steady state is the same when production rate is decreased (upper graph), but is shortened when fractional turnover rate is increased (lower graph). The rate of attainment of the new steady state is related to its new value; the lower the value, the more quickly it is achieved, as shown in the lower graph of the figure.

The rate of decline in pool size, on decreasing turnover rate, is limited by the fractional turnover rate itself. The decline in clotting factors, on administering warfarin, serves as a good example. This system is examined in greater detail, as it is representative of many other such systems in the body.

INTERPRETATION OF NONSTEADY-STATE OBSERVATIONS

Frequently, it is necessary to interpret data under nonsteady-state conditions. This arises following the acute administration of endogenous drugs and when one of the turnover parameters is acutely perturbed.

Administration of Endogenous Drug

Some marketed drugs are endogenous to the body. Examples are testosterone and L-thyroxine. The number of such drugs is increasing rapidly with developments in biotechnology that enable the expression and production of recombinant human polypeptides and proteins, such as follicle-stimulating hormone and erythropoietin. With many of these, a basal concentration in plasma exists that must be taken into account when attempting to define the pharmacokinetics of the administered compound. The approach that follows is successful when the basal turnover rate is unaffected by the additional material. Sometimes, this is not so because of feedback control systems that adjust the endogenous turnover rate to maintain homeostasis.

Table 23–2. Calculated Turnover Time and Half-Life of Creatinine when Renal Function is Decreased

RENAL FUNCTION (PERCENT OF "NORMAL")[a]	TURNOVER TIME (hr)	HALF-LIFE (hr)
100	6	4
50	12	8
33	18	12
25	24	17
20	30	21
10	60	42

[a]Based on an expected creatinine clearance of 7 L/hr for a 20-year-old, 70-kg male and a creatinine volume of distribution of 0.6 L/kg.

Figure 23–9A shows the serum concentrations of erythropoietin after i.v. bolus administration of epoetin alfa, a recombinant human erythropoietin, and placebo. Notice the decay of erythropoietin to its basal value. The equation defining the concentration during the decay, $C(t)$, is the sum of two concentrations, the basal concentration and that associated with the bolus dose, C_{bolus}. The difference between $C(t)$ and the basal concentration is seen to be approximated by a monoexponential equation, characterized by C_{bolus} (units/L) $= 1800 \, e^{-0.12t}$, with time in hours (Fig. 21–9B). The corresponding pharmacokinetic parameters are $V = 4$ L/70 kg; $CL = 0.5$ L/hr/70 kg and $t_{1/2} = 5.8$ hr.

Estimation of Creatinine Clearance in Acute Renal Impairment

In patients with acute renal dysfunction, it is not always possible or practical to wait for the serum creatinine to rise to a new steady state to estimate creatinine clearance from serum creatinine, particularly when renal function becomes very low and creatinine half-life becomes correspondingly very long. Creatinine clearance can still be estimated, however, from two (or more) serum creatinine values on the approach to plateau. The principle behind the method is the same as that used when considering the rise (or fall) in plasma concentration on going from one steady state to another following a change in its rate of constant input (Chap. 6). Namely, as depicted in Fig. 23–10, that the observed creatinine concentration is the sum of two concentrations: (1) that associated with what remains in

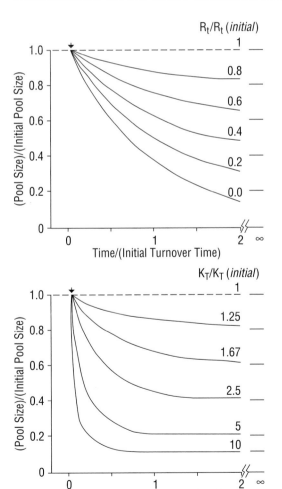

Fig. 23–8. *Upper graph,* Pool size decreases to a new steady state that corresponds to the factor R_t/R_t *(initial),* by which the turnover rate decreases. The new steady state is approached with the same half-life when (at arrow) input decreases. *Lower graph,* Pool size also decreases when (at arrow) fractional turnover rate increases by the factor k_t/k_t *(initial),* but the time (half-life) to achieve the new steady state is shortened.

the body from the time of the first observation and (2) the rising concentration that is due to the continual production of creatinine. That is, the serum creatinine concentration at any time after t_1 is given by

$$C(t) = C(t_1)e^{-k(d)t} \qquad + \qquad \frac{R_t}{CL_{CR}(d)}[1 - e^{-k(d)t}]$$

Concentration associated with   Concentration associated with
what remains of creatinine in   continual production of creatinine
body from time of first   at turnover rate R_t
observation

7

where $C(t_1)$ is the concentration at time t_1, $CL_{CR}(d)$ is the creatinine clearance in the patient

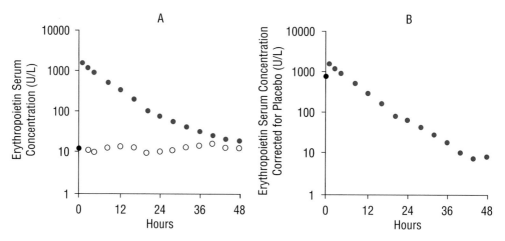

Fig. 23–9. *A*, Serum erythropoietin concentration with time plotted semilogarithmically after i.v. bolus administration of epoetin alfa (100 units/kg) (●) and placebo (○). *B*, Semilogarithmic plot of the difference between the erythropoietin concentration after the dose of epoetin alfa and the basal value (10 units/L), taken as the average over the period of study following the placebo. Mean data for 21 subjects. (From Halstenson, C.E., Macres, M., Katz, S.A., Schnieders, J.R., Watanabe, M., Sobota, J.T., and Abraham, P.A.: Comparative pharmacokinetics and pharmacodynamics of epoetin alfa and epoetin beta. Clin. Pharmacol. Ther., 50:702–712, 1991.)

Fig. 23–10. When renal function suddenly deteriorates, creatinine clearance immediately falls to a new value $CL_{CR}(d)$. Serum creatinine then rises toward a new steady state if renal function remains constant. At any time t_2, beyond a previous time t_1, interval t, the concentration may be regarded as the sum of that remaining from the amount in the body at t_1, $C(t_1)e^{-k(d)\cdot t}$, and that associated with the continual input of creatinine (both in color),

$$\frac{R_t}{CL_{CR}(d)}[1 - e^{-k(d)\cdot t}],$$

where $k(d) = CL_{CR}(d)/V$ and R_t is the turnover rate of creatinine, which is generally unaltered in acute renal impairment.

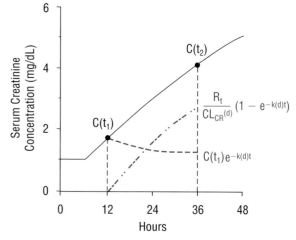

with renal function impairment, and $k(d)$ is the corresponding elimination rate constant. As shown in Appendix I–H, an estimate of $CL_{CR}(d)$ can also be obtained from concentrations at times t_1 and t_2 as follows:

$$CL_{CR}(d) = \frac{2R_t}{[C(t_1) + C(t_2)]} + \frac{2 \cdot V \cdot [C(t_1) - C(t_2)]}{\Delta t \cdot [C(t_1) + C(t_2)]} \qquad 8$$

where $C(t_2)$ is the creatinine concentration at the second observation and Δt is the time interval between observations, i.e., $t_2 - t_1$.

Although V and R_t, the turnover time (production rate) of creatinine, are not thought to change in acute renal impairment, being a function of total body water and muscle mass respectively, the specific values in the individual patient are generally not known. The value of V is taken to be total body water, given by 60% body weight in an otherwise normal subject. The value of R_t depends on body weight, age, gender, and whether the patient is emaciated, as discussed in Chap. 16, Disease. Based on the relationships given in Table 16–2 for adult patients who are not emaciated or obese,

$$\text{Males: } R_t \text{ (mg/day)} = \frac{(140 - \text{Age (years)}) \times \text{weight (kg)}}{5} \qquad 9$$

$$\text{Females: } R_t \text{ (mg/day)} = \frac{(140 - \text{Age (years)}) \times \text{weight (kg)}}{5.9} \qquad 10$$

To illustrate the method, consider the data in Fig. 23–10 obtained in a 20-year-old 60-kg male patient with acute renal function impairment. The serum concentrations are 1.9 mg/dL and 4.5 mg/dL measured 48 hr apart. The expected values of V and R_t (Eq. 9) are 36 L and 1440 mg/day or 60 mg/hr, respectively. Substituting these values and those of creatinine concentration (expressed in milligrams per liter, to ensure equality of units) into Eq. 8, gives a CL_{CR} of 0.6 L/hr, or 10 mL/min.

Equation 8 should be applied judiciously. Apart from the problems of estimating R_t and V in emaciated and obese patients, there are also issues surrounding the concentration data. The method provides a poor estimate of creatinine clearance when the difference between the two measurements is small (and the associated percentage error is large), unless, of course, they represent the steady-state value. The likelihood of this situation can generally be deduced from the values and the time difference between them. For example, if two values taken 24 hr apart are 3 and 3.3 mg/dL, respectively, they are likely to represent the steady-state value, in which case $CL_{CR}(d)$ can be estimated directly, $CL_{CR}(d) = R_t/C_{ss}$. The reasoning is as follows. With a normal serum creatinine of around 1 mg/dL, a steady-state concentration of about 3 mg/dL would correspond to approximately 30% of normal renal function (Eq. 16–12), with an expected creatinine half-life of 12 hr (Table 23–2). The 24-hr interval between the two measurements would therefore represent approximately 2 half-lives, enough time for the concentration to have approached steady state. Moreover, had renal function been much lower, the rise in serum creatinine over 24 hr would have been much greater than that observed.

A particular problem in the application of Eq. 8 arises when creatinine clearance is very low and at least one of the measurements is far from steady state. The extreme is the situation of measurements taken soon after almost total renal shutdown. Creatinine clearance, although obviously low, is very poorly estimated, as the slope of the concentration–time relationship is then approximately R_t/V (Fig. 23–4). Also, when renal function approaches zero, the normally insignificant nonrenal component becomes a substantial function of creatinine clearance, such that creatinine clearance is no longer solely a measure of renal function.

Finally, implicit in the method is that the estimate of creatinine clearance applies at all times within the period of measurement. Obviously, extrapolation to other times is dangerous when renal function is unstable.

Anticoagulant Effect of Warfarin

In common with other endogenous substances, the amount of each clotting factor in the body, A, is a result of a difference between its rate of synthesis, R_{syn}, and degradation, $k_t A$. And, at any moment, whether at steady state or not,

$$\frac{dA}{dt} = R_{syn} - k_t \cdot A \qquad\qquad 11$$

$$\underset{\substack{\text{Rate of change} \\ \text{of clotting factor}}}{} \qquad \underset{\substack{\text{Rate of} \\ \text{synthesis}}}{} \qquad \underset{\substack{\text{Rate of} \\ \text{degradation}}}{}$$

where k_t is the degradation rate constant (fractional turnover rate) of the clotting factor. Normally, the system is at steady state, $dA/dt = 0$, with synthesis matching degradation. However, in the presence of warfarin, the synthesis is inhibited without affecting k_t. The clotting factor concentration (or amount) then falls at a rate that depends on both the degree of inhibition of synthesis and k_t.

Either a steady-state or a nonsteady-state approach can be used to assess the more direct relationship between synthesis rate and plasma warfarin concentration. Each approach has its own merits. With the steady-state approach, the entire clotting system is allowed to reach a new steady state in the presence of a constant concentration of warfarin. Then, once again $dA/dt = 0$, so that $A_{ss} = R_{syn}/k_t$ and, as k_t is unaffected by warfarin, the steady-state amount is directly proportional to R_{syn}. The procedure is then repeated for different plateau concentrations of warfarin to elucidate the relationship between R_{syn} and plasma warfarin concentration. Although this approach appears simple, there is a practical problem. Recall that the time required to go from one plateau to another depends solely on the elimination half-life of the substance. As the degradation half-life of the clotting factors affected by warfarin vary from hours to days, with an average effective half-life (for prothrombin complex activity) of about 1 day, it takes nearly a week to reach each new steady state. Such a study therefore takes as long as a month to complete.

The nonsteady-state approach, which uses data obtained following a single bolus dose, is more rapid but requires an estimate of k_t. This value can be obtained by giving a dose of warfarin that completely blocks synthesis initially ($R_{syn} = 0$). The prothrombin complex activity then falls exponentially (Eq. 11), so that a semilogarithmic plot of the prothrombin complex activity against time gives a straight line with a slope of k_t (Fig. 23–3). Subsequently, as the plasma concentration of warfarin falls, the degree of inhibition of clotting factor synthesis decreases and the concentration of the prothrombin complex rises (see Fig. 5–6), eventually returning to its pre-warfarin value. The change in synthesis rate, R_{syn}, with time is calculated from simultaneous measurement of warfarin and prothrombin complex activity on return to the pre-warfarin value, as follows.

If A_1 and A_2 are the prothrombin complex activities at the beginning and end of a time interval, Δt, then the rate of change of activity is estimated from $(A_2 - A_1)/\Delta t$ and the average activity within the interval is given by $(A_1 + A_2)/2$. R_{syn} is then calculated from rearrangement of Eq. 11.

$$R_{syn} = (A_2 - A_1)/\Delta t + k_t \cdot (A_1 + A_2)/2 \qquad 12$$

The percent inhibition of synthesis is then approximated by

$$\text{Percent inhibition of synthesis} = 100 \cdot [(R_{syn}(n) - R_{syn})/R_{syn}(n)] \qquad 13$$

where $R_{syn}(n)$ is the normal prewarfarin synthesis rate. The normal rate is given by $k_t \cdot A(n)$, where $A(n)$ is the normal activity of the clotting factor. A plot of the percent inhibition of synthesis against logarithm of the warfarin concentration gives the classic response versus concentration relationship, as shown in Fig. 23–11.

Responses to standard doses of warfarin change in disease states and following coadministration of other drugs. By ascertaining the relationship between plasma concentration and direct effect, distinctions can be made between changes in pharmacokinetics of warfarin and changes in responsiveness of the clotting system to this drug. For example, the diminished response to warfarin, when coadministered with heptabarbital, is caused solely by increased clearance, there is no change in the direct response to the drug (Fig. 23–11).

Problem of Single-Time Measurement

The problem of using a plasma creatinine concentration to assess renal function when function changes acutely has been presented. Similarly, the prothrombin activity 5 hr after a dose of warfarin is hardly a measure of the effect of the drug in blocking the synthesis of the clotting factors. To further illustrate the interpretation of non-steady-state observations, consider the following situation:

A study is conducted to see if the drug metabolizing enzymes X and Y are inducible by phenobarbital. Homogenates of rat livers are obtained from untreated rats and from rats pretreated with phenobarbital to attain and maintain a constant concentration. The activity of each of the enzymes is determined in both groups of rats 5 hr after initiating phenobarbital administration. The average activity of enzyme X is increased to 280% of control. The average activity of enzyme Y is about 135% of control, but the value is not statistically different from the control value.

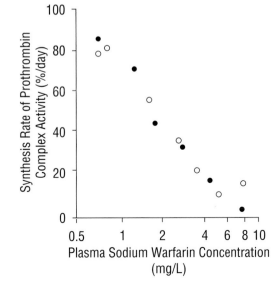

Fig. 23–11. Pretreatment with heptabarbital (400 mg daily for 15 days, starting 10 days before warfarin) decreased the response to a standard dose of warfarin but failed to alter the linear relationship between synthesis rate of prothrombin complex activity and logarithm of the concentration of warfarin in a 21-year-old normal subject; control experiment (O), with heptabarbital (●) (1 mg/L = 3.0 μM). (From Levy, G., O'Reilly, R.A., Aggeler, P.M., and Keech, G.M.: Pharmacokinetic analysis of the effect of barbiturate on the anticoagulant action of warfarin in man. Clin. Pharmacol. Ther., *11*:372–377, 1970.)

There is a tendency to conclude that enzyme X is induced whereas enzyme Y is not. Actually, enzyme Y may have been more induced than enzyme X. This condition is shown in Fig. 23–12. Although induction is virtually instantaneous on administering phenobarbital, the enzymes have different turnover characteristics. Consequently, on sampling at 5 hr, t_1 in the figure, one sees a larger change in enzyme X activity because this enzyme has a shorter half-life. Enzyme Y takes much longer to express its increased synthesis rate because it normally turns over slowly. Had the phenobarbital treatment continued to t_2, the degree of induction would have appeared to be equal, whereas at t_3 a more accurate estimate of actual degree of induction would have been obtained. Clearly, time of sampling is critical to any interpretation. Furthermore, had different steady-state concentrations of phenobarbital been studied, the threefold increase in the synthesis of enzyme X might have been the maximum value possible, whereas enzyme Y might have been maximally induced to a value 10 times the normal one.

TURNOVER IN MULTICOMPARTMENTAL SYSTEMS

Endogenous compounds, like drugs, show distribution kinetics within the body (Chap. 19). This distribution is not apparent from the plasma concentration measurement of the endogenous compound under the usual steady-state conditions, but becomes so when a *tracer* dose of the compound, in an isotopically labeled form, is administered. In the analysis of the tracer data, two major assumptions are often made. First, the disposition of the tracer is identical to that of the endogenous substance. Second, both input (formation) and elimination occur in the initial dilution volume. Unlike for most drugs, these restrictions are more problematic for body constituents that are often formed and destroyed in tissues and that do not equilibrate rapidly between tissue and plasma.

Mean Residence Time

When the two assumptions above hold, then a tracer molecule, on average, resides in the body the same length of time as a new endogenous molecule. This time is called the *mean residence time (MRT)*; it is identical to the turnover time (t_t) of the endogenous substance.

There are two procedures (Appendix I–D) to estimate *MRT*. One method uses the area-under-the-(first)-moment-versus-time curve, $\int_0^\infty t \cdot C_V^\star \cdot dt$, denoted as *AUMC*, and *AUC*. Namely,

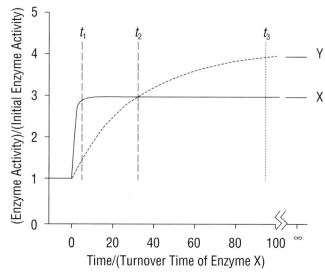

Fig. 23–12. Induction of enzyme X (solid line) by a factor of three and enzyme Y (dotted line) by a factor of four occurs. The turnover time of enzyme Y is 20 times that of enzyme X. The relative enzyme levels at the times indicated (dashed lines) are different, because of differences in the turnover times of the two enzymes. Time is expressed in terms of the turnover time of enzyme X.

$$MRT = \frac{AUMC^*}{AUC^*} \qquad 14$$

where $*$ refers to the labeled tracer. In the other method, MRT is obtained from urinary excretion of the unchanged tracer. Provided that fe remains constant with time, MRT (turnover time) is then

$$MRT = \frac{\int_0^\infty (Ae_\infty^* - Ae^*)dt}{Ae_\infty^*} \qquad 15$$

where Ae_∞^* and Ae^* are the cumulative amounts of labeled tracer excreted to time infinity and to any specified time, respectively.

Steady-State Volume of Distribution

Remembering that MRT (turnover time) is the ratio of pool size to turnover rate (p. 425), it follows that

$$MRT = \frac{A_{ss}}{R_t} = \frac{V_{ss} \cdot C_{ss}^*}{CL \cdot C_{ss}^*} \qquad 16$$

Thus, one arrives at the conceptually important relationship.

$$MRT = V_{ss}/CL \qquad 17$$

This relationship is analogous to the one derived for a drug based on constant-rate input (Eq. 8, Chap. 6). The value of V_{ss} can be estimated using the plasma tracer concentration, realizing that $CL = Dose^*/AUC^*$ and combining Eq. 14 with Eq. 17, to give

$$V_{ss} = \frac{Dose^*}{AUC^*} \cdot \frac{AUMC^*}{AUC^*} \qquad 18$$

To illustrate the use of a tracer to determine turnover parameters and V_{ss} of an endogenous substance, consider the following biexponential equation, which summarizes the experimental observations after a 10-mega-Becquerel i.v. bolus dose of a radiolabelled tracer.

$$C^* = 1.2\, e^{-1.2t} + 0.2\, e^{-0.01t} \qquad 19$$

where C^* is the plasma concentration in units of megaBecquerels/L and t is in minutes. One Becquerel equals one disintegration/second. The AUC is

$$AUC^* = \int_0^\infty C^* \cdot dt = \frac{1.2}{1.2} + \frac{0.2}{0.01} = 21 \text{ megaBecquerel-mins/L}$$

and that of $AUMC$ (Appendix I–D) is

$$AUMC = \int_0^\infty t \cdot C^* \cdot dt = \frac{1.2}{(1.2)^2} + \frac{0.2}{(0.01)^2} = 2{,}001 \text{ megaBecquerel-min}^2/\text{L}$$

Accordingly, the MRT (Eq. 14) is 95 min, and V_{ss} (Eq. 18) is 45 L.

Calculation of turnover rate requires knowledge of the concentration of the endogenous substance, for example 9 mg/L. The amount in the body (pool size) is then 9 mg/L $\times$ 45 L = 405 mg, and from turnover time, turnover rate (A_{ss}/MRT) is 4.3 mg/min, and fractional turnover rate is 0.01 min^{-1}. The turnover of this substance is now completely quantified.

STUDY PROBLEMS

(Answers to Study Problems are in Appendix II.)

1. Define the following terms:
   Turnover   Fractional turnover rate
   Turnover rate   Mean residence time
   Turnover time
2. Examination of the data in Fig. 23–9 indicates that the normal (basal) plasma concentration of erythropoietin is 10 units/L. Using the values of the parameters obtained following the i.v. administration of epoetin alfa (V = 4 L/70 kg; CL = 0.5 L/hr/70 kg), calculate the following parameters for erythropoietin, assuming that epoetin alfa behaves identically to erythropoietin.
   a. Turnover rate
   b. Turnover time
   c. Fractional turnover rate
3. To characterize the turnover of ascorbic acid, Kallner et al. (Kallner A., Hartmann, D., and Hornig D.: Steady-state turnover and body pool of ascorbic acid in man. Am. J. Clin. Nutr., 32:530–539, 1979) orally administered a radiolabeled tracer dose together with relatively low doses (30 to 180 mg) of this vitamin daily to 20- to 45-year-old male subjects who were on an ascorbic acid-deficient diet. The following information was obtained in one subject receiving 30 mg daily of ascorbic acid until a steady state was achieved: C_{ss} = 4.1 mg/L, V_{ss} = 234 L, CL = 6.3 L/day. From this information, calculate the following parameters for ascorbic acid:
   a. Pool size.
   b. The time needed for input to equal the amount in the body.
   c. The mean residence time.
   d. The fraction of the orally administered dose absorbed.
4. The "usual" plasma concentrations of urea and creatinine are 15 mg/100 mL (2.5 mM) and 1 mg/100 mL (0.09 mM), respectively, in young adult patients with normal renal function. The renal clearances of the two compounds are 70 mL/min and 120 mL/min, respectively; the volumes of distribution at steady state are about the same (42 L). Both compounds are eliminated only by renal excretion.
   a. Calculate the "usual" fractional turnover rates of both compounds.
   b. Were the rates of production of these compounds to remain "usual," how long would it take for the plasma urea concentration to increase by 30 mg/100 mL (5.0 mM) and the plasma creatinine concentration to increase by 2 mg/100 mL (0.18 mM) in an anephric patient?
   c. Urea is an end product of protein metabolism. Its formation can be reduced by decreasing protein in the diet. What is the total amount of urea ingested and produced in the body in 24 hr under steady-state conditions?
5. If the turnover time of an enzyme is 4 days and its synthesis rate is instantly increased to a constant value that is three times the normal rate, how long will it take for the enzyme activity (concentration) to double?
6. Consider two enzymes, A and B, both suspected of being subject to induction by a steroid hormone. Administration of the steroid to give nearly constant plasma concen-

trations for 24 hr results in a doubling of the activity of enzyme A, but enzyme B activity increases insignificantly (less than 20%). Based on this observation, the following statement is made, "The steroid has a much greater effect on the synthesis of enzyme A than on the synthesis of enzyme B." Is this conclusion warranted? Briefly discuss.

7. a. Prior to an episode of acute renal failure, a patient (Height, 165 cm; Weight, 60 kg) had a daily renal excretion of 1.6 g (14.2 mmoles) of creatinine and a plasma concentration of 1 mg/100 mL (0.9 mM). During acute renal failure, the plasma creatinine concentration rose by 3 mg/100 mL (0.27 mM)/day and the daily renal excretion of creatinine was virtually nil—anuria. Calculate the "normal" mean residence time (*MRT*) of creatinine in this patient.

   b. Had acute renal insufficiency resulted in an immediate drop in creatinine clearance to 10% of normal and had this functional state continued for an indefinite period of time, how long would it take for the plasma creatinine concentration to reach a value within 10% of the difference between that reflecting the degree of renal dysfunction and the initial value?

8. The turnover of albumin has been studied using tracer techniques (Sterling, K., J. Clin. Invest., *30*: The turnover rate of serum albumin in man as measured by ^{131}I-tagged albumin. 1228–1237, 1951). In one of the subjects, who received 6.75 megaBecquerels of ^{131}I-labeled albumin intravenously the concentration of radioactivity was observed to decline according to the following relationship (1 Becquerel = 1 disintegration per second):

$$C \atop \text{(in megaBecquerels/L)} = 1.5\,e^{-1.4t} + 1.2\,e^{-0.06t} \atop (t \text{ in days})$$

Knowing that the plasma albumin concentration was 42 g/L in this subject and making the assumption that both labeled and unlabeled albumin show the same kinetic behavior (observed to be a good approximation using other techniques), calculate the following:

a. The turnover time and fractional turnover rate of albumin.

b. The amounts of albumin in intravascular (initial dilution volume) and extravascular fluids.

c. The synthesis rate of albumin.

9. A drug acts directly by inhibiting the synthesis of an endogenous substance (e.g., uric acid production); the effect of the drug is measured indirectly, namely, by measurement of the plasma concentration of the endogenous substance, *S*. The scheme of events can be depicted as follows:

$$\xrightarrow[\text{Synthesis}]{} \boxed{A_s} \xrightarrow[\text{Elimination}]{k_s}$$

where A_s is the amount of *S* in the body and k_s is the elimination rate constant. In this scheme, the rate of synthesis of *S* responds instantaneously to changes in the concentration of drug.

The times and corresponding plasma concentrations of drug and *S* when a subject is challenged with a 100 mg i.v. bolus dose of drug are presented in Table 23–3. The pharmacokinetics of the drug are characterized by a one-compartment model in which $k = 0.05\ \text{hr}^{-1}$ and $V = 10\ \text{L}$. As expected, there is a delay in the maximum lowering of the plasma concentration of *S*.

Table 23-3.

TIME (hr)	0	2	4	6	8	10	12	16	24	30	36	48	60	72	84
Plasma concentration of drug (mg/L)	10	9.0	8.2	7.4	6.7	6.1	5.5	4.5	3.0	2.2	1.7	0.91	0.5	0.27	0.15
Plasma concentration of endogenous substance, S (% of normal)	100	72	53	40	31	25	21.5	19.1	24.5	32	48	72	88	96	99

Challenging the subject with a 200-mg bolus dose on another occasion did not shorten the time taken for the concentration of S to initially fall by 50%; it did, of course, cause a deeper and more prolonged depression in the plasma concentration of S.

a. Plot the time course of S on linear graph paper.

b. Based on the scheme above and the information given, construct a direct response (inhibition of synthesis) versus plasma drug concentration curve. (Hint. Write the rate equation for S and rearrange it to express the synthesis rate of S as a function of its plasma concentration and its elimination rate constant; you will need to estimate k_s to solve the problem.)

c. From the curve drawn in part "b", estimate the EC_{50} value and comment on the most likely value of γ in the relationship

$$E = \frac{E_{max}C^{\gamma}}{EC_{50}^{\gamma} + C^{\gamma}}$$

d. If a concentration of S, 30% of the normal value, is needed to achieve a desired therapeutic response, design a schedule of the drug (composed of a bolus dose and a constant-rate infusion) that will, as rapidly as possible, achieve this objective. For the purposes of these calculations, let the bolus dose promptly achieve the desired plateau plasma concentration of the drug.

DIALYSIS

OBJECTIVES

The reader will be able to:

1. Define dialysis, hemodialysis, extracorporeal dialysis, continuous ambulatory peritoneal dialysis, dialysis clearance, dialyzer, dialyzer efficiency, clinical dialyzability and hemofiltration.

2. Calculate the changes in clearance and half-life of a drug and predict the kinetic events brought about by hemodialysis, continuous ambulatory peritoneal dialysis, or hemofiltration given the clearance by the procedure, the total (body) clearance, and the half-life in the absence of the treatment.

3. Given dialysis clearance and the pharmacokinetic parameters of a drug in the absence of the dialysis procedure, anticipate if a supplementary dose is desirable immediately after dialysis. Also determine what the supplementary dose should be.

4. Distinguish among the following techniques: hemodialysis, hemofiltration, and hemoperfusion.

5. Given a drug with known physicochemical properties and pharmacokinetic behavior, discuss how well each of the procedures listed in objective 4 may remove drug from the body in an overdose situation.

Dialysis and related procedures have become established treatments for patients with end-stage renal disease. These procedures are designed to remove toxic waste products that accumulate in patients with this disease. However, they also remove drugs. Thus, such procedures may require adjustment of drug administration in these patients. This chapter provides information needed to decide when and how to make such an adjustment. Continuous ambulatory peritoneal dialysis is also discussed, because it is regarded as the treatment of choice for many patients. Hemofiltration, although not strictly a dialysis procedure, is also covered. The last part of the chapter is devoted to the use of hemodialysis, hemofiltration, and another nondialysis modality, hemoperfusion, to treat overdosed patients.

HEMODIALYSIS

Basically, *dialysis* involves separation of diffusible from less diffusible substances by the use of a semipermeable membrane with little or no net movement of fluid across the membrane. When the semipermeable membrane is that of the peritoneal cavity, the dialysis is termed *peritoneal dialysis*. The common dialysis technique, *hemodialysis*, involves passage of blood through a system containing an artificial semipermeable membrane. Because of the large area of membrane required, such a system is, by necessity, outside the body. Accordingly, this method is termed *extracorporeal dialysis*. The dialysis system itself is called a *hemodialyzer* or an *artificial kidney*. One prevalent kind of system used today is the hollow-fiber dialyzer. It contains hundreds of hollow fibers bundled within a compact cylinder. Blood flows through the semipermeable hollow fibers while dialysate fluid flows outside the fibers in a countercurrent direction. These systems are small, efficient, relatively easy to use, and are sometimes reusable. In the following discussion on quantitative procedures, *dialysis* and *dialyzer* are terms used to describe the general method and the apparatus of hemodialysis, respectively.

A typical period of dialysis is 2 to 4 hr. Even shorter times (1 to 2 hr) are used for the most efficient systems. The actual time required is a compromise between the time needed to adequately remove fluids and metabolic waste products and the comfort and convenience to patients in general. The efficiency of the dialyzer is a major determinant of both.

A variety of hemodialysis systems are in use today. The ability of a dialysis system to remove drugs from the body depends on many factors. These include drug characteristics (molecular weight, protein binding, volume of distribution); mechanical properties of the dialysis system (surface area and thickness of membrane, porosity, geometry of the system, e.g., whether blood and dialysate flows are countercurrent or concurrent); and dialysis conditions (e.g., blood and dialysate flow rates). Because of the variety of systems and conditions, quantitative extrapolation of data from one study to another may be difficult. Nonetheless, a body of principles applies to all systems and to the removal of both endogenous substances and drugs from the body by them. These principles and considerations of possible adjustment in drug administration in patients undergoing these procedures follow.

Dialysis Clearance

As with many other applications of pharmacokinetics, the most useful concept when dealing with dialysis of drugs is clearance. *Dialysis clearance* is a measure of how effectively a dialyzer can remove a drug from blood. It is the rate of removal relative to the concentration in the blood entering the dialyzer. The use of the concentration in blood, rather than in plasma, has an advantage in relating blood clearance to blood flow and in relating rate of removal to rate of presentation to the dialyzer, principles previously developed for hepatic and renal extraction (Chap. 11).

To appreciate how dialysis clearance is measured, consider the schematic representation of a dialyzer shown in Fig. 24–1. At steady state, i.e., when there is no net change in the amount of drug in the dialyzer, the rate of its removal from blood can be determined in several ways.

Extraction From Blood. One method is by taking the difference between the rates at which the substance enters ($Q_{b,in} \cdot C_{b,in}$) and leaves ($Q_{b,out} \cdot C_{b,out}$) the dialyzer, where $Q_{b,in}$ and $Q_{b,out}$ are the blood flows and $C_{b,in}$ and $C_{b,out}$ are the concentrations in the arterial blood entering and venous blood leaving the dialyzer.

Dialysis blood clearance, CL_{bD}, is then given by

$$CL_{bD} = \frac{(Q_{b,in} \cdot C_{b,in} - Q_{b,out} \cdot C_{b,out})}{C_{b,in}} \qquad 1$$

Dialysis clearance, CL_D, based on drug concentration in plasma entering the dialyzer, C_{in}, can be determined from $CL_D = CL_{bD} \cdot C_{b,in}/C_{in}$.

The values of $Q_{b,in}$ and $Q_{b,out}$ are not exactly equal, as there is often a 2- to 3-L loss of fluid during a typical 3- to 4-hr dialysis period. The value of $Q_{b,in}$ is now determined accurately with flow sensors. The value of $Q_{b,out}$ is calculated by multiplying $Q_{b,in}$ by the ratio of hematocrit values across the dialyzer.

Rate of Recovery in Dialysate. A second method uses the net rate at which the substance leaves in the dialysate fluid, $Q_{D,out} \cdot C_{D,out} - Q_{D,in} \cdot C_{D,in}$, where $Q_{D,out}$ and $Q_{D,in}$ are the dialysate flows leaving and entering the dialyzer, and $C_{D,out}$ and $C_{D,in}$ are the respective concentrations.

$$CL_{bD} = \frac{(Q_{D,out} \cdot C_{D,out} - Q_{D,in} \cdot C_{D,in})}{C_{b,in}} \qquad 2$$

Loss of water to the dialysate is accounted for here. With the common nonrecirculating (single-pass) dialysis systems, $C_{D,in} = 0$. Equation 2 then reduces to

$$CL_{bD} = \frac{Q_{D,out} \cdot C_{D,out}}{C_{b,in}} \qquad 3$$

Amount Recovered in Dialysate. A third, and generally the most accurate, method of determining dialysis clearance is to calculate the ratio of amount recovered in the dialysate ($V_D \cdot C_D$) to the area under the arterial blood concentration-time curve within the collection period, τ. That is,

$$CL_{bD} = \frac{V_D \cdot C_D}{\int_0^\tau C_{b,in} \cdot dt} \qquad 4$$

where V_D is the volume of dialysate collected during the interval, τ, and C_D is the drug concentration in the dialysate after mixing.

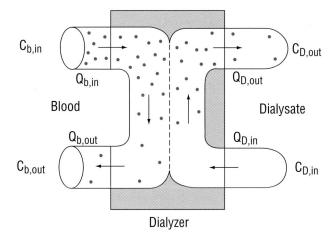

Dialyzer

Fig. 24–1. Schematic representation of a hemodialysis system in which drug is passively transferred across a semipermeable membrane (---) from blood to dialysate. Drug is delivered to the system at rate $Q_{b,in} \cdot C_{b,in}$ and is returned to the body at rate $Q_{b,out} \cdot C_{b,out}$. The difference between these rates is the net rate of loss into the dialyzing fluid. This rate of removal is the same as the difference between the rates leaving, $Q_{D,out} \cdot C_{D,out}$, and entering $Q_{D,in} \cdot C_{D,in}$, the dialyzer in the dialysate. Within the dialyzing system, blood and dialysate flows may be essentially concurrent, countercurrent, or crosscurrent, depending on the system design. Flows in the most common dialyzer, hollow fiber, are countercurrent, as shown. $C_{b,in}$; $C_{b,out}$ = drug concentrations in blood entering and leaving dialyzer, respectively. $C_{D,in}$; $C_{D,out}$ = drug concentrations in dialysate entering and leaving dialyzer, respectively. $Q_{b,in}$; $Q_{b,out}$ = blood flows (usually 200 to 400 mL/min) entering and leaving the dialyzer. $Q_{D,in}$; $Q_{D,out}$ = dialysate flows (usually 300 to 600 mL/min) entering and leaving the dialyzer.

Dialysis clearance depends on the dialysis system, the fraction unbound in blood, and the molecular size of the substance. A likely value can be predicted from

$$\frac{\text{Blood dialysis}}{\text{clearance}} = \frac{\text{Dialysis clearance}}{\text{of creatinine}} \cdot \sqrt{\frac{113}{\text{M.W.}}} \cdot fu_b \qquad 5$$

or

$$\frac{\text{Plasma}}{\text{dialysis}} = \frac{\text{Dialysis clearance}}{\text{of creatinine}} \cdot \sqrt{\frac{113}{\text{M.W.}}} \cdot fu$$
$$\text{clearance}$$

where fu_b is the fraction unbound in blood (fu is the fraction unbound in plasma), and M.W. is the molecular weight of the substance (a measure of molecular size).

Because protein binding is often altered in dialysis patients, a more useful parameter than blood or plasma dialysis clearance is

$$\frac{\text{Unbound}}{\text{dialysis clearance}} = \frac{\text{Dialysis clearance}}{\text{of creatinine}} \cdot \sqrt{\frac{113}{\text{M.W.}}} \qquad 6$$

The dialysis clearance of creatinine, a readily dialyzable endogenous compound not bound to plasma proteins, is a means of assessing the capability of a given dialysis system to remove drug from the body. With current dialyzers, dialysis clearance values for creatinine are usually between 80 and 200 mL/min. The unbound dialysis clearance for drugs and most other substances is usually lower than this because their molecular weights are greater than that of creatinine (M.W. = 113 g/mole) and, in the case of (total) dialysis clearance, because they are often bound to plasma proteins or blood cells.

The predictions of dialysis clearance based on concentrations in whole blood, plasma, or plasma water (Eqs. 5 and 6) tend to be underestimates of the respective clearances of drugs in systems with high flux membranes. This underestimation occurs because the dialysis clearance of creatinine, a low molecular weight endogenous substance, is limited by and approaches blood flow. The greater the efficiency of the dialyzer, the more this last statement applies. In addition, for drugs with higher molecular weight, the tendency for clearance to be blood-flow limited is less.

There is usually little, if any, correlation of dialysis clearance with either ionization or lipophilicity because the membranes used are porous rather than lipoidal barriers.

A large range of dialysis clearance values have been observed (Fig. 24–2). Part of this variability is caused by differences in binding of drug to plasma proteins, as shown in Fig. 24–2. Molecular weight differences, even though relatively small in the range observed for most drugs, also contribute to this variability. When both of these sources are accounted for, there is still considerable variability in dialysis clearance, owing, in large part, to the wide range of dialyzers and dialysis conditions used to acquire the information shown. Relating dialysis clearance to that of creatinine for each dialyzer should adjust for more of this remaining variability. In the absence of such information, Eqs. 5 and 6 can be used but should be treated as rough approximations.

Extraction Coefficient

Under steady-state conditions, rate of removal relative to the rate of presentation is a measure of the *efficiency* of a dialysis system. By this definition, efficiency is the dialyzer extraction ratio, or more commonly, the *extraction coefficient*. Its value can be calculated from the dialysis blood clearance and blood flow. That is,

$$\frac{\text{Extraction}}{\text{Coefficient}} = \frac{CL_{bD}}{Q_{b,in}} \qquad\qquad 7$$

where CL_{bD} is estimated from Eqs. 1, 2, or 4. Dialysis clearance and efficiency are measures of the ability of the dialyzer to remove drug from blood, but they do not indicate how readily it is removed from the body. A measure of the latter is the fraction of drug initially in the body removed during a period of dialysis treatment. This value is a measure of the *clinical dialyzability* of the drug.

Pharmacokinetic evaluation of hemodialysis and related procedures requires information on the parameters CL_b, CL_{bD}, and V_b (or the corresponding sets of values based on unbound drug CLu, CLu_D, and Vu; or on drug in plasma CL, CL_D, and V) and the duration of the procedure. In the following derivation and throughout the remainder of this chapter, for convenience, the set of parameter values based on measurement of unbound drug is emphasized.

Drug Elimination

During dialysis, drug is removed by the dialyzer and by the body's own elimination mechanisms, therefore,

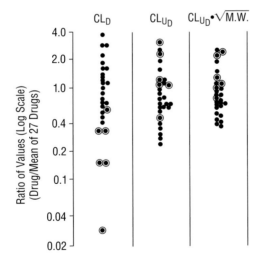

Fig. 24–2. Plasma dialysis clearance and unbound dialysis clearance with an adjustment for molecular size for 27 different drugs show considerable variability. Variability is greatest for (total) dialysis clearance CL_D. On correcting for protein binding to give unbound dialysis clearance, CLu_D, variability is decreased, and those drugs that are highly bound (⊙) are brought into the range of unbound dialysis clearance values of the other drugs. Correction of unbound dialysis clearance with the square root of the molecular weight (M.W.) appears to diminish variability further, but prediction using both molecular weight and fraction unbound is still not too accurate. Presumably, further adjustment for dialyzer and dialysis conditions by relating dialysis clearance of the drug to that of creatinine should be helpful. The data in this figure were obtained before the advent of systems with greater efficiencies and the use of high flux membranes. Because the results are expressed relative to the mean of the values obtained, the observations on more recent systems would probably remain similar to those shown here. However, the dispersion of the values due to the different systems may not be as great. For comparative purposes, in each column the value for a drug has been expressed relative to the average value for all 27 drugs on a logarithmic scale. (Data from Lee, C.C., and Marbury, T.C.: Drug therapy in patients undergoing haemodialysis: Clinical pharmacokinetic considerations. Clin. Pharmacokinet., 9:42–66, 1984.)

$$\begin{array}{l}\text{Rate of elimination from} \\ \text{body during dialysis}\end{array} = (CLu + CLu_D) \cdot Cu \qquad\qquad 8$$

If the clearance values are constant with time then, on integration, the unbound concentration at any time t after starting dialysis is

$$Cu = Cu(0) \cdot e^{-k_D t} \qquad\qquad 9$$

where $Cu(0)$ is the unbound drug concentration in blood at the start of dialysis and k_D is the elimination rate constant $[(CLu + CLu_D)/Vu]$ during dialysis. Thus, $e^{-k_D \tau}$ is the fraction of drug remaining at the end of a dialysis period τ, and so

$$\begin{array}{l}\text{Fraction lost from body} \\ \text{during a dialysis period}\end{array} = 1 - e^{-k_D \tau} \qquad\qquad 10$$

The contribution of dialysis to total drug elimination remains to be determined. Of the total drug eliminated during a dialysis period, the fraction removed by dialysis, f_D, is

$$f_D = \frac{CLu_D}{(CLu + CLu_D)} \qquad\qquad 11$$

Fraction of total elimination
occurring by dialysis

The fraction of drug in the body at the start of dialysis that is eliminated by the dialysis procedure depends on the fraction of total elimination that dialysis represents, Eq. 11, and the fraction of drug lost by all routes of elimination, Eq. 10. Therefore,

$$\begin{array}{l}\text{Fraction of drug initially in} \\ \text{body eliminated by dialysis}\end{array} = f_D \cdot [1 - e^{-k_D \cdot \tau}] \qquad\qquad 12$$

Effectiveness of Procedure

Figure 24–3 demonstrates the effectiveness of hemodialysis as a function of unbound clearance and unbound volume of distribution (Eq. 12) for a typical 3-hour dialysis period. An unbound dialysis clearance of 150 mL/min, a common value for drugs with high-flux dialyzers is used. It is apparent from this figure that hemodialysis is ineffective (less than 20% of drug initially in body is removed by dialysis treatment) if the unbound volume of distribution is large (greater than 120 L). Also, if CLu is much greater than the unbound dialysis clearance, dialysis becomes less effective in eliminating the drug. Indeed, when CLu is 400 mL/min or greater, the amount removed by the treatment must be less than 20% (the value of f_D) of the amount initially present, regardless of the value of Vu.

The effectiveness of dialysis may also be evaluated by comparing the half-lives during $(t_{1/2,during})$ and between $(t_{1/2})$ dialysis treatments. During dialysis

$$t_{1/2,during} = \frac{0.693 \cdot Vu}{(CLu + CLu_D)} \qquad\qquad 13$$

and, between dialysis treatments

$$t_{1/2} = \frac{0.693 \cdot Vu}{CLu} \qquad\qquad 14$$

The change in the half-life during dialysis is a function of how much dialysis clearance contributes to the body's own clearance of a drug, that is,

$$\frac{t_{1/2,during}}{t_{1/2}} = \frac{Clu}{(Clu + Clu_D)} = 1 - f_D \qquad\qquad 15$$

A dramatic reduction in half-life during dialysis does not guarantee that the procedure effectively removes drug during a single dialysis treatment. Take, for example, phenobarbital in a 70-kg end-stage renal disease patient whose pharmacokinetic parameters are $Vu = 77$ L, $CLu = 0.4$ L/hr, $k = 0.005$ hr^{-1} and $t_{1/2} = 137$ hr. Using a value of 150 mL/min (9 L/hr) for unbound dialysis clearance, the half-life of phenobarbital is reduced to 5.7 hr during dialysis. Thus, dialysis accounts for 96% of drug elimination (Eq. 11); but only 29% (Eq. 12) of the drug present in the body at the start of dialysis is removed during a 3-hr dialysis period. Even though the half-life of phenobarbital is decreased 24-fold, the fraction removed in the 3-hr dialysis period is small, because the half-life during dialysis is still considerably longer than the period of treatment.

DRUG ADMINISTRATION IN HEMODIALYSIS PATIENTS

One approach to dosage adjustment is to replace the amount lost in the dialysate during the treatment period. This amount can be calculated from Eq. 12, knowing the amount in the body at the start of dialysis, $V \cdot C(0)$. A more appealing approach is to restore the amount in the body at the end of dialysis to the value that would have occurred had the patient not been dialyzed; this procedure permits the patient's existing regimen to be maintained (Fig. 24–4). The amount to be replaced is calculated as follows. The amount remaining in the body at time τ had no dialysis been employed is $V \cdot C(0)^{-k \cdot \tau}$: the corre-

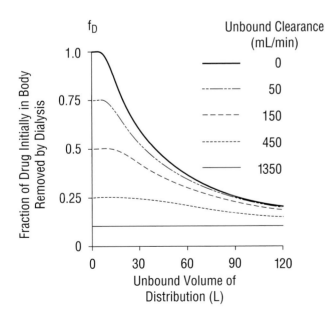

Fig. 24–3. Displayed is the fraction of drug in the body at the start of dialysis that is eliminated by 3 hr of dialysis treatment as a function of unbound clearance (nondialysis elimination) and unbound volume of distribution. The unbound dialysis clearance is set at 150 mL/min, a common value for drugs in high flux systems. The y-axis is f_D, the fraction of total elimination occurring by dialysis. Each line represents the expected fraction eliminated at a given unbound clearance as a function of the unbound volume of distribution. Clearly, either a small f_D ($CLu > CLu_D$) or an unbound volume of distribution greater than about 120 L would produce a recovery in the dialysate during a 3-hr dialysis treatment with the high flux system of less than 20% of the original amount in the body. The unbound volume of distribution has a lower limit, that of the extracellular volume (about 16 L). Only those conditions in which Vu is greater than 16 L therefore apply.

sponding amount when dialysis is employed is $V \cdot C(0)e^{-k_D \cdot \tau}$. The difference between these two terms provides an estimate of the supplemental dose needed to achieve the objective.

$$\text{Supplementary dose} = V \cdot C(0)[e^{-k\tau} - e^{-k_D\tau}] \qquad\qquad 16$$

This kinetic approach toward dosage adjustment is subsequently illustrated with gentamicin and phenobarbital.

The pharmacokinetic parameters of gentamicin in the typical 55-year-old, 70-kg patient are (Table 18–4): $CL = 5.1$ L/hr, $V = 15$ L, $t_{1/2} = 2$ hr, $fe > 0.95$. As fe is greater than 0.95 and probably close to 1.0, the kinetics of this drug are drastically altered in a patient without renal function. From the relationship $t_{1/2}(d) = t_{1/2}(t) \cdot Vu(d)/Vu(t) \cdot 1/R_d$ (Eq. 9, Chap. 16), and given that $Vu(d) = Vu(t)$, the half-life of this drug in anephric patients is greater than 40 hr. Needless to say, administration of this drug to an anephric patient requires extreme caution. For purposes of the example below, assume a half-life of 72 hr in an individual anephric patient on gentamicin alone. This half-life corresponds to a clearance of 2.4 mL/min; the rate of administration to maintain the same average steady-state concentration should therefore be 36 times less than usual. A common regimen of gentamicin for a patient with normal renal function is 80 mg (1.2 mg/kg), intramuscularly or intravenously, every 8 hr; the initial dose and the maintenance doses are the same. But a strong argument exists for reducing the initial dose for an anephric patient, when the dosing interval is much shorter than the half-life (Chap. 16, p. 260). Accordingly, a recommendation for an anephric patient might be a 40-mg loading dose followed by 12 mg every other day. As previously discussed (Chap. 5, Therapeutic Response and Toxicity), appropriateness of large and infrequent versus small and frequent doses is not settled for aminoglycosides, especially for patients with compromised renal function.

The expected amount in the body with time following this recommended regimen, in the absence of dialysis, is shown as Curve A in Fig. 24–5. The anephric patient is dialyzed for 4 hr on days 2, 4 and 6 between doses on days 1, 3 and 5. Consideration of a supple-

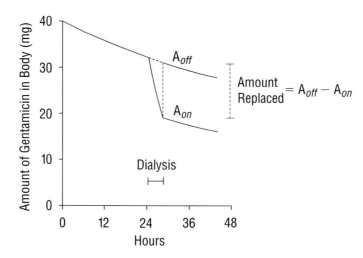

Fig. 24–4. The dose of gentamicin needed to return the amount in the body at the end of dialysis to the value that would have been present at that time, had the patient not been dialyzed, is the difference between the amounts in the body at the end of the interval in the absence (A_{off}) and presence (A_{on}) of dialysis. The replacement dose (12 mg) in this example of an anephric patient is close to the amount in the dialysate because little has been lost by the body's own mechanisms during the dialysis interval.

mentary dose requires an estimate of the fraction lost in the dialysate during each treatment period. The dialysis clearance of gentamicin, a drug not bound in plasma, in a common dialyzer is 30 mL/min. The combined clearance in this patient is therefore 32.4 mL/min. The corresponding elimination rate constant, k_D, is 0.13 hr^{-1} ($t_{1/2}$ = 5.3 hr). Using Eq. 10, the fraction lost during a 4-hr dialysis period is 0.4.

Thus, hemodialysis every 2 or 3 days would result (1 week later) in very little gentamicin being in the anephric patient (Curve B, Fig. 24–5) if the suggested regimen above were not adjusted. Clearly, a supplementary dose at the end of each dialysis period is needed.

The supplementary dose should be sufficient to return the amount in the body to the value that would have occurred had the patient not been dialyzed, the condition simulated in Curve C of Fig. 24–5. The amount continues to decline with dialysis every other day after a loading dose of 40 mg. The amount in the body at the time of the first dialysis on day 2 ($40 \times e^{-0.693 \times 24/72}$) is 32 mg. The supplementary dose is then 12 mg (Eq. 16). Table 24–1 shows representative drugs for which supplementary doses might be considered.

For a drug that is readily dialyzed and is required by the patient at all times, consideration might be given to administering it during dialysis treatment. Another approach is to use a therapeutic (unbound) concentration of the drug in the dialysate. Although theoretically more logical, the latter approach may be very expensive. The total volume used is

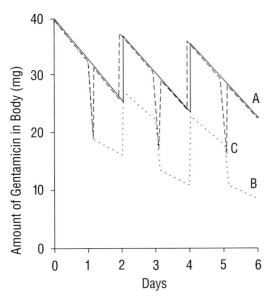

Fig. 24–5. Sketch of amount of gentamicin in the body with time in an anephric patient on an i.m. dosage regimen of 40 mg initially and 12 mg every other day. Curve A (——)—patient not dialyzed. Curve B (·····)—patient undergoing dialysis (for 4 hr) on days 2, 4, and 6. Curve C (----)—patient undergoing dialysis is given a supplementary dose of 12 mg just after each dialysis period. A one-compartment model with instantaneous absorption is used.

Table 24–1. Representative Drugs for Which Supplemental Doses Postdialysis May Be Required in Patients Undergoing Hemodialysis[a]

Aminoglycosides	Cephalosporins	Penicillins
Amikacin	Cefamandole	Amoxycillin
Gentamicin	Cefazolin	Ampicillin
Kanamycin	Cefsulodin	Carbenicillin
Tobramycin	Cephalexin	Penicillin-G
Other Antimicrobial Agents	Immunosuppressive Agents	Miscellaneous
Chloramphenicol	Cyclophosphamide	Disopyramide
Isoniazid	5-Fluorouracil	Phenobarbital
Flucytosine	Methotrexate	Theophylline

[a]Modified from Lee, C.-S.C., and Marbury, T.C.: Drug therapy in patients undergoing haemodialysis: Clinical pharmacokinetic considerations. Clin. Pharmacokinet., 9:42–66, 1984.

144 L when a typical dialysate flow rate of 600 mL/min is continued for 4 hr. For gentamicin, a therapeutic concentration of 2 mg/L in the dialysate would therefore require the addition of almost 300 mg. If the drug is an antibiotic, one might argue that doing this would help to prevent infection.

Although only about 29% of phenobarbital initially present was previously calculated to be removed in a single 3-hr session with a high-flux dialysis system, the steady-state phenobarbital concentration may be considerably reduced during repeated sessions. The amount of phenobarbital in a patient who has a half-life of 5.5 days and a volume of distribution of 38 L is decreased by 12% ($e^{-CL \cdot \tau/V}$) during the dosing interval (1 day). The additional loss of 29% every other day (on dialysis) would more than double the average percent lost (12%/day between dialysis treatments and about 40% on dialysis day). In this patient, the dosage would have to be doubled to keep the same average amount in the body at steady state. Clearly, the effect of dialysis should also be examined at steady state, the therapeutically relevant situation for phenobarbital.

PERITONEAL DIALYSIS

Peritoneal dialysis is accomplished by introducing dialyzing fluid into the peritoneal cavity via a catheter. After a period, the *dwell time*, the fluid is drained and discarded. Table 24–2 lists three kinds of chronic peritoneal dialysis procedures used clinically. The one that has become the most common is *continuous ambulatory peritoneal dialysis* CAPD. The subsequent discussion is largely restricted to this dialysis modality.

Dialysis Clearance

In CAPD, dialysis clearance, CL_{PD}, is most frequently expressed as the amount of a drug or substance recovered in the drained dialysate relative to the AUC during the dwell time, τ, after administration by any route. Analogous to Eq. 4 and with the subscript *PC* meaning peritoneal cavity,

$$CL_{PD} = \frac{C_{PC} \cdot V_{PC}}{\int_0^\tau C \cdot dt} \qquad 17$$

where V_{PC} is the dialysate volume in the peritoneal cavity. The plasma and dialysate concentrations of the cephalosporin, cefsulodin, during a commonly employed 5-hr dwell time, after intravenous (i.v.) and intraperitoneal (i.p.) administrations are shown in Fig. 24–6. At the end of the dwell time, the peritoneal concentration approaches that of plasma after i.v. administration, and the plasma concentration approaches that of dialysate after i.p. admin-

Table 24–2. Chronic Peritoneal Dialysis Procedures

PROCEDURE	VOLUME EXCHANGED PER DAY (L/day)	NUMBER OF EXCHANGES PER DAY	DWELL TIMES (hr)	TOTAL DIALYSIS TIME PER DAY (hr)
Continuous procedures				
Continuous ambulatory peritoneal dialysis	6–12	3–5	4–12	24
Continuous cycling peritoneal dialysis	8–20	4–8	1–12	24
Discontinuous procedures				
Nocturnal peritoneal dialysis	10–30	5–15	0.3–1.5	12
Intermittent peritoneal dialysis	40–70	20–30	0.2–0.5	12

istration. Clearance, obtained by Eq. 17, then reflects the net movement of the drug during the dwell time. This clearance term is not strictly a measure of the ability of a drug to pass from blood into the peritoneal cavity as its value decreases with dwell time. This situation is in contrast to the clearance term for nonrecirculating hemodialysis for which sink conditions are maintained. A unidirectional measure can be obtained for peritoneal dialysis if the dialysate is exchanged at sufficient frequency to ensure that sink conditions are approximated.

The unbound (peritoneal) dialysis clearance value for most drugs lies between 2 and 7 mL/min. The reason for this low value can be explained as follows. There is negligible protein in the dialysate fluid (1 to 2 g/2 L) at the end of the dwell time. Consequently, when equilibrium is achieved ($C_{PC} = Cu$), the amount in the dialysate is $Cu \cdot V_{PC}$, where Cu is the unbound concentration in plasma and C_{PC} is the unbound concentration in dialysate. If the plasma concentration is constant with time, then the unbound AUC is $Cu \cdot \tau$. Thus, the unbound dialysis clearance value is $Cu \cdot V_{PC}/Cu \cdot \tau$ or V_{PC}/τ. With a usual dialysate volume of 2000 mL and a τ of 300 min, the net clearance value is 6.7 mL/min. This low clearance means that drug elimination by peritoneal dialysis is not a major consideration for patients on CAPD. When CAPD is the only route of elimination and drug is distributed in extracellular fluids (0.25 L/kg, the smallest volume possible for unbound drug), the half-life is then 1810 min ($t_{1/2} = 0.693$ [250 mL/kg $\times$ 70 kg]/6.7 mL/min) or 1.26 days. Clearly, other routes of elimination or therapeutic maneuvers to remove drug are generally of greater importance than CAPD.

Dialysis clearance values for intermittent peritoneal dialysis and continuous cycling peritoneal dialysis can be 10 to 40 mL/min, values much greater than those for CAPD, because sink conditions tend to be maintained when using short dwell times. For this reason, removal of a significant fraction of drug in the body can occur during a treatment period just as with hemodialysis, but dialysis is then not continuous. The methods of analysis and prediction of drug removal are the same, except that the intermittent nature of the modality must be incorporated.

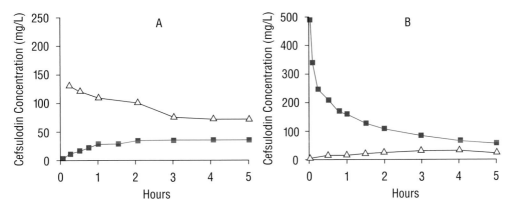

Fig. 24–6. The plasma ($\triangle$) and dialysate ($\blacksquare$, color) concentrations of cefsulodin, a cephalosporin antibiotic that is virtually unbound in plasma, after i.v. administration (A) and i.p. administration (B) to a patient with end-stage renal disease tend to approach an equilibrium within a 5-hr dialysate dwell time. The concentration in plasma after i.v. administration does not decline much because of the patient's renal disease and because the amount distributing into the 2-L dialysate volume from the 16-L extracellular fluid volume of distribution is small. In contrast, the concentration in the dialysate drops dramatically as it distributes from the 2-L volume into the 16-L volume (1 mg/L = 1.9 µM). (Data from Brouard, R., Tozer, T.N., Merdjan, H., Guillemin, A., and Baumelou, A.: Transperitoneal movement and pharmacokinetics of cefotiam and cefsulodin in patients on continuous ambulatory peritoneal dialysis. Clin. Nephrol., *30*:197–206, 1988.)

Route of Administration

Although little drug is lost into the peritoneal cavity during CAPD after parenteral administration, most (more than 60%) of a dose administered into the peritoneal cavity is absorbed into the body during a typical 3- to 6-hr dwell time. Because of the continuous nature of CAPD, this route of administration has a potential application for systemic purposes, especially for drugs that cannot be absorbed when taken orally, due to poor intestinal permeability, as is the case for many antibiotics. Dwell time becomes particularly important here as a determinant of systemic bioavailability. Not all of the drug instilled into the cavity reaches the systemic circulation. This is shown in Fig. 24–7 for teicoplanin, a glycopeptide antibiotic. Bioavailability increases with dwell time and is about 78% at 5 hr. The data also indicate a much greater coefficient of variation in bioavailability at earlier times. Thus, to ensure consistent absorption, a short dwell time is not recommended.

Peritonitis is the major drawback to CAPD. A major question here is whether direct administration of an antibiotic into the peritoneal cavity to treat peritonitis might be more effective than systemic administration. Although intraperitoneal administration would appear to be superior, drug may be delivered to the site of infection more readily via the capillaries than through the peritoneum. In some situations, a combination of both intraperitoneal and other routes of administration may be advantageous.

HEMOFILTRATION

Another technique used to treat patients with end-stage renal disease is *hemofiltration*. With this technique, endogenous compounds are removed by filtering plasma water from blood under pressure (pump). Blood cells are returned to the body; the filtered plasma water is replaced by an equal volume of physiologic fluid administered intravenously. For systems in which both dialysis and filtration contribute extensively, the term *hemodiafiltration* is applied.

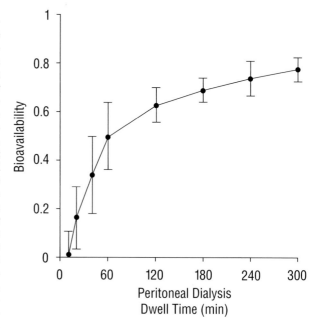

Fig. 24–7. Relationship between systemic bioavailability (mean ± SD of five patients) and dwell time when teicoplanin is administered intraperitoneally. Two liters of peritoneal dialysis solution were instilled into the peritoneal cavity for 5 hr in patients undergoing continuous ambulatory peritoneal dialysis. Bioavailability was calculated by comparison of *AUC* values following single i.p. and i.v. doses as well as from the amount of drug remaining within the peritoneal cavity with time. At 5 hr (300 min), the bioavailability was about 0.78 by both methods. The coefficient of variation (SD/mean) was much greater at early than at late times. Longer dwell times therefore give more complete and less variable bioavailability. (Redrawn from Brouard, R.J., Kapusnik, J.E., Gambertoglio, J.G., Schoenfeld, P.Y., Sachdeva, M., Freel, K., and Tozer, T.N.: Teicoplanin pharmacokinetics and bioavailability during peritoneal dialysis. Clin. Pharmacol. Ther., 45:674–681, 1989. With permission.)

As with hemodialysis, there are many variations in hemofiltration techniques. The principles of drug removal are similar, but not the same. In hemodialysis, molecular size influences dialysis clearance by determining diffusion across the membrane. In hemofiltration, filtration is generally not affected by molecular weight as long as the size remains below the exclusion limit, the value of which depends on the membrane used. Binding to plasma proteins is also a determinant as the size of most proteins is above the exclusion limit so that only drug in plasma water is filtered. The rate of filtration is then approximated by the relationship

$$\text{Rate of filtration} = fu \cdot Q_f \cdot C = Q_f \cdot Cu \qquad\qquad 18$$

where Q_f is the rate of filtrate flow, often in the 50- to 150-mL/min range. Because of the dependence of dialysis on molecular size, hemofiltration often removes large (M.W. >500 g/mole) molecules better than hemodialysis.

DIALYSIS AND FILTRATION IN DRUG OVERDOSE

Assessment of the contribution of hemodialysis or hemofiltration to the reduction of the morbidity and mortality of drug intoxication is facilitated by quantitative information on drug removal. Measurement of the amount of drug in the dialysate or filtrate alone is inadequate. For example, a recovery of 10 g may be unimportant if more than 100 g were in the body at the start of the procedure. Information on the fraction of the amount initially in the body that is eliminated by the procedure is needed.

Several factors associated with the overdosed patient may affect the pharmacokinetics of a drug, e.g., anoxia, metabolic acidosis, carbon dioxide retention, hypotension, depressed renal function, and hypothermia. Furthermore, complications may arise because of slow tissue distribution of a drug (Chap. 19) and because of the concentrations of drug and active metabolites attained (Chap. 21). Comments on a few of these complications are in order.

Drug Redistribution

An important consideration in evaluating the potential use of hemodialysis or hemofiltration in an overdose situation is drug redistribution. For certain drugs, the procedure may remove drug more readily from the plasma than it can be replaced from tissue stores, thereby resulting in a rebound of the plasma drug concentration when the procedure is stopped. Two primary mechanisms account for this slow return: slow diffusion through membranes and limited vascular perfusion (Chap. 10) of the tissues in which drug is stored.

Lithium (Fig. 24–8) is an example of a drug that exhibits postdialysis rebound due to slow diffusion from cells. Dialysis clearance adds substantially to the total body clearance (virtually all renal clearance) of this drug. Lithium disappears rapidly from plasma during dialysis, and a large fraction in the body is expected to be removed into the dialysate. The slow return from tissue stores, however, limits the total amount removed and produces a rebound in the concentration upon stopping dialysis treatment. In this case, assessment of the fraction of the initial amount of drug removed by dialysis is relatively simple, since virtually all the drug eliminated by the body is excreted into the urine. The fraction is the amount recovered in the dialysate divided by the sum of the amounts in the dialysate and the urine during the dialysis period.

Another method of assessing the contribution of dialysis to total elimination is to extrapolate the terminal part of the curve, when equilibrium has been reestablished, back to the beginning of dialysis (see Fig. 24–8). The difference between the initial concentration

(3.0 mg/L) and the extrapolated value (1.6 mg/L) relative to the initial value is the fraction eliminated by dialysis.

Concentration-Dependent Kinetics

An additional consideration in the dialysis of drugs in the overdose situation is concentration-dependent kinetics (Chap. 22), whereby either the volume of distribution or the total clearance, or both, depends on the concentration of drug in plasma. Ethchlorvynol shows such concentration-dependent kinetic behavior (Fig. 24–9). At normal therapeutic doses, the half-life is 25 hr; in overdose cases it is increased to more than 100 hr, probably because of a decreased metabolic clearance at the higher concentrations. Similar to lithium, ethchlorvynol also shows plasma rebound after dialysis. The redistribution here is a consequence of the high affinity of the drug for fat, a poorly perfused tissue.

Fig. 24–8. During 6.5 hr of hemodialysis (solid bar) of a patient poisoned with lithium, the plasma concentration of lithium (●) dropped dramatically; however, on discontinuing dialysis the plasma concentration rose with redistribution of drug from tissue cells to plasma, so that only about one-half of the lithium initially in the body was removed by dialysis. A rough estimate of fraction lost can be obtained by extrapolating (----) the terminal curve back to the time dialysis was started. A semilogarithmic plot should be used for the extrapolation in those situations in which the postdialysis concentration declines linearly on such a plot. (Redrawn from data of Amdisen, A., and Skjoldborg, H.: Haemodialysis for lithium poisoning. Lancet, 2:213, 1969.)

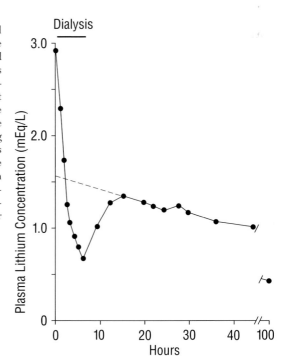

Fig. 24–9. The overall decline of ethchlorvynol concentration in blood on this semilogarithmic plot shows concentration dependence in an intoxicated patient. During each 8-hr dialysis period (⊢——⊣), the concentration (●——●) was reduced but tended to rise again when dialysis was discontinued, indicative of redistribution (1 mg/L = 6.9 μM). (Redrawn from Tozer, T.N., Witt, L.D., Gee, L., Tong, T.G., and Gambertoglio, J.: Evaluation of hemodialysis for ethchlorvynol (Placidyl) overdose. Am. J. Hosp. Pharm., *31*:986–989, 1974. Original data from Gibson, P.F., and Wright, N.: Ethchlorvynol in biological fluids: Specificity of assay methods. J. Pharm. Sci., *61*:169–174, 1972.)

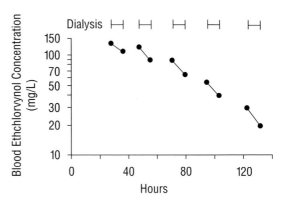

As stated in Chap. 22, concentration-dependent kinetics is perhaps more the rule than the exception in drug overdose. Assessment of the dialyzability of drugs under this circumstance is more difficult than at therapeutic concentrations.

Toxic Metabolites

Little correlation may exist between the drug concentration and the patient's clinical status for drugs for which a metabolite is primarily responsible for toxicity. Clinical response is then expected to be more closely related to the blood concentration of the metabolite. The removal of active metabolite, as well as unchanged drug, should be considered. Often, there is a paucity of information of this nature.

Other Considerations

Determination of the overall benefit-to-risk ratio of hemodialysis or hemofiltration requires weighing of many factors. The severity of the poisoning, the value of other procedures such as forced diuresis (Chap. 11), the control of urine pH, and the risks of the procedure to the patient, in addition to other clinical variables must all be considered. Table 24–3 lists representative substances for which extracorporeal methods may be of potential value in treating severely intoxicated patients.

HEMOPERFUSION

A final system, which operates on principles different from those of peritoneal dialysis, hemofiltration, and hemodialysis, is *hemoperfusion*. In this system, whole blood is passed through a charcoal or resin bed. Molecules that are adsorbed are retarded; blood cells and plasma proteins readily pass through. This system can have a high efficiency for removing certain drugs. As virtually all the drug can be extracted from the blood and, blood flows through the hemoperfusion cartridge can be 200 to 400 mL/min, clearances of greater than 200 mL/min can be obtained for substances that strongly adsorb to the system. This method appears to have potential in the treatment of drug overdose. It is, however, not without its own set of limitations, including the removal of platelets, white blood cells, various endogenous steroids, and other substances. The pharmacokinetic principles discussed for assessing the effectiveness of hemodialysis also apply here, except that drug removed by hemoperfusion is determined from the amount within the cartridge instead of the amount recovered in the dialysate.

Table 24–3.   Representative Substances for Which Extracorporeal Methods (Hemodialysis, Hemofiltration, and Hemoperfusion) May Be of Potential Value in Treating Severe Intoxication[a]

Acetaminophen		
Aminoglycosides	Diazepam	Methyprylon
Amobarbital	Ethanol	Paraquat
Butabarbital	Ethchlorvynol	Pentobarbital
Bromide ion	Ethylene glycol	Procainamide
Carbamazepine	Glutethimide	Salicylic acid
Chloral hydrate	Lithium	Secobarbital
(Trichlorothanol)	Methanol	Theophylline

[a]Cutter, R.E., Forland, S.C., Hammond, P.G.S.J., and Evans, J.R: Extracorporeal removal of drugs and poisons by hemodialysis and hemoperfusion. Ann. Rev. Pharmacol. Toxicol., *27*:169–191, 1987. Gossel, T.A., and Bricker, J.D.: Principles of Clinical Toxicology. 2nd ed., Raven Press, New York, 1990, pp. 50–55. Pond, S.M.: Extracorporeal techniques in the treatment of poisoned patients. Med. J. Aust., *154*:617–622, 1991.

STUDY PROBLEMS

(Answers to Study Problems are in Appendix II.)

1. Define dialysis, extracorporeal dialysis, hemodialysis, hemofiltration, continuous ambulatory peritoneal dialysis, dialysis clearance, dialyzer, dialyzer efficiency, and clinical dialyzability of a drug.

2. a. Complete Table 24–4 by estimating unbound and total dialysis clearance values, the ratio of half-lives between and during dialysis treatments, and the half-life between dialysis treatments for each of the three drugs listed. Use a creatinine dialysis clearance of 150 mL/min and a one-compartment model.

Table 24–4. Pharmacokinetic Information and Estimated Unbound Dialysis Clearances and Half-Life Ratios (During/Between Dialysis Treatments) During Hemodialysis of Specific Patients With End-Stage Renal Disease

	V (L)	f_u	Cl (L/hr)	UNBOUND DIALYSIS CLEARANCE (L/hr)	DIALYSIS CLEARANCE (L/hr)	$\left(\dfrac{t_{1/2}}{t_{1/2,during}}\right)$	$t_{1/2}$ (hr)
S-Naproxen (M.W. = 230 g/mole)	11	0.003	0.55				
Tobramycin (M.W. = 468 g/mole)	23	0.95	0.3				
Verapamil (M.W. = 455 g/mole)	350	0.10	105				

b. Using Eq. 12 and Fig. 24–3, assess the *clinical dialyzability* of the three compounds listed in Table 22–4 using a 4-hr dialysis treatment. For any drug of questionable dialyzability, briefly discuss the one kinetic property that is most likely responsible for its being a poor candidate for removal by dialysis.

3. In a study of the removal of phenytoin by hemodialysis (Adapted from Martin, E., Gambertoglio, J.G., Adler, D.S., Tozer, T.N., Roman, L.A., and Grausz, H.: Removal of phenytoin by hemodialysis in uremic patients. JAMA, 238:1750–1753, 1977), the following data were obtained in one of the subjects. Sodium phenytoin (350 mg of acid form of drug) was administered intravenously over 30 min 2 hr before hemodialysis treatment. The average blood and dialysate flows through the dialyzer were 305 and 267 mL/min, respectively. The plasma phenytoin concentration dropped from 3.9 to 3.5 mg/L during the 6-hr dialysis treatment. The fraction unbound was 0.21, and the amount of phenytoin collected in the 6-hr dialysate was 14 mg. The dialysis clearance of creatinine was 83 mL/min. The concentrations in blood and plasma were virtually identical.

a. Calculate the dialysis clearance of phenytoin.

b. What is the efficiency (extraction coefficient) of the dialyzer used?

c. The blood concentrations into and out of the dialyzer could have been used to determine dialysis clearance. If they had been used, what would the ratio (out/in) have been to give the clearance observed in "a"? Assume no net loss of fluid from the body into the dialysate. Do you think clearance could have been determined accurately from the blood concentrations into and out of the dialyzer?

d. Calculate the fraction of drug initially in the body that is eliminated by dialysis.

e. Is the observed dialysis clearance of phenytoin (M.W. = 252 g/mole) close to the value predicted by Eq. 5 in the text?

4. The data in Table 24–5 on vancomycin were acquired in patients receiving CAPD treatment. Vancomycin was given intravenously and intraperitoneally in doses of 10

mg/kg on separate occasions. The first dwell time after vancomycin administration was
4 hr. Two additional 4-hr exchanges and an overnight 12-hr dwell time were used.

Table 24–5.[a]

ROUTE OF ADMINISTRATION	CLEARANCE[b] (mL/min)	PERITONEAL DIALYSIS CLEARANCE (mL/min)
Intravenous	9	1.5[c]
Intraperitoneal instillation	15	2.5[d]

[a]Data from Bunke, C.M., Aronoff, G.R., Brier, M.E., Sloan, R.S., and Luft, F.C.: Vancomycin kinetics during continuous ambulatory peritoneal dialysis.
Clin. Pharmacol. Ther., 34:631–637, 1983.
[b]Includes peritoneal dialysis clearance. Calculated from Dose/AUC.
[c]Amount in dialysate between 0 and 72 hr divided by AUC within the same interval.
[d]Amount in dialysate between 4 and 72 hr divided by AUC within the same interval.

    a. The authors claim that the value of vancomycin peritoneal dialysis clearance, cal-
culated after i.p. instillation, differs from that after i.v. administration. Do you agree?
Defend your answer.

    b. Can you explain the differences observed in the estimates of clearance from the
two routes of administration?

5. Table 24–6 contains the value of several pharmacokinetic parameters and the recommended dosage regimen for adults with normal renal function for digitoxin and theophylline. In addition, their approximate values for dialysis clearance are given.

**Table 24–6. Selected Pharmacokinetic Parameters, Dosage Regimens,
and Dialysis Clearances of Digitoxin and Theophylline**[a]

PARAMETERS	DIGITOXIN	THEOPHYLLINE
Half-life (hr)	160	8
Volume of distribution, plasma (L)	38	35
Fraction excreted unchanged	0.3	0.13
Route of administration	Oral	Oral
Usual maintenance dosage regimen	0.1 mg daily	240 mg every 6 hr
Dialysis clearance, plasma (L/hr)[b]	<0.1	2.5
Fraction unbound	0.03	0.44

[a]In patients with normal renal function.
[b]Estimates from Eq. 5. Dialysis clearance of creatinine on the dialyzer used is assumed to be 120 mL/min.

In answering the questions below, the following apply: metabolites are inactive and
nontoxic; nonrenal clearance, volume of distribution, and bioavailability in normal and
anuric patients are the same; the pharmacokinetic parameter values are independent
of concentration; and distribution to the tissues is instantaneous. Also, theophylline is
thought by the clinician to be essential to the therapeutic management of this anephric
(no renal function) patient who is undergoing repeated hemodialysis treatment every
other day.

    a. Based on pharmacokinetic principles, indicate whether or not a supplementary dose
might be appropriate at the end of a 4-hr dialysis period with the dialyzer used.
Show how you come to your conclusion.

    b. What supplemental dose would you suggest for postdialysis administration?

    c. Fully delineate the dosage regimen that you would recommend for initiating and
maintaining theophylline therapy in the anephric patient undergoing hemodialysis?

6. From a pharmacokinetic point of view, is digitoxin (see Table 24–6) a candidate for
hemodialysis (24-hr duration) detoxification of a severely overdosed patient with normal
renal function?

7. Cisapride, a new drug for treating disorders of gastrointestinal motility was studied in end-stage renal disease patients undergoing hemodialysis (problem adapted from data in Gladziwa, U., Bares, R., Klotz, U., Dakshinamurty, K.V., Ittel, T.H., Seiler, K.U., and Sieberth, H.-G.: Pharmacokinetics and pharmacodynamics of cisapride in patients undergoing hemodialysis. Clin. Pharmacol. Ther., 50:675–681, 1991). The kinetics of cisapride in these patients (while not on hemodialysis) after oral administration of 20 mg is summarized as follows:

$$t_{1/2} = 9.6 \text{ hr} \quad V/F = 350 \text{ L} \quad F = 0.8$$

During a 5-hr dialysis period, the $AUC_{0-\tau}$ was 242 µg-hr/L, and the amount recovered in the dialysate was 0.36 mg.
Calculate the following:
a. Dialysis clearance.
b. Total clearance $(CL + CL_D)$ during dialysis.
c. Recovery in dialysate as a fraction of that eliminated by all pathways during dialysis treatment (f_D).
d. Fraction of drug initially in body that is lost in the dialysate during dialysis treatment.

8. Since the introduction of membranes with high molecular weight cutoff values, high dialysis clearances of relatively large molecules have been possible. Vancomycin (M.W. = 1448 g/mole) is an example of a drug that had been shown to be essentially non-dialyzable with previous conventional membranes. Böhler et al. examined the dialyzability of vancomycin with high-flux, high molecular weight cutoff membranes. Table 24–7 lists the plasma concentrations of vancomycin with time in one patient following i.v. infusion of 1 g over 1 hr. Blood samples were taken at the times (after end of infusion) indicated.

Table 24–7. Plasma Vancomycin Concentration at Various Times Over 1 Week in a Patient Who Received an i.v. Infusion of 1 g Over 1 hr and Who Was Hemodialyzed on Days 3, 5, and 7[a]

TIME (hr)	VANCOMYCIN CONCENTRATION (mg/L)
0.17	43.0
1.0	31.3
4.0	22.0
6.0	18.7
24	12.5
66[b]	10.0
66.5	8.65
67.5	8.02
70	6.40
71	8.01
73	8.50
76	8.74
110[b]	7.33
114	5.22
120	6.72
158[b]	5.64
162	3.74
167	4.75

[a]Adapted from data in Böhler, J., Reetze-Bonorden, P., Keller, E., Kramer, A., and Schollmeyer, P.J.: Rebound of plasma vancomycin levels after hemodialysis with highly permeable membranes. Br. J. Clin. Pharmacol., 42:635–640, 1992.
[b]Periods of hemodialysis: 66–70 hr, 110–114 hr, and 158–162 hr.

a. Prepare a semilogarithmic plot of the data.
b. What is the half-life of vancomycin during dialysis?
c. Five to six hours after the end of each dialysis period, the plasma concentration had recovered most of the decline observed during dialysis. Give an explanation for this observation.

d. Vancomycin is usually given only once a week to hemodialysis patients. Maintenance of a plasma concentration above 5 mg/L is desired. Does dialysis three times a week with the dialyzer used appear to suggest the need for additional doses of vancomycin?

e. This patient was dialyzed using a blood flow of about 125 mL/min. Would you expect the removal of vancomycin to be increased if the blood flow to the dialyzer were increased to 220 mL/min, a value used for other patients in the study? Focus your answer on the apparent distribution of the drug.

9. Cefprozil, a broad-spectrum oral cephalosporin antibiotic, is composed of cis and trans geometric isomers in an approximate ratio of 9:1. Both isomers are primarily excreted unchanged in urine in patients with normal renal function. Table 24–8 lists selected pharmacokinetic parameters of the cis isomer after a 1000-mg single oral dose of the mixture in subjects with varying degrees of renal function, including a group (Group V) undergoing intermittent hemodialysis. The kinetic behavior of the trans isomer was virtually identical to that of the cis. Hemodialysis was performed with (what appears to be) a high-flux dialyzer for 3 hr approximately 18 hr after administration of the drug. The half-life during dialysis was 2.05 hr. The average amount of the mixture recovered in the 3-hr dialysate was 30 mg, during which time the AUC was 5.75 mg-hr/L.

Table 24–8. Mean Pharmacokinetic Parameters and Observations of the Cis Isomer of Cefprozil After a Single 1000-mg Oral Dose in Patients With Varying Degrees of Renal Function[a]

	GROUP				
	I	II	III	IV	V
Creatinine clearance (mL/min)	>90	61–90	31–60	<31	Hemodialysis[b]
Parameter/observation					
C_{max} (mg/L)	13.3[c]	16.1	22.6	30.4	36.7
	(1.61)	(3.1)	(2.4)	(9.5)	(6.2)
T_{max} (hr)	2.1	1.8	2.7	3.7	4.0
	(0.7)	(0.3)	(0.8)	(1.0)	(1.3)
$t_{1/2}$ (hr)	1.7	2.1	3.4	5.2	5.9
	(0.6)	(0.6)	(1.1)	(1.1)	(1.1)
$AUC_{0-\infty}$ (mg-hr/L)	46	72	117	260	373
	(7)	(17)	(14)	(96)	(51)

[a]Shya, W.C., Pittman, K.A., Wilber, R.B., Matzke, G.R., and Barbhaiya, R.H.: Pharmacokinetics of cefprozil in healthy subjects and patients with renal impairment. J. Clin. Pharmacol., 31:362–371, 1991.
[b]Patients with low renal function who regularly received intermittent hemodialysis.
[c]Mean (SD).

a. Explain why C_{max} and t_{max} tend to increase on going from Group I to Group V.

b. Calculate the hemodialysis clearance of cis cefprozil.

c. What fraction of drug (cis isomer) in the body at the beginning of dialysis is removed during a 3-hr procedure?

d. Predict the dialysis clearance (based on plasma concentration) expected from knowledge of the drug's molecular weight (407 g/mole), its protein binding ($fu = 0.7$) and the dialysis clearance of creatinine (158 mL/min).

e. How well does the hemodialysis clearance of cefprozil (part "b") agree with your prediction (part "d")? If they are not in agreement, suggest a reason for the discrepancy.

10. The pharmacokinetics of ranitidine, a well-known H_2-receptor antagonist used in treating peptic ulcers, was studied in end-stage renal disease patients undergoing hemofiltration (problem adapted from data in Gladzivoa, U., Krishna, D.R., Klotz, U., Ittel, T.H., Schunkert, H., Glockner, W.M., and Mann, H.: Pharmacokinetics of ranitidine

in patients undergoing haemofiltration. Eur. J. Clin. Pharmacol., 35:427–430, 1988). The drug was administered intravenously (50 mg) immediately after the start of a 3.5-hr period of hemofiltration using a blood flow of 348 mL/min and an average filtrate flow of 86 mL/min. Ranitidine (MW = 351 g/mole) is only weakly bound to plasma protein (fu = 0.85). The concentration of ranitidine in the total filtrate volume collected was 0.47 mg/L. The AUC from time zero to 3.5 hr was 2.11 mg-hr/L. The clearance (in the absence of hemofiltration) in these patients averaged 298 mL/min, and the half-life was 2.6 hr.

a. Calculate the hemofiltration clearance of ranitidine.

b. Given that the blood-to-plasma concentration ratio is close to 1.0, estimate the efficiency (extraction coefficient) of the hemofiltration system in extracting ranitidine from blood.

c. Determine the contribution of hemofiltration to total elimination during treatment.

d. The recommendation for ranitidine in patients with severe renal function impairment and on intermittent hemodialysis is to reduce dosage (for renal function impairment) to 150 mg every 24 hr and to adjust dosing so that the timing of a scheduled dose coincides with the end of hemodialysis. Do you think this recommendation would work for hemofiltration as well? Briefly discuss.

SELECTED READING

BOOKS AND SELECTED ARTICLES

Selected references to monographs and journal articles containing material related to topics of this book follow. The references are listed by topic area. Many of the references could be listed in multiple areas, particularly the general ones that survey the field. To avoid repetition, references are listed in only one category even though they may contain material pertinent to several others.

General

Benet, L.Z., Massoud, N., and Gambertoglio, J.G. (eds.): Pharmacokinetic Basis for Drug Treatment. New York, Raven Press, 1984.

Evans, W.E., Schentag, J.J., and Jusko, W.J. (eds.): Applied Pharmacokinetics. 3rd Ed. San Francisco, Applied Therapeutics, 1992.

Ferraiolo, B.L., Mohler, M.A. and Gloff, C.A. (eds.): Pharmaceutical Biotechnology. Vol. 1. Protein Pharmacokinetics and Metabolism. New York, Plenum, 1992.

Garzone, P.D., Colburn, W.A., and Motokoff, M. (eds.): Pharmacokinetics and Pharmacodynamics. Vol. 3. Peptides, Peptoids, and Proteins. Cincinnati, OH, Harvey Whitney, 1994.

Gibaldi, M.: Biopharmaceutics and Clinical Pharmacokinetics. 4th Ed. Philadelphia, PA, Lea & Febiger, 1991.

Gibaldi, M., and Perrier, D.: Pharmacokinetics, 2nd Ed. New York, Marcel Dekker, 1982.

Hull, C.J.: Pharmacokinetics for Anesthesia. Butterworth-Heinemann, Oxford, 1991.

Kutt, H.: Overview of the pharmacokinetics of antiepileptic drugs. In Drugs Control Epilepsy. Edited by C.L. Faingold and G.H. Fromm. Boca Raton, FL, CRC, 1994, pp. 361–374.

Levy, R.H., and Shand, D.G.: Clinical implications of drug-protein binding. Proceedings of a symposium. Clin. Pharmacokinet., 9:51–104, 1984.

Murphy, J.E. (ed.): Clinical Pharmacokinetics: Pocket Reference. American Society of Hospital Pharmacists, 1993.

Rowland, M., and Tucker, G. (eds.): Pharmacokinetics: Theory and Methodology. Oxford, Pergamon Press, 1986.

Schoenwald, R.D.: Pharmacokinetics in ocular drug delivery. In Biopharm. Ocul. Drug Delivery. Edited by P. Edman. Boca Raton, FL, CRC, 1994, pp. 159–191.

Stanski, D.R., and Watkins, W.D.: Drug Disposition in Anesthesia. Grune & Stratton, New York, 1982.

Vree, T.B., and Hekster, Y.A.: Clinical Pharmacokinetics of Sulfonamides and their Metabolites: An Encyclopedia. Basel, S. Karger, 1987.

Wagner, J.: Pharmacokinetics for the Pharmaceutical Scientist. Lancaster PA, Technomic, 1993.

Wester, R.C., and Maibach, H.I.: Percutaneous absorption of drugs. Clin. Pharmacokinet., 23:253–266, 1992.

Welling, P., and Tse, H.: Pharmacokinetics: Regulatory-Industrial-Academic Perspectives. (Drugs and the Pharmaceutical Sciences Ser., No. 33). New York, Marcel Dekker, 1988.

Welling, P.G., and Tse, F.L.S.: Pharmacokinetics of Cardiovascular, Central Nervous System, and Antimicrobial Drugs. London, Royal Society of Chemistry, 1985.

Williams, R.L., Brater, D.C., and Mordenti, J. (eds.): Clinical Pharmacology. Vol. 16. Rational Therapeutics: A Clinical Pharmacologic Guide for the Health Professional. New York, Marcel Dekker, 1990.

Therapeutic Regimens

Ansel, H.C., and Popovich, N.G.: Pharmaceutical Dosage Forms and Drug Delivery Systems, 5th Ed. Philadelphia, Lea & Febiger, 1990.

DeVane, C.L., and Jusko, W.J.: Dosage regimen design. Pharmacol. Ther., 17:143–164, 1982.

Goodman, L.S., and Gilman, A.: The Pharmacological Basis of Therapeutics. Vol. 1. 8th Ed. New York, McGraw-Hill, 1992.

Heilmann, K.: Therapeutic Systems. Rate-Controlled Drug Delivery: Concept and Development. 2nd Rev. Ed. New York, Thieme-Stratton, 1983.

Liliemark, J., and Peterson, C.: Pharmacokinetic optimisation of anticancer therapy. Clin. Pharmacokinet., 21:213–231, 1991.

Theeuwes, F.: Drug delivery systems. Pharmacol. Ther., 13:149–192, 1981.

Physiologic Concepts and Kinetics

Lin, J.H., Cocchetto, D.M., and Duggan, D.E.: Protein binding as a primary determinant of the clinical pharmacokinetic properties of nonsteroidal anti-inflammatory drugs. Clin. Pharmacokinet., 12:402–432, 1994.

Pacifici, G.M., Viani, A.: Methods of determining plasma and tissue binding of drugs: Pharmacokinetic consequences. Clin. Pharmacokinet., 23:449–468, 1994.

Pond, S.M., and Tozer, T.N.: First-pass elimination: Basic concepts and clinical consequences. Clin. Pharmacokinet., 9:1–25, 1984.

Steinberg, I., and Zaske, D.E.: Body composition and pharmacokinetics. Rep. Ross Conf. Med. Res., 6:96–102, 1985.

Tillement, J.-P., and Lindenlaud, E. (eds.): Protein Binding and Drug Transport. Symposia Medica Hoechst, 20. New York, F.K. Schattauer Verlag, 1986.

Individualization
General

Brune, K.: Pharmacokinetic factors as causes of variability in response to nonsteroidal anti-inflammatory drugs. Agents Actions Suppl., 17:59–63, 1994.

Dahl, S.G., and Hals, P.A.: Pharmacokinetic and pharmacodynamic factors causing variability in response to neuroleptic drugs. Psychopharmacol. Ser., 3:266–275, 1994.

Dayer, P., Merier, G., Perrenoud, J.J., Marmy, A., and Leemann, T. Interindividual pharmacokinetic and pharmacodynamic variability of different beta blockers. J. Cardiovasc. Pharmacol., 8(Suppl. 6):S20–S24, 1994.

Rowland, M., and Aarons, L. (eds.): New Strategies in Drug Development and Clinical Evaluation. The Population Approach. Luxembourg, Commission of the European Communities, 1992.

Rowland, M., Sheiner, L.B., and Steimer, J.-L. (eds.): Variability in Drug Therapy. New York, Raven Press, 1985.

Welling, P.G., and Tse, F.L.S.: Factors contributing to variability in drug pharmacokinetics. I. Absorption. J. Clin. Hosp. Pharm., 9:163–179, 1984.

Whiting, B., Kelman, A.W., and Grevel, J.: Population Pharmacokinetics: Theory and Clinical Application. Clin. Pharmacokinet., 11:387–401, 1986.

Wilson, K.: Sex-related differences in drug disposition in man. Clin. Pharmacokinet., 9:189–202, 1984.

Genetics

Kalow, W., Goedde, W.H., and Agarwal, D.P.: Ethnic Differences in Reactions to Drugs and Xenobiotics. New York, Alan R. Liss, 1986.

Price Evans, D.A.: Genetic Factors in Drug Therapy. Cambridge, Cambridge University Press, 1993.

Tucker, G.T.: Clinical implications of genetic polymorphism in drug metabolism. J. Pharm. Pharmacol., 46:417–424, 1994.

Weber, W.: Acetylator Genes and Drug Response. New York, Oxford University Press, 1987.

Age and Weight

Blouin, R.A., Kolpek, J.H., and Mann, H.J.: Influence of obesity on drug disposition. Clin. Pharm., 6:706–714, 1994.

Cheymol, G.: Clinical pharmacokinetics of drugs in obesity. An update. Clin. Pharmacokinet., 25:103–114, 1993.

Greenblatt, D.J., Harmatz, J.S., and Shader, R.I.: Clinical pharmacokinetics of anxiolytics and hypnotics in the elderly. Therapeutic considerations. Part I. Clin. Pharmacokinet., 21:165–177, 1991.

Greenblatt, D.J., Harmatz, J.S., and Shader, R.I.: Clinical pharmacokinetics of anxiolytics and hypnotics in the elderly. Therapeutic considerations Part II. Clin. Pharmacokinet., 21:262–273, 1991.

Krauer, B., and Dayer, P.: Fetal drug metabolism and its possible clinical implications. Clin. Pharmacokinet., 21:70–80, 1991.

Norman, T.R.: Pharmacokinetic aspects of antidepressant treatment in the elderly. Prog. Neuro-psychopharmacol. Biol. Psychiatry, 17:329–344, 1994.

Ritschel, W.: Gerontokinetics: Pharmacokinetics of Drugs in the Elderly. Telford Press, 1989.

Wallace, S.M., and Verbeeck, R.K.: Plasma protein binding of drugs in the elderly. Clin. Pharmacokinet., 12:41–72, 1987.

Woodhouse, K.: Drugs and the liver. Part III: Ageing of the liver and the metabolism of drugs. Biopharm. Drug Dispos., 13:311–320, 1994.

Disease

Bennett, W.M., Aronoff, G.R., Morrison, G., Golper, T.A., Pulliam, J., Wolfson, M., and Singer, I.: Drug prescribing in renal failure:

Dosing guidelines for adults. Am. J. Kidney Dis., 3:155–191, 1983.

Bickley, S.K.: Drug dosing during continuous arteriovenous hemofiltration. Clin. Pharm., 7:198–206, 1994.

Brenner, B.M., and Rector, F.C., Jr. (eds.): The Kidney. Vols. I and II. 3rd Ed. Philadelphia, PA, W.B. Saunders, 1986.

Gubbins, P.O., and Bertch, K.E.: Drug absorption in gastrointestinal disease and surgery. Clinical pharmacokinetic and therapeutic implications. Clin Pharmacokinet., 21:431–447, 1991.

Hiddemann, W., Buchner, T., Keating, M., Plunkett, W., Wormann, B., and Andreeff, M. (eds.): Acute Leukemias—Pharmacokinetics: Pharmacokinetics and Management of Relapsed and Refractory Disease. New York, Springer-Verlag, 1992.

McLean, A.J., and Morgan, D.J.: Clinical pharmacokinetics in patients with liver disease. Clin. Pharmacokinet., 21:42–69, 1991.

Reetze-Bonorden, P., Bohler, J., and Keller, E.: Drug dosage in patients during continuous renal replacement therapy. Pharmacokinetic and therapeutic considerations. Clin. Pharmacokinet., 24:362–379, 1993.

Williams, R.L., Brater, D.C., and Mordenti, J. (eds.): Drug Administration in Disease States. New York, Marcel Dekker, 1988.

Workman, P., and Graham, M.A. (eds.): Pharmacokinetics and Cancer Chemotherapy. (Cancer Surveys Ser., Vol. 17.) Cold Spring Harbor, NY, Cold Spring Harbor Laboratory Press, 1993.

Interacting Drugs

Hansten, P.D.: Drug Interactions. Clinical Significance of Drug–Drug Interactions. Philadelphia, Lea & Febiger, 1990.

Hansten, P.D., and Horn, J.R.: Drug Interactions and Updates. Philadelphia, Lea & Febiger, 1993.

Shinn, A.F., and Shrewsbury, R.P.: American Pharmaceutical Association, Professional Drug Systems. In Evaluations of Drug Interactions. 3rd Ed. St. Louis, MO, C.V. Mosby, 1985.

Welling, P.G.: Interactions affecting drug absorption. Clin. Pharmacokinet., 9:404–434, 1984.

Wood, M.: Pharmacokinetic drug interactions in anaesthetic practice. Clin. Pharmacokinet., 21:285–307, 1991.

Monitoring

Burton, M.E., Vasko, M.R., and Brater, D.C.: Comparison of drug dosing methods. Clin. Pharmacokinet., 10:1–37, 1985.

Koda-Kimble, M.A., Young, L.Y., Guglielmo, J., Jr., and Kradjan, W.A.: Handbook of Applied Therapeutics. 2nd ed. Spokane, WA, Applied Therapeutics, 1992.

Lin, E.T., and Sadee, W.: Drug Level Monitoring: Analytical Techniques, Metabolism and Pharmacokinetics. Vol. 2. New York, Wiley & Sons, 1986.

Musa, M.N. (ed.): Pharmacokinetics and Therapeutic Monitoring of Psychiatric Drugs. Springfield, IL, Charles C. Thomas, 1993.

Nahata, M.C.: Intravenous infusion conditions. Implications for pharmacokinetic monitoring. Clin. Pharmacokinet., 24:221–229, 1993.

Peck, C., Conner, D.P., and Murphy, M.G.: Bedside Clinical Pharmacokinetics: Simple techniques for individualizing drug therapy. Spokane, WA, Applied Therapeutics, 1989.

Rugstad, H.E.: Immunosuppressive drugs. The need for therapeutic drug monitoring. In Immunopharmacol. Autoimmune Dis. Transplant. Edited by H.E. Rugstad, L. Endresen, and F. Oeystein. New York, Plenum, 1994, pp. 233–244.

Sunshine, I. (ed.): Recent Developments in Therapeutic Drug Monitoring and Clinical Toxicology. New York, Dekker, 1994.

Winter, M.E.: Basic Clinical Pharmacokinetics, 3rd Ed. Spokane, WA, Applied Therapeutics, 1994.

Selected Topics
Distribution Kinetics

Gibaldi, M., and Perrier, D.: Pharmacokinetics. 2nd Ed., New York, Marcel Dekker, 1982.

Shafer, S.L., and Stanski, D.: Improving the clinical utility of anesthetic drug pharmacokinetics. Anesthesiology 76:327–330, 1992.

Pharmacologic Response

Hennis, P.J., and Stanski, D.R.: Pharmacokinetic and Pharmacodynamic Factors That Govern the Clinical Use of Muscle Relaxants. In Seminars in Anesthesia. Vol. 4. Edited by R.L. Katz. New York, Grune & Stratton, 1985.

Holford, N.H.G., and Sheiner, L.B.: Kinetics of pharmacologic response. Pharmacol. Ther., 16:143–166, 1982.

Metabolite Kinetics

Eadie, M.J.: Formation of active metabolites of anticonvulsant drugs: A review of their pharmacokinetic and therapeutic significance. Clin. Pharmacokinet., 21:27–41, 1994.

Ebihara, A., and Fujimura, A.: Metabolites of antihypertensive drugs. An updated review of their clinical pharmacokinetic and therapeutic implications. Clin. Pharmacokinet., 21:331–343, 1994.

Garattini, S.: Active drug metabolites: An overview of their relevance in clinical pharmacokinetics. Clin. Pharmacokinet., *19*:216–227, 1985.

Houston, J.B.: Kinetics of disposition of xenobiotics and their metabolites. Drug Metab. Drug Interact., 6:47–83, 1994.

Pang, K.S.: A review of metabolic kinetics. J. Pharmacokinet., Biopharm., *13*:633–662, 1985.

Dose and Time Dependencies

Labrecque, G., and Belanger, P.M.: Time-dependency in the pharmacokinetics and disposition of drugs. *In* Topics in Pharmaceutical Sciences. Edited by D.D. Breimer and P. Speiser. Amsterdam, Elsevier, 1985, pp. 167–178.

Lemmer, B.: Implications of chronopharmacokinetics for drug delivery: Antiasthmatics, H_2-blockers and cardiovascular active drugs. Adv. Drug Delivery Rev., 6:83–100, 1994.

Van Rossum, J.M., Van Lingen, G., and Burgers, J.P.T.: Dose-dependent pharmacokinetics. Pharmacol. Ther., *21*:77–100, 1983.

Turnover Concepts

Rescigno, A., and Segre, G.: Turnover. *In* Drug and Tracer Kinetics. Waltham, MA, Blaisdell, 1966.

Shipley, R.A., and Clark, R.E.: Tracer Methods for In Vivo Kinetics: Theory and Applications. New York, Academic Press, 1972.

Dialysis

Gokal, R.: Continuous Ambulatory Peritoneal Dialysis: Edinburgh, Churchill Livingstone, 1986.

Gotch, F.A.: Kinetics of hemodialysis. Art. Org., *10*:272–281, 1986.

Henderson, L.W., Quellhorst, E.A., Baldamus, C.A., and Lysaght, M.J. (eds.): Hemofiltration. New York, Springer-Verlag, 1986.

Pond, S.M.: Extracorporeal techniques in the treatment of poisoned patients. Med. J. Aust., *154*:617–622, 1991.

Sieberth, H.G., Mann, H., and Stummvoll, H.K.: Continuous Hemofiltration. 2nd International Conference on Continuous Hemofiltration. Baden Austria, Sept. 10–11, 1990. New York, 1991.

ADDITIONAL CONCEPTS
AND DERIVATIONS

ASSESSMENT OF AUC

Several methods exist for measuring the area under the plasma concentration-time curve (AUC). One method, to be discussed here, is the simple numeric estimation of area by the *trapezoidal rule*. The advantage of this method is that it only requires a simple extension of a table of experimental data. Other methods involve either greater numeric complexity or fitting of an equation to the observations and then calculating the area by integrating the fitted equation.

General Case: Consider the blood concentration-time data, first two columns of Table A–1, obtained following oral administration of 50 mg of a drug. What is the total AUC?

Figure A–1 is a plot of concentration against time after drug administration. If a perpendicular line is drawn from the concentration at 1 hr (7 mg/L) down to the time-axis, then the area bounded between zero time and 1 hr is a trapezoid with an area given by the product of average concentration and time interval. The average concentration is obtained by adding the concentrations at the beginning and end of the time interval and dividing by 2. Since, in the first interval, the respective concentrations are 0 and 7 mg/L and the time interval is 1 hr, it follows that:

$$AUC_1 = \frac{0 + 7}{2} \text{ mg/L} \qquad \times 1 \text{ hr}$$

| Area of trapezoid within the first time interval | Average concentration over the first interval | First time interval |

or,

$$AUC_1 = 3.5 \text{ mg-hr/L}$$

In this example, the concentration at zero time is 0. Had the drug been given as an intra-

Table A–1. Calculation of Total AUC Using the Trapezoidal Rule

TIME (hr)	BLOOD CONCENTRATION (mg/L)	TIME INTERVAL (hr)	AVERAGE CONCENTRATION (mg/L)	AREA (mg·hr/L)
0	0	—	—	—
1	7	1	3.5	3.5
2	10	1	8.5	8.5
3	5	1	7.5	7.5
4	2.5	1	3.75	3.75
5	1.25	1	1.88	1.88
6	0.6	1	0.93	0.93
7	0.2	1	0.4	0.4
8	0	1	0.1	0.1
			Total Area =	26.60

venous (i.v.) bolus, the concentration at zero time might have been the extrapolated value, $C(0)$.

The area under each time interval can be obtained in an analogous manner to that outlined above. The total AUC over all times is then simply given by

$$\text{Total } AUC = \text{Sum of the individual areas}$$

Usually, *total AUC* means the area under the curve from zero time to infinity. In practice, infinite time is taken as the time beyond which the area is insignificant.

The calculations used to obtain the AUC, displayed in Fig. A–1, are shown in Table A–1. In this example the total AUC is 26.6 mg-hr/L.

SPECIAL CASE

An Intravenous Bolus. When a drug is given as an i.v. bolus and the decline in plasma concentration is monoexponential, total AUC is calculated most rapidly by dividing the extrapolated zero-time concentration ($C(0)$) by the elimination rate constant (k). For example, if $C(0)$ is 100 mg/L and k is 0.1 hr^{-1}, then the total AUC is 1000 mg-hr/L.

Proof: The total AUC is given by

$$\text{Total } AUC = \int_0^\infty C \cdot dt \qquad\qquad 1$$

But $C = C(0) \cdot e^{-kt}$, and since $C(0)$ is a constant, it follows that

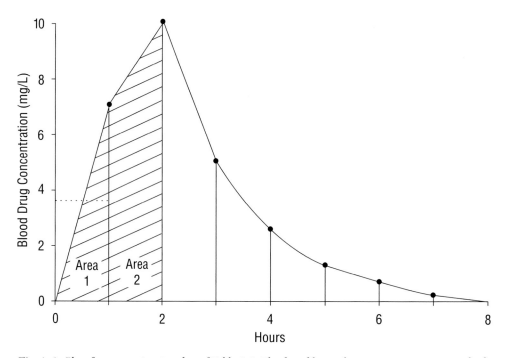

Fig. A–1. Plot of concentration-time data of Table A–1. The dotted line is the average concentration in the first interval.

$$\text{Total } AUC = C(0) \int_0^\infty e^{-kt} \cdot dt \qquad 2$$

which on integrating between time zero and infinity yields

$$\text{Total } AUC = \frac{C(0)}{-k} [e^{-kt}]_0^\infty = \frac{C(0)}{-k} [0 - 1] = \frac{C(0)}{k} \qquad 3$$

When Decline Is Logarithmic. The numeric method used to calculate AUC by the trapezoid rule assumes a linear relationship between observations. Frequently, especially during the decline of drug concentration, the fall is exponential. Then a more accurate method for calculating area during the decline can be used, the *log trapezoidal rule*, as follows.

Consider, for example, two consecutive observations $C(t_i)$ and $C(t_{i+1})$ at times t_i and t_{i+1}, respectively. These observations are related to each other by

$$C(t_{i+1}) = C(t_i) \cdot e^{-k_i \cdot \Delta t_i} \qquad 4$$

where k_i is the rate constant that permits the concentration to fall exponentially from $C(t_i)$ to $C(t_{i+1})$ in the time interval $t_{i+1} - t_i$, that is, Δt_i. The value of k_i is given by taking the logarithm on both sides of Eq. 4 and rearranging, so that

$$k_i = \frac{\ln[C(t_i)/C(t_{i+1})]}{\Delta t_i} \qquad 5$$

Now the AUC during the time interval Δt_i, AUC_i, is the difference between the total areas from t_i to ∞ and from t_{i+1} to ∞, respectively. It therefore follows from events after an i.v. bolus that

$$AUC_i = \frac{C(t_i) - C(t_{i+1})}{k_i} \qquad 6$$

and, by appropriately substituting for k_i in Eq. 6, one obtains

$$AUC_i = \frac{[C(t_i) - C(t_{i+1})] \cdot \Delta t_i}{\ln[C(t_i)/C(t_{i+1})]} \qquad 7$$

This calculation is then repeated for all observations that lie beyond the peak concentration.

In practice, a large discrepancy arises between the method above and that using the (linear) trapezoidal rule only when consecutive observations differ by more than twofold.

STUDY PROBLEMS

1. The following data (Table A–2) were obtained following the ingestion of 50 mg of a drug.

Table A–2.

Time (hr)	0	0.5	1	1.5	2	3	4	6	8	12
Plasma concentration (mg/L)	0	0.38	0.6	0.73	0.85	0.95	0.94	0.87	0.66	0.37

Estimate the total *AUC*. It should be noted that the last sample was taken before the concentration had fallen to an insignificant value. (Hint: To estimate the *AUC* beyond the last observation, imagine that this last measurement was the zero-time concentration following an i.v. bolus and that the disposition kinetics of the drug does not change beyond the last observation.)

2. Estimate the total *AUC* for the data set in Table A–3 obtained after an i.v. dose.

Table A-3.

TIME (hr)	0	2	4	6	8	10	12	16	20	24
Plasma concentration (mg/L)	10^a	6.3	4.0	2.5	1.6	1.0	0.63	0.25	0.10	0.04

^{a}Estimated by extrapolation on a semilogarithmic plot to zero time.

3. The set of data displayed in Fig. A–1 is unusual in that the time between collection of blood samples is constant, in this case, 1 hr. Prove in this special case that

$$\text{Total } AUC = \frac{\text{Time}}{\text{interval}} \left[\left(\frac{\text{First + last concentrations}}{2} \right) + \left(\begin{array}{c} \text{Sum of all other} \\ \text{concentrations} \end{array} \right) \right]$$

Use the data in Table A–1 to confirm that this simple method works satisfactorily.

4. The concentration of a drug declines exponentially according to the equation C (mg/L) $= 64\, e^{-0.173t}$ (t in hours). Complete Table A–4 to show the errors, if any, in each of the *AUC* calculations over the interval given.

Table A-4.

	AUC WITHIN TIME INTERVAL		
TIME INTERVAL (hr)	CALCULATED AUC	TRAPEZOIDAL RULE	LOG TRAPEZOIDAL RULE
	$\dfrac{(64 - C(t))}{k}$		
0–2			
0–4			
0–8			
0–12			

ESTIMATION OF ELIMINATION HALF-LIFE
FROM URINE DATA

Consider the urine data in Table B–1, obtained following a 50-mg i.v. bolus dose of a drug. These are the same data as presented in Table 3–1. The observations are times of urine collection, volumes collected, and concentrations of unchanged drug in each sample. These data are treated to derive further information. Of special interest are rate-time profile and cumulative amount excreted. The amount excreted in each time interval is the product of volume of urine collected and concentration, e.g., the amount in Sample 1 is 120 mL times 133 µg/mL or 16 mg; therefore, the average rate of excretion over the first 2-hr period is 8 mg/hr. The cumulative amount excreted up to any time is the sum of all drug excreted up to that time. By 24 hr, the cumulative amount excreted is 39.1 mg, and since 37.2 mg was excreted in the first 12 hr and only another 1.9 mg over the next 12 hr, 39.1 mg approximates the ultimate amount of drug excreted.

Excretion rate data are occasionally displayed as a bar histogram, but this form of presentation is not as useful as one in which the rate data are plotted against the midpoint of the collection interval on semilogarithmic paper (Fig. B–1). The time for the excretion rate to fall in half (e.g., from 5 mg/hr to 2.5 mg/hr) is the elimination half-life of the drug (2.8 hr). The reason for using midpoint time was given in Chap. 3, namely, the measured urinary excretion rate reflects the average plasma concentration during the collection interval.

Formal proof of the observation of elimination half-life is not difficult to derive. Using Eq. 21 of Chap. 3,

$$\text{Excretion rate} = CL_R \cdot C \qquad\qquad 1$$

If $\text{Dose} \cdot e^{-kt}$ is substituted for C,

Table B–1. Urine Data Obtained Following an i.v. Bolus Dose of Drug

	OBSERVATION			TREATMENT OF DATA			
SAMPLE	TIME OF COLLECTION (hr)	VOLUME OF URINE (mL)	CONCENTRATION OF UNCHANGED DRUG IN URINE (µg/mL)	AMOUNT EXCRETED IN TIME INTERVAL (mg)	EXCRETION RATE (mg/hr)	CUMULATIVE AMOUNT EXCRETED (mg)	AMOUNT REMAINING TO BE EXCRETED (mg)
0	0		—		—	0	39.1
1	0–2	120	133	16.0	8	16.0	23.1
2	2–4	180	50	9.0	4.5	25.0	14.1
3	4–6	89	63	5.6	2.8	30.6	8.5
4	6–8	340	10	3.4	1.7	34.0	5.1
5	8–12	178	18	3.2	0.8	37.2	1.9
6	12–24	950	2	1.9	0.16	39.1	—

$$\text{Excretion rate} = \frac{CL_R}{V} \cdot \text{Dose} \cdot e^{-kt} \qquad\qquad 2$$

and taking logarithms

$$\ln(\text{excretion rate}) = \ln\left[\frac{CL_R}{V} \cdot \text{Dose}\right] - k \cdot t \qquad\qquad 3$$

The slope of the curve is $-k$, the rate constant for elimination of drug by all routes. Even if renal excretion were only a small fraction of total drug elimination, the excretion rate would still decline with time in parallel with concentration. Concentration is the driving force for renal excretion; as concentration declines, so does rate of excretion.

In practice, uncertainty of complete bladder emptying and need to collect urine over short intervals, relative to the elimination half-life of the drug, pose limitations on the quality of excretion rate data. When complete urine recovery of drug is ensured, estimates of elimination half-life and elimination rate constant can also be made by analyzing cumulative excretion data. The cumulative excretion plots (Fig. B–2) generally tend to be smoother than the corresponding excretion rate plots.

The cumulative amount excreted up to any time t, $Ae(t)$, is obtained by summing the amount excreted unchanged in each time interval up to that time. For example, by 8 hr,

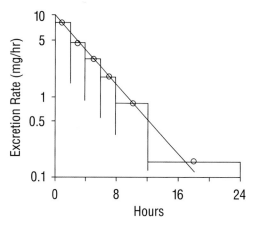

Fig. B–1. Semilogarithmic plot of the rate of excretion against the midpoint time of urine collection. The period over which the average excretion rate was obtained is superimposed. Data from Table B–1.

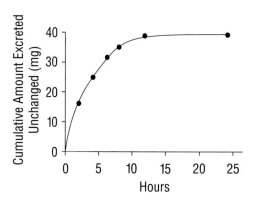

Fig. B–2. The amount of drug excreted unchanged in the urine accumulates asymptotically toward a limiting value, Ae_∞, following an i.v. bolus dose. Half that limiting amount is excreted in one half-life.

34.0 mg have been excreted. Initially, large amounts are excreted, but as the amount of drug in the body falls, so does the excretion rate; by 24 hr, a limiting amount (39.1 mg) has been excreted (Fig. B–2). Small amounts continue to be excreted beyond 24 hr, since theoretically the amount of drug in the body approaches but never falls to zero. However, these additional amounts do not substantially alter the 24 hr value. Accordingly, 39.1 mg can be taken to be an estimate of the total amount of drug to be excreted unchanged (Ae_∞). Half this amount (approximately 20 mg) is excreted by 2.6 hr (Fig. B–2). Interestingly, again, this is the value for the half-life of this drug, estimated from plasma concentration and urinary excretion rate data. As the following analysis shows, this is more than a mere coincidence.

The rate of excretion at any time is given by

$$\frac{dAe}{dt} = CL_R \cdot C \qquad\qquad 4$$

The amount excreted up to time t is obtained by integrating the rate equation.

$$Ae(t) = CL_R \int_0^t C \cdot dt \qquad\qquad 5$$

Since the drug was given as an i.v. bolus, $C = \dfrac{\text{Dose}}{V} \cdot e^{-kt}$, so that

$$Ae(t) = \frac{CL_R}{V} \int_0^t \text{Dose} \cdot e^{-kt} \cdot dt \qquad\qquad 6$$

or

$$Ae(t) = \frac{CL_R}{V} \cdot \text{Dose} \left[\frac{e^{-kt}}{-k} \right]_0^t \qquad\qquad 7$$

Remembering that $e^{-0} = 1$, the preceding equation reduces to

$$Ae(t) = \frac{CL_R \cdot \text{Dose}}{V \cdot k} [1 - e^{-kt}] \qquad\qquad 8$$

but since $e^{-\infty} = 0$, and $V \cdot k = CL$, the amount excreted by infinite time (Ae_∞) must be given by

$$Ae_\infty = \frac{CL_R \cdot \text{Dose}}{CL} \qquad\qquad 9$$

which when substituted into the preceding equation yields

$$Ae(t) = Ae_\infty (1 - e^{-kt}) \qquad\qquad 10$$

Rearrangement of Eq. 10 gives

$$Ae_{\infty} - Ae(t) = Ae_{\infty} \cdot e^{-kt} \qquad\qquad 11$$

and taking logarithms

$$\ln(Ae_{\infty} - Ae(t)) = \ln Ae_{\infty} - k \cdot t$$

Thus, a semilogarithmic plot of $Ae_{\infty} - Ae(t)$ against time should give a straight line with a slope of $-k$.

As the difference, $Ae_{\infty} - Ae(t)$, is the amount remaining to be excreted (ARE), the resulting plot is sometimes called an ARE plot. In practice, the value of ARE at each time is obtained by subtracting the cumulative amount excreted up to that time from the total amount excreted. These values are presented in the last column of Table B–1 and the corresponding semilogarithmic plot of ARE versus time is shown in Fig. B–3. The elimination half-life, taken as the time for the ARE to fall by one-half, is 2.8 hr. Hence, $k = 0.25\ hr^{-1}$.

Several points should be noted. First, at zero time the value for ARE is Ae_{∞}. Second, the value of ARE is plotted against the actual time of urine collection, e.g., the time at which 5.1 mg remains to be excreted is 8 hr (Table B–1). In this last respect, the ARE plot has a distinct advantage over the excretion rate plot, in which the excretion rate is plotted against the midpoint of the urine collection interval. Recall that the use of the midpoint time was necessary because the excretion rate is an average value over the period of collection.

Although the ARE plot tends to smooth out the data, it is not used as frequently as the excretion rate plot for four reasons: (1) It requires an accurate estimate of Ae_{∞}, since an underestimation of Ae_{∞} tends to grossly underestimate the true ARE values as $Ae(t)$ approaches Ae_{∞}. This means that there has to be complete urine collection for at least four half-lives, which in clinical practice is often difficult to ensure. The rate method does not require urine to be collected until no more drug is excreted. (2) $Ae(t)$ values are usually obtained by summing the amount excreted in each collection period. Hence, assay errors are accumulated, while failure to obtain a complete urine collection produces a systematic error in all subsequent estimates of $Ae(t)$. The excretion rate analysis does not contain these

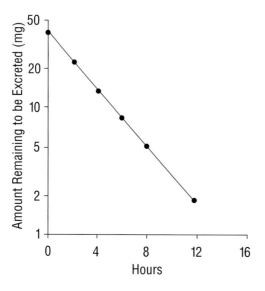

Fig. B–3. The amount remaining to be excreted (ARE), following an i.v. bolus dose of drug, declines exponentially with time. In one half-life, the ARE falls by one-half.

sources of error. (3) Smoothing out data can obscure important information. Urinary pH and urine flow fluctuate throughout the day. If the renal clearance of a drug is sensitive to these factors (Chap. 11), it is readily apparent in an excretion rate plot but tends to be lost in the *ARE* plot. (4) When the drug is administered extravascularly, e.g., orally, delays in excretion caused by absorption produce distortions of the *ARE* plot, frequently making analysis difficult. In contrast, the excretion rate plot can be readily analyzed.

STUDY PROBLEMS

1. Swintosky et al. (Sulfaethylthiadiazole II. Distribution and disappearance from the tissues following intravenous injection. J. Am. Pharm. Assoc., *46*:403–411, 1957) studied the disposition kinetics of the sulfonamide, sulfaethylthiadiazole. Table B–2 contains a list of the amounts of drug excreted unchanged with time following an i.v. bolus dose of 2.0 g sulfaethylthiadiazole to a subject (weight 81 kg).

Table B–2.

Time interval (hr)	0–3	3–6	6–9	9–12	12–15	15–24	24–48
Amount excreted unchanged (mg)	534	436	181	139	110	202	195

    a. Estimate graphically the elimination half-life of sulfaethylthiadiazole from a semilogarithmic plot of excretion rate against the midpoint time of urine collection.

    b. Given that the cumulative amount excreted unchanged up to 48 hr represents a good estimate of Ae_∞, calculate the fraction of the dose excreted unchanged.

    c. Estimate the elimination half-life of sulfaethylthiadiazole from cumulative excretion data, and compare the answer with that obtained from the excretion rate data.

2. a. Suppose that the urine sample collected over the 3- to 6-hr interval in problem 1 was inadvertently discarded. Using both the excretion rate and *ARE* methods, determine the elimination half-life of the drug. Briefly discuss the problems encountered.

    b. From the answers to problem 1, estimate how much unchanged drug in the body remains to be excreted at 48 hr.

ESTIMATION OF ABSORPTION KINETICS

FROM PLASMA CONCENTRATION DATA

Two methods are presented to calculate absorption kinetics from plasma concentration-time data following an extravascular dose. The first method applies when absorption is a first-order process. The second, a numeric and more general method, makes no assumption about the nature of the absorption process. It relies on mass balance considerations and is commonly referred to as the *Wagner-Nelson method*. Both methods require that one-compartment linear disposition kinetics apply. Other less restrictive but generally more complex numeric methods exist to deal with more complicated situations. Finally, if an equation exists that adequately defines both absorption and disposition, it can be fitted directly to the observations to estimate the parameter values characterizing the absorption kinetics.

FIRST-ORDER ABSORPTION

Consider the plasma data in Table C–1, obtained following a 100-mg oral dose of a drug. Figure C–1 is a semilogarithmic plot of the same data. The half-life, estimated from the linear portion of the decline phase, is 5 hr. Giving the drug intravenously confirmed that this is the elimination half-life of the drug. Hence, disposition rate-limits drug elimination.

A graphic procedure to test whether or not absorption is a first-order process and, if so, to determine the absorption half-life, is known as the *method of residuals*. The procedure is as follows: (1) Back extrapolate the log linear portion of the decline phase. Let $\overleftarrow{C}$ denote the plasma concentration along this extrapolated line. (2) Subtract the observed plasma concentration (C) from the corresponding extrapolated value at each time point. These calculations are shown in Table C–1. (3) Plot the residuals $(\overleftarrow{C} - C)$ against time on the same semilogarithmic graph paper.

Table C–1. Plasma Concentration-Time Data Following Oral Administration of a 100-mg Dose of a Drug

	OBSERVATION		TREATMENT OF DATA	
TIME (hr)	PLASMA CONCENTRATION C,(mg/L)		EXTRAPOLATED PLASMA CONCENTRATION $\overleftarrow{C}$, (mg/L)	DIFFERENCE IN CONCENTRATIONS $\overleftarrow{C} - C$, (mg/L)
1	0.38		1.90	1.52
2	0.73		1.65	0.92
3	0.91		1.40	0.49
4	0.97		1.23	0.26
5	0.97		1.07	0.10
6	0.92		0.95	0.03
8	0.71		0.71	—
10	0.53		0.53	—
12	0.40		0.40	—
14	0.30		0.30	—

If, as in this example, the residual plot is a straight line, then absorption is a first-order process. The absorption half-life, taken as the time for the residual value to diminish by one-half, is 1.3 hr. The corresponding absorption rate constant, ka, is 0.693/1.3 or 0.53 hr^{-1}.

Theoretically, absorption half-life can also be estimated from urinary excretion data. When renal clearance is essentially constant, excretion rate parallels plasma concentration. The method of residuals should, therefore, be equally applicable to excretion rate data. In practice, however, estimates of absorption half-life from urinary data are usually poor. The half-life of many absorption processes is 30 min or less. Incomplete bladder emptying and inability to collect samples frequently enough to characterize such absorption processes are two major sources of error. Consequently, analysis of plasma data is the preferred method for estimating absorption kinetics.

Let us examine the underlying basis of the method of residuals. At any time the plasma concentration following extravascular administration is given by

$$C = \left(\frac{F \cdot \text{Dose} \cdot ka}{V(ka - k)}\right)(e^{-k \cdot t} - e^{-ka \cdot t})\qquad 1$$

where all terms are as previously defined in the body of the book. The proof of Eq. 1 is involved and beyond the scope of this book. When (as is most frequently the case) absorption is a more rapid process than elimination $(ka > k)$, the value of $ka \cdot t$ is always greater than $k \cdot t$, and hence $e^{-ka \cdot t}$ approaches zero more rapidly than does $e^{-k \cdot t}$. At some point past the peak plasma concentration, $e^{-ka \cdot t}$ is essentially zero, absorption is over and the extrapolated line is given by

$$\overleftarrow{C} = \left(\frac{F \cdot \text{Dose} \cdot ka}{V(ka - k)}\right) e^{-k \cdot t}\qquad 2$$

Subtracting C from $\overleftarrow{C}$ therefore yields

Fig. C–1. By the method of residuals, an estimate can be made of both the absorption half-life (from slope of colored line) and the lag time (noted by arrow), following oral administration of a drug.

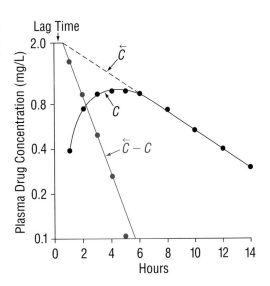

$$\overleftarrow{C} - C = \left(\frac{F \cdot Dose \cdot ka}{V(ka - k)} \right) e^{-ka \cdot t} \tag{3}$$

and taking natural logarithms

$$\ln \left(\overleftarrow{C} - C \right) = \ln \left(\frac{F \cdot Dose \cdot ka}{V(ka - k)} \right) - ka \cdot t \tag{4}$$

Hence, if absorption is a first-order process, a semilogarithmic plot of the residual value against time yields a straight line with a slope of $-ka$. When this residual line is not log linear, absorption is not a simple first-order process, and other methods are needed to calculate how absorption varies with time.

Lag Time: Examination of Eqs. 2 and 3 suggests a simple graphic method for estimating lag time, that is, the time between administration and start of absorption. By definition, absorption begins when the extrapolated and residual curves intersect. This must be so since only at that time, $t = 0$, when $e^{-ka \cdot t} = e^{-kt} = 1$, are the values of the two equations the same, and equal to $(F \cdot Dose \cdot ka)/[V(ka - k)]$. It is seen from Fig. C–1 that in the present example the lag time is approximately 30 min.

Events at the Peak: The peak concentration, C_{max}, and the time of its occurrence, t_{max}, are often important factors influencing drug therapy. Together, they can sometimes also provide a simple measure of the speed of drug absorption for a given dose of drug. However both C_{max} and t_{max} are also influenced by the disposition kinetics of the drug, and questions sometimes arise concerning the impact of changes in absorption and disposition on these values. The answers to such questions are most readily provided by solving Eq. 1 for the condition at the peak. It is seen that if t_{max} is known, C_{max} can be calculated. The value of t_{max} is determined as follows. At that time, rate of absorption is matched by rate of elimination, and hence rate of change of plasma concentration is zero, i.e., $dC/dt = 0$. So, to determine t_{max}, we must first determine dC/dt, which by differentiation of Eq. 1, is

$$\frac{dC}{dt} = \frac{F \cdot Dose \cdot ka}{V(ka - k)} \left(-k \cdot e^{-k \cdot t} + ka \cdot e^{-ka \cdot t} \right) \tag{5}$$

At t_{max}, when $dC/dt = 0$, it follows from Eq. 5 that

$$t_{max} = \frac{1}{(ka - k)} \ln \left(\frac{ka}{k} \right) \tag{6}$$

Equation 6 clearly shows that only the rate constants for absorption and elimination influence t_{max}. Thus, for a given value of k, t_{max} can be calculated for various values of ka. Note, however, that if t_{max} and k are known, ka can be determined only by substituting values for ka into the right-hand side of Eq. 6 until the calculated t_{max} equals the observed value. Finally, when there is a lag time, C_{max} occurs at $t_{max} + t_{lag}$.

WAGNER-NELSON METHOD

At any time, the amount absorbed is given by the familiar mass balance equation

$$\begin{array}{ccc} Aab & = A & + \; Ael \\[4pt] \text{Amount} & \text{Amount} & \text{Amount} \\ \text{absorbed} & \text{in body} & \text{eliminated} \end{array} \tag{7}$$

Now $A = V \cdot C$ and $Ael = CL \cdot \int_0^t C \cdot dt$, which on substitution into Eq. 7, gives

$$Aab = V \cdot C + CL \cdot \int_0^t C \cdot dt \qquad 8$$

Hence, if CL and V are known from i.v. data, changes in Aab with time can then be calculated. The value rises until absorption stops. Then, $Aab = F \cdot$ Dose, allowing bioavailability to be determined. Notice that no assumption is made regarding the nature of the absorption process; it could be simple or complex. Indeed, the calculated absorption-time profile can be analyzed further to characterize the absorption process.

Often, no i.v. dosage form is available, and then Eq. 1 must be modified to allow assessment of absorption kinetics. This is accomplished by noting that $CL = k \cdot V$, so that division of Eq. 1 by V yields

$$\frac{Aab}{V} = C + k \cdot \int_0^t C \cdot dt \qquad 9$$

Thus, knowing the elimination rate constant, k, the ratio Aab/V can be determined from the plasma concentration-time data, with AUC to each time estimated by the appropriate numeric method (Appendix I–A).

Ultimately, the value calculated using Eq. 9 reaches an upper limit, signifying that absorption has stopped. This limiting value is therefore $F \cdot$ Dose$/V$, which also equals $k \cdot \int_0^\infty Cdt$, as $F \cdot$ Dose $= k \cdot V \int_0^\infty Cdt$. Accordingly, the fraction of bioavailable dose that is absorbed with time can be estimated; it is given by

$$\begin{matrix} \text{Fraction of} \\ \text{bioavailable} \\ \text{drug absorbed} \end{matrix} = \frac{C + k \cdot \int_0^t C \, dt}{k \cdot \int_0^\infty C \, dt} \qquad 10$$

To illustrate the method, consider the concentration-time data listed in Fig. C–2 and

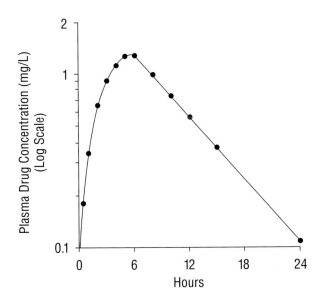

Fig. C–2.

displayed semilogarithmically in Fig. C–2 following the oral administration of a 100-mg dose of drug. First, k is estimated from the declining concentration-time data; it is 0.14 hr^{-1} ($t_{1/2}$ = 5 hr). Next, the AUC to each time point is calculated; the values, calculated using the trapezoidal rule, are also listed in Table C–2. The product $k \cdot \int_0^t C\,dt$ is then calculated and added to the plasma concentration to yield Aab/V. For example, the value of $k \cdot AUC$ at the first sampling time of one hour is 0.14 hr^{-1} × 0.045 mg-hr/L or 0.006 mg/L which when added to 0.18 mg/L gives 0.186 or 0.19 mg/L for Aab/V. The values of Aab/V with time are listed in Table C–2 and displayed in Fig. C–3. They show that absorption proceeds almost linearly with time for much of the absorption process, but abruptly stops at about 6 hr, suggesting that absorption may be close to zero-order. Fur-

Table C–2. Estimation of Cumulative Amount of Bioavailable Drug Absorbed With Time

OBSERVATION		TREATMENT OF DATA			
TIME(hr)	PLASMA DRUG CONCENTRATION, C(mg/L)	AUC (mg-hr/L)	k · AUC (mg/L)	C + k · AUC (mg/L) [Aab/V]	FRACTION OF BIOAVAILABLE DRUG ABSORBED
0	0	0	0	0	0
0.5	0.18	0.045	0.006	0.19	0.095
1	0.35	0.178	0.025	0.38	0.19
2	0.66	0.683	0.096	0.75	0.38
3	0.91	1.468	0.210	1.12	0.56
4	1.12	2.483	0.35	1.47	0.78
5	1.27	3.678	0.52	1.79	0.90
6	1.28	4.953	0.693	1.97	0.99
8	0.99	7.223	1.011	2.00	1.00
10	0.75	8.963	1.254	2.00	1.00
12	0.57	10.283	1.439	2.01	1.00
15	0.38	11.708	1.638	2.01	1.00
24	0.11	13.912	1.946	2.05	1.00

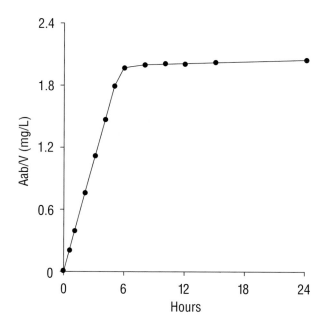

Fig. C–3.

thermore, statements can be made about the fraction of the bioavailable drug that is absorbed at various times (also shown in Table C–2) but, obviously, not the amount absorbed.

Finally, a word of caution is needed here. Critical to the method is an accurate estimate of k. Problems arise when the decline of plasma concentration is absorption rate-limited. Then, no reliable estimate of k can be made. This problem often arises when evaluating controlled-release products. A possible solution is to use an estimate of k in the subject, obtained following administration of a rapid-release dosage form on a separate occasion. The assumptions, often reasonable, are that the decline in plasma concentration is now limited by elimination and that the disposition kinetics (both V and CL) in the subject to not vary significantly from one occasion to another.

STUDY PROBLEMS

1. The following plasma concentrations (Table C–3) were observed in a patient who took a 100 mg tablet of a drug.

Table C–3.

Time (hr)	0.25	0.5	1	2	3	4	6	8	10	12
Plasma concentration (mg/L)	1.6	2.7	3.7	3.5	2.7	2.0	1.02	0.49	0.26	0.12

a. Prepare a semilogarithmic plot of the data and determine the rate constants for absorption and elimination.
b. Estimate when absorption began.
c. Given that absorption is complete (100%), calculate: (1) clearance; (2) volume of distribution.

2. The absorption kinetics of a drug, known to be acid labile, was studied in two groups: group A, patients with normal gastric function; group B, patients with achlorhydria (a condition in which little or no acid is secreted into the stomach). Each group received the same dose of drug. Analysis of the plasma concentration-time curves yielded the following estimates: group A, $F = 0.30$, $ka = 1.15$ hr^{-1}, group B, $F = 0.90$; $ka = 0.39$ hr^{-1}. The investigators proposed that the longer half-life for absorption in patients with achlorhydria was caused by a slower gastric emptying in this group. Suggest an alternative proposal that is consistent with all the observations.

3. A 500-mg controlled-release oral formulation was tested against a solution (500 mg) of a drug in 18 healthy volunteers. A previous study demonstrated that the drug is rapidly and completely absorbed when given in solution. Subjects took a single dose of each formulation on a fasted stomach on separate occasions.

Plasma drug concentration-time data following oral ingestion of the controlled-release product are listed in Table C–4 for one subject. Following administration of the oral solution, the AUC and half-life of the drug in the subject were 86.6 mg-hr/L and 5 hr, respectively.

Table C–4. Plasma Concentration and *AUC* Data Following a 500-mg Controlled-Release Product

TIME (hr)	PLASMA CONCENTRATION (mg/L)	AREA (mg·hr/L)	Aab/V (mg/L)
0	0.00	0.00	
0.5	0.76	0.19	
1	1.42	0.73	
2	2.48	2.68	
3	3.24	5.54	
4	3.75	9.03	
6	4.27	17.05	
8	4.31	25.63	
10	4.09	34.03	
12	3.72	41.84	
18	2.46	60.38	
24	1.45	72.11	
36	0.43	83.39	
48	0.11	86.63	

    a. Using the Wagner-Nelson method, complete Table C–4 by calculating *Aab/V* with time, following administration of the controlled release dosage form. In your calculation use the half-life obtained in this subject following administration of the solution.

    b. What assumptions have you made in applying the Wagner-Nelson method?

    c. What is the bioavailability of the drug in the subject from the controlled-release product relative to that from the oral solution?

    d. By an appropriate graphical analysis of the absorption data, ascertain whether absorption of drug from the controlled-release product *in vivo* is first-order, and if so, the half-life of the absorption process.

4. In problem 5, Chap. 6, plasma concentration time data are provided during and following a 24-hr i.v. constant-rate infusion and a rectal delivery device of droperidol.

    a. Given a half-life of 1.9 hr estimated from the declining concentration after stopping the i.v. infusion, apply the Wagner-Nelson method to the plasma concentration-time data to calculate the absorption kinetics of droperidol following administration of the rectal device.

    b. The device is intended to deliver the drug at a constant rate for 15 hr. Do the absorption kinetics *in vivo* meet this expectation?

MEAN RESIDENCE TIME

A dose of drug comprises many millions of molecules. For example, even a dose as small as 1 mg for a drug with a molecular weight of 300 g/mole contains close to 2×10^{18} molecules $[(10^{-3} \text{ g}/300) \times 6.023 \times 10^{23}$ (Avogadro's number)]. On administration, these drug molecules spend different times within the body. Some are eliminated rapidly, others stay for a long time. A few may remain for a lifetime. The result is a distribution of residence times that can be characterized by a mean value.

The *mean residence time (MRT)* is the average time the number of molecules introduced (N) reside in the body, that is,

$$MRT = \sum_{j=1}^{N} t_j/N \qquad\qquad 1$$

where t_j is the residence time of the jth molecule (time between its input and its elimination from the body). Individual molecules cannot be counted, of course, but groups of them can. Letting n_1 be the number of molecules with an average time in the body of t_1, the total residence time accumulated by this group of molecules is $t_1 \cdot n_1$, and the value

$$\frac{(t_1 \cdot n_1) + (t_2 \cdot n_2)}{n_1 + n_2} \qquad\qquad 2$$

is the mean residence time of two such groups of molecules. Extending this concept to account for all molecules administered, the mean residence time becomes

$$MRT = \frac{\displaystyle\sum_{i=1}^{m} t_i \cdot n_i}{\displaystyle\sum_{i=1}^{m} n_i} = \frac{\displaystyle\sum_{i=1}^{m} t_i \cdot n_i}{N} \qquad\qquad 3$$

where n_i is the number of molecules in the ith group; t_i is their average time in the body; m is the number of groups; and the denominator is the total number of molecules introduced.

The *MRT* is determined more readily after an i.v. bolus dose than after any other mode of drug administration. Here all the molecules of the dose start their residence in the body at the same time; thus, for each group, t_i is the time between drug administration and elimination. When the number of molecules eliminated in each group (dn) approaches a relatively small value, the mean residence time can be expressed in integral notation,

$$MRT = \frac{\displaystyle\int_0^N t \cdot dn}{N} \qquad\qquad 4$$

The limits correspond to the number of molecules eliminated at zero and infinite times. None of the molecules has been eliminated at time zero; at infinite time all have been eliminated. The number of molecules eliminated by all pathways can be expressed in terms of the amounts eliminated, Ael. That is, $Ael = n \cdot$ (molecular weight)/(Avogadro's number). So that

$$MRT = \frac{\int_0^{Ael_\infty} t \cdot dAel}{Ael_\infty} \qquad 5$$

The denominator of Eq. 5 is the dose of drug administered. Integration of Eq. 5, by parts, leads to

$$MRT = \frac{\int_0^\infty (Dose - Ael)dt}{Dose} \qquad 6$$

where Ael is the amount eliminated up to a given time t.

The MRT after an i.v. bolus dose can be estimated from either urinary excretion or plasma drug concentration data as follows.

Excretion Data: When the fraction excreted unchanged, fe, remains constant with time, the amount of drug excreted unchanged in the urine, Ae, equals $fe \cdot Ael$ and Ae_∞ equals $fe \cdot Dose$. On substituting these values into Eq. 6, it is apparent that MRT can be determined from urinary excretion data using the relationship

$$MRT = \frac{\int_0^\infty (Ae_\infty - Ae(t))dt}{Ae_\infty} \qquad 7$$

Figure D–1 shows the cumulative amount excreted unchanged, $Ae(t)$, at various times and the amount ultimately excreted unchanged, Ae_∞. The area between these curves (shaded) is the numerator in Eq. 7. For a given amount excreted unchanged, it is apparent that the area and, therefore, the MRT are increased when drug remains longer in the body.

Plasma Concentration Data: When clearance is constant with time, the rate of elimination is proportional to the plasma concentration, that is, $dAel/dt = CL \cdot C$. Substituting $CL \cdot C \cdot dt$ for $dAel$ and $CL \cdot \int_0^\infty Cdt$ for Ael_∞ into Eq. 5 gives

$$MRT = \frac{\int_0^\infty tCdt}{\int_0^\infty Cdt} \qquad 8$$

The product $t \cdot C$ is called the *first-moment* of the concentration, because concentration is multiplied by time raised to the power of 1. Therefore, the numerator is called the area under the (first)-moment versus time curve ($AUMC$), whereas the denominator is the area under the plasma concentration-time curve (AUC). The time course of both the plasma concentration and its first-moment are shown in Fig. D–2.

The MRT concept is equally applicable to measurement of the turnover of an endogenous substance, using a tracer, and determination of the mean time a drug resides in the body. As an example, let us examine the measurement of MRT after an i.v. bolus dose of a drug from both the urinary and plasma data contained in Table D–1. The value of AUC can be estimated as shown in Appendix I–A. The value of $AUMC$ is calculated from the first-moment (column 3) in a manner similar to that of AUC, but the extrapolated area after last point (C_{last} at t_{last}) is different. In this case the area remaining can be shown to be

$$\int_{t_{last}}^{\infty} t \cdot C \cdot dt = \frac{C_{last} \cdot t_{last}}{\lambda_z} + \frac{C_{last}}{\lambda_z^2}$$

   9

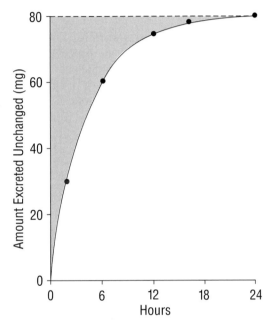

Fig. D–1. The difference between amount excreted unchanged (solid line) and amount ultimately excreted (dashed line) is the amount remaining to be excreted. The area under the amount remaining-to-be-excreted-time curve (shaded), relative to total amount excreted (Eq. 7 in text), is a measure of mean residence time of a substance in the body. Data from Table D–1.

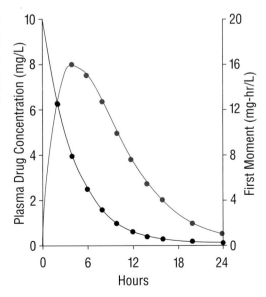

Fig. D–2. After an i.v. bolus dose, the plasma concentration (black curve) declines with time. The first-moment (colored curve), product of time and concentration, rises to a peak and declines with time. The area beyond the last sampling time is much greater for the first-moment time curve than for the concentration-time curve. Data from Table D–1.

where λ_z is the rate constant of the terminal decay of the plasma drug concentration. When the entire concentration-time profile can be described by a sum of exponentials, the area under the first-moment curve can be determined directly from the coefficients and exponential coefficients defining the equation. For example, if $C = C_1 e^{-\lambda_1 t} + C_2 e^{-\lambda_2 t}$ then

$$AUMC = \frac{C_1}{\lambda_1^2} + \frac{C_2}{\lambda_2^2} \qquad\qquad 10$$

In the example considered, the calculated *AUC*, *AUMC*, and area under the amount remaining to be excreted versus time curve are 44.2 mg-hr/L, 17.7 mg-hr^2/L and 340 mg-hr, respectively. The areas remaining under the first two curves after the last time point are 0.17 mg-hr/L and 4.9 mg-hr^2/L respectively. Figures D–1 and D–2 contain the data from Table D–1. The calculated *MRT* values from Eqs. 7 (urinary data) and 8 (plasma data) are then 4.25 hr and 4.0 hr, respectively. The simulated value is 4.3 hr. The differences arise from approximations introduced by the use of the trapezoidal rule to calculate area.

The *MRT*, calculated by either Eq. 7 or 8, is a measure of the average time a substance spends in the body after an i.v. bolus dose. When a drug is given by a constant-rate i.v. infusion or by an extravascular route, the drug spends additional time in the syringe or at the site of administration (e.g., gastrointestinal tract, muscle, or subcutaneous tissues). The observed time, estimated from Eq. 7 or 8, is then the sum of the mean times at these sites and in the body. Table D–1 shows the mean input times (*MIT*) and observed mean total residence times for three common modes of drug input.

Following extravascular administration of a drug solution, the observed total *MRT* is the sum of the *MRT* in the body and the *mean absorption time*. The mean absorption time can be determined from the difference between the *MRT* values (calculated from Eq. 7 or Eq. 8), after extravascular and i.v. bolus doses given on separate occasions. After giving a solid dosage form, the mean input time includes time for disintegration, deaggregation, dissolution, and absorption from solution. Gastric emptying, intestinal motility, and other physiologic and physicochemical factors influence the mean absorption time as well.

Table D–1.   Mean Residence Times for Selected Modes^a of Drug Input

MODE OF ADMINISTRATION	MODEL^b	MEAN INPUT TIME	OBSERVED MEAN RESIDENCE TIME
Single intravenous bolus dose	$\triangledown \xrightarrow{\ k\ }$	0	$1/k$
Constant-rate intravenous infusion	$\xrightarrow{R_o} \bigcirc \xrightarrow{\ k\ }$	$t_{inf}/2^c$	$1/k + t_{inf}/2$
Single extravascular dose	$\triangledown \xrightarrow{\ ka\ } \bigcirc \xrightarrow{\ k\ }$	$1/ka$	$1/k + 1/ka$

^{a}Disposition is assumed to be first-order from a one-compartment model.
^{b}The symbol ∇ denotes a bolus dose into the compartment.
$^c t_{inf}$ is the duration of the infusion.

STUDY PROBLEMS

1. Using the definition of *MRT* in Eq. 8 and an equation for the time-course of plasma drug concentration after an i.v. bolus dose, prove mathematically that the observed *MRT* given in Table D–2 for this route of administration is correct for a one-compartment model.

Table D-2. Plasma Concentration-Time, and Urinary Excretion-time Data Following an i.v. 200-mg Bolus Dose of a Drug

TIME (hr)	PLASMA DRUG CONCENTRATION (mg/L)	FIRST-MOMENT OF PLASMA CONCENTRATION (mg·hr/L)	CUMULATIVE AMOUNT EXCRETED (mg)	AMOUNT REMAINING TO BE EXCRETED (mg)
0	10^a	0	0	80^b
2	6.3	12.6	30	50
4	4.0	16.0	48	32
6	2.5	15.0	60	20
8	1.6	12.8	67	13
10	1.0	10.0	72	8
12	0.63	7.6	75	5
14	0.39	5.5	—	—
16	0.25	4.0	78	2
20	0.10	2.0	—	—
24	0.04	0.96	80	0

^{a}Estimated by extrapolation on a semilogarithmic plot to zero time.
^{b}The cumulative amount excreted at infinite time.

2. Prove that the mean time that a drug is in a syringe during a constant-rate i.v. infusion is equal to $t_{inf}/2$, where t_{inf} is the duration of the infusion.
3. The observed mean total residence times in an individual subject, calculated from plasma concentration-time data (Eq. 8) following an i.v. bolus dose, an i.v. infusion, and an oral dose, on separate occasions, were 8, 10, and 12 hr, respectively.
    a. Assuming a constant-rate input, determine the duration of the infusion.
    b. Assuming a first-order oral input, determine the absorption half-life.
4. Using Eq. 1 in Appendix I–C and Eq. 8 of this appendix, prove mathematically that the value of *AUMC/AUC* after extravascular administration depends on neither the dose nor bioavailability.
5. In problem 5, Chap. 6 (p. 80), plasma concentration-time data are provided during and following a 24-hr i.v. constant-rate infusion and a rectal delivery device of droperidol.
    a. From the i.v. data, calculate the ratio of *AUMC/AUC* and hence *MRT* of droperidol. (Note: The extrapolated *AUMC* beyond the last concentration measurement is given by Eq. 9).
    b. How does your estimate of *MRT* compare with the calculated value of 1.44 $t_{1/2}$, where $t_{1/2}$ (1.9 hr) is the half-life after stopping the infusion, and what conclusion do you draw from the comparison?
    c. Calculate the ratio *AUMC/AUC* associated with the rectal delivery device, and hence the mean input time.
    d. Assessed *in vitro*, the mean release time of the rectal delivery device is 9 hr. If this time also applied *in vivo*, what is the mean absorption time of droperidol from solution in the rectum, once released from the device. For this calculation, release and subsequent transfer across the rectal epithelium are taken to be sequential processes.

AMOUNT OF DRUG IN BODY ON

ACCUMULATION TO PLATEAU

Accumulation of drug in the body is addressed here for multiple i.v. and extravascular doses of fixed size and dosing interval.

MULTIPLE INTRAVENOUS DOSES

Accumulation. Consider the situation in which a dose of drug is given as an i.v. bolus every dosing interval, τ. Recall that after each dose the fraction remaining at time, t, is e^{-kt}. The fraction of drug remaining at the end of a dosing interval τ, therefore, is $e^{-k\tau}$. When time is equal to 2τ, the fraction remaining is $e^{-2k\tau}$. The amount of drug in the body following multiple doses is simply the sum of the amounts remaining from each of the previous doses. The amount of drug in the body just after the next dose is shown in Table E–1 for four successive equal doses given every τ.

It is apparent from the table that the maximum amount of drug in the body just after the fourth dose, $A_{max,4}$, is the fourth dose plus the sum of the amounts remaining from each of three previous doses (sum of terms in row 4 of Table E–1). That is, letting $r = e^{-k\tau}$,

$$A_{4,max} = \text{Dose}(1 + r + r^2 + r^3) \qquad 1$$

Just after the Nth dose the amount in the body is

$$A_{N,max} = \text{Dose}(1 + r + r^2 + r^3 \ldots + r^{N-2} + r^{N-1}) \qquad 2$$

Multiplying by r,

$$A_{N,max} \cdot r = \text{Dose}(r + r^2 + r^3 + r^4 \ldots + r^{N-1} + r^N) \qquad 3$$

Subtracting Eq. 3 from Eq. 2,

Table E-1. Drug in Body Just After Each of Four Successive Doses

TIME	1st DOSE	AMOUNT REMAINING IN BODY FROM EACH DOSE 2nd DOSE	3rd DOSE	4th DOSE
0	Dose			
τ	Dose $\cdot\ e^{-k\tau}$	Dose		
2τ	Dose $\cdot\ e^{-2k\tau}$	Dose $\cdot\ e^{-k\tau}$	Dose	
3τ	Dose $\cdot\ e^{-3k\tau}$	Dose $\cdot\ e^{-2k\tau}$	Dose $\cdot\ e^{-k\tau}$	Dose

$$A_{N,max} \cdot (1 - r) = \text{Dose}(1 - r^N) \qquad 4$$

Therefore,

$$A_{N,max} = \text{Dose} \frac{(1 - r^N)}{(1 - r)} \qquad 5$$

Hence the amount of drug in the body at any time t during a dosing interval, after the Nth dose, $A_N(t)$ is

$$A_N(t) = A_{max,N} \cdot e^{-kt} \qquad 6$$

At the end of the dosing interval, when $t = \tau$, it follows that the minimum amount in the body after the Nth dose, $A_{N,min}$ is

$$A_{N,min} = A_{N,max} \cdot r = \text{Dose} \frac{(1 - r^N) \cdot r}{(1 - r)} \qquad 7$$

Steady State. As the number of doses, N, increases, the value of r^N approaches zero, since r is always a value less than 1. The maximum and minimum amounts of drug in the body during an interval approach upper limits. Then, the amount lost in each interval equals the amount gained, the dose. For this reason drug in the body is then said to be at *steady state* or at *plateau*. Here the maximum, $A_{ss,max}$, the minimum, $A_{ss,min}$, and the amount in the body at any time during the dosing interval, $A_{ss}(t)$, are readily obtained by letting $r^N = 0$ in Eqs. 5 and 7

$$A_{ss,max} = \frac{\text{Dose}}{1 - r} \qquad 8$$

$$A_{ss,min} = \frac{\text{Dose} \cdot r}{1 - r} = A_{ss,max} - \text{Dose} \qquad 9$$

$$A_{ss}(t) = \frac{\text{Dose}}{1 - r} \cdot e^{-kt} \qquad 10$$

or expressed in terms of the dose,

$$\frac{A_{ss,max}}{\text{Dose}} = \frac{1}{1 - r} \qquad 11$$

$$\frac{A_{ss,min}}{\text{Dose}} = \frac{r}{1 - r} = \frac{1}{1 - r} - 1 \qquad 12$$

and

$$\frac{A_{ss}(t)}{\text{Dose}} = \frac{e^{-kt}}{1 - r} \qquad 13$$

Time to Reach Steady-State. The time to approach plateau, whether defined with respect to the maximum or minimum amount of drug in the body, depends solely on the half-life of the drug. The proof of this statement is readily apparent by dividing the equations that define the respective amounts after the Nth dose by the equations that define the respective amounts at plateau,

$$\frac{A_{N,max}}{A_{ss,max}} = \frac{A_{N,min}}{A_{ss,min}} = 1 - r^N \tag{14}$$

As r^N equals $e^{-Nk\tau}$, $N \cdot \tau$ is the time elapsed. Thus, in one half-life the fraction remaining equals 0.5, and half the plateau value is reached; in two half-lives, three-quarters of the plateau value is reached, and so on. A similar conclusion is drawn when relating the average amount during each dosing interval with the average amount at plateau.

MULTIPLE EXTRAVASCULAR DOSES

Accumulation. From Eq. 1 in Appendix I–C and knowing that $A = V \cdot C$, it is apparent that the amount in the body after a single dose is simply the algebraic sum of two exponential terms with a common coefficient, that is

$$\text{Amount in body} = \frac{F \cdot Dose \cdot ka}{(ka - k)} (e^{-kt} - e^{-kat}) \tag{15}$$

Using the principles of additivity and letting $r = e^{-k \cdot \tau}$ and $s = e^{-ka \cdot \tau}$, the amount in the body at the time the Nth dose is administered becomes

$$A_{N,min} = \frac{F \cdot Dose \cdot ka}{(ka - k)} \left[\frac{(1 - r^N)}{(1 - r)} - \frac{(1 - s^N)}{(1 - s)} \right] \tag{16}$$

Steady State. The amount in the body at the beginning ($A_{ss}(0)$) and end ($A_{ss}(\tau)$) of each dosing interval at steady state (r^N and s^N approach zero) is

$$A_{ss}(0) = A_{ss}(\tau) = \frac{F \cdot Dose \cdot ka}{(ka - k)} \left[\frac{1}{(1 - r)} - \frac{1}{(1 - s)} \right] \tag{17}$$

The amount in the body at any time within the dosing interval at steady state is

$$A_{ss}(t) = \frac{F \cdot Dose \cdot ka}{(ka - k)} \left[\frac{e^{-kt}}{(1 - r)} - \frac{e^{-kat}}{(1 - s)} \right] \tag{18}$$

and the time when the peak concentration is reached is

$$t_{peak(multiple\ dose)} = \frac{\ln \left[\dfrac{k \cdot (1 - r)}{ka \cdot (1 - s)} \right]}{(ka - k)} \tag{19}$$

Time to Reach Steady State. The time to reach steady-state is a function of both the absorption and elimination half-lives and the dosing interval. This can be seen by examining the ratio $A_{N,min}/A_{ss,min}$. On dividing Eq. 16 by Eq. 17 and rearranging, the amount in the body at the time of the Nth dose is

$$\frac{A_{N,min}}{A_{ss,min}} = \frac{(1 - r^N)(1 - s) - (1 - s^N)(1 - r)}{r - s} \qquad 20$$

Note: To calculate relationships for plasma concentration, each of the equations above for amount in the body should be divided by V.

STUDY PROBLEMS

Note: The accumulation equations derived in this appendix, particularly those following multiple i.v. doses, are applied in the study problems of Chap. 7, Multiple-Dose Regimens.
1. Prove the identity of the two functions in Eq. 12.
2. Equation 17 for the amount in the body at the end of a dosing interval at steady state can also be written as

$$A_{ss}(\tau) = \frac{F \cdot Dose \cdot ka}{(ka - k)} \cdot \left[\frac{r}{(1 - r)} - \frac{s}{(1 - s)} \right]$$

Prove that these two equations are identical.

DISTRIBUTION OF DRUGS EXTENSIVELY
BOUND TO PLASMA PROTEINS

The distribution of the plasma protein to which a drug binds is a major determinant of the distribution of a drug with a small (less than 0.2 L/kg) volume of distribution. This gives rise to kinetic consequences that are different from those expected for a drug with a large volume of distribution when binding to the plasma protein is altered.

Using albumin as a prototypic binding protein, the body can be represented as having three aqueous compartments, as shown in Fig. F–1. The amount of drug in plasma is the product of volume of plasma and plasma drug concentration. The amount of drug in extracellular fluids outside plasma is the product of the aqueous volume of this space and the average concentration within it. The amount outside the extracellular space (in or on cells or bound to connective elements) is accounted for by the product of the aqueous volume into which drug distributes outside the extracellular fluids and an average concentration in this compartment.

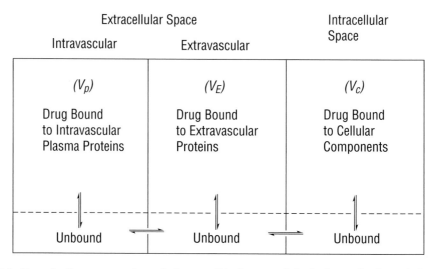

Fig. F–1. Drug distributes among plasma (volume = V_P), the extracellular fluids outside plasma (volume = V_E), and the remainder of the body water (volume = V_R). Equilibrium is achieved when unbound concentrations in the three spaces are the same. The bound concentrations in the three spaces are functions of the affinities of drug for the substances in these spaces to which the drug binds. Throughout the extracellular fluids (V_P and V_E), drug is bound to the same protein(s).

Using the symbols defined in Table F–1,

$$
\underset{\substack{\text{Amount} \\ \text{in body}}}{V \cdot C} = \underset{\substack{\text{Amount} \\ \text{in plasma}}}{V_p \cdot C} + \underset{\substack{\text{Amount in} \\ \text{extracellular} \\ \text{fluids outside} \\ \text{plasma}}}{V_E \cdot C_E} + \underset{\substack{\text{Amount in} \\ \text{the remainder} \\ \text{of the body}}}{V_R \cdot C_R} \tag{1}
$$

Defining fu_R as Cu/C_R, fu as Cu/C, and Cb_E as the average concentration of bound drug in the extracellular space outside plasma and dividing by C yields

$$
V = V_P + V_E \cdot fu \cdot \frac{(Cu + Cb_E)}{Cu} + V_R \cdot \frac{fu}{fu_R} \tag{2}
$$

To be useful, it is necessary to solve for Cb_E in Eq. 2. This is accomplished as follows. For a given protein with one class of binding sites, the law of mass action gives

$$
Ka = \frac{Cb_P}{Cu \cdot (P)_P} = \frac{Cb_E}{Cu_E \cdot (P)_E} \tag{3}
$$

where Cb_P and Cb_E are the bound drug concentrations and $(P)_P$ and $(P)_E$ are the concentrations of unoccupied protein binding sites in plasma and in other extracellular fluids, all expressed in equivalent units, respectively, and Ka is the association or affinity constant between drug and protein. If unbound drug concentrations are identical in both fluids ($Cu_E = Cu$), then

$$
\frac{Cb_P}{(P)_P} = \frac{Cb_E}{(P)_E} \tag{4}
$$

Table F-1. Symbols and Their Definitions

SYMBOL	DEFINITION
C	Total concentration of drug in plasma
Cb_P	Concentration of bound drug in plasma
Cb_E	Average concentration of bound drug in extracellular fluids outside plasma
Cb_R	Average concentration of drug bound outside the extracellular fluids
C_E	Average total concentration of drug in extracellular fluids outside plasma
C_R	Average total concentration of drug outside the extracellular fluids
Cu	Concentration of unbound drug in plasma and, presumably, throughout aqueous spaces into which drug distributes
fu	Fraction unbound to protein in plasma, Cu/C
fu_R	Fraction unbound outside the extracellular fluids, Cu/C_R
Ka	Association or affinity constant between drug and protein
$(P)_P$	Concentration of available binding sites on protein in plasma
$(P)_E$	Average concentration of available binding sites on plasma protein in extracellular fluids outside plasma
$(Pt)_P$	Total concentration of binding sites on protein in plasma
$(Pt)_E$	Average concentration of binding sites on protein in extracellular fluids outside plasma
$R_{E/I}$	Ratio of the total binding sites (or amount of protein) in the extracellular fluids outside plasma to the total binding sites in plasma
V	Apparent volume of distribution of drug
V_{bw}	Volume of total body water, average value = 42 L/70 kg
V_P	Plasma volume, average value = 3 L/70 kg
V_E	Extracellular fluid volume minus plasma volume, average value = 12 L/70 kg
V_R	Aqueous volume outside extracellular fluids into which drug distributes

Also,

$$(Pt)_P = (P)_P + Cb_P \qquad\qquad 5$$

and

$$(Pt)_E = (P)_E + Cb_E \qquad\qquad 6$$

where $(Pt)_P$ and $(Pt)_E$ are the average total concentrations of binding sites in plasma and in other extracellular fluids, respectively. It follows that $(Pt)_P/(P)_P = (Pt)_E/(P)_E$ (obtained by dividing Eq. 5 by $(P)_P$ and Eq. 6 by $(P)_E$). Consequently,

$$Cb_E = Cb_P \cdot \frac{(Pt)_E}{(Pt)_P} \qquad\qquad 7$$

or

$$Cb_E = Cb_P \cdot R_{E/I} \cdot \frac{V_P}{V_E} \qquad\qquad 8$$

where $R_{E/I}$ is the ratio of total number of binding sites, or amount of protein, in extracellular fluids outside plasma (extravascular) to that in plasma (intravascular). This relationship, Eq. 8, can also be shown to be valid when more than one class of binding sites exist on a protein or when saturation is approached. Substituting Eq. 8 into Eq. 2 gives

$$V = V_P + fu \cdot \left[\frac{V_E \cdot Cu + Cb_P \cdot V_P \cdot R_{E/I}}{Cu} \right] + \frac{V_R \cdot fu}{fu_R} \qquad\qquad 9$$

However, since by dividing by C,

$$Cb_P/Cu = (1 - fu)/fu \qquad\qquad 10$$

then

$$V = V_P(1 + R_{E/I}) + (V_E - V_P \cdot R_{E/I}) \cdot fu + \frac{V_R \cdot fu}{fu_R} \qquad\qquad 11$$

The volume of the extracellular fluids outside plasma is, on average, 12 L and the plasma volume is 3 L in a normal 70-kg man. Furthermore, as about 60% of the total body albumin is usually found outside plasma (Table 10–5), its extravascular/intravascular distribution ratio, $R_{E/I}$, is approximately 1.5. Using these typical values, Eq. 11 becomes

$$V = 7.5 + 7.5 \cdot fu + V_R \cdot \frac{fu}{fu_R} \qquad\qquad 12$$

or

$$V = 7.5 + \left[7.5 + \frac{V_R}{fu_R} \right] \cdot fu \qquad\qquad 13$$

These last two equations show that if a drug is distributed only in the extracellular fluids, e.g., if it cannot enter the cells $(V_R = 0)$, the smallest apparent volume of distribution it can have is

$$V = 7.5 + 7.5 \cdot fu \qquad\qquad 14$$

Thus, at distribution equilibrium, the observed apparent volume of distribution cannot be less than 7.5 L, the volume of distribution of albumin, no matter how tightly the drug is bound to albumin. For a drug that is restricted to the extracellular fluids only $(V_R = 0)$ and is not plasma protein bound $(fu = 1)$, the apparent volume of distribution is limited to the value of the total extracellular fluid volume, 15 L. Furthermore, it is apparent from Eqs. 13 and 14 that the volume of distribution varies linearly with fu whether drug is bound in tissue $(fu_R$ less than 1; $V_R = 27$ L$)$ or restricted to extracellular space $(V_R = 0)$.

The volume of distribution based on unbound drug, Vu, by definition is V/fu. Thus, from Eq. 12

$$Vu = \frac{7.5}{fu} + 7.5 + \frac{V_R}{fu_R} \qquad\qquad 15$$

Note that the smallest value of Vu possible is 15 L, a value expected for a drug that is not bound to plasma proteins $(fu = 1)$ or tissue components $(fu_R = 1)$ and does not enter cells. If it does readily enter cells $(V_R = 27$ L$)$, but does not bind anywhere, the unbound volume is that of total body water, 42 L. Increased binding $(fu$ decreased$)$ to plasma proteins increases the unbound volume of distribution. In contrast, increased binding to plasma proteins decreases the volume of distribution based on the total drug concentration in plasma (Eqs. 12 through 14). These changes in V and Vu with fraction unbound are shown in Fig. F–2 for three drugs with normal fu values of 0.01, 0.05, and 0.1.

DISTRIBUTION IN BODY

The model expressed by Eq. 11 and schematically shown in Fig. F–1 can be used to analyze the distribution of a drug in the body. Relationships, listed in Table F–2, for the fractions

Table F–2. Relationships and Their Approximations for Analyzing Drug Distribution

FRACTION OF DRUG IN BODY	RELATIONSHIPS	APPROXIMATION[a]
In plasma	V_P/V	$3/V$
Unbound in body water	$\dfrac{V_{bw} \cdot fu}{V}$	$\dfrac{42 \cdot fu}{V}$
Unbound in extracellular fluids	$\dfrac{(V_P + V_E) \cdot fu}{V}$	$\dfrac{15 \cdot fu}{V}$
In extracellular fluids	$\dfrac{V_P(1 + R_{E/I}) + fu(V_E - V_P \cdot R_{E/I})}{V}$	$\dfrac{7.5(1 + fu)}{V}$
Outside extracellular fluids	$\dfrac{V - V_P(1 + R_{E/I}) - fu(V_E - V_P \cdot R_{E/I})}{V}$	$\dfrac{V - 7.5(1 + fu)}{V}$
Bound to proteins in plasma	$\dfrac{V_P \cdot (1 - fu)}{V}$	$\dfrac{3(1 - fu)}{V}$
Bound to extracellular proteins	$\dfrac{V_P}{V}(1 - fu)(1 + R_{E/I})$	$\dfrac{7.5(1 - fu)}{V}$
Bound outside the extracellular fluids	$\dfrac{V - V_{bw} \cdot fu - V_P(1 - fu)(1 + R_{E/I})}{V}$	$\dfrac{V - 35 \cdot fu - 7.5}{V}$

[a]Applies to drugs that bind to albumin and distribute throughout total body water; approximations of V_P, V_{Ex}, and V_R are 3, 12, and 27 L, respectively; and $R_{E/I}$ equals 1.5.

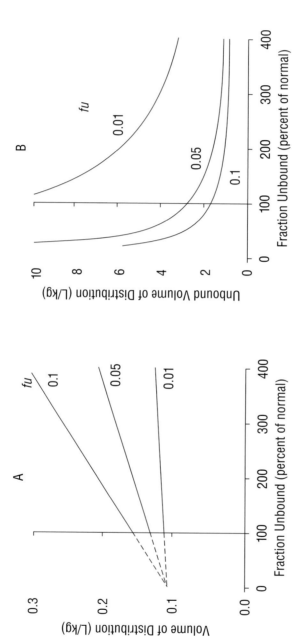

Fig. F–2. An increase in fraction unbound in plasma, expressed here as percent of the normal value, has only a minor effect on (total) volume of distribution (*A*), but dramatically decreases unbound volume of distribution (*B*) for three hypothetical drugs. These drugs bind only to albumin (*fu*$_R$ = 1), distribute throughout body water, and have normal fractions unbound in plasma of 0.1, 0.05 and 0.01. Note that with this model (Eq. 13) the (total) volume of distribution approaches a limiting value of 0.11 L/kg, the apparent volume of distribution of the binding protein, albumin, as *fu* approaches zero. On the other hand, the unbound volume of distribution (Eq. 15) approaches a large value as *fu* approaches zero.

of total drug in body that are in the three compartments in the form of total, unbound, and bound drug are derived as follows:

The fraction of drug in plasma is simply

$$\text{Fraction in plasma} = \frac{V_P}{V} \qquad 16$$

and that outside plasma is

$$\text{Fraction outside plasma} = \frac{V - V_P}{V} \qquad 17$$

The fraction of drug in the body unbound in the total body water, V_{bw}, is

$$\frac{(V_P + V_E + V_R)Cu}{V \cdot C} = \frac{V_{bw} \cdot fu}{V} \qquad 18$$

and that unbound in extracellular fluids is

$$\text{Fraction unbound in extracellular fluids} = \frac{(V_P + V_E)}{V} \cdot fu \qquad 19$$

Since

$$\begin{array}{ll}
\text{Amount bound} \\
\text{to extracellular} = V \cdot C & - (V_P + V_E)Cu - V_R \cdot C_R \\
\text{protein}
\end{array}$$

$$\begin{array}{lll}
\quad\quad\quad\quad \text{Amount} & \text{Amount} & \text{Amount in} \qquad\qquad 20\\
\quad\quad\quad\quad \text{in body} & \text{unbound in} & \text{remainder} \\
& \text{extracellular} & \text{of body} \\
& \text{fluids}
\end{array}$$

it follows that

$$\begin{array}{l}
\text{Fraction of drug in body} \\
\text{bound to extracellular protein}
\end{array} = \frac{V \cdot C - (V_P + V_E)Cu - V_R \cdot C_R}{V \cdot C} \qquad 21$$

Knowing that $V_R \cdot C_R = V_R \cdot fu \cdot C/fu_R$, solving Eq. 1 for $V_R \cdot C_R$, and substituting these relationships and Eq. 9 into Eq. 21 gives

$$\begin{array}{l}
\text{Fraction bound to} \\
\text{extracellular protein}
\end{array} = \frac{V_P(1 - fu)(1 + R_{E/I})}{V} \qquad 22$$

The fraction of drug bound outside the extracellular fluids is 1 minus the sum of the fractions of drug in the total body water (Eq. 18) and bound to extracellular proteins (Eq. 22). That is,

$$\begin{array}{l}
\text{Fraction bound outside} \\
\text{extracellular fluids}
\end{array} = \frac{V - V_{bw} \cdot fu - V_P(1 - fu)(1 + R_{E/I})}{V} \qquad 23$$

Similar relationships for the fractions inside and outside the extracellular fluids can be derived; these too are listed in Table F–2.

The relationships summarized in Table F–2 have a potential utility in identifying, analyzing, and predicting alterations in the apparent volume of distribution of any drug when there is an alteration either in the unbound fraction in plasma or in the unbound fraction outside the extracellular fluids, or when there is a change in the extravascular/intravascular distribution ratio of the binding protein as occurs, e.g., in severe burns, after surgery or trauma, in the nephrotic syndrome, and in pregnancy.

DISTRIBUTION OF PROTEIN

When virtually all the drug in the body is bound to a single plasma protein, the apparent volume of distribution of the drug is identical with the apparent volume of distribution of that binding protein. In this situation, Eq. 11 simplifies to

$$V = V_P(1 + R_{E/I})$$ 24

If V_P is known or is measured, the value of $R_{E/I}$ can be calculated.

The principles above for distribution of drug and its binding protein may also be applied to other plasma proteins. α_1-Acid glycoprotein, the protein that binds many basic drugs, appears to have an extravascular/intravascular distribution ratio that is the inverse of that of albumin, i.e., its value of $R_{E/I}$ is about 0.7 rather than 1.5.

STUDY PROBLEMS

1. a. Given the information in Table F–3 complete Table F–4 by replacing the dashes with values.

Table F–3. Distribution Parameters of Selected Drugs[a]

| DRUG | VOLUME OF DISTRIBUTION | | FRACTION UNBOUND IN PLASMA |
	(L/kg)[b]	L	
Nafcillin	0.35	24.5	0.11
Naproxen	0.16	11.2	0.003
Nitrazepam	1.90	133	0.13

[a]Data from Appendix II, Benet, L.Z., and Williams, R.L.: The Pharmacological Basis of Therapeutics. 8th Ed., Edited by A.G. Gilman, T.W. Rall, A.S. Nies, and P. Taylor. Macmillan, New York, 1993.
[b]For this problem, assume that the unbound form of each drug distributes evenly throughout total body water and that albumin is the only protein to which each drug binds in plasma. The extravascular/intravascular distribution ratio of albumin is 1.5.

Table F–4. Analysis of the Distribution of Nafcillin, Naproxen, and Nitrazepam[a]

PERCENT OF DRUG IN BODY THAT IS . . .	NAFCILLIN	NAPROXEN	NITRAZEPAM
In Plasma	12	27	—
Unbound	—	—	4
In extracellular fluids	34	—	—
Outside extracellular fluids	—	33	94
Bound to protein in plasma	11	27	2
Bound intracellularly (in or on tissue cells, including blood cells)	54	32	—

[a]For a 70-kg person.

b. For which one of the drugs in Table F–3 would a twofold increase in the fraction unbound in plasma give the greatest (percent) change in the apparent volume of distribution?

2. The information contained in Table F–5 summarizes the effect of acute viral hepatitis on the disposition of tolbutamide, a drug that is eliminated almost exclusively by hepatic metabolism. Explain the apparent differences in tolbutamide disposition between these two groups. What is the cause of the shorter half-life in the subjects with acute viral hepatitis?

Table F–5. Effect of Acute Viral Hepatitis on Tolbutamide Disposition[a]

SUBJECTS	HALF-LIFE (hr)	VOLUME OF DISTRIBUTION (L/kg)	CLEARANCE (mL/hr/kg)	FRACTION OF DRUG IN PLASMA UNBOUND
Healthy	5.8	0.15	18	0.06
Acute viral hepatitis	4.0	0.15	26	0.10

[a]Data from Williams, R.L., Blaschke, T.F., Meffin, P.J., Melmon, K.L., and Rowland, M.: Influence of acute viral hepatitis on disposition and plasma binding of tolbutamide. Clin. Pharmacol. Ther., *21*:301–309, 1977.

BLOOD-TO-PLASMA
CONCENTRATION RATIO

The interrelationships among extraction ratio, blood flow, and blood clearance of drugs require measurement of drug concentration in whole blood. Because plasma is the usual site of measurement, knowledge of how blood concentration and plasma concentration are related can be useful.

At equilibrium the ratio of blood-to-plasma concentrations depends on plasma protein binding, partitioning into blood cells, and the volume occupied by blood cells. This dependence is, perhaps, most readily appreciated from mass balance considerations, as follows:

$$C_b \cdot V_B = C \cdot V_P + C_{bc} \cdot V_{bc}$$

| Amount in blood | Amount in plasma | Amount in blood cells | 1 |

where C_b = blood concentration of drug
V_B = blood volume
C = plasma concentration of drug
V_P = plasma volume
C_{bc} = blood cell concentration of drug
V_{bc} = volume occupied by blood cells

The ratio of concentration in blood cells to that unbound in plasma, Cu, is a measure of the affinity of blood cells for drug. Using ρ for this ratio and since $Cu = fu \cdot C$,

$$C_{bc} = \rho \cdot Cu = \rho \cdot fu \cdot C \qquad 2$$

The volume occupied by blood cells is a function of hematocrit, H, and blood volume, i.e.

$$V_{bc} = H \cdot V_B \qquad 3$$

The plasma volume is related to hematocrit by

$$V_P = (1 - H)V_B \qquad 4$$

Substituting Eqs. 2 to 4 in Eq. 1

$$C_b \cdot V_B = (1 - H) \cdot V_B \cdot C + fu \cdot \rho \cdot H \cdot V_B \cdot C \qquad 5$$

Finally, dividing by $V_B \cdot C$, and simplifying,

$$\frac{C_b}{C} = 1 + H[fu \cdot \rho - 1] \qquad 6$$

This relationship clearly shows how the ratio of concentrations, blood/plasma, varies with hematocrit, plasma protein binding, and affinity of drug for blood cells. The ratio can be calculated if these parameters are known. If hematocrit and affinity are constant, a plot of the ratio against fu gives a straight line with an intercept of $1 - H$ and a slope of $H \cdot \rho$. This correlation is useful in situations in which plasma protein binding is variable, such as for certain drugs in uremia, in hypo- and hyperalbuminemic states, and in displacement interactions. In situations in which the plot is not linear, affinity of the blood cells or hematocrit is also changing.

If Eq. 6 is rearranged to solve for ρ, a useful means of determining affinity of blood cells for the drug is obtained, namely,

$$\rho = \frac{H - 1 + (C_b/C)}{fu \cdot H} \qquad 7$$

Determination of ρ requires measurement of hematocrit, concentration ratio, and fraction of drug in plasma unbound to proteins.

STUDY PROBLEM

The ratio of concentration of a drug in blood to that in plasma usually averages about 2.35 in a typical patient who has a hematocrit of 0.45 and a fraction unbound in plasma of 0.1.

a. Calculate the ratio of concentration in blood cells to that unbound in plasma (ρ).

b. In an anemic patient hematocrit is decreased to 0.27, but serum concentration of albumin, the protein to which this drug binds, remains normal, 4.3 g/dL. Calculate the expected ratio of drug concentrations in blood and plasma in this patient.

c. Predict the ratio of plasma and blood clearances in a patient with the nephrotic syndrome in whom the hematocrit is normal but the fraction unbound in plasma is increased to 0.32, a secondary consequence of the loss of plasma proteins into urine.

ESTIMATION OF CREATININE CLEARANCE

UNDER NONSTEADY-STATE

CONDITIONS *

Consider the relationship given in Chap. 23 (Eq. 7) that applies to creatinine when renal function deteriorates acutely and creatinine clearance falls immediately to a new stable value, $CL_{CR}(d)$.

$$C = C(t_1)e^{-k(d) \cdot t} + \frac{R_t}{CL_{CR}(d)} [1 - e^{-k(d) \cdot t}] \qquad 1$$

where C is the creatinine concentration at time t after the first measurement $C(t_1)$, at time t_1, $k(d)$ is the new (and lower) elimination rate constant of creatinine $(CL(d)/V)$; and R_t is its turnover rate.

Integration of Eq. 1 between time t_1 and the next observation $C(t_2)$ at time t_2, with interval $\Delta t = (t_2 - t_1)$, gives

$$\begin{aligned} AUC(\Delta t) = \int_{t_1}^{t_2} C(t)dt = \frac{C(t_1)}{k(d)} [1 - e^{-k(d)\Delta t}] \\ + \frac{R_t}{CL_{CR}(d)} \left[\Delta t - \frac{1}{k(d)} (1 - e^{-k(d) \cdot \Delta t}) \right] \end{aligned} \qquad 2$$

which on rearrangement yields

$$AUC(\Delta t) = \frac{C(t_1)}{k(d)} + \frac{R_t \cdot \Delta t}{CL_{CR}(d)} - \frac{1}{k(d)} \left[C(t_1)e^{-k(d)\Delta t} + \frac{R_t}{CL_{CR}(d)} (1 - e^{-k(d)\Delta t}) \right] \qquad 3$$

But, from Eq. 1, it is seen that

$$C(t_2) = C(t_1) e^{-k(d)\Delta t} + \frac{R_t}{CL_{CR}(d)} (1 - e^{-k(d)\Delta t}) \qquad 4$$

which, when substituted into Eq. 3, recognizing that $CL_{CR}(d) = V \cdot k(d)$ and collecting terms, results in

---

*This appendix was adapted and expanded from Chiou, W.L., and Hsu, F.H.: Pharmacokinetics of creatinine in man and its implications in the monitoring of renal function and in dosage regimen modifications in patients with renal insufficiency. J. Clin. Pharmacol., 15:427–434, 1975.

$$CL_{CR}(d) = \frac{R_t \cdot \Delta t + [C(t_1) - C(t_2)] \cdot V}{AUC(\Delta t)} \qquad 5$$

Now $AUC(\Delta t)$ can be approximated by a trapezoid (Appendix I–A)

$$AUC(\Delta t) = \frac{[C(t_1) + C(t_2)]}{2} \cdot \Delta t \qquad 6$$

so that

$$CL_{CR}(d) = \frac{2R_t}{[C(t_1) + C(t_2)]} + \frac{2 \cdot V \cdot [C(t_1) - C(t_2)]}{\Delta t \cdot [C(t_1) + C(t_2)]} \qquad 7$$

STUDY PROBLEMS

1. A 33-year-old 60-kg woman entered hospital in shock with suspected acute renal impairment. The serum creatinine concentrations soon after admission and 48 hr later were 2.6 and 4.2 mg/dL, respectively.
   a. Estimate the expected turnover rate and volume of distribution of creatinine in the patient.
   b. Estimate the creatinine clearance in the patient.
   c. Comment on the accuracy of your estimate of creatinine clearance.
2. A 67-year-old 55-kg man with end-stage renal disease was on hemodialysis for 3 hr. At the end of dialysis treatment, the serum creatinine concentration was 5.8 mg/dL (58 mg/L). Seventy-two hours later, the serum creatinine had risen to 8.6 mg/dL (86 mg/L).
   a. Estimate the creatinine clearance in the patient between dialysis treatments.
   b. The dialysis clearance of creatinine in the dialyzer used is 120 mL/min. Is the serum creatinine concentration of 5.8 mg/dL at the end of the dialysis period consistent with the estimated pharmacokinetic parameters of creatinine in the patient?

ANSWERS TO PROBLEMS

ANSWERS TO STUDY PROBLEMS (CHAP. 2)

1. *Pharmacokinetics*—quantitation of the time-course of a drug and its metabolites in the body.

   Intravascular administration—parenteral injection of a drug directly into the circulatory system, either arterial or venous.

   Extravascular administration—administration by any route other than directly into the circulatory system.

   Absorption—process by which a drug proceeds from the site of administration to the site of measurement within the body.

   Disposition—all the processes that occur subsequent to the absorption of a drug.

   Distribution—reversible transfer of a drug to and from the site of measurement.

   Metabolism—irreversible conversion to another chemical species.

   Excretion—irreversible loss of the chemically unchanged drug.

   First-pass effect—following oral administration, a drug must first cross the gastrointestinal membranes and pass through the liver to be absorbed systemically. Removal of drug on this first passage into the general circulation is the *first-pass effect*. The term may also apply to other extravascular sites of administration, e.g., intramuscular and subcutaneous.

   Enterohepatic cycling—the secretion of drug into bile followed by reabsorption from the intestines completing a cycle. The drug may also recycle through a metabolite. The metabolite is excreted into bile, converted in the intestine to drug which is reabsorbed into the body.

   Compartment—a component of a kinetic model denoting a specific location of drug or metabolite (a chemically different molecule). A compartment is defined kinetically and does not necessarily reflect a physical space.

2. Absorption or disposition, or both, can be different for R- and S-isomers. Measurement of the sum of the two isomers can therefore give erroneous information following administration of a racemic mixture. The overall kinetic profile is then not that of either isomer. The difference in the kinetics becomes particularly important in therapy when the isomers have different pharmacologic and toxic activities.

3. A poor correlation may result whenever the drug and metabolite do not change proportionally. For example, if drug is rapidly converted to an inactive metabolite that persists in the body, the effect would disappear even though the assay would continue to give a high value. Under these conditions, concentration and response would not be simply correlated.

4. No. By measuring radioactivity, no distinction is made between drug and metabolite(s). The drug may have been degraded in the gut lumen, on passage across the gut wall, or in the liver, with the products being fully excreted into the urine. Only specific measurement of unchanged drug permits one to assess its absorption.

5. a. It must, since the amount ultimately excreted equals the dose. An exception might be renal excretion of an unstable metabolite which, during storage of urine or under assay conditions, reverts back to the original drug. In this case, excretion of unchanged drug is not being measured; the observation is an artifact.

   b. When rate of elimination equals rate of absorption. Prior to that time, rate of absorption exceeds rate of elimination, subsequently the converse is true after a single oral dose.

   c. Yes, if amount in body and amount eliminated are both known.

   d. When rate of absorption is zero. This is the case following intravascular administration or following extravascular administration when absorption has stopped.

   e. When the rate of elimination is zero. This condition exists when there is virtually no drug in the body. It occurs initially following extravascular administration and is essentially the case during most of the absorption phase, if absorption is much faster than elimination.

ANSWERS TO STUDY PROBLEMS (CHAP. 3)

1. a. Correct. $k = 0.693/t_{1/2} = 0.693/4$ hr.

   b. Incorrect. 16 hr is 4 half-lives; in 4 half-lives, 0.925 $(1 - 1/2 \times 1/2 \times 1/2 \times 1/2)$, or 92.5%, has been eliminated from the body.

   c. Correct. It takes 2 half-lives to eliminate 0.375 g following a 0.5-g bolus dose; it takes 1 half-life to eliminate 0.5 g following a 1-g dose.

   d. Incorrect. By 12 hr (3 $t_{1/2}$), only 87.5% of Ae_∞ is excreted; to gain a good estimate of Ae_∞, urine should be collected for 5 half-lives, i.e., up to approximately 24 hr.

   e. Generally correct. For many drugs, within the therapeutic dose range, the pharmacokinetic parameters do not change with dose. Occasionally, one or more of the parameters do.

2. a. Fraction remaining $= 0.71$. $k = 0.693/6$ hr $= 0.1155$ hr^{-1}. Hence fraction remaining in 3 hr $= e^{-kt} = e^{-0.1155 \text{ hr}^{-1} \times 3\text{hr}}$.

   b. $t_{1/2} = 1.6$ hr. Fraction remaining at 4 hr $= 0.18 = e^{-k \times 4\text{hr}}$. Taking antilogarithms and rearranging gives

$$k = 0.43 \text{ hr}^{-1}$$

$$t_{1/2} = 0.693/0.43 \text{ hr}^{-1}$$

3. First determine the half-life $(0.693/0.347 = 2 \text{ hr})$. On a semilogarithmic plot place a point of 0.9 mg/L at zero time and another point, 0.45 mg/L at one half-life (2 hr). Connect and extend the straight line joining these two points.

4. See Fig. II–1.

   Notes: a. Plasma data: Two half-lives have elapsed during the 1 hr for the concentration to fall from 10 to 2.5 mg/L. Hence, the half-life is 0.5 hr, which allows the concentration to be calculated at all other times.

   b. Urine data: In 1 half-life (0.5 hr) the cumulative amount excreted is 0.5 Ae_∞, or 30 mg. At two half-lives (1 hr), it is 0.75 Ae_∞, or 45 mg, and so on.

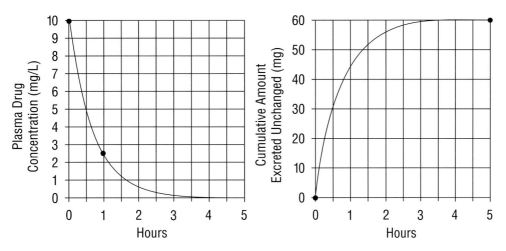

Fig. II–1.

5. a. 77.2%. The fraction eliminated by 3 hr = $AUC(0 \text{ to } 3)/AUC(0 \text{ to } \infty)$ = (5.1 mg-hr/L)/(22.4 mg-hr/L) = 0.228 or 22.8%. Hence percent remaining in the body as drug at 3 hr is 77.2%.

 b. CL = 2.2 L/hr. CL = Dose/AUC = 50 mg/ 22.4 mg-hr/L.

 c. CL_R = 0.49 L/hr. $CL_R = Ae_\infty/AUC$ = 11 mg/22.4 mg-hr/L.

 d. fe = 0.22. $fe = Ae_\infty$/Dose = 11 mg/50 mg. Alternatively, $fe = CL_R/CL$ = 0.49 L/hr/2.2 L/hr.

6. a. V = 14 L. V = Dose/$C(0)$ = 100 mg/7.14 mg/L.

 b. $t_{1/2}$ = 4.0 hr. $t_{1/2}$ = 0.693/k = 0.693/0.173 hr^{-1}.

 c. Total AUC = 41.3 mg-hr/L. total AUC = $C(0)/k$ = 7.14 mg/L/0.173 hr^{-1} (see Appendix I–A for derivation of relationship).

 d. CL = 2.4 L/hr. CL = Dose/AUC = 100 mg/41.3 mg-hr/L.

 e. C = 16.9 mg/L.

$$C = (Dose/V)e^{-kt}$$

$$= \left(\frac{250 \text{ mg}}{14 \text{ } L}\right) e^{-0.173 \text{ hr}-1 \times 20\text{min}/60\text{min}/\text{hr}}$$

7. a. Half-life = 27 hrs. Plot of data is not shown.

 b. Using the relationship $AUC = C(0)/k$, AUC = 5.5 × 10^3 mg-hr/L. Using the trapezoidal rule and remembering that at zero time the concentration is $C(0)$, AUC = 5.7 × 10^3 mg-hr/L. The slightly higher value using the trapezoidal rule arises because, at any time, the concentration along the straight line connecting two data points is always greater than the corresponding concentration on the declining exponential curve. A closer correspondence between $C(0)/k$ and AUC calculated numerically is obtained by using the log linear trapezoid approximation (Appendix I–A).

 c. Clearance = 33 mL/hr.

 d. Volume of distribution = 1.3 L. This is a newborn infant of 3.7 kg (184 mg divided by 50 mg/kg). Thus, the volume of distribution is 0.35 L/kg.

8. a. Plot of data on semilogarithmic paper is not shown.

   b. Half-life = 0.7 hr. Clearance = 1.4×10^2 L/hr.
      Calculated from:

$$CL = \frac{Dose}{AUC}. \text{ For the i.v. bolus case only: } AUC = C(0)/k.$$

   c. Volume of distribution = 1.9 L/kg.

ANSWERS TO STUDY PROBLEMS (CHAP. 4)

1. "c" and "d."

   a. The slower the absorption process, the *lower* is the peak plasma concentration after a single dose.

   b. In some situations, there may be an increase in bioavailability and a shortening of the peak time (ka ↑), but they do not necessarily go together. For example, the bioavailability may be increased in hepatic disease for a drug extensively metabolized during the first pass through the liver, but the rate-time profile for drug reaching the liver may not be affected.

2. a. From AUC analysis, $F = 0.76$; $F_{rel} = 0.95$
      From Ae_∞ analysis, $F = 0.83$; $F_{rel} = 0.95$
      AUC Analysis

$$F = \frac{[AUC/Dose]_{oral}}{[AUC/Dose]_{i.v.}} = \frac{[(19.9 \text{ mg-hr/L})/1000 \text{ mg}]}{[(13.1 \text{ mg-hr/L})/500 \text{ mg}]}$$

$$F_{rel} = \frac{[AUC/Dose]_2}{[AUC/Dose]_1} = \frac{[(19.9 \text{ mg-hr/L})/1000 \text{ mg}]}{[(20.9 \text{ mg-hr/L})/1000 \text{ mg}]}$$

Urine Analysis

$$F = \frac{[Ae_\infty/Dose]_{oral}}{[Ae_\infty/Dose]_{i.v.}} = \frac{(554 \text{ mg}/1000 \text{ mg})}{(332 \text{ mg}/500 \text{ mg})}$$

$$F_{rel} = \frac{[Ae_\infty/Dose]_2}{[Ae_\infty/Dose]_1} = \frac{(554 \text{ mg}/1000 \text{ mg})}{(586 \text{ mg}/1000 \text{ mg})}$$

Assumptions made are:

   1. CL and fe do not vary between treatments.
   2. Estimates of AUC and Ae_∞ are accurate (e.g., no missed urine collections, correct extrapolations to infinity).

   b. Time interval of 48 hr is adequate to ensure a good estimate of Ae_∞. With half-life of about 2.7 hr, 48 hr corresponds to 18 half-lives. The high percent of the dose excreted unchanged ($fe = 332$ mg/500 mg = 0.66) indicates that urine analysis is appropriate for assessment of bioavailability of procainamide.

   c. CL_R values (Ae_∞/AUC) are 25, 28, and 28 L/hr for the i.v., formulation 1, and formulation 2 treatments, respectively. These differences are small and probably insignificant (only mean data shown).

3.

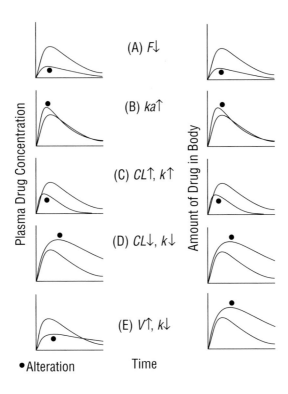

(A) $F\downarrow$

(B) $ka\uparrow$

(C) $CL\uparrow, k\uparrow$

(D) $CL\downarrow, k\downarrow$

(E) $V\uparrow, k\downarrow$

● Alteration   Time

Fig. II–2.

4. a. $CL = 0.8$ L/hr; $V = 7.7$ L.

$$CL = \frac{Dose_{i.v.}}{AUC} = \frac{60 \text{ kg} \times 40 \text{ units/kg}}{3010 \text{ unit-hr/L}}$$

$$V = \frac{CL}{k} = \frac{0.8 \text{ L/hr}}{0.693/6.7 \text{ hr}}$$

b. 0.46. The drug is probably, in large part, absorbed through the lymphatic system (because of molecular size) and metabolized there.

$$F = \frac{AUC_{s.c.}}{AUC_{i.v.}} = \frac{1371 \text{ unit-hr/L}}{3010 \text{ unit-hr/L}} = 0.46$$

c. Two explanations:
   1. F only 0.46
   2. Absorption from subcutaneous site rate-limits ($t_{1/2}$ now 16 hr) the elimination of the drug.

5. a. A delayed esophageal transit profoundly affects the rapidity, but not the extent, of absorption of acetaminophen. The peak concentration is much lower (delayed transit group, 3.9 mg/L; normal transit group, 6.3 mg/L) and delayed (90 min vs. 40 min), but the AUC values (990 vs. 999 mg-hr/L) are comparable. AUC remaining after last time point is calculated from C_{last}/k; $k = 0.0048$ min^{-1} for both groups.

  b. Drug disposition is the rate-limiting step; displayed semilogarithmically, the declining plasma concentrations for the two groups are parallel. The slopes would probably be divergent if absorption had been the rate-limiting step.
  c. To ensure rapid absorption, acetaminophen should be taken while upright with plenty of water.
6. a. Yes, absorption appears to be rate-limiting for either subcutaneous administration into the thigh or for administration at both sites. Semilogarithmic plots of the data show different terminal slopes. If elimination were always rate-limiting, then the same terminal half-life should be observed.
  b. 0.54. The relative bioavailability is not well determined because of the lack of data beyond 12 hr. The value calculated was determined using the trapezoidal rule to 12 hr and C_{last}/k to estimate the area remaining under each curve.

$$F_{rel} = \frac{AUC_{s.c.}(\text{thigh})}{AUC_{s.c.}(\text{abdomen})} = \frac{0.310 \text{ unit-hr/L}}{0.577 \text{ unit-hr/L}} = 0.54$$

  c. 0.72. The AUC expected for $F = 1$ is Dose/CL or 4 units/5 L/hr = 0.8 unit-hr/L.

$$F = \frac{AUC_{s.c.}}{AUC_{i.v.}} = \frac{0.577 \text{ unit-hr/L}}{0.8 \text{ unit-hr/L}}$$

  Alternatively, $F = CL \cdot AUC_{s.c.}/\text{Dose}$
  $\qquad\qquad = 5 \text{ L/hr} \times 0.577 \text{ unit-hr/L/4 units}$
7. a. 16.7 hr. Estimated from slope of semilogarithmic plot of data following i.v. administration (not shown). $k = 0.0415 \text{ hr}^{-1}$
  b. $AUC_{i.v.} = 217 \text{ mg-L/hr}$; $AUC_{oral} = 191 \text{ mg-L/hr}$. Estimated by trapezoidal rule up to 48 hr, with extrapolation given by $C(48)/k$.
  c. $CL = 2.3 \text{ L/hr}$; $V = 55 \text{ L}$. $CL = \text{Dose}/AUC_{i.v.} = 500 \text{ mg}/217 \text{ mg-hr/L}$. $V = CL/k = 2.3 \text{ L/hr}/0.0415 \text{ hr}^{-1}$
  d. $F = 0.88$. $F = (AUC/\text{Dose})_{oral}/(AUC/\text{Dose})_{i.v.}$

$$= 191 \text{ mg-L/hr}/217 \text{ mg-L/hr}$$

  e. $CL_R = 1.86 \text{ L/hr}$. $CL_R = fe \cdot CL = 0.81 \times 2.3 \text{ L/hr}$.
8. a. Absorption rate limits griseofulvin elimination for 24 to 40 hr. This time corresponds to the normal transit time of food in the gut. Thereafter, unabsorbed drug is expelled from the gut, and the plasma concentration of griseofulvin then falls parallel to that following the i.v. dose.
  b. Griseofulvin is incompletely absorbed in this subject. A cursory examination of the data plotted on regular graph paper indicates that, based on AUC corrected for dose, griseofulvin is poorly bioavailable (F approximately 0.4). Griseofulvin, sparingly soluble in water (10 mg/L), is difficult to dissolve.
9. a. Bioavailability = 1.01.
  Using the trapezoid rule (Appendix I–A),

$$F = \frac{[AUC/\text{Dose}]_{i.m.}}{[AUC/\text{Dose}]_{i.v.}} = \frac{[(275.8 \text{ mg-hr/L})/500 \text{ mg}]}{[(136.3 \text{ mg-hr/L})/250 \text{ mg}]}$$

b. A semilogarithmic plot shows that decline in plasma concentration after i.m. administration is slower than that following i.v. administration, indicating that absorption from the i.m. site rate-limits the elimination of phenytoin from the body.

c. First-order process. When plotted on regular graph paper, the amount absorbed does not increase at a constant rate, as expected if absorption was zero-order, but approaches the total amount absorbed asymptotically, as expected if absorption is a first-order process. The first-order nature of the absorption process is confirmed by a semilogarithmic plot of the amount remaining to be absorbed against time; the decline is a straight line, with a half-life of 20 hr.

ANSWERS TO STUDY PROBLEMS (CHAP. 5)

1. a. An *all-or-none response* is a drug effect that is measured in on/off or yes/no units. Death, induction of sleep, and lowering of blood pressure by 25 mm Hg are examples.

   b. A *graded response* is a drug effect that is scaled or graded. Examples here are extent of contraction of a muscle in an *in vitro* preparation, change in heart rate, and increase in urine flow.

   c. The *therapeutic window* is the region of plasma drug concentrations within which the probability of achieving therapeutic success is high.

   d. A *utility curve*, as used here, is a curve that incorporates the incidence of both desired and undesired effects and the relative importance of these "good" and "bad" effects, as a function of the plasma drug concentration.

   e. *Tolerance* denotes a diminished pharmacologic response to a drug with time.

2. A dose does not take into account the time-course of absorption and disposition of a drug. Concentration of plasma, presumably a reflector of the concentration at the site(s) of action, does do so.

3. a. Presence of active metabolite. Here the response is a function of both drug and metabolite. There is even a possibility that the drug disappears before the active metabolite does. Correlation of response to drug concentration would then be nonsense.

   b. Tolerance. When tolerance is caused by a change in response at a given amount in the body or at a given plasma concentration, one expects to see a poor concentration-response relationship, unless time is considered.

   c. Measured response is an indirect effect of drug. There may be a number of steps between the direct action of the drug and the response actually measured, producing time delays and a poor correlation between measured response and concentration.

   d. Measured response related to duration of exposure. The effect of the drug may be more closely related to the duration of inhibition of a process or to the *AUC* than to the concentration at any one time.

4. See Table 5–2. The therapeutic windows of these drugs will be referred to again in subsequent chapters.

5. One situation is when response is directly related to plasma concentration for a drug with a narrow therapeutic window. An example is theophylline. Too large a fluctuation in plasma concentration, associated with relatively infrequent administration, leads to periods of either undermedication or excessive toxicity. Another situation is when acute tolerance to the drug occurs, e.g., with nitroglycerin. A sustained plasma concentration of this drug produces tolerance to peripheral vasodilatation. Other examples are found with antibacterial agents, such as cephalosporins and aminoglycosides, as discussed in this chapter.

1. b.
   a. The approach to plateau depends on half-life.
   b. By definition of CL, the steady-state concentrations must be the same if R_0 is the same $(R_0 = CL \cdot C_{ss})$.
   c. Only if the volumes of distribution of the drugs are also the same. Otherwise, the half-lives are different.
   d. It can if the elimination rate constants (CL/V) are the same. The amount at steady state is R_0/k (Eq. 3 in text).

2. 3.5 and 35 min. At plateau, infusion rate $(R_0) = k \cdot A_{ss}$, or $t_{1/2}$ is given by $0.693 \cdot A_{ss}/R_0$. For succinylcholine, $A_{ss} = 20$ mg, so that when $R_0 = 0.4$ mg/min, $t_{1/2} = 35$ min and when $R_0 = 4$ mg/min, $t_{1/2} = 3.5$ min. The wide range in the half-life of succinylcholine arises from differences in the amount and type of pseudocholinesterase, the enzyme responsible for succinylcholine hydrolysis and inactivation. The longer half-life is only rarely encountered.

3. See Fig. II–3 on p. 524.

4. a. $CL = 1.2$ L/min, $t_{1/2} = 1.6$ hr; $V = 164$ L; $MRT = 137$ min. $CL = R_0/C_{ss}$. The half-life is estimated from the slope of a semilogarithmic plot of the declining plasma concentration observed on stopping the infusion. The volume of distribution is obtained by dividing clearance by the elimination rate constant $(0.693/t_{1/2})$. $MRT = V/CL$.
   b. Yes. Half the plateau value, 10.5 µg/L, should be reached by 1.6 hr and 14.5 µg/L reached by 2 hr. More precisely, using the equation $C = C_{ss} (1 - e^{-kt})$, the expected values at 1, 2, 4, and 6 hr are 7.4, 12, 17, and 19.6 µg/L, which are in reasonably close agreement with the observed values.
   c. Plasma concentrations expected are 14.8, 24, and 42 µg/L. Doubling the infusion rate results in a doubling of the concentration at all times.
   d. Loading dose = 6.9 mg. Dose = $V \cdot C(0) = 164$ L × 42 µg/L.

5. a. $t_{1/2} = 1.9$ hr. Estimated from semilogarithmic plot of the plasma concentration against time after stopping the i.v. infusion (not shown).
   b. $MRT = 2.74$ hr. $MRT = 1/k = 1.44 \, t_{1/2}$.
   c. $F = 0.50$. Calculated from AUC considerations.

$$AUC_{i.v.} = AUC(0\text{--}30 \text{ hr}) + C(30 \text{ hr})/k = 69.6 + 1.0 = 70.6 \, \mu\text{g-hr/L}$$

$$AUC_{rectal} = AUC(0\text{--}30 \text{ hr}) + C(30 \text{ hr})/k = 34.8 + 0.3 = 35.1 \, \mu\text{g-hr/L}$$

where AUC (0–30 hr) is estimated by trapezoidal approximation (Appendix I–A).

$$F = (AUC/Dose)_{rectal}/(AUC/Dose)_{i.v.} = \frac{((35.1 \, \mu\text{g-hr/L})/3 \text{ mg})}{((70.6 \, \mu\text{g-hr/L})/3 \text{ mg})}$$

   d. $CL = 42$ L/hr. $CL = Dose/AUC_{i.v.} = 3000 \, \mu\text{g}/70.6 \, \mu\text{g-hr/L}$.
   e. $V = 116$ L. $V = CL \times MRT = 42$ L/hr × 2.74 hr.

6. a. 12.8 µg/hr. Over the interval 12 to 24 hr, the plasma concentration is essentially constant, average value 1.53 µg/L, signifying the attainment of plateau. At plateau, rate of absorption = rate of elimination, therefore,

$$\text{Rate of absorption} = CL \cdot C_{ss}$$
$$= 8.4 \text{ L/hr} \times 1.53 \, \mu\text{g/L}$$

b. 330 μg. The amount absorbed equals the amount eliminated, that is,

$$\text{Amount absorbed} = CL \cdot AUC$$

Calculating the AUC from the trapezoidal rule and estimating the remaining area from $C(30)/k$,

$$\text{Amount absorbed} = 8.4 \text{ L/hr} \times 39.3 \text{ } \mu\text{g-hr/L}$$

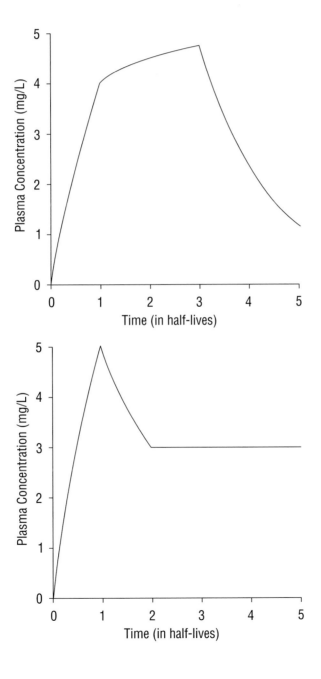

Fig. II–3.

   c. No. There is an apparent lag time ($\sim$2 hr) in the appearance of drug in the systemic circulation, a common observation with transdermal devices.

TIME (hr)	0	1	2	4	6	8	∞
Concentration (mg/L)							
Expected[a]	0	0.33	0.59	0.97	1.2	1.35	1.6
Observed	0	0	0.05	0.8	1.1	1.5	1.6

[a] $C = C_{ss}(1 - e^{-kt})$

7. $V = 22$ L, $k = 0.28$ hr^{-1} $t_{1/2} = 2.5$ hr, and $CL = 6.2$ L/hr. From postinfusion data, $t_{1/2} = 2.5$ hr ($k = 0.28$ hr^{-1}). Clearance is best estimated from the relationship $CL = $ Dose/AUC, where Dose is 50 mg/hr $\times$ 7.5 hr and the total area under the curve, calculated by the trapezoidal rule, is 60.4 mg-hr/L.

$$V = \frac{CL}{K} = \frac{6.2 \text{ L/hr}}{0.28 \text{ hr}^{-1}}$$

The answers might also have been obtained from data during the infusion. At $t_{1/2}$ during the infusion,

$$C = \frac{1}{2} \cdot \frac{R_0}{k \cdot V} = \frac{C_{ss}}{2} = 4 \text{ mg/L}$$

$$CL = \frac{R_0}{C_{ss}} = \frac{50 \text{ mg/hr}}{8 \text{ mg/L}}$$

Note: The second method, dependent on interpolation at one time point, provides a less reliable estimate of clearance.

8. $V = 25$ L, $k = 0.1$ hr^{-1}, $t_{1/2} = 7$ hr, and $CL = 2.5$ L/hr.

$$V = \frac{\text{Dose}}{C(0)} = \frac{250 \text{ mg}}{10 \text{ mg/L}} \quad \text{and} \quad CL = R_0/C_{ss} = (10 \text{ mg/hr})/(4 \text{ mg/L})$$

$$k = \frac{CL}{V} = (2.5 \text{ L/hr})/(25 \text{ L}).$$

9. a. 0.42 of a half-life.

$$(1/2)^n = \frac{C_{ss} - C}{C_{ss} - C(0)} = \frac{15}{20}$$

$$n = \log(15/20)/\log(0.5).$$

   b. 4.74 half-lives.

$$(1/2)^n = \frac{C_{ss} - C}{C_{ss} - C(0)} = \frac{-15}{-400}$$

$$n = \log(15/400)/\log(0.5).$$

ANSWERS TO STUDY PROBLEMS (CHAP. 7)

1. a. True. The process of accumulation always occurs on multiple dosing.
   b. False. The less frequently a drug is given, the lower its extent of accumulation.
   c. False. The time to reach plateau depends on the elimination half-life.
   d. Only true if $F = 1$.
   e. False. $C_{ss,av}$ is independent of volume of distribution.
   f. False. $C_{ss,av}$ is independent of the absorption kinetics, unless absorption becomes so protracted as to affect bioavailability.
2. a. Relative bioavailability (from AUC) = 0.93 (Eq. 27); relative bioavailability (from urine) = 1.00 (Eq. 29).

   Note: These calculations are based on steady state having been reached. As procalinamide has a half-life of 2.7 hr, such must be the case.
   b. Renal clearance (Eq. 28) = 29.4 or 31.6 L/hr. $CL_R = Ae_{\tau,ss}/AUC_{ss}$.
3. a. 1. $A_{ss,max}$ = 100 mg; $A_{ss,min}$ = 68 mg.
      2. Accumulation ratio = 3.1.
      3. $C_{ss,min}$ = 0.24 mg/L.
      4. Time to reach 50% of plateau in 1.8 days $(t_{1/2})$.
   b. Table II-1.

Table II-1.

Dose	1	2	3	4	5	6	7	∞
$A_{N,max}$ (mg)[a]	32	54	69	79	85	90	93	100
$A_{N,min}$ (mg)[b]	22	37	47	53	58	61	63	68

$$^a A_{N,max} = \frac{F \cdot Dose(1 - e^{-Nk\tau})}{(1 - e^{-k\tau})}$$
$$^b A_{N,min} = A_{N,max} \cdot e^{-k\tau}$$

   c. Sketch should be scaled as follows: Amount to 100 mg $(A_{ss,max})$ and time to 7 days (5 half-lives) at least.
   d. Loading dose = 150 mg $(A_{ss,max}/F)$.
4. Several possibilities, no single solution. Three 100-mg tablets to start, then either three 100-mg tablets every 8 hr or two 200-mg tablets every 12 hr, if given as a controlled-release product.

   Regimen Design

$$t_{1/2} = \frac{0.693 \cdot V}{CL} = 8.7 \text{ hr}$$

$$\tau_{max} = 1.44 \cdot t_{1/2} \cdot \log(C_{max}/C_{min}) = 8.7 \text{ hr}$$

$$D_{M,max} = \frac{V}{F}(C_{max} - C_{min}) = \begin{array}{l} 5 \text{ mg/kg or} \\ 300 \text{ mg of theophylline} \end{array}$$

$$\text{Dosing rate} = \frac{D_{M,max}}{\tau_{max}} = \begin{array}{l} 34 \text{ mg/hr, 204 mg/6hr} \\ 272 \text{ mg/8hr, 408 mg/12 hr} \end{array}$$

Table II-2. Possible Maintenance Regimens

Regimens	$C_{ss,max}$[a]	$C_{ss,min}$[b]	Comment
One 200-mg tablet every 6 hr[c]	14.9	9.2	Under
Two 200-mg tablets every 8 hr	24	12.7	Over
Three 100-mg tablets every 8 hr[c]	18	9.5	Under[d]
Two 200-mg tablets every 12 hr	18.4	7.1	Under

$$^a C_{ss,max} = \frac{F \cdot D}{V(1 - e^{-k\tau})}$$
$$^b C_{ss,min} = C_{ss,max} \, e^{-k\tau}$$
[c]One 200-mg tablet = 170 mg theophylline.
[d]Probably satisfactory and convenient if orally administered—especially as a controlled-release preparation.

Loading Dose

$$D_L = \frac{V}{F} \cdot C_{ss,max} = \frac{30}{1} \times 15 \text{ mg/L} = 450 \text{ mg}$$

That is, approximately three tablets of 170 mg of theophylline (200 mg of aminophylline)

5. a. Oral maintenance dosing rate = 6.2 mg/hr.

$$F \cdot Dose_{single} = CL \cdot AUC_{single}$$

$$F \cdot D_M/\tau = CL \cdot C_{ss,av}$$

$$\frac{D_M}{\tau} = Dose_{single} \cdot \frac{C_{ss,av}}{AUC_{single}} = 50 \text{ mg} \times \frac{10 \text{ mg/L}}{80.6 \text{ mg-hr/L}}$$

b. 1. Maintenance dose = 75 mg (12 hr × 6.2 mg/hr).
2. At plateau, the trough plasma concentration at 12 hr is 5.4 mg/L. The trough concentration at plateau is the sum of the concentrations at 12, 24, 36, 48 hr, etc., after a single dose of 75 mg. Concentrations associated with a 75-mg oral dose are 1.5 times those obtained with a 50-mg oral dose. At plateau, one can ignore contributions from doses that are given more than 5 half-lives previously, that is, five times 8 hr or 40 hr. Hence,

$$C_{ss}(12 \text{ hr}) = 1.5 \, [C(12) + C(24) + C(36) + C(48)]$$

$$= 1.5 \, [2.8 + 0.6 + 0.14 + 0.03]$$

Note: Although helpful, it is not essential to know the half-life of the drug. One includes concentration values until they become insignificant, which can be judged directly from the concentration-time curve following the single oral dose.

6. a. 70 mg. Situation analogous to a constant-rate infusion. Amount in formulation = $k \cdot A_{ss} \cdot n$, where n is time desired to maintain A_{ss}. Amount = (0.693/4 hr) × 50 mg × 8 hr.
b. Immediately. Loading dose (50 mg) + sustaining dose (70 mg).
c. Total dose for day 1 = 260 mg; total dose for day 2 = 210 mg.
d. See Table II–3.

7. a. Release from the CR product. This conclusion follows from the terminal half-life following the CR product (5.5 hr) being much longer than after the IR product (2.2 hr).
b. Yes. The time taken to reach plateau is essentially determined by the half-life associated with the terminal decline phase. For the IR product ($t_{1/2}$ = 2.2 hr), a plateau is expected to be reached by 3.3 $t_{1/2}$ or 7.3 hr. That is, by the second dose

Table II–3. Amount in Body (mg)

TIME (hr)	0	4	8	12	16	20	24	28	32	36
Regimen										
Every 4 hr	0	25	63	81	91	95	98	99	99.5	100
Every 8 hr	0	25	38	44	47	49	49	50	50	50
Every 12 hr	0	25	38	19	34	42	21	36	43	22

of the 8-hourly regimen. For the CR product ($t_{1/2}$ = 5.5 hr), a plateau should be reached by 18 hour. That is, by the third dose of the 12-hourly regimen. In the multiple-dose study, both preparations were administered for 7 days.

c. Yes.

For IR product: 40 mg every 8 hr

$$AUC_{ss}(0\text{–}24 \text{ hr})_{expected} = 3 \times AUC(single)_{40 \text{ mg}} = 3 \times 0.57 \text{ mg-hr/L}$$
$$= 1.71 \text{ mg-hr/L}$$

$$AUC_{ss}(0\text{–}24 \text{ hr})_{observed} = 1.72 \text{ mg-hr/L}$$

For CR product: 60 mg every 12 hour

$$AUC_{ss}(0\text{–}24 \text{ hr})_{expected} = 2 \times AUC(single)_{60 \text{ mg}} = 2 \times 0.88 \text{ mg-hr/L}$$
$$= 1.76 \text{ mg-hr/L}$$

$$AUC_{ss}(0\text{–}24 \text{ hr})_{observed} = 1.57 \text{ mg-hr/L}$$

d. For single-dose, F_{rel} = 1.03; on multiple dosing, F_{rel} = 0.91.

Single dose

$$F_{rel} = \frac{[AUC/Dose]_{CR}}{[AUC/Dose]_{IR}} = \frac{[0.88 \text{ mg-hr/L/60 mg}]}{[0.57 \text{ mg-hr/L/40 mg}]}$$
$$= 1.03$$

Multiple dosing

$$F_{rel} = \frac{[AUC_{ss}/Dose]_{CR}}{[AUC_{ss}/Dose]_{IR}} = \frac{[1.57 \text{ mg-hr/L/120 mg}]}{[1.72 \text{ mg-hr/L/120 mg}]}$$
$$= 0.91$$

e. Yes. Generally, t_{max} after multiple dosing is shorter than after single-dose administration. This arises because, with accumulation, the condition when rate of elimination = rate of absorption is met earlier with multiple dosing. In the specific case of adinazolam, the t_{max} values following single doses of the IR and CR products are 1.0 and 2.5 hr, respectively, which are already short relative to the multiple-dosing intervals of 8 hr and 12 hr, respectively, for these products. Hence, following multiple dosing, the durations over which the plasma concentration are expected to decline are at least 7 hr and 9.5 hr for the IR and CR products, respectively. These times are at least 3 expected terminal half-lives for the IR product and close to 2 expected terminal half-lives for the CR product. Obviously, for the CR product it would be better to determine the half-life after stopping administration. Clearly, difficulties in estimating the terminal half-life within the dosing interval would be expected had the CR product been given 8 hourly.

f. Degree of accumulation is 1.27 for the IR product and 1.78 for the CR product.

$$\text{Degree of accumulation} = \frac{AUC(0 - \tau)_{ss}}{AUC(0 - \tau)_{single}}$$

For both IR and CR products, information provided concerns the AUC over 24 hour at plateau ($AUC(0\text{–}24 \text{ hr})_{ss}$). That is over three dosing intervals for IR product and two dosing intervals for the CR product. Hence,

For IR product

$$\text{Degree of accumulation} = \frac{(1.72 \text{ mg-hr/L})/3}{0.45 \text{ mg-hr/L}}$$

For CR product

$$\text{Degree of accumulation} = \frac{(1.57 \text{ mg-hr/L})/2}{0.44 \text{ mg-hr/L}}$$

ANSWERS TO STUDY PROBLEMS (CHAP. 8)

1. *Passive diffusion*—Tendency for molecules to move down a concentration gradient.
   Passive facilitated diffusion—Enhanced tendency to move down a concentration gradient but showing capacity-limited properties, presumably caused by a limited amount of a "carrier."
   Active transport—A form of facilitated transport in which movement against a concentration gradient, expenditure of energy, as well as a capacity limitation are evident.
   Permeability—A measure of the ease with which a substance moves across a membrane. Its value depends on the properties of both drug and membrane. The rate of movement also depends on surface area and the concentration gradient driving the reaction. Permeability has units of distance/time.
2. a. True. The perfusion limitation exists because, functionally, there is no diffusional barrier.
   b. False. Permeability is a property of the membrane. The rate of movement through the membrane depends on surface area, permeability, and concentration gradient across the membrane.
   c. False. Diffusion in both directions continues. Only the net rate of movement is zero.
   d. False. Carrier-mediated transport may or may not be coupled with an energy-consuming reaction.
   e. False. Permeability is a property of the membrane. Binding in the aqueous phase does not appear to affect this property.
3. Doubling the molecular weight from 100 to 200 reduces the permeability by about 0.5 log units (factor of 3.2). Doubling from 200 to 400 reduces permeability by about 1.1 log units (factor of 12.6), while doubling from 400 to 800 reduces permeability by 2.6 log units (factor of 400). Clearly, molecular size has a major effect on permeability. Indeed, compounds with a partition coefficient of 1 and a molecular weight of 200 are expected to show greater permeability than compounds with a partition coefficient of 10^6 and a molecular weight of 1000.
4. The ionized forms of drugs, be they acids or bases, do not appear to cross most membranes readily. If lipophilic, the un-ionized form does penetrate membranes. Thus, the degree of ionization can be a controlling factor in determining the rate of movement across membranes.

5. a. 0.45 L/hr.

$$CL \text{ (during treatment)} = \frac{0.693 \times 38.5 \text{ L}}{36 \text{ hr}} = 0.74 \text{ L/hr}$$

$$CL \text{ (no treatment)} = \frac{0.693 \times 38.5 \text{ L}}{93 \text{ h}} = 0.29 \text{ L/hr}$$

By difference, CL (charcoal treatment) = 0.45 L/hr

b. $t_{1/2}$ (absorption) = 0.62 hr.

$$ka \cdot Va = CL \text{ (charcoal treatment)}$$

where Va is the volume of fluid in the intestinal lumen (0.4 L).

$$ka = \frac{0.45 \text{ L/hr}}{0.4 \text{ L}} = 1.125 \text{ hr}^{-1}$$

$$t_{1/2} \text{ (absorption)} = \frac{0.693}{1.125} = 0.62 \text{ hr}$$

ANSWERS TO STUDY PROBLEMS (CHAP. 9)

1. Insufficient time for absorption, competing reactions in the gastrointestinal tract, and extraction during the first pass through the liver.
2. a. True. Small lipophilic drugs in solution are very rapidly absorbed across the small intestine, and when these drugs are given orally, absorption is rate-limited by delivery from the stomach into the small intestine.
   b. False. When intestinal absorption is rate-limited by membrane permeability, absorption kinetics—and hence the plasma concentration-time profile—is relatively insensitive to changes in dissolution kinetics. For rapidly dissolving products of such drugs, most of the drug has dissolved before appreciable absorption has occurred.
   c. False. Polar drugs primarily traverse the small intestine via the paracellular pathway; they have great problems traversing across the relatively lipophilic cell membranes.
   d. True. Administered intramuscularly, large protein drugs have great difficulty permeating the capillary membranes. Such drugs enter the systemic circulation primarily via the lymphatic system so that, because lymph flow is low, absorption occurs slowly.
   e. True. Gastric emptying of large nondisintegrating tablets or dosage units is, on average, greatly delayed, especially after a heavy meal.
3. Any six of the drugs listed in Table 9–3.
4. Surface area, solubility, pH, and stirring.
5. This statement is generally true. An exception arises with large polar drugs, such as gentamicin, which traverse the capillary membrane of muscle much more readily than the small intestine epithelium. Other exceptions are drugs that precipitate at the injection site, from which dissolution is very slow.
6. a. Much faster (solubility of solid has greater effect than pH of medium.)

    b. At essentially the same rate (dissolution relatively insensitive to pH of solution).

    c. In divided doses during the day (solubility problem).

    d. Drug A (solubility problem).

7. a. Small intestine. Based on comparison of AUC as a measure of the amount absorbed, little drug is absorbed from the large intestine (ascending and descending colon). And, absorption of drugs from the stomach is always much slower than from the small intestine.

    b. Duodenum. Jejunal delivery results in only 26% absorption compared to gastric delivery ($AUC_{duodenal}/AUC_{gastric}$ = 0.38 mg-L/hr/1.48 mg-L/hr). As drugs are poorly absorbed across the gastric epithelium, and the duodenum separates the stomach from the jejunum, the duodenum is likely to be a primary site of absorption for ciprofloxacin.

    c. Poor. For dosage forms that readily empty from the stomach (e.g., those comprising small multipelleted units), within 6 hr of administration the dosage form would be in the large intestine where, because of poor absorption characteristics, rate control from the delivery system is likely to be lost. A possible solution is to use a large controlled-release nondisintegrating product, which, when taken on a full stomach, is retained there and delivers drug continuously to the more permeable small intestine. In addition, it would be important for release of drug from the delivery system to be independent of such factors as pH, stirring rate, and electrolyte composition, which can vary markedly in the stomach.

ANSWERS TO STUDY PROBLEMS (CHAP. 10)

1. *Apparent volume of distribution*—Parameter that relates the amount in the body to the plasma concentration.

    Fraction unbound—Ratio of unbound and total concentrations in plasma.

    Tissue-to-blood equilibrium distribution ratio—Ratio of concentrations in whole tissue and blood when there is no net transfer of drug to or from the tissue. It is best determined under steady-state conditions.

    Perfusion and permeability limitations in drug distribution—Conditions in which the rate of distribution to a tissue from blood, or the converse, is limited by the flow of blood and the ability to cross cell membranes, respectively.

2. a. 0.025 mg/L (Dose/V)

    b. 600 mg ($V \cdot C$).

    c. 1. 99.993% [$(V - V_p)/V$]

        2. 0.020% [$7.5(1 + fu)/V$]

        3. 99.97% [$(V - 35 \cdot fu - 7.5)/V$]

3. a. and b.

4. a. See Fig. II–4 on p. 523. In the presence of Drug B, which significantly (two-fold change) displaces drug from tissue binding sites only.

Parameter:	CL	CLu	AUC	$AUCu$	V	Vu	$t_{1/2}$
Anticipated Change:	↔	↔	↔	↔	↓	↓	↓

Note: This drug has a large volume of distribution (V = Dose/$C(0)$ = 500 mg/5 mg/L = 100 L).

    b. See Fig. II–5 on p. 523. At a subsequent time when the patient's serum albumin is reduced from 42 to 21 g/L (e.g., when a patient develops nephrotic syndrome). Binding to other constituents in the body is unaffected.

Parameter:	CL	CLu	AUC	$AUCu$	V	Vu	$t_{1/2}$
Anticipated Change:	↑	↔	↓	↔	↑	↔	↔

5. a. True. The volume of the liver is 2.3% of body weight; therefore at distribution equilibrium the minimum volume of distribution (consisting only of plasma and liver) = $V_P + 50 \cdot V_T = [3 + (50 \times 1.6)]$ L = 83 L.
   b. True. It would take much longer to equilibrate if the drug primarily distributed into poorly perfused tissues.
6. Times (min): Lungs, 0.07; Kidneys, 0.7; Heart, 3.5; Liver, 13; and Skin, 347.
   Calculated from:

$$\begin{array}{l}\text{Time to reach}\\ \text{50\% of} \\ \text{equilibrium}\end{array} = t_{1/2} = \frac{0.693 \cdot K_p}{Q/V_T}$$

7. Fraction of digitoxin unbound in extracellular fluids = 0.012.
   Calculated from:

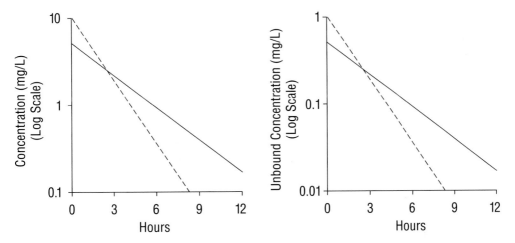

Fig. II–4. Solid line represents control; dashed line, presence of drug B.

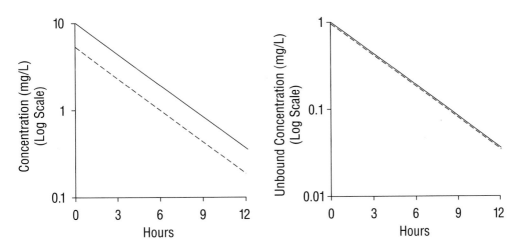

Fig. II–5. Solid line represents control; dashed line, presence of drug B.

$$\text{Fraction of drug in body unbound in extracellular fluids} = \frac{15 \cdot fu}{V} = \frac{15 \times 0.03}{38}$$

8. Digitoxin ($fu_R = 0.027$) is more tightly tissue bound than digoxin ($fu_R = 0.039$). *Calculated from* rearangement of Eq. 25.

$$\text{Fraction unbound in intracellular fluids } (fu_R) = \frac{27 \cdot fu}{V - 7.5 - 7.5 \cdot fu}$$

9. a. 0.0172.

$$\frac{fu'}{fu} \approx \frac{P_t}{P_t'} = \frac{43}{12.5}$$

b. 14 L.
   Given under control conditions, $V = 9.4$ and $fu = 0.005$. Hence, by substitution into Eq. 25, $fu_R = 0.0725$. Accordingly, in patients with nephrotic syndrome,

$$V' = 7.5 + \left(7.5 + \frac{27}{fu_R}\right) fu' = 7.5 + \left(7.5 + \frac{27}{0.0725}\right) 0.0172$$

   where fu' (0.0172) is from "a" above.
c. Yes. The shortening of half-life is expected from the minor increase in V compared to the large increase in CL.

ANSWERS TO STUDY PROBLEMS (CHAP. 11)

1. Theophylline (CL_R of 10 mL/min < $fu \cdot GFR$ of 60 mL/min) is filtered and reabsorbed; secretion cannot be ruled out. Phenytoin (CL_R of 0.15 mL/min = $fu \cdot$ (urine flow)) is filtered and reabsorbed to equilibrium if compound is not ionized (with a pKa of 8.3, it is not). Cefonicid (CL_R of 20 mL/min > $fu \cdot GFR$ of 2.4 mL/min) is filtered and secreted. Reabsorption cannot be discounted, although like cephalosporins, in general, cefonicid should be relatively polar.
2. a. 2, 4.
   1. Incorrect. No pH sensitivity in renal clearance is expected unless the drug is reabsorbed.
   2. Possible. pKa lies in the range in which the fraction un-ionized varies substantially with changes in urine pH.
   3. Incorrect. Clearance and volume of distribution relate to different processes.
   4. Possible—if pKa lies in the range of 3.5 to 7.0 and un-ionized compound is lipophilic. However, changes in urine pH do not affect the total amount of drug excreted unchanged as $fe = 1$.
   b. 2.
   1. Incorrect. If polar, it is unlikely to be reabsorbed in the kidneys, an essential requirement for forced diuresis to be effective.
   2. Correct. Both tubular reabsorption and excretion of a substantial percent by the route of elimination, especially during intoxication, are essential conditions for diuresis to materially affect elimination.
   3. See 1. above.

    4. Incorrect. This compound is not secreted and not reabsorbed; its unbound clearance equals the renal clearance of creatinine, a measure of *GFR*.

  c. 1.

    1. Correct. Renal clearance exceeds *GFR*, even without correcting for *fu*.

    2. Incorrect. Its renal extraction ratio is 0.52

$$\left(E_R = CL_{R,b}/Q_R = \frac{0.567 \text{ L/min}}{1.1 \text{ L/min}} \right)$$

    3. Uncertain. Without knowing total clearance as well as renal clearance, an estimate of the importance of renal excretion to total elimination cannot be made unambiguously.

    4. Not necessarily so. Many drugs highly bound to plasma proteins have a high renal clearance; they are efficiently handled by a secretory transport system.

  d. 3.

    1. Not necessarily so. Although a high renal clearance is likely to be relatively constant, there is no guarantee this will be so.

    2. Incorrect. Condition occurs when equilibrium exists between drug in urine and that in blood. Then renal clearance varies proportionately with changes in urine flow.

    3. Correct. Renal clearance is constant with time, because a fixed rate of excretion results from a given plasma concentration when a constant fraction of filtered and secreted drug is reabsorbed.

3. a. Alcohol is reabsorbed in the nephron virtually to the same extent as water.

  b. No. The excretion rate is calculated by multiplying urine flow by urine concentration. Thus, at a given plasma alcohol concentration, excretion rate is flow dependent. Because of typical variability in urine flow, excretion rate only roughly correlates with the plasma alcohol concentration.

4. a. 1. Tocainide. Only for this drug is the pKa in the correct range and its un-ionized form nonpolar, enabling tubular reabsorption to occur.

    2. Nafcillin. CL_R $(0.693 \cdot fe \cdot V/t_{1/2}) = 4.7$ L/hr; the CL_R values of the other drugs are lower.

    3. Nafcillin. Being polar, it will have great difficulty crossing the placenta to the fetus.

    4. Tocainide. This drug is extensively reabsorbed in the kidneys (CL_R of 1.46 L/hr $< fu \cdot GFR$, 6.8 L/hr), and a substantial fraction is excreted unchanged even under normal conditions ($fe = 0.14$). This fraction is likely to increase in intoxication owing to saturation of metabolic enzymes, which frequently occurs. Nafcillin is not reabsorbed, and for cyclosporine, renal excretion is a minor pathway of elimination ($fe < 0.01$), even if renal clearance increases markedly during diuresis.

    5. Nafcillin. It has the smallest volume of distribution.

    6. Tocainide. It has the lowest clearance ($0.693 V/t_{1/2} = 10.4$ L/hr).

  b. 1. Increase—because the renal clearance of nafcillin, 4.7 L/hr, is low compared to either renal blood flow (66 L/hr) or renal plasma flow (40 L/hr).

    2. Alkalinization—because the drug tocainide is an amine for which tubular reabsorption is likely to be more extensive at higher pH values, at which the fraction un-ionized is greater.

    3. Is not—because nafcillin would have to have a volume of distribution of 15 L and be unbound in plasma.

    4. Metabolism—because *fe* is very low. Cyclosporine could be eliminated primarily by biliary excretion, but being nonpolar, this is unlikely and in fact is not the case.

5. Can—because a large volume of distribution only indicates that the affinity of tissues for drug is much greater than that of plasma. The value of fu for cyclosporine is 0.05.

6. 99%—because percent outside plasma $[(V - V_p)/V]$ for tocainide is 98.5%.

c. 1. Tocainide. Fraction remaining $= e^{-kt}$, $k = 0.693/t_{1/2} = 0.05$ hr^{-1}, $t = 24$, $e^{-kt} = 0.30$.

2. Tocainide. $R_{acc} = 1/(1 - e^{-k\tau})$. The R_{ac} values for nafcillin, tocainide, and cyclosporine given every 8 hr are 1.00, 3.06, and 2, respectively.

3. Cyclosporine. $C_{ss} = R_0/CL$. The values of CL (0.693 $V/t_{1/2}$) for nafcillin, tocainide, and cyclosporine are 17 L/hr, 10 L/hr, and 21 L/hr, respectively. Thus, cyclosporine with the highest CL will achieve the lowest value of C_{ss}.

4. Tocainide. $AUC = $ Dose/CL. For nafcillin, $AUC = 15$ mg-hr/L (250 mg/17 L/hr); tocainide, $AUC = 40$ to 60 mg-hr/L (400 to 600 mg/10 L/hr); cyclosporine, $AUC = 17$ mg-hr/L (350 mg/21 L/hr).

5. Nafcillin.

$$C = \frac{R_0}{CL}(1 - e^{-kt}).$$

At 8 hr, the respective values for nafcillin, tocainide, and cyclosporine are 1.2 mg/L, 0.65 mg/L, and 0.48 mg/L.

5. All the loss of bioavailability can be explained by hepatic first-pass elimination.

$$CL = 42 \text{ L/hr (Answer to Problem 5 of Chap. 6)}$$

$$\text{Blood-to-plasma concentration ratio} = 1$$

Hence

$$CL_b = 42 \text{ L/hr} = CL_{b,H} \text{ (as } fe \sim 0)$$

$$Q_H = 81 \text{ L/hr}$$

Hence, value of F if all rectally absorbed drug passes through liver

$$= 1 - \frac{CL_{b,H}}{Q_H} = 1 - \frac{42 \text{ L/hr}}{81 \text{ L/hr}} = 0.48$$

In practice, a part of the blood supply to the rectum bypasses the liver and enters the vena cava directly.

6. a. From plasma $F = 0.114$: from urine $F = 0.116$.
From Plasma

$$F = \frac{\left[\dfrac{AUC}{Dose}\right]_{oral}}{\left[\dfrac{AUC}{Dose}\right]_{i.v.}} = \frac{[0.22 \text{ mg-hr/L/100 mg}]}{[1.93 \text{ mg-hr/L/100 mg}]}$$

From Urine

$$F = \frac{\left[\dfrac{Ae_\infty}{Dose}\right]_{oral}}{\left[\dfrac{Ae_\infty}{Dose}\right]_{i.v.}} = \frac{[1.22 \text{ mg/100 mg}]}{[10.5 \text{ mg/100 mg}]}$$

b. Probably only partly, $F \approx 0.11$, $F_H = 0.24$.

$$F_H = 1 - \frac{E_H}{Q_H} = 1 - \frac{CL_{b,H}}{Q_H}$$

$$CL_{b,H} = (1 - fe) \cdot CL_b = (1 - fe) \cdot \left(\frac{CL}{R}\right)$$

where R = blood-to-plasma drug concentration ratio.
Now

$$fe = \left[\frac{Ae_\infty}{Dose}\right]_{i.v.} = 10.5 \text{ mg/100 mg} = 0.105$$

$$CL = \left[\frac{Dose}{AUC}\right]_{i.v} = 100 \text{ mg/1.93 mg-hr/L}$$

$$= 51.8 \text{ L/hr}$$

$$CL_b = \frac{51.8 \text{ L/hr}}{0.77} = 67.2 \text{ L/hr}$$

$$Q_H = \left(\frac{81 \text{ L/hr}}{70 \text{ kg}}\right) \times \frac{68}{70} = 79 \text{ L/hr}$$

So that

$$F_H = 1 - \frac{(1 - 0.105) \times 67.2 \text{ L/hr}}{79 \text{ L/hr}} = 0.24$$

Conclusion: The discrepancy between $F_H = 0.24$, and observed $F = 0.11$ suggests that appreciable losses may have occurred within the gastrointestinal tract.
Possibilities: Incomplete dissolution, destruction within the gastrointestinal epithelium, chemical instability, destruction by intestinal microflora.
Note: The calculated F_H is sensitive to the value of Q_H. Had the true value of Q_H in the subject been 67 L/hr, instead of the assumed 79 L/hr, $F_H = 0.105$. Thus, first-pass may still fully account for the low F.

ANSWERS TO STUDY PROBLEMS (CHAP. 12)

1. A list of examples of such physiologic variables is contained in Table 12–1.
2. See Table II–4.
   The key equations used to analyze the changes are

$$CL_H = \frac{Q_H \cdot fu_b \cdot CL_{int}}{Q_H + fu_b \cdot CL_{int}}$$

$$V_b = V_B + V_T \cdot \frac{fu_b}{fu_T}$$

$$t_{1/2} = \frac{0.693 \cdot V_b}{CL_H}$$

$$F_H = 1 - \frac{CL_b}{Q_H}$$

3. See Fig. II–6 on p. 529.

4. a.

	BEFORE	AFTER
CL (L/min) $= \dfrac{Dose_{i.v.}}{AUC_{i.v.}}$	$\dfrac{800}{1207} = 0.66$	$\dfrac{800}{1405} = 0.57$
$F = \dfrac{AUC_{p.o.}}{AUC_{i.v.}}$	$\dfrac{142}{1207} = 0.12$	$\dfrac{716}{1405} = 0.51$

   b. The blood clearance is 1.1 L/hr $(CL \cdot C/C_b)$. This value indicates the probability of high first-pass effect. Inhibition of metabolism of 6-mercaptopurine increases bioavailability with only a small decrease in clearance, because of its high extraction ratio.

5. a. 1. CL: $(+)$-isomer $= 68$ L/hr; $(-)$-isomer $= 112$ L/hr.

	d-isomer	l-isomer
$CL = \dfrac{Dose_{i.v.}}{AUC}$	$\dfrac{10,000\ \mu g}{148\ \mu g\text{-hr/L}}$	$\dfrac{10,000\ \mu g}{89\ \mu g\text{-hr/L}}$

    2. F: $(+)$-isomer $= 0.20$; $(-)$-isomer $= 0.04$.

	$(+)$-isomer	$(-)$-isomer
$F = \dfrac{AUC_{p.o.}}{AUC_{i.v.}} \cdot \dfrac{Dose_{i.v.}}{Dose_{oral}}$	$\dfrac{120\ \mu g\text{-hr/L}}{148\ \mu g\text{-hr/L}} \times \dfrac{10\ mg}{40\ mg}$	$\dfrac{15\ \mu g\text{-hr/L}}{89\ \mu g\text{-hr/L}} \times \dfrac{10\ mg}{40\ mg}$

    3. V: $(+)$-isomer $= 589$ L; $(-)$-isomer $= 583$ L

Table II-4.

HEPATIC EXTRACTION RATIO	HEPATIC BLOOD FLOW	FRACTION IN BLOOD UNBOUND	FRACTION IN TISSUE UNBOUND	TOTAL CLEARANCE[a]	VOLUME OF DISTRIBUTION[a]	HALF-LIFE	ORAL BIOAVAILABILITY
High	↑	↔	↔	↑	↔	↓	↑
High	↔	↓	↔	↔	↓	↓	↑
High	↔	↔	↑	↔	↓	↓	↔
Low	↑	↔	↔	↔	↔	↔	↔
Low	↔	↔	↑	↔	↓	↓	↔
Low	↔	↑	↑	↑	↔	↓	↔

[a]Based on drug concentration in blood.

$$V = \frac{CL \cdot t_{1/2}}{0.693} \qquad \frac{68 \times 6}{0.693} \qquad \frac{112 \times 3.6}{0.693}$$

(+)-isomer $\qquad$ (−)-isomer

b. The bioavailability of the (−)-isomer is much less than that of the (+)-isomer. As the plasma clearances of both drugs approach hepatic blood flow (insufficient data to calculate blood clearances), one possible explanation is a major difference in first-

Altered Binding to Plasma Proteins

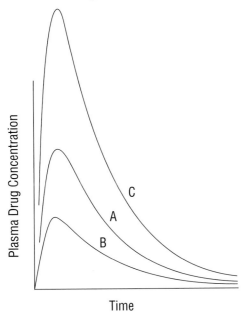

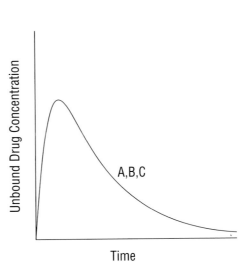

Altered Tissue Binding

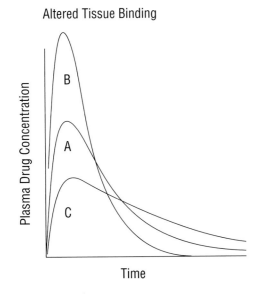

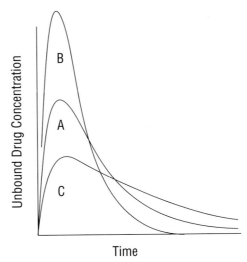

Fig. II–6.

pass hepatic metabolism. Clearance for the $(-)$-isomer is not much higher than that for the $(+)$-isomer because clearance approaches hepatic blood flow.

The elimination half-life is shorter for the $(-)$-isomer, a result of greater clearance; volume of distribution is the same for both isomers.

c. 0.2; Yes, the $(-)/(+)$ plasma concentration ratio will decrease further with time. The ratio of amounts absorbed systematically is the ratio of the F values.

$$\frac{F((-)\text{-isomer})}{F((+)\text{-isomer})} = \frac{0.04}{0.20}$$

The liver acts as a filter; the filtrate is enriched in the $(+)$-isomer relative to the $(-)$-isomer.

The $(-)/(+)$ plasma concentration ratio will decrease with time as the $(-)$-isomer is eliminated more rapidly $(t_{1/2} = 3.9$ hr$)$ than the $(+)$-isomer $(t_{1/2} = 5.7$ hr$)$.

6. a. $CL = 154$ L/hr; $CL_b = 77$ L/hr; $V_b = 120$ L; and $t_{1/2} = 1.1$ hr.

$$CL_b = Q_H \cdot E_H = 81 \text{ L/hr} \times 0.95$$

$$CL = \frac{CL_b \cdot C_b}{C} = 77 \text{ L/hr} \times 2$$

$$\frac{C_b}{C} = \frac{fu}{fu_b} = \frac{0.01}{0.005} = 2$$

$$V_b = \frac{V}{C_b/C} = \frac{240 \text{ L}}{2}$$

$$t_{1/2} = \frac{(0.693 \cdot V)}{CL} = \frac{(0.693 \times 240 \text{ L})}{154 \text{ L/hr}}$$

b. Yes; tissue binding is decreased.

$$\frac{fu_T(\text{uremic})}{fu_T(\text{normal})} = 5.2$$

$$fu_T(\text{normal}) = \frac{V_T \cdot fu}{V - V_P}$$

$$= \frac{V_T \times 0.01}{240 - 3}$$

$$fu_T(\text{uremic}) = \frac{V_T \times 0.03}{140 - 3}$$

c. A sixfold increase. Blood clearance should not change, therefore the total plateau concentration is unaltered, but the unbound concentration increases from 0.5% to 3% of the total.

7. Minimum oral maintenance dose $= 220$ mg.
The renal clearance is 128 mL/min,

$$CL_R = fe \cdot CL = 0.8 \times 160 \text{ mL/min}$$

The plasma ampicillin concentration when the urine concentration is 50 mg/L is 0.39 mg/L,

$$C = \frac{(\text{Urine flow}) \cdot (\text{Urine drug concentration})}{CL_R}$$

$$= \frac{1 \text{ mL/min} \times 50 \text{ mg/L}}{128 \text{ mL/min}}$$

The steady-state trough plasma concentration must be 0.39 mg/L. The maintenance dose required to achieve this value is 220 mg,

$$C_{ss,min} = \frac{F \cdot \text{Dose}}{V} \cdot \frac{e^{-k\tau}}{(1 - e^{-k\tau})}$$

$$\text{Dose} = \frac{C_{ss,min} \cdot V(1 - e^{-k\tau})}{F \cdot e^{-k\tau}}$$

$$k = 0.48 \text{ hr}^{-1}; \tau = 6 \text{ hr}; V = 20 \text{ L}; \text{ and } F = 0.6.$$

8. Yes. The high-protein meal, which causes an increased portal blood flow, produces a 70% increase in oral bioavailability. This is accompanied by a 38% increase in clearance and an insignificant change in AUC after an oral dose. Propranolol is a drug with a high hepatic extraction ratio ($CL_b = 1$ L/min). For such a drug, an increase in hepatic blood flow is expected to produce increases in bioavailability and clearance. The observation of different extents of increase may be explained by the increased blood flow being primarily restricted to early times when the food given is digested and absorbed. Absorption of drug occurs during this period, while elimination of absorbed drug ($t_{1/2} \approx 3.6$ hr, data not given) occurs predominantly thereafter. The small change in AUC is a consequence of similar changes in both CL_b and F.

ANSWERS TO STUDY PROBLEMS (CHAP. 13)

1. a. Any three of the following examples: genetics, disease, age, drugs and noncompliance.
   b. See Table 13–2.
2. How much a pharmacokinetic parameter varies within the population is as important to drug therapy as is its mean value. Together with information on the therapeutic window, information on the distribution of the pharmacokinetic parameter values helps in deciding the number of dose strengths needed to treat a patient population.
3. Bioavailability. Variable hepatic drug extraction on the first pass through the liver is most likely responsible. Estimates of the ratio CL/F [from Dose/($\tau \cdot C_{ss,av}$)] range from 0.25 to 2.5 L/min. Therefore either high clearance, low F, or both are responsible for the high values of CL/F. Since nortriptyline is stable in the gastrointestinal tract and lipophilic, high clearance in the liver is the probable explanation. Being of high clearance, most of the variability in intrinsic clearance, CL_{int}, is expressed in variability in oral bioavailability.
4. Either the patient population sampled was biased, or this patient represents an extreme of the whole patient population. Recall that the patient was not part of the population from which the population pharmacokinetic values were obtained.
5. a. Clearance. Reference to Table 13–2 indicates that clearance is the most variable pharmacokinetic parameter among patients; F and V vary relatively little.

b. Renal Function. Lithium is eliminated almost entirely by urinary excretion, i.e., $CL = CL_R$, and as with, e.g., ceftazidine (Fig. 13–11), renal clearance is expected to be highly correlated with renal function, a continuous characteristic.

6. Wide differences in hepatic metabolic activity. Alprenolol is highly cleared by the liver. Accordingly, differences in hepatic enzyme activity do not produce much variability in clearance, which is perfusion rate-limited; but these small differences in clearance may cause wide differences in bioavailability ($F_H = 1 - E_H$).

7. a. Most variable is fu_T, least variable is CLu.

Table II–5.

SUBJECT:	1	2	3	4	5	RANGE MEAN
Clu^a	80	84	76	84	79	0.10
fu	0.1	0.15	0.09	0.16	0.11	0.57
fu_T^b	0.024	0.057	0.083	0.033	0.043	1.23

$^a Clu$ calculated from $\dfrac{R_0}{C_{ss} \cdot fu}$.

$^b fu_T$ calculated from $V = \dfrac{Clu \cdot fu}{k}$ and $fu_T = \dfrac{V_{TW} fu}{V - V_P}$ (Eq. 22, Chap. 10) as V is >50 L.

b. The lack of variability in the unbound clearance means that the unbound concentration and presumably the drug effect at plateau are highly predictable from the rate of administration. There are, however, differences in the total concentration. Also, the time to achieve the plateau is variable because of large differences in the half-life, which is primarily a result of variability in tissue binding.

8. There is the danger of not being able to define a clear dose–response relationship. The fourfold range in dose is less than the fivefold range in clearance, so that some patients of low clearance receiving the low-dose regimen will have similar average plasma concentrations to those of high clearance receiving the high-dose regimen, thereby potentially introducing considerable variability in the dose–response relationship. One solution is to use very large numbers of patients in each group. If feasible in clinical practice, a more efficient design, requiring less patients to test for a dose–response relationship, involves exposing each patient to two, and preferably all three, doses of the drug. Refer to the section Defining the Dose–Response Relationship in this chapter for further discussion.

ANSWERS TO STUDY PROBLEMS (CHAP. 14)

1. Inherited variability in pharmacokinetics is seen with isoniazid and metoprolol. Examples of inherited variability in pharmacodynamics are seen in the resistance to the oral anticoagulant warfarin and in drug-induced hemolytic anemia, caused by nitrofurantoin. See Tables 14–1 and 14–2 for additional examples.

2. *Genotype* is the assortment of genes in an individual. *Phenotype* is a characteristic expression of an individual. *Genetic polymorphism* is the occurrence of distinguishable differences in a given characteristic under genetic control.

3. An inherited source of variability in a pharmacokinetic parameter is suggested by a polymodal distribution of the parameter value within the population and by comparative studies between identical and nonidentical twins. It is characterized by familial studies and by correlation studies with other drugs which are known to exhibit genetically determined polymorphism in their pharmacokinetics.

4. The optimal dosage regimen of the drug may vary among different ethnic groups. The frequency of slow acetylators varies being relatively high in Caucasians and blacks, and

low in Japanese and Chinese. The therapeutic implication depends on whether activity/toxicity resides in drug, N-acetylated metabolite, or both. The implication is clear. Due regard to ethnicity should be taken in the prescribing of drugs.

5. The poor correlation of atenolol pharmacokinetics with debrisoquine oxidation phenotype is expected; atenolol is primarily excreted unchanged. The strong correlations seen with metoprolol and timolol indicate that they are predominantly eliminated either via a major metabolic pathway or via several pathways that involve debrisoquine hydroxylase (CYP2D6). Propranolol is predominantly metabolized; the weak correlation with this compound suggests that the major metabolic pathways involved (e.g., formation of naphthoxylactic acid, p. 372, Chap. 21) are not under the debrisoquine type of control.

6. a. Nortriptyline, dextromethorphan. See Table 14–1 for additional examples.
   b. 1. Normally, flecainide is predominantly excreted unchanged, so that variation in the formation of the metabolite via CYP2D6 has little effect on total clearance and hence dosage requirements. In patients with severe renal impairment, however, little drug is excreted unchanged, and formation of the metabolite is the major route of drug elimination. Under such circumstances, genetic polymorphism is of increasingly therapeutic importance.
      2. The minor metabolite of dapsone is N-acetyldapsone, a less active antitubercular compound than dapsone. In contrast, morphine, the minor metabolite of codeine, is a potent analgesic agent. There is some question whether codeine per se has any substantial analgesic activity.
      3. Quinidine is a specific inhibitor of debrisoquine hydroxylase, effectively converting extensive metabolizers to poor metabolizer status. For drugs for which genetic polymorphism involving debrisoquine hydroxylase normally has a therapeutic implication, co-administration of quinidine is likely to produce a clinically significant drug interaction.

7. Frequencies of slow and fast oxidizers are 2.25% and 97.75%, respectively. Frequency of allele associated with slow oxidation $(p) = 0.15$; frequency of allele associated with fast oxidation $(q) = 0.85$. Hence, the frequency of (p^2) of homozygous slow oxidizers is 0.0225; while 0.9775 $(2pq + q^2)$ is the frequency of heterozygous and homozygous fast oxidizers.

ANSWERS TO STUDY PROBLEMS (CHAP. 15)

1. a. False. Oral biovailability is independent of body weight; there is no rational basis to consider otherwise.
   b. True. V/(Body weight) tends to be independent of body weight. An exception concerns distribution of polar compounds in the obese, where volume of distribution correlates better with ideal body weight than body weight.
   c. True. In children, CL tends to vary in direct proportion to body surface area (or $W^{0.7}$). As age increases, so does body weight, and as surface area/body weight decreases with increasing size, so does CL/body weight.
   d. False. Renal function tends to decrease by approximately 1%/year, beyond 20 years of age.
   e. False. Half-life tends to be shortest in children around 1 to 2 years of age.
2. a. No. As a first approximation, the volume of distribution normalized for body weight (V/kg) is expected to be independent of body weight and age. The observed values of V/body weight are 18, 15, and 10 L/kg for children, young adults, and elderly adults, respectively. Possible explanations include variations in plasma and tissue protein binding with age.

b. Yes, for the elderly, no for children. First, consider the adults. Assuming a 1%/year decline in clearance, the expected clearance in the elderly adults (age 69 years) based on the data in young adults (age 32 years; clearance 98 L/hr) is 61 L/hr, which is reasonably close to the observed clearance, 50 L/hr. Second, consider the data in children. The observed clearance (93 L/hr) is much higher than that expected. Thus, assuming a 1% decline in clearance beyond 20 years,

$$\text{Expected clearance in a 20-year-old} = 1.14 \times CL_{\text{32-year-old}} = 1.14 \times 98 \text{ L/hr}$$

$$= 112 \text{ L/hr}$$

$$\text{Expected child's clearance} = \left(\frac{Wt_{\text{child}}}{Wt_{\text{20-year-old}}}\right)^{0.7} \times CL_{\text{20-year-old}}$$

$$= \left(\frac{32 \text{ kg}}{70 \text{ kg}}\right)^{0.7} \times 112 \text{ L/hr} = 65 \text{ L/hr}$$

There is no obvious explanation for this higher than expected clearance in the children.

3. 7 mg/day. By application of Eq. 5,

$$\text{Child's maintenance dosage} = 1.4 \times \left[\frac{10 \text{ kg}}{70 \text{ kg}}\right]^{0.7} \times 20 \text{ mg/day}$$

Because of an expected shorter half-life in the child, than in adults, the child may need to be given the drug twice daily instead of once daily.

4. a. 24 mg (1.6 mg/kg) gentamicin administered intramuscularly every 8 hr. Calculation made using Eq. 6. *Note*: The manufacturer's recommended dose of gentamicin for a child is 2 to 2.5 mg/kg every 8 hr. The age of the adult patient population was not given. If, as likely, those adults with severe infections requiring gentamicin are more elderly, then assuming a mean age of 55 years is reasonable.

b. 36 mg (0.58 mg/kg) gentamicin administered intramuscularly every 8 hr, or possibly 54 mg (0.87 mg/kg) administered every 12 hr. The half-life is longer in this elderly patient compared with a 55-year-old patient; both have normal renal function for their age. Calculation made using Eq. 6.
Note: There is a relatively small difference in the maintenance dosing rate (mg/8 hr) between the 4-year-old child in part "a" and in this elderly patient, despite the large difference in body weight.

c. 1.2 mg every 8 hr.
From the relationship CL_{cr} (mL/hr) $= 0.0045\, e^{+0.16 \times \text{age (weeks)}}$
For a conceptional age of 36 weeks
$CL_{cr} = 0.0045\, e^{+0.16 \times 36} = 1.5$ mL/min
To maintain the same average plasma concentration as a typical adult

$$\text{Dosage rate in infant} = \frac{1.5 \text{ mL/min}}{85 \text{ mL/min}} \times \text{Adult dosing rate}$$

$$= 0.0176 \times \frac{70 \text{ mg}}{8 \text{ hr}}$$

Note: Because of a longer half-life in the premature infant, a dosing interval of 12 or 24 hr may be more appropriate (same daily dose).

5. a. The observations in broad agreement with the expectations for a drug primarily excreted, suggest that biliary excretory function follows a trend similar to that of renal function. The low clearance per square meter of body surface area in the neonate and the elder reflects depressed excretory function at both extremes of life. Between 1 and 20 years, clearance per square meter is expected to be relatively constant; the data in this age range are too few to draw a firm conclusion.

   b. The half-life should be at a minimum at around 2 years of age, and should be greater than the minimum by a factor of 2 to 3 at the extremes of age. This conclusion is based on the relationship $t_{1/2} = 0.693\ V/CL$; volume of distribution does not vary much on a weight basis, but clearance per square meter of body surface area is at a maximum around 2 years of age. As clearance per square meter varies by a factor of 3 (Fig. 15–12), so should half-life.

   c. Dosing rate needs to be reduced in neonates and in patients over 70 years of age, even when correcting for weight. Perhaps dosing can be less frequent than in the typical adult patient.

6. a. Much depends on the therapeutic window of the drug. For felodopine it is relatively narrow, and it would seem appropriate to consider adjusting dose for age. It is noted, however, that hypertensive patients are generally middle-aged or older and with only modest increase in $AUC(0–12\ \text{hr})_{ss}$, 12 hr between those in the age groups 40 to 59 and 60 to 80 years, dose adjustment for age might not be needed. An increase in the usual adult dose might be appropriate if felodopine is used to treat young adults with hypertension.

   b. There is no trend of volume of distribution with age. The estimated mean values of $V\ (= 1.44 \cdot CL \cdot t_{1/2})$ are 17 L/kg, 15 L/kg, and 15 L/kg for the age groups 20 to 39, 40 to 59, and 60 to 80 years, respectively. Given the inherent interpatient variability of this, and other pharmacokinetic parameters, the changes in V with age are not significant.

   c. $F = 0.14, 0.16, 0.14$ for the age groups 20–39, 40–59, and 60–80 years, respectively. At steady state: $F \cdot Dose = CL \cdot AUC_{ss,\tau}$. Note that $AUC_{ss,\tau}$ has been normalized to a 10-mg twice-daily regimen.

$$F_{20\text{–}39\ \text{years}} = \frac{(0.82\ \text{L/min} \times 60\ \text{min/hr}) \times 0.028\ \text{mg-hr/L}}{10\ \text{mg}}$$

$$F_{40\text{–}59\ \text{years}} = \frac{(0.64\ \text{L/min} \times 60\ \text{min/hr}) \times 0.041\ \text{mg-hr/L}}{10\ \text{mg}}$$

$$F_{60\text{–}80\ \text{years}} = \frac{(0.45\ \text{L/min} \times 60\ \text{min/hr}) \times 0.052\ \text{mg-hr/L}}{10\ \text{mg}}$$

   d. First-pass hepatic loss. The clearance of felodopine is high, and with little excreted unchanged in urine, the most likely explanation for the low bioavailability in all age groups is first-pass hepatic metabolism.

   e. Clearance. $AUC(0 - \tau)_{ss} = F \cdot Dose/CL$. With F does not change with age, the decrease in CL explains the increase in $AUC(0 - \tau)_{ss}$ with advancing age.

   f. A decrease in hepatic blood flow with increasing age. For drugs for which a low oral bioavailability is due to first-pass hepatic loss, $F \approx 1 - E_H = 1 - CL_{b,H}/Q_H$. For F not to change, the ratio of $CL_{b,H}/Q_H$ must remain constant. But, as CL (a reflector of $CL_{b,H}$) decreases with increasing age, Q_H would also need to decrease in parallel for F to remain constant.

7. a. Differences among theophylline, digoxin, and diazepam can be explained by differences in the partition of these drugs into fat. Obese subjects for a given height primarily differ from normal subjects in the much greater preponderance of fat; the body water space is essentially unchanged. Both theophylline and digoxin are poorly lipophilic and so, for these drugs, volume of distribution does not increase with the increase in body fat. In contrast, diazepam is lipophilic, and so its volume of distribution increases in the obese subject, both on absolute and weight-corrected bases.

b. The information has relevance to the loading dose and the degree of fluctuation in plasma concentration on chronic dosing, but not to the maintenance dose requirement, which depends on clearance. No weight correction in the loading dose is needed for either digoxin or theophylline. Diazepam is administered intravenously over 1 to 4 min as a sedative, for relief of muscle spasm, and as an anticonvulsant. Under these circumstances, because fat is poorly perfused, there may be little difference in the initial concentrations in plasma and in highly perfused tissues, such as the brain, in obese patients compared with normal weight patients. Accordingly, there may be little need to adjust the intravenous dose of diazepam in the obese patient. A loading dose is not used with oral diazepam regimens. However, associated with the larger volume distribution is a longer half-life of diazepam in the obese patient. Even so, because the half-life of diazepam in normal weight subjects is already long (approximately 40 hr), there should be no need to adjust the usual recommended dosing regimen of diazepam in obese patients, although there will be less fluctuation in the plasma concentration at plateau.

ANSWERS TO STUDY PROBLEMS (CHAP. 16)

1. Cirrhosis, uremia, congestive cardiac failure, Crohn's disease, thyroid disease, and pneumonia. See Table 16–1 for other examples and brief comments.

2. a. $B > D > C > E > A$. Calculated from Eq. 7 for a typical 55-year-old, 70-kg patient.
   b. B and perhaps C and D.

3. a. For both pentazocine and meperidine, the blood clearance in control subjects is sufficiently high to expect hepatic bioavailabilities $(1 - CL_b/Q_H)$ of about 8% and 33%, respectively, if elimination occurs only in the liver and the hepatic blood flow is 1.35 L/min. For both drugs, cirrhosis appears to decrease clearance by about 35% to 37% and to increase bioavailability by 278% and 81%, respectively. Decreased blood flow would explain the decreased clearance but would not explain the increased bioavailability. Decreased metabolic activity or shunting of portal blood would explain both effects. The latter has been shown to occur in cirrhosis and is probably the major mechanism.

   b. The bioavailability of pentazocine is more extensively affected by cirrhosis than that of meperidine, because it has the higher hepatic extraction ratio. The higher the extraction ratio, the lower is the bioavailability and the greater is the effect of a decrease in metabolic activity or shunting on bioavailability.

4.

Patients:	S.W.	B.J.	D.A.	B.T.
a. Estimated Creatinine Clearance (ml/min)[a]:	134	16	10	27
b. Relative Renal Function (RF):	1.58	0.19	0.12	0.32

[a]See Table 16–2 for equations.

5. a. $C_{ss,max} = 48$ mg/L; $C_{ss,min} = 12$ mg/L

$$V = 0.4 \times 70 = 28 \text{ L}$$

$$C_{ss,max} = \frac{D}{V}\left(\frac{1}{1 - e^{-k\tau}}\right)$$

$$= \frac{1000 \text{ mg}}{28 \text{ L}}\left(\frac{1}{1 - e^{-12 \times 0.693/6}}\right) = 48 \text{ mg/L}$$

$$C_{ss,min} = C_{ss,max} - D/V = 12 \text{ mg/L}$$

b. Loading dose = 243 mg [(17/70) × 1000 mg]; Maintenance dose = 100 mg/12 hr.

Creatinine clearance expected in child is

$$\frac{(0.48 \times 108)}{2.7} \times \left(\frac{17}{70}\right)^{0.7} = 7.1 \text{ mL/min}$$

Creatinine clearance in a typical patient (55-year-old) is 85 mL/min

$$RF \text{ (child)} = \frac{7.1 \text{ mL/min}}{85 \text{ mL/min}} = 0.082; \ fe(n) = 0.95$$

$$R_d = RF \cdot fe(t) + [1 - fe(t)]\left[\frac{(140 - \text{Age}) \times \text{Weight}^{0.7}}{1660}\right] = 0.078 + 0.030;$$

$R_d = 0.108$ (decrease of nine- to tenfold in adult regimen).

Suggest reducing maintenance dose tenfold to achieve a tenfold reduction in dosing rate. It could be 100 mg every 12 hr or 200 mg every 24 hr. For demonstrative purposes, a dosing interval of 12 hr is used for the subsequent calculations.

c. Parameters in child: $CL = 7.1$ mL/min or 0.43 L/hr, $V = 6.8$ L (0.4 L/kg × 17 kg); $k = 0.063 \text{ hr}^{-1}$; and $t_{1/2} = 11$ hr.

   1. Dose: 600 mg every 12 hr, regimen adjusted for age and weight only.

$$\frac{D_m}{\tau} \text{ (child)} = \frac{(140 - \text{Age}) \times \text{Weight}^{0.7}}{1660} \cdot \frac{D_M}{\tau} \text{ (reference patient)}$$

$$= 0.59 \times 1000 \text{ mg/12 hr}$$

$$\approx 600 \text{ mg every 12 hr.}$$

   2. Dose: 100 mg every 12 hr, adjusted for age, weight, and renal function.

$$\frac{D_M}{\tau} \text{ (child)} = Rd \cdot \frac{D_M}{\tau} \text{ (reference patient)}$$

$$= 0.108 \times 1000 \text{ mg/12 hr}$$

$$\approx 100 \text{ mg/12 hr}$$

   3. Table II–6 lists the calculated maximum and minimum amounts in the body in the child on approach to steady state on giving the maintenance regimen given in 1 and 2. To plot the data the appropriate scales are

$$\text{Scale time to 4 to 5 half-lives} \approx 48 \text{ hr.}$$

Scale amount in body to $A_{ss,max}$ on regimen of 600 mg every 12 hr

$$= 600 \cdot \frac{1}{(1 - e^{-0.063 \times 12})} \approx 1200 \text{ mg}$$

6. a. 1. Oral bioavailability increased 2.3-fold.

$$\frac{F_{cirrhotic}}{F_{healthy}} = \frac{\dfrac{AUC_{oral}}{AUC_{i.v.}} \cdot \dfrac{Dose_{i.v.}}{Dose_{oral}} \text{ (cirrhotic)}}{\dfrac{AUC_{oral}}{AUC_{i.v.}} \cdot \dfrac{Dose_{i.v.}}{Dose_{oral}} \text{ (healthy)}} = \frac{\dfrac{3.36}{1.14} \times \dfrac{100}{400}}{\dfrac{0.52}{0.41} \times \dfrac{100}{400}}$$

2. Volume of distribution is virtually unchanged (282 L vs. 266 L).

$$V = \frac{CL \cdot t_{1/2}}{0.693} = \frac{Dose_{i.v.} \cdot t_{1/2}}{AUC_{i.v.} \cdot 0.693}$$

$$V \text{ (cirrhotic)} = \frac{100 \text{ mg}}{1.14 \text{ mg-hr/L}} \times \frac{2.1 \text{ hr}}{0.693} = 266 \text{ L}$$

$$V \text{ (healthy)} = \frac{100 \text{ mg}}{0.41} \times \frac{0.8}{0.693} = 282 \text{ L}$$

3. Clearance is decreased by a factor of 0.36. Half-life is increased from 0.8 to 2.1 hr.

	Cirrhotic	Healthy
$CL = \dfrac{Dose_{i.v.}}{AUC_{i.v.}}$	$\dfrac{100 \text{ mg}}{1.14 \text{ mg-hr/L}}$	$\dfrac{100 \text{ mg}}{0.41 \text{ mg-hr/L}}$
	88 L/hr	244 L/hr

b. The plasma clearance in the healthy subjects exceeds hepatic blood. No data were given on the ratio of blood and plasma concentrations, but the data suggest a high first-pass metabolism in the liver and, perhaps, even high clearance in extrahepatic tissues. The increased F in cirrhotic patients may be explained by a large fraction of portal blood flow bypassing the functional cells of the liver in cirrhosis. No change in volume of distribution was apparent. Clearance may be decreased because of decreased blood flow to functional liver tissue, although other processes may also be affected.

7. a. Control: $C_{ss,max} = 50 \, \mu g/L$; $C_{ss,min} = 33 \, \mu g/L$.
   Tetraplegic: $C_{ss,max} = 68 \, \mu g/L$; $C_{ss,min} = 52 \, \mu g/L$

Table II-6. Maintenance Regimen

TIME (hr)	0	12	12+[a]	24	24+	36	36+	48
Amount in Body (mg)								
600 mg/12 hr	600	282	882	414	1014	476	1076	505
100 mg/12 hr	100	47	147	69	169	79	179	84

[a]The plus sign (+) means just after the dose.

$$C_{ss,max} = \frac{F \cdot Dose}{V} \cdot \frac{1}{(1 - e^{-k\tau})} \qquad C_{ss,min} = C_{ss,max} - \frac{F \cdot Dose}{V}$$

Controls

$$C_{ss,max} = \frac{0.9 \times 2,000 \, \mu g}{1.5 \, L/kg \times 70 \, kg} \cdot \frac{1}{1 - e^{-0.693 \times 12hr/20hr}}$$

$$C_{ss,min} = 50 \, \mu g/L - \frac{0.9 \times 2000 \, \mu g}{1.5 \, L/kg \times 70 \, kg}$$

Tetraplegics

$$C_{ss,max} = \frac{0.9 \times 2000 \, \mu g}{1.6 \, L/kg \times 70 \, kg} \cdot \frac{1}{1 - e^{-0.693 \times 12 \, hr/31 \, hr}}$$

$$C_{ss,min} = 68.3 - \frac{0.9 \times 2000 \, \mu g}{1.6 \, L/kg \times 70 \, kg}$$

    b. 1. Decreased hepatic blood flow, by itself, seems unlikely to be an explanation. Clearance is only 76 mL/min/1.8 m² in the controls. A change in blood flow should not directly affect CL or $t_{1/2}$ of a low extraction ratio drug.

        2. Decreased enzyme activity is a possibility based on the kinetic changes.

        3. This is a possibility. Lorazepam undergoes hepatic recycling through its glucuronide, which is cleaved in the colon. The released drug is reabsorbed. Biliary dyskinesia, more common to these patients, may result in less recycling and an apparent decrease in clearance (increase in half-life).

        4. Changes in protein binding are unlikely to explain the alterations, as the volume of distribution is unaffected. An equivalent increase in tissue binding would also have to be involved.

  8. Yes. Clearance is more variable. If the ratio of the highest and lowest values are compared (11.7/6.2 = 1.9 in healthy subjects and 5.8/1.1 = 5.3 in cirrhotics), the increase in variability is apparent. Variability in the half-life is certainly increased as well.

ANSWERS TO STUDY PROBLEMS (CHAP. 17)

  1. a. True. The patient is often stabilized on one drug and, by adding the second, a change in intensity of response is produced (erythromycin → theophylline). Similarly, a patient may be stabilized on two drugs and withdrawal of one precipitates a clinical problem (pentobarbital → warfarin).

    b. Generally true. One should realize that Drug B must bind to the same (or an indirectly affected) site on the same protein as Drug A.

    c. True. The major problem with most displacement reactions is the interpretation of the plasma concentration observed. Seldom is there a therapeutic consequence of the displacement.

    d. True. Of all the kinds of interactions, this mechanism and enzyme induction are generally of greatest therapeutic concern.

    e. True. The graded nature of the response depends on whether the interaction is *unindirectional, bidirectional,* or *mutual* in nature.

2. a. *fu* increased. See Fig. II–7. Dashed colored line is new value.
   b. CL_{int} decreased. See Fig. II–8. Dashed colored line is new value.
3. a. See Fig. II–9 on p. 541. Dashed colored line is new value.

WITHOUT KETOCONAZOLE	WITH KETOCONAZOLE
$V(L)^a$ = 22.5	22.5
$CL(L/hr)^b$ 1.63	0.90

^aV = Dose/$C(O)$.
^bCL = $V \cdot k$ = $V \cdot 0.693/t_{1/2}$.

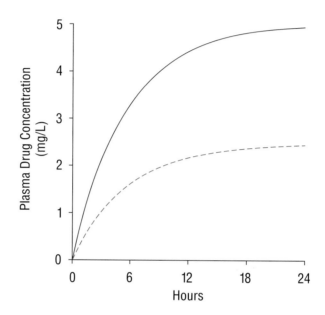

Fig. II–7.

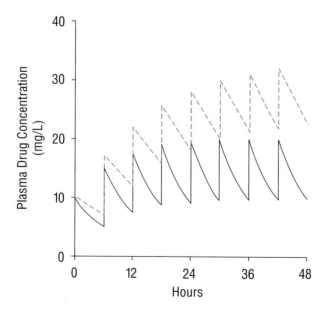

Fig. II–8.

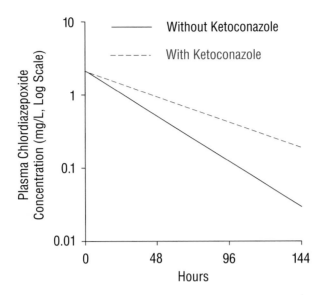

Fig. II–9.

b. CL_{int} decreased. Low extraction ratio drug $(CL/Q_H = 1.63$ L/hr/81 L/hr$) = 0.02$. Volume of distribution did not change. Clearance decreased, and the half-life lengthened. A decrease in intrinsic clearance is a logical conclusion. Another possible explanation is an increase in both plasma and tissue binding so that volume of distribution did not change. This would decrease clearance and lengthen half-life. The former has been found to be the mechanism of interaction.

4. a. CL_{int} decreased, fu decreased. Decreased intrinsic clearance (metabolism) would cause the trough concentration to increase during mexiletine coadministration. No information is given here on protein binding, but increased binding to plasma proteins could also explain the results. The binding of this drug in plasma is only 60% ($fu = 0.4$, see Fig. 10–5). Therefore, this is not a likely explanation. In addition, because theophylline binds to albumin, such an increase in binding due to an increase in serum albumin is most unlikely.

b. Mexiletine is a competitive inhibitor of theophylline metabolism. Other consistent answers include inhibition of biliary excretion, or decreased renal clearance (change in urine pH or competitive inhibition of secretion). Although consistent, in reality, neither of these additional proposals is likely to explain the magnitude of the effect of mexiletine. Little theophylline is excreted in bile or urine.

5. a. Drug A is secreted and reabsorbed. Renal clearance/$(fu \cdot GFR)$ is 2.1 in the absence and 0.3 in the presence of Drug B.

b. Displacement from plasma and tissue binding sites and either inhibition of tubular secretion or enhanced tubular reabsorption, e.g., by a change in urine pH. The threefold increase in the unbound fraction of Drug A in the presence of Drug B should increase the renal clearance threefold; instead the renal clearance decreased from 1.5 L/hr to 0.6 L/hr.

The extrarenal clearance increased approximately threefold. For Drug A alone,

$$CL \text{ (nonrenal)} = \frac{25 \text{ mg/hr}}{10 \text{ mg/L}} - 1.5 \text{ L/hr}$$

$$= 1.0 \text{ L/hr}$$

and in the presence of Drug B,

$$CL \text{ (nonrenal)} = \frac{25 \text{ mg/hr}}{6.7 \text{ mg/L}} - 0.60 \text{ L/hr}$$

$$= 3.1 \text{ L/hr}$$

By calculation ($V = 1.44 \cdot CL \cdot t_{1/2}$), the volume of distribution of Drug A, 43 L, is seen to not change during coadministration with Drug B. As displacement from plasma proteins occurs, so must displacement occur in tissues to keep the volume of distribution unchanged.

c. The plateau unbound concentration ($fu \cdot C_{ss}$) of Drug A increases from 1 mg/L in the absence to 2 mg/L in the presence of Drug B. This suggests that the response produced by Drug A is increased, perhaps excessively. No information is given on A → B.

6. a. The change in distribution must occur by a decrease in tissue binding (fu_T ↑). Quinidine decreases the volume of distribution of digoxin but does not appear to alter plasma protein binding.

   b. Twofold reduction in loading dose. If the range of therapeutic plasma concentrations of digoxin remains unchanged in the presence of quinidine, then the digitalizing dose will need to be reduced, on average, about twofold (500/240) to compensate for the change in volume of distribution. To achieve a concentration of 1.5 μg/L requires only 360 μg of digoxin intravenously. For digoxin tablets, with an availability of about 0.75, the requirement is about 500 μg.

   c. Because of quinidine's relatively short half-life, its accumulation is rapid. By 24 hr it has reached its plateau and, presumably, its maximum effect on the distribution and elimination of digoxin. Associated with the reduction in its volume of distribution, the concentration of digoxin doubles during this period and stays there, since clearance is reduced to one-half of its normal value. The converse occurs when quinidine is discontinued. Because of its relatively short half-life, the plasma concentration of quinidine falls rapidly before much digoxin is eliminated. The fall in quinidine concentration produces a redistribution of digoxin from plasma back into the tissues, with an associated fall in the digoxin concentration in plasma. Then, because the clearance of digoxin returns to its prequinidine value, so does the digoxin concentration.

   d. Yes. Nonrenal clearance (total − renal) in the absence of quinidine is 39 mL/min. In the presence of quinidine, it is reduced to 21 mL/min (total clearance of 72 mL/min minus renal clearance of 51 mL/min). This change would then require that the dosing rate of digoxin be reduced in a patient with renal insufficiency.

7. a. $CL_{int} \cdot fu = 289$ L/hr in absence and 27 L/hr in presence of fluoxetine. From the *well-stirred* model,

$$CL_H = \frac{Q_H \cdot fu_b \cdot CL_{int}}{Q_H + fu_b \cdot CL_{int}}$$

$$F_H = \frac{Q_H}{Q_H + fu_b \cdot CL_{int}}$$

so that $CL_H/F_H = fu \cdot CL_{int}$

   b. Inhibition of desipramine metabolism. The value of Dose/AUC (CL/F) is 289 L/hr for desipramine alone. This value greatly exceeds hepatic blood flow (81 L/hr), indicating that either F is extremely low or clearance is high and first-pass metabolism occurs. The drug is extensively metabolized, as supported by an fe of 0.03. If metabolism primarily occurs in the liver, both a low F and a high clearance are expected. The coadministration of fluoxetine then results in diminished metabolism and consequently an increase in F and a decrease in CL.

c. The change in CL/F directly reflects a change in $fu \cdot CL_{int}$ irrespective of whether the drug has a high or low hepatic extraction ratio. For a high extraction drug, however, CL and half-life are relatively less sensitive to a change in CL_{int} (see first equation in part "a" above). Half-life is increased by a factor of 4.12 (0.693 V/CL (fluoxetine present)/0.693 $\cdot V/CL$ (fluoxetine absent)). The value of CL/F is decreased by a factor of 10.7 (CL/F (fluoxetine present)/CL/F (fluoxetine absent)).

d. Without reducing dosage, there is an increased likelihood of a greater incidence and intensity of adverse effects. The AUC of desipramine after a single dose is increased about 11-fold in the presence of fluoxetine. On chronic administration, the average steady-state concentration should be increased correspondingly.

8. See Table II–7.

Table II–7.

	CLEARANCE	VOLUME OF DISTRIBUTION	HALF-LIFE	FRACTION EXCRETED UNCHANGED	ORAL BIOAVAILABILITY
			OBSERVATION		
Drug A	↓	↔	↑	↓	↔
Drug B	↑	↔	↓	↔	↔
Drug C	↔	↔	↔	↔	↔
Drug D	↔	↑	↑	↑	↓
Drug E	↔	↓	↓	↔	↔
Drug F	↑	↑	↔	↔	↔
Drug G	↔	↔	↔	↔	↔

9. a. $C_{ss,av} = 38$ mg/L; $t_{90\%} = 19$ hr, i.e., by time of third dose (24 hr).

$$C_{ss,av} = \frac{F \cdot \text{Dose}}{CL \cdot \tau} = \frac{1.0 \times 500 \text{ mg}}{1.1 \text{ L/hr} \times 12 \text{ hr}} = 38 \text{ mg/L}$$

$$t_{90\%} = 3.3 \times t_{1/2} = 3.3 \times \frac{0.693 \times V}{CL} = \frac{3.3 \times 0.693 \times 9 \text{ L}}{1.1 \text{ L/hr}} = 19 \text{ hr}$$

b. 1. $C_{ss,av} = 245$ mg/L

The plateau concentration of inhibitor:

$$C_{ss,av,inhibitor} = \frac{1.0 \times 1000 \text{ mg}}{0.6 \text{ L/hr} \times 12 \text{ hr}} = 139 \text{ mg/L}$$

$$Cu_{ss,av,inhibitor} = fu \cdot C_{ss,av,inhibitor}$$

$$= 0.03 \times 139 \text{ mg/L} = 4.2 \text{ mg/L}$$

Clearance of tolbutamide in the presence of the inhibitor:

$$CL_{inhibited} = \frac{fm \cdot CL_{tolbutamide}}{1 + \dfrac{Cu_{ss,av,inhibitor}}{K_I}} + CL_{R,tolbutamide}$$

$$= \frac{0.97 \times 1.1 \text{ L/hr}}{1 + \dfrac{4.2 \text{ mg/L}}{0.6 \text{ mg/L}}} + 0.03 \times 1.1 \text{ L/hr}$$

$$= 0.17 \text{ L/hr}$$

Hence, the expected new plateau concentration of tolbutamide in presence of plateau concentration of inhibitor is

$$C_{ss,av} = \frac{F \cdot Dose}{CL_{inhibited} \cdot \tau} = \frac{1.0 \times 500 \text{ mg}}{0.17 \text{ L/hr} \times 12 \text{ hr}} = 245 \text{ mg/L}$$

That is, the average plateau concentration of tolbutamide will increase by 6.5-fold.

2. $t_{90\%} = 5.2$ days. The new half-life of tolbutamide in the presence of plateau concentration of inhibitor is

$$t_{1/2,inhibited} = \frac{CL_{normal}}{CL_{inhibited}} \times t_{1/2,normal}$$

$$= 6.5 \times 5.8 \text{ hr} = 38 \text{ hr}$$

Hence, $t_{90\%} = 3.3 \times t_{1/2,inhibited} = 125$ hr or 5.2 days

Note: In practice, the rise to the new plateau takes longer than calculated above. This occurs because during the accumulation of the inhibitor, the degree of inhibition, and corresponding half-life of tolbutamide increases continuously. And, only after a plateau of inhibitor has been reached does the new half-life of tolbutamide stabilize. So, as a first approximation, the time for tolbutamide to reach new plateau is $3.3 \times (t_{1/2,inhibited}) = 3.3 \times (12 \text{ hr} + 38 \text{ hr})$, or 165 hr (6.9 days).

3. 1/4 tablet (125 mg) daily. To maintain the normal average concentration of tolbutamide (38 mg/L), the dosing rate needed in the presence of the inhibitor is

$$CL_{inhibited} \cdot C_{ss,av} = 0.17 \text{ L/hr} \times 38 \text{ mg/L}$$
$$= 6.5 \text{ mg/hr}$$

This is 6.5-fold lower than the normal rate. With $t_{1/2,inhibited}$ of 38 hr, once-a-day dosing is appropriate. Hence, daily dose = 6.5 mg/hr $\times$ 24 hr = 156 mg. The nearest practical approximation is 1/4 tablet daily. Clearly, there is likely to be uncertainty in the actual dose taken each day, even though the tablet is scored. In this situation, it is difficult to predict accurately individual dosage requirements. Generally, such situations should be avoided by not giving both drugs together or by substituting another drug.

ANSWERS TO STUDY PROBLEMS (CHAP. 18)

1. The criteria for performing drug concentration monitoring are discussed in the section on Target Concentration Strategy (pp. 293–296).

2. a. $CL = 82$ mL/min or 4.9 L/hr; $V = 19$ L; $k = 0.26$ hr^{-1}; and $t_{1/2} = 2.7$ hr.

$$CL = CL_{cr} = \frac{(140 - 42) \times 85}{85 \times 1.2} = 82 \text{ mL/min}$$

$$V = 85 \text{ kg} \times 0.22 \text{ L/kg}$$

  b. 5.4 and 1 mg/L. At the time of the first sample, 32 hr has elapsed, i.e., over 10 half-lives. Hence steady-state equations are appropriate. At 45 min after end of infusion, $C = 5.4$ mg/L. Just before the next dose, $C = 1.0$ mg/L.

$$C = \frac{120}{0.75} \times \frac{(1 - e^{-k \cdot t_{inf}})}{4.9} \cdot \frac{1}{(1 - e^{-k \cdot \tau})} \cdot e^{-k(t - t_{inf})}$$

where $t_{inf} = 0.75$ hr, $t_{post} = 0.75$ hr, $\tau = 8$ hr, so that at $t = 1.5$, $C = 5.4$ mg/L, and at $t = 8$, $C = 1.0$ mg/L.

3. a. $CL = 3.51$ L/hr, $V = 21.5$ L, $t_{1/2} = 4.3$ hr.

    Half-life

        $C(t_1)$ is sampled 1.5 hr after the start of the infusion.

        $C(t_2)$ is sampled just before the next dose.

$$k = \frac{\ln(C(t_1)/C(t_2))}{t} = \frac{\ln(7.2/2.5)}{6.5 \text{ hr}} = 0.163 \text{ hr}^{-1}$$

$$t_{1/2} = \frac{0.693}{k} = 4.3 \text{ hr}$$

    Clearance

$$C = \frac{Ro}{CL} \frac{(1 - e^{-kt_{inf}})}{(1 - e^{-k\tau})} \cdot e^{-k(t - t_{inf})}$$

$$CL = \frac{120 \text{ mg}/0.75 \text{ hr}}{2.5 \text{ mg/L}} \frac{(1 - e^{-0.163 \times 0.75})}{(1 - e^{-0.163 \times 8})} \cdot e^{-0.163 \times 6.5} = 3.51 \text{ L/hr}$$

    Volume

$$V = \frac{CL}{k} = \frac{3.51 \text{ L/hr}}{0.163 \text{ hr}^{-1}} = 21.5 \text{ L}$$

  b. No. A 20% reduction in dose would give a peak concentration of 5.78 mg/L and trough of 2.0 mg/L. Clearly, the rules given in Table 18–4 for the therapeutic window need to be modified for patients with compromised renal function (especially those with severe function impairment).

4. Using Eq. 9 and the expected values of F, S, CL, and k, the predicted plasma theophylline concentrations are 3.4, 11.6, and 14.5 mg/L in the three patients, respectively. Clearly, patient 2 has a lower than average value of clearance, and patient 3 has a much higher than average value. By an iterative procedure and using Eq. 9, the values of clearance in the three patients are 0.031, 0.016 and 0.107 L/hr/kg, and the values of

the half-life are 11, 22, and 3 hr, respectively. In patient 1 the sampling time is so short that one has virtually no confidence in the clearance or half-life estimate; a wide range of clearance values gives essentially the same concentration. In patient 2, the clearance is low, and indeed from the estimated clearance and half-life, the value of 18 is far from the estimated steady-state concentration, 40 mg/L. Clearly, the rate of administration of aminophylline in this patient should be reduced, probably about fourfold. A subsequent sample, obtained about 48 to 72 hr later, would then be appropriate. In patient 3, the estimated value of the half-life is such that a good estimate of clearance is obtained. Here, the rate of administration must be doubled to achieve a concentration within the therapeutic range of 10 to 20 mg/L.

5. a. $CL = 0.04 \times 0.4 \times 1.6 \times 70 = 1.79$ L/hr; $V = 0.5 \times 70 = 35$ L; $k = 0.051$ hr^{-1}, $t_{1/2} = 13.5$ hr; $F = 1.0$; and $S = 0.85$.
   b. 14.9 mg/L.

$$C = (0.85/35) \cdot [400 \cdot e^{-0.051 \times 24} + 200 \cdot e^{-0.051 \times 20}$$
$$+ 300 \cdot e^{-0.051 \times 10} + 300 \cdot e^{-0.051 \times 6}]$$

   c. 14.9 mg/L predicted versus 18 mg/L observed.
   d. Observed and predicted concentrations are fairly close. However, because the sample is obtained at not much more than 1 half-life after starting therapy and the patient is on an unequal-dose-equal-interval regimen, one has little confidence in revising the parameters. It might be prudent to recommend a lowering of the dose, as the quantity metabolized (amount absorbed minus amount in body) in the 24 hr period is only about 400 mg [0.85 × total dose given (400 + 200 + 300 + 300)— amount in body at time of sampling (35 × 18)].

6. a. *Evaluation*:
   1. *Expected parameter values*:
      $CL = 0.27$ L/hr or 6.5 L/day (0.0037 L/hr/kg × 74 kg); $V = 0.55$ L/kg × 74 kg = 41 L; $k = 0.0067$ hr^{-1} or 0.16 day^{-1}; $t_{1/2} = 104$ hr or 4.3 days; $F = 1$; and $S = 1$.
   2. *Estimation of concentrations at times of sampling*: 30 and 12 mg/L (compliance is assumed, and because $t_{1/2}$ is much greater than τ and the first blood sample is obtained in the middle of the dosing interval after prolonged treatment, the plasma concentration expected at the first sampling time is well approximated by $C_{ss,av}$).

$$C_{ss,av} = F \cdot \frac{Dose}{CL \cdot \tau} = \frac{200\ mg}{0.27\ \frac{L}{hr} \times 24\ \frac{hr}{day} \times 1\ day} = 30\ mg/L$$

$$C(6\ days\ later) = 30\ e^{-0.16\ day^{-1} \times 6\ days} = 12\ mg/L$$

   3. *Comparison of concentrations (mg/L)*:

DATE	JAN. 10	JAN. 16
Predicted	30	12
Observed	56	16

4. a. *Estimation of parameter values in individual:* $k = 0.21$ day^{-1}; $t_{1/2} = 3.3$ days; $CL = 86$ L/day

Half-life. This parameter is the most accurately estimated one in this case.

$$k = \frac{\log(56/16)}{6 \text{ days}}$$

$$= 0.21 \text{ day}^{-1} \text{ and } t_{1/2} = 3.3 \text{ days.}$$

Clearance: From k value (greater than expected) and usual volume of distribution,

$$CL = 0.21 \text{ day}^{-1} \times 41 \text{ L} = 8.6 \text{ L/day}$$

b. Recommendation. With an estimated clearance higher than that expected and since a change in volume of distribution cannot explain the high concentration observed (fluctuation is small at steady state for a drug with a 3.3-day half-life), the likely explanation for the 56 mg/L value is that the patient has taken more than prescribed. Phenobarbital therapy should be resumed on January 11.

The following relationship $\left(F \cdot \dfrac{\text{Dose}}{\tau} = CL \cdot C_{ss,av} \right)$ can be used as a guide for dosing.

$$\text{Daily dose (mg)} = 8.6 \text{ L/day} \times \text{Plasma concentration (mg/L)}$$

The clinician can decide whether he wishes to have a steady-state concentration toward the higher or lower end of the therapeutic window, 10 to 30 mg/L. A daily dose of 200 mg is expected to give a steady-state concentration in the 20 to 25 mg/L range. Patient education is in order.

7. Step 1. *Estimation of Expected Parameter Values:*

$F = 1$, $S = 0.8$ for i.v. aminophylline and 0.85 for oral aminophylline (hydrate)

$$V = 0.5 \text{ L/kg} \times 70 \text{ kg} = 35 \text{ L}$$

$$CL = 0.04 \text{ L/hr/kg} \times 0.4 \times 70 \text{ kg} = 1.12 \text{ L/hr}$$

$$k = \frac{CL}{V} = \frac{1.12 \text{ L/hr}}{35 \text{ L}} = 0.032 \text{ hr}^{-1}$$

$$t_{1/2} = \frac{0.693}{k} = \frac{0.693}{0.32} = 21.7 \text{ hr}$$

Step 2. *Estimation of Expected Concentration at Time of Sampling:* 15.5 mg/L.

$$C(\text{mg/L}) = \frac{0.8 \times 300 \text{ mg}}{35 \text{ L}} e^{-0.032 \times 28} + \frac{0.8 \times 30 \text{ mg/hr}}{1.12 \text{ L/hr}} (1 - e^{-0.032 \times 28})$$

Step 3. *Comparison of Observed and Expected Concentrations*:
The measured concentration was 20 mg/L. Revision of parameter estimates would appear to be in order.

Step 4. *Revision of Parameter Values*:
Clearance

$$C \text{ (mg/L)} = \frac{0.8 \times 300 \text{ mg}}{35 \text{ L}} e^{-Cl \cdot 28/35} + \frac{0.8 \times 30 \text{ mg/hr}}{CL \text{ L/hr}} (1 - e^{-Cl \cdot 28/35})$$

$$20 = 6.86 \, e^{-0.8 \cdot Cl} + \frac{24}{Cl} (1 - e^{-0.8 \cdot Cl})$$

Solving iteratively,

Cl (L/hr)	C predicted (mg/L)
1.0	16.3
0.8	17.8
0.6	19.4
0.5	20.4
0.56	19.9

Half-life

$$\text{Half-life} = \frac{0.693 \cdot V}{Cl} = \frac{0.693 \times 35 \text{ L}}{0.56 \text{ L/hr}} = 43 \text{ hr}$$

Volume is not revised as it does not vary much (See discussion on p. 305).

Step 5. *Recommendation/Future Action*:
Note that the steady-state concentration expected on a 30-mg/hr infusion is

$$C_{ss} = \frac{Ro}{Cl} = \frac{0.8 \times 30 \text{ mg/hr}}{0.56 \text{ L/hr}} = 43 \text{ mg/L}$$

Whereas the value following the suggested oral dose is

$$C_{ss,av} = \frac{S \cdot D}{Cl \cdot \tau} = \frac{0.85 \times 200 \text{ mg}}{0.56 \text{ L/hr} \times 6 \text{ hr}} = 51 \text{ mg/L}$$

The blood sample was obtained too early to get a good estimate of clearance in the patient. Nevertheless, the measured concentration indicates that the dosage is excessive. The oral dosing rate should be decreased by a factor of approximately 3 (e.g., to 150 mg every 12 hr, approximately the same as two 100-mg tablets twice daily).

The continued infusion to 9:00 on April 11 (15 hr later) would cause the concentration to continue to rise. A concentration of 25 mg/L is calculated based on the *CL* estimate above.

$$C = C(t_1) e^{-k \cdot t} + \frac{Ro}{Cl} (1 - e^{-kt})$$

$$= 24.9 \text{ mg/L}$$

The oral dose at 13:00 adds further to the plasma concentration ($S \cdot D/V = 4.9$ mg/L). It may be prudent to take another plasma sample either late in the day on April 11 or the following morning. The information obtained may then allow the patient's dosing requirements to be better estimated. At a minimum, the current dosage needs to be reduced to avoid the likely development of toxicity.

ANSWERS TO STUDY PROBLEMS (CHAP. 19)

1. *Initial dilution volume (V_1)*—is the volume that a drug appears to occupy initially following an i.v. dose; its value is given by dividing dose by concentration at zero time, a value predicted from an equation that fits the plasma concentration-time data.
   Volume of distribution during terminal phase (V)—is the apparent volume of distribution that a drug occupies after distribution equilibrium has been achieved following one or more discrete doses of drug or after stopping an infusion.
   Volume of distribution at steady state (V_{ss})—is given by the ratio of the amount of drug in the body at steady state and the corresponding plasma concentration.

2. a. True. The extent of distribution outside blood may be small and the rate of distribution very rapid, in which case frequent sampling at early times after a bolus dose would be needed to observe the kinetics of distribution.
   b. This is a reasonable representation for most drugs, as the kidneys and the liver are the major organs of elimination, and both organs are highly perfused. Some drugs are metabolized by many tissues, e.g., nitroglycerin, and for them the proposition that elimination takes place only in the central compartment is questionable.
   c. This statement is true provided the terminal phase is correctly identified. If the majority of the area under the plasma concentration-time curve is associated with the initial phase, then most of the drug is eliminated before distribution equilibrium is achieved and the terminal phase is reached. In this case, the statement is conservative.

3. a. $C_1 = 90$ mg/L, $\lambda_1 = 0.24$ min^{-1}, $C_2 = 29$ mg/L, $\lambda_2 = 0.046$ min^{-1}. Initial half-life = 2.9 min, terminal half-life = 17 min. See Fig. II–10.

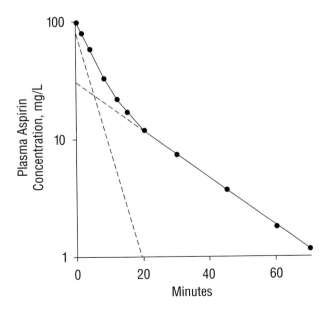

Fig. II–10.

b. $CL = 0.65 \ L/min$, $V_1 = 5.5$ L, $V = 14$ L.

$$CL = \frac{\text{Dose}}{AUC} = \frac{\text{Dose}}{\left(\dfrac{C_1}{\lambda_1} + \dfrac{C_2}{\lambda_2}\right)} = \frac{650 \text{ mg}}{\left(\dfrac{90}{0.24} + \dfrac{29}{0.046}\right) \text{mg-hr/L}}$$

$$V_1 = \frac{\text{Dose}}{C(0)} = \frac{\text{Dose}}{(C_1 + C_2)} = \frac{650 \text{ mg}}{(90 + 29) \text{ mg/L}}$$

$$V = \frac{CL}{\lambda_2} = \frac{0.65 \text{ L/min}}{0.046 \text{ min}^{-1}}$$

c. $C(10) = 26.5$ mg/L, $C(50) = 2.9$ mg/L, $C(70) = 1.2$ mg/L. Values obtained by appropriate substitution into the equation

$$C \text{ (mg/L)} = 90 \ e^{-0.24t} + 29 \ e^{-0.046t}, \ t \text{ in min.}$$

d. 9.3 mg/L. The measured concentration is the sum of the contributions from each dose. In this case, at 60 min after the first dose and 30 min after the second dose, the values are 1.8 and 7.5 mg/L, respectively.

4. a. Slow acetylator: $C_1 = 1.59$ mg/L; $C_2 = 0.65$ mg/L, $\lambda_1 = 5.5 \ \text{hr}^{-1}$; $\lambda_2 = 0.11 \ \text{hr}^{-1}$
   Fast acetylator: $C_1 = 1.57$ mg/L; $C_2 = 0.42$ mg/L; $\lambda_1 = 4.2 \ \text{hr}^{-1}$; $\lambda_2 = 0.40 \ \text{hr}^{-1}$
   Plots not shown.

   b. Slow acetylator: $CL = 12$ L/hr; $V_1 = 33$ L; $V = 110$ L
   Fast acetylator: $CL = 53$ L/hr; $V_1 = 38$ L; $V = 132$ L
   The major difference between fast and slow acetylators is in clearance.

   c. Yes. The initial dilution space (33 and 38 L) must include some well-perfused tissues.

   d. Slow acetylator: $CL = 12.7$ L/hr; $V = 115$ L.
   Fast acetylator: $CL = 71$ L/hr; $V = 178$ L.
   In addition to differences in clearance, one might have concluded that differences in distribution (V) also existed, which is not so (see b).

   e. $f_2 = 0.95$ (slow acetylator), 0.74 (fast acetylator).

   f. Yes. Since f_2 approaches 1.0 for both subjects, the terminal half-life primarily determines the time for the plasma concentration to reach plateau.

5. a. For halazepam, the fluctuation at plateau primarily reflects a balance between the kinetics of absorption and distribution; the 8-hr dosing interval is too short to permit distribution equilibrium to be achieved.

   b. Not well, and certainly not within a dosing interval, which is too short relative to the terminal half-life. Theoretically, the terminal half-life could be measured from the rising trough concentration on approach to plateau, but in practice this measurement has too much error to provide a reliable estimate of terminal half-life. The most reliable estimate is gained on stopping drug administration and following the decline in plasma drug concentration.

6. a. $V_1 = 18.2$ L; $CL = 2.8$ L/hr; $V = 295$ L; and $V_{ss} = 70.9$ L.

$$V_1 = \frac{\text{Dose}}{C_1 + C_2} \qquad V = \frac{CL}{\lambda_2}$$

$$CL = \frac{Dose}{\left(\dfrac{C_1}{\lambda_1} + \dfrac{C_2}{\lambda_2}\right)} \qquad V_{ss} = \frac{Dose}{\left(\dfrac{C_1}{\lambda_1} + \dfrac{C_2}{\lambda_2}\right)} \cdot \frac{\left(\dfrac{C_1}{\lambda_1^2} + \dfrac{C_2}{\lambda_2^2}\right)}{\left(\dfrac{C_1}{\lambda_1} + \dfrac{C_2}{\lambda_2}\right)}$$

b. Only glomerularly filtered.

$$CLu_R = CL_R/fu = \frac{2.8}{0.37} \, L/hr = 7.6 \, L/hr \, (\approx GFR)$$

and being polar, the drug is not expected to be reabsorbed. Since the glomerular filtrate comes directly from arterial blood, a model in which elimination occurs from the central compartment only is reasonable.

c. $V > V_{ss}$. Elimination of drug from plasma increases the ratio of drug concentration in slowly equilibrating tissue to that in plasma during the terminal phase. The slower the distribution of drug between plasma and the slowly equilibrating tissues, the greater is the difference between V and V_{ss}.

d. $f_1 = 0.8$; $f_2 = 0.2$. The half-lives of the corresponding exponential coefficients are 3.6 and 73 hr, respectively. The half-lives reflect a composite of distribution and elimination kinetics. In the present case the majority of drug is eliminated before distribution equilibrium is achieved, and so with respect to elimination, the first half-life is of particular importance. Here, the terminal half-life is only of importance if interest lies in the slowly equilibrating tissues. For most drugs, the majority of drug is eliminated during the terminal phase, that is $f_2 > f_1$.

e. 1. 5 and 72 hr to reach 50% and 90% of plateau, respectively. See Table II–8. Cannot solve for time explicitly; it is estimated iteratively by successive approximations.

$$\frac{C}{C_{ss}} = f_1(1 - e^{-\lambda_1 t}) + f_2(1 - e^{-\lambda_2 t})$$

$$= 0.8 \, (1 - e^{-0.19t}) + 0.2 \, (1 - e^{-0.0095t})$$

Note that 50% of the plateau value is reached in approximately one initial half-life (3.8 hr; $0.693/\lambda_1$), but that the rise to the 90% value becomes increasingly determined by the long terminal half-life, 73 hr. Under these circumstances, the statement that it takes one half-life to reach 50% of plateau and 3.3 half-lives to reach plateau is misleading.

2. A pronounced biexponential curve is observed on stopping the infusion at steady state, because the rate of movement of drug from the slowly equilibrating tissues initially does not match the rapid elimination of drug from plasma. Eventually, decline of drug in plasma becomes controlled by movement of drug from the slowly equilibrating tissues to the central compartment.

Table II-8.

Time (hr)	2	4	5	6	12	24	48	72	96
C/C_{ss}	0.26	0.43	≈0.50	0.55	0.74	0.83	0.87	0.90	0.92

   3. Now $f_2 = 0.83$, signifying that distribution equilibrium occurs before much drug
      is eliminated. Under this circumstance, although there will still be a biexponential
      fall on stopping the infusion, the first phase will be very shallow because drug
      rapidly moves from the tissues as it is eliminated from plasma. Given the general
      inability to distinguish two concentrations that differ by 10% and have the usual
      variation in plasma concentrations, it is unlikely that the first phase can be seen;
      the postinfusion decay would then appear monoexponential, with rate constant
      λ_2.
   7. The observation in Figure 19–16 is explained by differences in the distribution kinetics
      of these drugs. For pancuronium, distribution equilibrium is achieved before much
      drug is eliminated in patients with both normal and impaired renal function; diminished
      renal clearance then causes a change in the terminal half-life. For d-tubocurarine, most
      drug is eliminated from the plasma (and the well-stirred pool) before much drug is
      eliminated in patients with both normal and impaired renal function; the terminal phase
      in both cases is primarily controlled by slow movement of drug out of the slowly
      equilibrating tissues. Diminished renal clearance is reflected by a smaller fall in d-tu-
      bocurarine concentration before the terminal phase is reached as less drug has been
      eliminated by that time than in a patient with normal renal function.
   8. a. Alfentanil: $f_1 = 0.072, f_2 = 0.206, f_3 = 0.722$
         Fentanyl: $f_1 = 0.080, f_2 = 0.128, f_3 = 0.792$
         Sulfentanil $f_1 = 0.116, f_2 = 0.332, f_3 = 0.552$
      b. For all three drugs, the plasma concentration has fallen by 50% of the value at the
         end of the 60-min infusion. Fig. II–11 shows the decline plasma concentration for
         each of the drugs.
      c. The terminal half-life has no utility in predicting the duration of action on stopping
         an infusion for drugs such as the i.v. anesthetics, which display pronounced distri-
         bution kinetics. For example, the durations of action of alfentanil, fentanyl, and
         sufentanil after stopping a 60-min infusion are much shorter at 24.5, 15.6, and 14.8
         min, respectively, than, and in the reverse order to, the terminal half-lives (111, 462
         and 577 min, respectively).

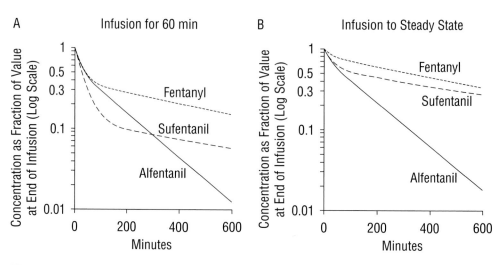

Fig. II–11.

d. Yes. The durations of action (and times for the plasma concentration to fall by 50%) on stopping an infusion at steady-state are 62, 307, and 106 min for alfentanil, fentanyl, and sufentanil, respectively.

e. The ranking of anticipated duration of action is sensitive to the duration of infusion. This is readily seen by comparing the times for the plasma concentration of alfentanil, fentanyl, and sufentanil to fall by 50% on stopping an infusion after 1 hr (24.5, 15.6, and 14.8 min, respectively) and at steady state (62, 307, and 106 min, respectively). Collectively, the answers to this question illustrate the need to consider all parameters defining disposition kinetics when predicting temporal events under a variety of input conditions.

9. a. $V_{ss} = 8.6$ L.

$$V_{ss} = \frac{\text{Dose}\left(\dfrac{C_1}{\lambda_1^2} + \dfrac{C_2}{\lambda_2^2}\right)}{\left(\dfrac{C_1}{\lambda_1} + \dfrac{C_1}{\lambda_2}\right)^2} = \frac{500 \text{ mg}\left(\dfrac{37}{0.17^2} + \dfrac{57}{0.0027^2}\right) \text{mg-hr}^2/\text{L}}{\left(\dfrac{37}{0.17} + \dfrac{57}{0.0027}\right)^2 (\text{mg-hr/L})^2}$$

b. $V_1 = 5.3$ L, $k_{12} = 0.064$ min^{-1}, $k_{21} = 0.104$ min^{-1}, $k_{10} = 0.0044$ min^{-1}.

$$V_1 = \frac{\text{Dose}}{C(0)} = \frac{\text{Dose}}{(C_1 + C_2)} = \frac{500 \text{ mg}}{(37 + 57) \text{ mg/L}}$$

$$C_1 = \frac{\text{Dose}}{V_1} \cdot \left(\frac{k_{21} - \lambda_1}{\lambda_2 - \lambda_1}\right)$$

so that

$$k_{21} = \frac{C_1 V_1 (\lambda_2 - \lambda_1)}{\text{Dose}} + \lambda_1$$

$$= \frac{37 \text{ mg/L} \times 5.3 \text{ L} \times (0.0027 - 0.17) \text{ min}^{-1}}{500 \text{ mg}} + 0.17 \text{ min}^{-1}$$

$$k_{10} = \frac{\lambda_1 \cdot \lambda_2}{k_{21}} = \frac{0.17 \text{ min}^{-1} \times 0.0027 \text{ min}^{-1}}{0.104 \text{ min}^{-1}}$$

$$k_{12} = (\lambda_1 + \lambda_2) - (k_{21} + k_{10})$$

c. $V_{ss} = 8.6$ L.

$$V_{ss} = V_1\left(1 + \frac{k_{12}}{k_{21}}\right) = 5.3 \text{ L}\left(1 + \frac{0.064 \text{ min}^{-1}}{0.104 \text{ min}^{-1}}\right)$$

d. $C(\text{mg/L}) = 36.6e^{-0.169t} + 57.7e^{-0.00136t}$, t in min.

$$\text{Clearance} = V \cdot k_{10}$$

$$\text{New clearance} = 5.31 \text{ L} \times 0.0044 \text{ min}^{-1}$$

New $\lambda_1 + \lambda_2 = k_{12} + k_{21} + k_{10} = 0.064 + 0.104 + 0.0022 = 0.1702 \text{ min}^{-1}$

New $\lambda_1 \cdot \lambda_2 = k_{21}k_{10} = 0.104 \times 0.0022 = 0.000229 \text{ min}^{-2}$

Hence,

$$\text{New } \lambda_1 = 0.5 \left[(k_{12} + k_{21} + k_{10}) + \sqrt{(k_{12} + k_{21} + k_{10})^2 - 4 \, k_{21} \, k_{10}} \right]$$

$$= 0.5 \left[0.1702 + \sqrt{0.1702^2 - 4 \times 0.000229} \right]$$

$$= 0.169 \text{ min}^{-1}$$

$$\text{New } \lambda_2 = 0.5 \left[(k_{12} + k_{21} + k_{10}) - \sqrt{0.1702^{-2} - 4 \times 0.000229} \right]$$

$$= 0.00136 \text{ min}^{-1}$$

$$C_1 = \frac{\text{Dose}}{V_1} \left[\frac{k_{21} - \lambda_1}{\lambda_2 - \lambda_1} \right] = \frac{500 \text{ mg}}{5.3 \text{ L}} \left[\frac{0.104 - 0.169}{0.00136 - 0.169} \right]$$

$$= 36.6 \text{ mg/L}$$

$$C_2 = \frac{\text{Dose}}{V_1} - C_1 = \frac{500 \text{ mg}}{5.3 \text{ L}} - 36.6 \text{ mg/L} = 57.7 \text{ mg/L}$$

ANSWERS TO STUDY PROBLEMS (CHAP. 20)

1. a. *False.* Considering even the simplest pharmacokinetic model ($C = D/V \cdot e^{-kt}$), for a given endpoint, with an associated concentration, C_{min}, the duration t_d is proportional to log Dose;

$$t_d = \frac{1}{k} \cdot \ln \left[\frac{\text{Dose}}{V \cdot C_{min}} \right]$$

   b. *True.* The concentration always decreases with time. Thus a complete "hysteresis" loop is not possible.
   c. *True.* In the equation, Effect $= E_{max} \cdot C^{\gamma}/(EC_{50}^{\gamma} + C^{\gamma})$, it is apparent that if $C = EC_{50}$, then Effect $= E_{max}/2$, irrespective of the value of γ.
   d. *True.* In this region, where Effect $\simeq (E_{max}/EC_{50}^{\gamma}) \cdot C^{\gamma}$, the Effect will be directly proportional to C only if $\gamma = 1$.
   e. *True.* Before distribution equilibrium is achieved, interpretation of plasma concentrations is complicated by temporal aspects.
2. $C_{20} = 5.7$ mg/L and $C_{80} = 17.4$ mg/L. On rearrangement of Eq. 20–1;

$$C = EC_{50} \cdot \left[\frac{\text{Effect}}{1 - \text{Effect}} \right]^{1/\gamma}$$

where Effect is expressed as a fraction of the maximum response. For $\gamma = 2.5$ and $EC_{50} = 10$ mg/L, $C_{20} = 5.7$ mg/L, and $C_{80} = 17.4$ mg/L.
3. a. See Fig. II–12 (p. 555).
   b. $E_{max} = 30$ beats/min; $EC_{50} = 3 \times 10^{-7}$ M; $\gamma = 1$. Response appears to approach a limit of 30 beats/min, and the concentration (EC_{50}) at which the response is one-

trations approximately 1/10 and 10 times the value of EC_{50}, respectively (open circles). The data appear to show this relationship, although the best fit of the model
using statistics may occur with a γ slightly greater than 1. The line shown in Fig. II–
12 has a γ of 1.0.

4. a. A_{min} = 0.38 mg/kg. From a plot of t_d versus ln dose.
   b. Data consistent. A_{min} still in body when second dose of 1 mg/kg is given; i.e., total
      effective dose is 1.38 mg/kg. This total dose, 1.38 mg/kg, on t_d versus ln dose graph
      gives t_d of about 8 min.

$$\text{Same answer by calculation, } t_d = \frac{1}{k} \cdot \ln\left(\frac{\text{Dose}}{A_{min}} + 1\right)$$

5. a. 11.4 hr [A_{min} = 320 mg; substitute into equation in 4b].
   b. 18.3 hr (11.4 hr + half-life).
   c. 1. 22.8 hr and 2. 8.9 hr.
   d. Doubling the dose increases the duration by 1 half-life. The effect of doubling the
      half-life depends on the mechanism of the change. A decreased clearance leads to
      a doubling of the duration of effect, whereas in this example, duration is decreased
      when the cause of the increased half-life is a doubling of the volume of distribution.
6. a. Counterclockwise hysteresis. See Fig. II–13 (p. 556). The sequence of observations
      with time is indicated by the arrows.
   b. No. Strong evidence of hysteresis is lacking in the plot of response versus saliva
      procainamide concentration. See Fig. II–14(p. 556). Apparently, the delay in drug
      reaching the saliva from plasma is similar to the delay in response relative to the
      concentration in plasma.
   c. Yes. This plot (Fig. II–15 p. 556) emphasizes the delay associated with drug distrib-
      uting to the saliva.
   d. This approach is useful in that it can account for delay in response compared to the
      measured concentration. The delay may be associated with distribution to the active
      site but may also be a result of other processes, e.g., the formation of an active

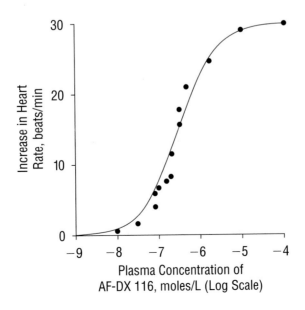

Fig. II–12.

metabolite or a sequence of pharmacodynamic events required to elicit the observed response. Whatever the cause of the delay, the model is useful for quantifying response with time after various methods of drug administration.

7. a. The increase in duration of action seen after the second, third, and fourth doses of pancuronium is a consequence of distribution kinetics. The effect of the first dose occurs during the distribution phase of the drug. On successive doses, because of a

Fig. II–13.

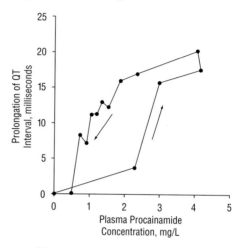

Fig. II–14.

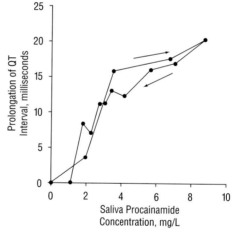

Fig. II–15.

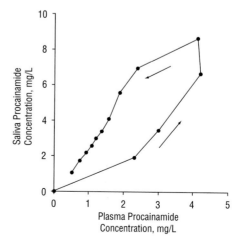

rising tissue concentration, the tendency of drug to move from plasma into tissues decreases, thereby prolonging the time before the plasma concentration reaches the predetermined value.

    b. No. The duration will reach a limiting value when the amount eliminated during the interval equals the dose of drug administered.

8. a. $t_{1/2} = 2.3$ hr. Calculated from: A linear plot of intensity of effect versus time, the slope $(m \cdot k) = 3.5\%/$hr; given that $m = 11.5\%$, then $k = 0.3$ hr^{-1}.

    b. 1. 6.3 hr and 2. 7.7 hr.

    After a 20-mg dose, the effect remains above 15% for 4 hr (Table 20–5).

    1. After a 40-mg dose, the duration is increased 1 half-life (total of 6.3 hr).

    2. After a 60-mg dose, the duration is increased an extra 3.7 hr

$$t_d = \frac{\ln(60/20)}{k} + 4 = 7.7 \text{ hr}$$

9. a. Counterclockwise. Example in problem 6.

    b. Clockwise. At early times the response is large relative to concentration. As time passes the response to a given concentration is diminished. Following an oral dose, clockwise hysteresis is expected.

    c. No hysteresis. Giving drug (same dose) by a controlled-release dosage form lowers peak concentration and increases peak time, but slower input, of itself, should not affect the response–concentration relationship.

ANSWERS TO STUDY PROBLEMS (CHAP. 21)

1. Only the clearance associated with the formation of N-acetylprocainamide and the total clearance of N-acetylprocainamide. This follows from the equation $C(m)_{ss,av}/C_{ss,av} = CL_f/CL(m)$. Note that in all patients in whom the ratio is greater than 1.0, the clearance of N-acetylprocainamide must be less than the clearance of procainamide.

2. a. only.

    a. Induction leads to an increase in CL_f.

$$\frac{AUC(m)}{AUC} = \frac{CL_f}{CL(m)}$$

    b. Ratio independent of V or $V(m)$.

    c. Ratio independent of Dose.

    d. If alternate pathway is reduced, f_m is increased in proportion to decrease in CL, but CL_f is unaffected.

3. Clearance of carbamazepine increases, at least partially due to an increase in the formation clearance of the 10,11-epoxide with increasing daily dose of carbamazepine. See Chap. 22, Dose and Time Dependencies (p. 414), for further discussion of this phenomenon.

Carbamazepine

$$CL = \frac{Dose/\tau}{C_{ss,av}}$$

where $\tau = 24$ hr, dose is in mg, and concentration is in mg/L.

DAILY DOSE (mg)	100	200	400	800	1200
CL (L/hr)	1.6	1.9	2.9	4.6	5.6

Carbamazepine-10,11-epoxide

$$\frac{C(m)_{ss,av}}{C_{ss,av}} = \frac{CL_f}{CL(m)}$$

As this ratio increases with increasing daily dose of carbamazepine, and $CL(m)$ does not change, CL_f must have increased.

4. Elimination of the trans-diol metabolite must be rate-limited by its formation from carbamazepine. The possibility of absorption of carbamazepine being the rate limiting step is doubtful, even in the absence of any other information; an absorption half-life of 30 hr is very uncommon, as very little drug would be absorbed within the usual gastrointestinal transit times, of 12 to 48 hr. Independent information (not presented), following oral and i.v. administration, indicates that carbamazepine is absorbed relatively rapidly.

5. The rate of excretion of salicyluric acid can be taken to be its rate of formation from salicylic acid. The rate of elimination of salicyluric acid is limited by, and hence essentially equal to, its rate of formation. However, the rate of elimination of salicyluric acid is its rate of excretion.

6. a. fm (2-mononitrate) = 0.25. The amount of metabolite formed after a 5-mg i.v. dose of isosorbide dinitrate is

$$CL(m) \cdot AUC(m) = 23 \text{ L/hr} \times 0.044 \text{ mg-hr/L} = 1.01 \text{ mg}$$

Hence

$$f_m = \frac{\text{Amount metabolite formed}}{\text{Dose of drug}} = \frac{1.01 \times \dfrac{236}{191} \text{ mg drug equivalents}}{5 \text{ mg}}$$

b. Assumptions are (i) $CL(m)$ after administration of metabolite equally applies after drug administration, and (ii) all metabolite formed enters the systemic circulation.

c. 99%. Percentages of drug converted to the 2- and 5-mononitrates are 25 and 74, respectively.

7. a. Conjugation of isoproterenol occurs primarily in the gut wall during absorption. Had sulfate conjugation occurred in the liver, some urinary excretion of this metabolite after i.v. administration would be expected, which was not the case. Furthermore, conjugation probably occurs intracellularly within the intestinal epithelium with subsequent substantial systemic absorption of the conjugate; the conjugate is probably too polar to be appreciably absorbed had it been formed in the gut lumen.

b. Yes. Had O-methylation occurred only systemically, one would have expected the ratio of O-methylated compound to its sulfate conjugate to be the same following both oral and i.v. administrations. In practice, the ratio is approximately 4 (5.6/1.3) when drug is taken orally, compared with 0.5 (13.0/24.8) when administered intravenously.

c. Much of the inhaled dose is swallowed. The possibility that pulmonary epithelium is metabolically very similar to intestinal epithelium cannot be excluded, given only the data in Table 21–8. However, a considerable body of data for other drugs clearly indicates that much of an inhaled dose, usually delivered as an aerosol, is swallowed.

8. a. $F_{oral} = 0.19$

$$F = \frac{\left[\dfrac{AUC}{Dose}\right]_{oral}}{\left[\dfrac{AUC}{Dose}\right]_{i.v.}} = \frac{\left[\dfrac{43 \text{ nmol-hr/L}}{10 \text{ mg}}\right]}{\left[\dfrac{229 \text{ nmol-hr/L}}{10 \text{ mg}}\right]}$$

b. Probably.

$$CL_b = \frac{CL_p}{\text{(Blood to plasma concentration ratio)}} = \frac{\dfrac{10 \text{ mg (or 35,000 nmol)}}{229 \text{ nmol-hr/L}}}{2.2}$$

$$= 69.5 \text{ L/hr}$$

If the liver is the only site for drug metabolism, the oral bioavailability expected due to first-pass hepatic loss is given by

$$F_H = 1 - E_H = 1 - \frac{CL_b(1 - fe)}{Q_H}$$

And, as $fe = 0.08$, $Q_H = 81$ L/hr

$$F_H = 1 - \frac{0.92 \times CL_b}{81 \text{ L/hr}} = 0.21$$

c. Yes. With very little morphine excreted unchanged ($fe = 0.08$), for the liver to be the sole site of metabolism, the expectation is that the value of $AUC(m)$ should be independent of the route of administration, oral or i.v. Reference to Table 21–8 for both the 3- and 6-glucuronides supports this expectation.

d. No. Based on AUC considerations, the systemic bioavailability of morphine is essentially the same whether given orally ($F = 0.19$) or sublingually ($F = 0.21$). Furthermore, the respective AUC values for morphine-3 glucuronide and morphine 6-glucuronide are the same following oral and sublingual administration, suggesting that all sublingually administered morphine is swallowed.

e. Given that morphine-6-glucuronide has analgesic activity, with comparable C_{max} and AUC values after oral and i.v. administration of morphine, adjustment of the i.v. dose, based on the oral bioavailability of morphine will tend to overestimate the oral dose of morphine needed to achieve comparable analgesic activity.

f. Because the volume of distribution of the more polar acidic glucuronide is likely to be much smaller than that of the more lipophilic and basic parent compound, morphine. Consequently, the value of C_{max} for the glucuronide will be much greater than that for morphine, for a comparable amount in the body.

g. Fraction of oral morphine converted to morphine-6-glucuronide is 0.06.

$$\text{Fraction converted} = CL\ (m) \times \frac{AUC\ (m)}{\text{Dose}}$$

$$= \frac{5.8\ \text{L/hr} \times 371\ \text{nmol-hr/L}}{35,000\ \text{nmol}}$$

9. A major fraction of 4-hydroxypropranolol is formed during the absorption of propranolol, which is subject to extensive first-pass hepatic elimination. This metabolite has a shorter half-life than propranolol, and so initially the plasma 4-hydroxypropranolol concentration falls faster than that of propranolol; the terminal decline of metabolite is parallel to that of drug because the elimination of metabolite formed from absorbed propranolol is formation rate-limited. The 4-hydroxypropranolol concentration peaks earlier than that of propranolol because it has the shorter half-life. Recall from Chap. 4, the peak is reached when rate of elimination matches the rate of absorption, and it occurs earlier the shorter the half-life of elimination.

10. a. Fraction of drug converted to metabolite = 0.90; formation clearance of metabolite = 8.4 L/hr. Disposition kinetics of metabolite: $t_{1/2} = 4.0$ hr, $k(m) = 0.17\ \text{hr}^{-1}$, $CL(m) = 2.9$ L/hr; $V(m) = 17$ L.

From a semilogarithmic plot, it can be seen that elimination of metabolite is disposition rate-limited. And, from respective decline phases $t_{1/2}$ (drug) = 1.3 hr, $t_{1/2}$ (metabolite) = 4.0 hr.

For drug

$$(F = 1),\ CL\ (\text{Dose/AUC}) = \frac{1000\ \text{mg}}{108\ \text{mg-hr/L}} = 9.3\ \text{L/hr}$$

and

$$V\ (\text{from } CL/k) = \frac{9.3\ \text{L/hr}}{0.53\ \text{hr}^{-1}} = 17\ \text{L}$$

For metabolite

1. $fm = \dfrac{AUC(m)}{AUC} \cdot \dfrac{CL(m)}{CL}$

And given that $V(m) = V$, then

$$fm = \frac{AUC(m)}{AUC} \cdot \frac{k(m)}{k}$$

$AUC(m) = 319$ mg-hr/L [by trapezoidal rule to 12 hr + $C(m, 12\ \text{hr})/k(m)$]

$\quad\quad\quad = 300$ mg drug equivalents-hr/L

Hence

$$fm = 0.90$$

2. $CL_f = fm \cdot CL = 8.4$ L/hr.
3. $V(m) = V = 17$ L.
4. $CL(m) = V(m) \cdot k(m) = 2.9$ L/hr.

b. 1. $C_{ss,av} = 13.5$ mg/L; $C(m)_{ss,av} = 40$ mg/L.

$$C_{ss,av} = \frac{AUC_{single}}{\tau} = \frac{108 \text{ mg-hr/L}}{8 \text{ hr}}; \text{ and}$$

$$C(m)_{ss,av} = \frac{AUC(m)_{single}}{\tau} = \frac{319 \text{ mg-hr/L}}{8 \text{ hr}}$$

2.

Table II-9.

TIME WITHIN DOSING INTERVAL (hr)	0	1	2	4	6	8
C(mg/L)	1.2	32	32	9	4	1.2
C(m) (mg/L)	21.3	39.5	59.0	43.3	32.6	21.3

For both drug and metabolite $C_{ss}(t) = C_1(t) + C_1(t + \tau) \ldots C_1(t + n \cdot \tau)$, where $C_1(t)$ refers to the concentration after a single dose, and n is a number of doses sufficiently large that the concentration associated with time, $t + n \cdot \tau$, is negligible compared with $C_1(t)$. In practice $n \cdot \tau = 5 \cdot t_{1/2}$, or n is equal to $5t_{1/2}/\tau$. For drug, n is less than 1. That is, there is negligible accumulation and so the concentrations within a dosing interval, at plateau, are essentially those obtained after a single dose. For metabolite, $n = 2.5$. The concentration at 1 h after dosing, at plateau, is

$$C_{ss}(1 \text{ hr}) = C_1(1) + C_1(9) + C_1(17) + C_1(25) + \ldots$$

The values at 9, 17, and 25 hr are calculated from the 8-hr value (16 mg/L), knowing the elimination rate constant, $k(m)$. Thus C (9) = C (8) $e^{-k(m) \times 1 \text{ hr}}$, C (17) = C (8) $e^{-k(m) \times 9 \text{ hr}}$, and so on. Which gives

$$C_{ss}(1 \text{ hr}) = 22 + 13 + 3.4 + 0.84 + 0.21 + 0.05$$

$$= 39.5 \text{ mg}$$

Similarly,

$$C_{ss} (8 \text{ hr}) = C_{ss} (0 \text{ hr}) = C_1(8) + C_1(16) + C_1(24) \ldots$$

$$= 21.3 \text{ mg/L}$$

3. For drug, steady state is reached within one dosing interval. With metabolite, it is reached by three dosing intervals.

11. a. Counterclockwise. The metabolite must be formed for the effect to be seen, but the drug must be present first to form metabolite. The requisite drug to metabolite sequence tends to make the drug-to-metabolite ratio decrease with time. This would produce counterclockwise hysteresis.

b. Clockwise. The metabolite would be formed in large amounts during the first pass. The metabolite so formed would disappear quickly compared to the absorbed drug.

The effect would be a clockwise hysteresis on relating response to drug concentration.

ANSWERS TO STUDY PROBLEMS (CHAP. 22)

1. a. 5.
    1. A *more* than proportional increase is expected.
    2. The apparent half-life is *longer* at high concentration.
    3. The rate increases as the amount in the body increases but approaches a limiting value, Vm.
   b. 3.
    1. Induction should produce a concentration *lower* than predicted, because of increased metabolic activity.
    2. A change in V should *not affect* the mean steady-state concentration.
   c. 1, 2, and 3.
    4. Increased V would *not* explain the lack of proportional increase in C_{ss}, unless an increase in *fu* occurred. In this case, *CL* would increase as well.
   d. 2 and 4.
    1. Saturable absorption would lead to a *less* than proportional increase in Ae_∞.
    3. Saturable active tubular secretion would result in a less than proportional increase in the amount excreted unchanged as the dose is increased.
2. Saturable first-pass metabolism produces dose dependence in bioavailability. It occurs by capacity-limited metabolism during first-pass of orally administered drug through the intestines and liver. It can occur without apparent saturable elimination after an equivalent i.v. dose, when the concentration entering the intestines or the liver after the oral dose greatly exceeds that after the i.v. dose. Factors favoring this condition include rapid absorption and a large volume of distribution.
3. a. The graph on the left (Fig. 22–22A) should be a horizontal line, as the y-axis is equivalent to F/CL, and no change is expected in either of these parameters with dose. The steady-state unbound concentration (graph on right) should increase in direct proportion to the dosing rate.
   b. Saturation of plasma protein binding. Since phenylbutazone was administered orally, the declining steady-state concentration with dosing rate could reflect either a decreased bioavailability, an increased clearance, or a change in both parameters. This conclusion is based on the relationship

$$\frac{C_{ss,av}}{(\text{Dose}/\tau)} = \frac{F}{CL}$$

where the symbols are as previously defined. Because only negligible amounts of drug are detected in urine or feces, it is tempting to conclude that absorption is always complete. However, bioavailability can decrease with an increased oral dose, even though no drug appears in the feces, if unabsorbed drug is degraded by the microflora in the lower intestines. Dose dependence in absorption could be proven by parenteral administration of the drug. One cause of an increased clearance, elevated organ blood flow, can be immediately excluded. Clearance, estimated by appropriately substituting the data in Fig. 22–22 into the relationship above, is low and so is not expected to change with blood flow. As drug was not detected in urine, a change in clearance must occur by an extrarenal route, presumably by (hepatic) metabolism. Another possible explanation for an increased clearance is an increased ability to metabolize the drug. This possibility might arise from enzyme activation, or from induction of the drug's own metabolic enzymes. The data do not permit distinction between these possibilities.

The actual cause of the dose-dependent observation is apparent when plasma protein binding is measured. Clearance is increased because of saturability of phenylbutazone binding to plasma proteins. The unbound clearance of phenylbutazone is constant (slope of unbound drug in Fig. 22–22B); the total clearance ((Dose/τ)/ $C_{ss,av}$) changes with the concentration. Furthermore, saturation of binding of this acidic drug to albumin is expected at bound (total minus unbound) concentrations of 80 to 120 mg/L or 0.3 to 0.4 mM (M.W. = 308 g/mole), values approaching the molar concentration typical of plasma albumin (0.6 mM).

4. a. I, III, and VI. From the relationship $F \cdot \mathrm{Dose} = CL_b \cdot AUC_b$, it is apparent that either F is increased or CL_b is decreased.

   b. I and III. At steady state, $R_0 = CL \cdot C_{ss}$. Clearance must decrease with increasing dosing rate.

   c. I and III. From the relationships $\mathrm{Dose} = V_b \cdot C_b(0)$ and $\mathrm{Dose} = CL_b \cdot AUC_b$ it is evident that volume of distribution is not changed and CL_b is decreased.

5. Glucose must be actively reabsorbed. At plasma concentrations above 2 g/L, the capacity of the reabsorption system is exceeded, as shown in Fig. II–16.

6. Saturable binding to plasma proteins, saturable reabsorption in renal tubules, or autoinduction. The ratio, infusion rate/C_{ss}, is equal to clearance. Calculation of the ratio shows that clearance increased with increasing infusion rate of disopyramide in both subjects. The increase in clearance could be a result of saturable binding to plasma proteins ($fu \uparrow$ with higher infusion rates). This conclusion is supported by its binding to a_1-acid glycoprotein. Drug concentrations in the 2- to 5-mg/L range (6–15 µM) are greater than 20% of the average plasma concentration (15 µM) of this protein. Saturable binding is the explanation: It can be proven by concurrent measurement of protein binding.

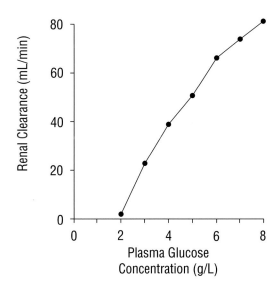

Fig. II–16.

Saturable reabsorption in the renal tubule is another possibility. This mechanism cannot be substantiated, as no further information was given on the route of elimination or whether the drug is reabsorbed by a facilitated mechanism in the renal tubule. Autoinduction is a third possibility. It would be an explanation if the degree of autoinduction varied greatly within the concentration range in which the observations were made.

7.

Table II–10. Disposition Kinetics and Total and Unbound Steady-State Blood Drug Concentrations as a Function of Dose Dependence in Each of Several Sources Following Oral and i.v. Administrations

SOURCE OF DOSE DEPENDENCY	DIRECTION OF CHANGE[a] WITH INCREASED TOTAL DAILY DOSE	VOLUME OF[b] DISTRIBUTION	CLEARANCE	HALF-LIFE	$\left[\dfrac{\text{CONCENTRATION}}{\text{RATE OF ADMINISTRATION}}\right]^c$ TOTAL	UNBOUND
Oral administration						
Bioavailability	↓	↔	↔	↔	↓	↓
Absorption						
Rate Constant	↓	↔	↔	↔[d]	↔	↔
Intravenous Administration						
Fraction unbound in blood						
Low extraction ratio drug	↑	↑	↑	↔	↓	↔
High extraction ratio drug	↑	↑	↔	↑	↔	↑
Fraction unbound in tissue	↑	↓	↔	↓	↔	↔
Metabolic clearance	↑	↔	↑	↓	↓	↓
Renal clearance	↓	↔	↓	↑	↑	↑

[a]Only one example of each direction of change is shown.
[b]A volume of distribution greater than 50 L.
[c]The average steady-state total and unbound blood drug concentrations relative to the rate of administration.
[d]Unless absorption rate limits elimination of drug, then the terminal half-life increases.

8.

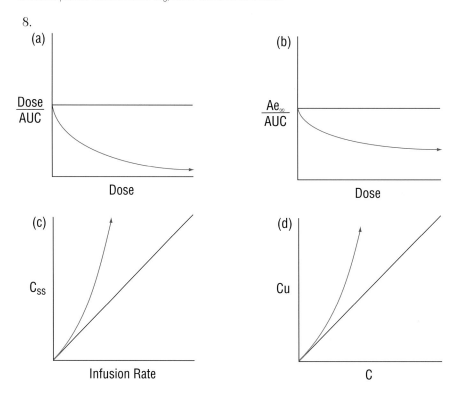

Fig. II–17.

9. No. The peak concentration of the drug after the 2-g dose is 60 mg/L or 120 μM. This is just the concentration (20% of albumin concentration, 600 μM) expected to produce a 20% increase in fu if there is one binding site per molecule. The effect of saturable binding is therefore not expected to be very great at the concentrations observed. Furthermore, if the value of fu is increased with time for the 2-g dose relative to the 1-g dose, then renal clearance should be increased, not decreased, as was observed.

10. a. See Fig. II–18.

   b. Yes. The slope is less ($t_{1/2}$ longer) at the higher dose. The intercepts suggest that the volume of distribution may increase slightly with dose. The AUC is increased suggesting a decrease in clearance with dose.

   c. No. With Michealis-Menten kinetics the slope is the same at a given concentration on a semilogarithmic plot.

$$-\frac{dC}{dt} = \frac{1}{V} \cdot \frac{Vm \cdot C}{Km' + C}$$

$$\text{Slope} = \frac{d \ln C}{dt} = \frac{-dC/dt}{C} = \frac{1}{V} \cdot \frac{Vm}{(Km' + C)}$$

   d. No. If all the components measured by the assay behaved linearly, then the curves should superimpose when normalized to dose. The data suggest nonlinear behavior for one or more of the components.

11. a. On administration of the racemate, the bioavailability of the (+)-isomer is approximately 10 to 20 times greater than that for the (−)-isomer (see Table 12–8). This is a consequence of greater first-pass metabolism of the (−)-isomer. Both isomers have clearance values close to hepatic blood flow. The extraction ratios for the (+)- and (−)-isomers appear to be 0.8 and 0.96. With comparable clearances and vol-

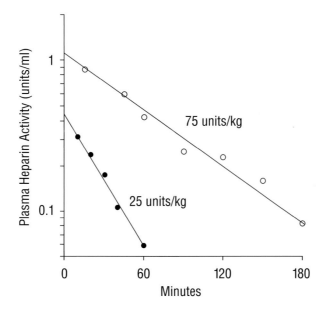

Fig. II–18.

umes of distribution (see Table 12–8 and answers to problem 5, Chap. 12) the half-lives should be nearly the same.

b. Yes. The metabolites are formed during the first pass through the liver and from drug that reaches the systemic circulation. With the same amount formed, the *AUC* value of these metabolites should be the same if their clearances are the same.

c. Similar half-lives of ritalinic acid metabolites as corresponding parent enantiomers. The amount of drug, especially (−)-methylphenidate, that is absorbed into the systematic circulation is small. As such, the decline in the metabolite concentration must be primarily rate-limited by metabolite elimination. Fortuitously, this half-life is comparable to that of both (+)- and (−)-methylphenidate.

d. Probably due to differences in extent of first pass metabolism. The bioavailability of (+)-methylphenidate is 0.20, while that of (−)-methylphenidate is approximately 0.04 (problem 5, Chap. 12). As a consequence, the amount of (−)-ritalinic acid formed during the first pass should be about 20% greater than that of (+)-ritalinic acid. Differences in distribution, plasma protein or tissue binding, could also be an explanation.

e. Saturable first-pass metabolism. At higher doses a greater fraction escapes metabolism during passage across the liver.

ANSWERS TO STUDY PROBLEMS (CHAP. 23)

1. *Turnover*—The process of renewal of substance in a pool at steady state.
   Turnover rate—The rate of input (production and transfer) into a pool.
   Turnover time—The time required to bring into a pool an amount equal to that in the pool.
   Fractional turnover rate—The ratio of turnover rate and pool size.
   Mean residence time—The average time a molecule resides in the body or in a pool.

2. a. Turnover rate = 5 units/hr.
   b. Turnover time = 8 hr.
   c. Fractional turnover rate = 0.125 hr^{-1}.

$$\text{Turnover rate} = CL \cdot C_{ss} = 0.5 \text{ L/hr} \times 10 \text{ units/L}$$

$$\text{Turnover time} = \frac{1}{k_t} = \frac{V}{CL} = \frac{4 \text{ L}}{0.5 \text{ L/hr}}$$

$$\text{Fractional turnover rate} = k_t = \frac{0.5 \text{ L/hr}}{4 \text{ L}}$$

3. a. A_{ss} = 960 mg.

$$\text{Pool size} = A_{ss} = C_{ss}V_{ss} = 4.1 \text{ mg/L} \times 234 \text{ L}$$

b. $t_t = MRT$ = 37 days.

$$\text{Turnover time } t_t = \frac{\text{Pool size } (A_{ss})}{\text{Turnover rate } (CL \cdot C_{ss})}$$

$$= \frac{960 \text{ mg}}{6.3 \text{ L/day} \times 4.1 \text{ mg/L}}$$

c. $t_t = MRT = 37$ days.

$$MRT = t_t$$

d. $F = 0.86$.

$$F = \frac{\text{Turnover rate}}{\text{Daily dosing rate}} = \frac{25.8 \text{ mg/day}}{30 \text{ mg/day}}$$

4. a. k_t (urea) $= 0.10 \text{ hr}^{-1}$; k_t (creatinine) $= 0.17 \text{ hr}^{-1}$.

$$k_t = \frac{CL \cdot C}{V \cdot C}$$

$$k_t \text{ (urea)} = \frac{4.2 \text{ L/hr}}{42 \text{ L}}$$

$$k_t \text{ (creatinine)} = \frac{7.2 \text{ L/hr}}{42 \text{ L}}$$

b. Urea $= 20$ hr; creatinine $= 11.7$ hr. For both compounds the time required is twice the turnover time. In an anephric patient with no elimination of either compound, the rate of increase in plasma concentration is R_t/V and the total increase over time t is $R_t \cdot t/V$.

$$t = \frac{\Delta C \cdot V}{CL \cdot C_{ss}} = \frac{\Delta C}{C_{ss}} \cdot t_t$$

For both urea and creatinine, $\dfrac{\Delta C}{C_{ss}} = 2$.

c. 15.2 g. Daily amount excreted in 1 day ($CL_R \cdot C_{ss} \cdot t$)

$$= \frac{4.2 \text{ L}}{\text{hr}} \times \frac{24 \text{ hr}}{\text{day}} \times \frac{150 \text{ mg}}{\text{L}} \times 1 \text{ day}.$$

5. 2.8 days. The enzyme activity (concentration) will increase to a steady state three times its normal value. The doubling of the concentration (half-way between 1 and 3) will occur at 1 half-life or $0.693 \times$ turnover time.

6. No. It depends on the fractional turnover rates of the two enzymes. Enzyme A may have reached its new steady state by 24 hr, while enzyme B may take a week or more to reach its new steady state, which may be more than double its normal value.

7. a. 8 hr. In this anuric patient, the amount of creatinine in the body (and the plasma concentration) doubles in a turnover time. With a rise of 3 mg/100 mL in 24 hr, the value must have increased by the normal value of 1 mg/100 mL in 8 hr.

b. 183 hr. With a normal turnover time of 8 hr, the normal half-life is 5.5 hr ($t_{1/2} = 0.693 \times t_t$). If renal function decreases 10-fold, the new half-life is 55 hr. Consequently, it takes 183 hr, or 7.6 days, to reach 90% of the full increase to the new steady state.

8. a. 15.9 days and 0.063 day^{-1}.

$$MRT = \frac{AUMC}{AUC}$$

$$= \frac{\dfrac{1.5}{1.4^2} + \dfrac{1.2}{0.06^2}}{\dfrac{1.5}{1.4} + \dfrac{1.2}{0.06}} = 15.9 \text{ days}$$

$$k_t = 1/t_t = 1/MRT$$

b. 105 g and 109 g.
   Intravascular

$$A = V_1 \cdot C(0)$$

$$V_1 = \frac{Dose}{C(0)^*} = \frac{6.75 \text{ megaBecquerels}}{2.7 \text{ megaBecquerels/L}} = 2.5 \text{ L}$$

$$A = 2.5 \text{ L} \times 42 \text{ g/L} = 105 \text{ g}$$

Total in body

$$A = V_{ss} \cdot C(0)$$

$$V_{ss} = MRT \cdot CL = MRT \cdot Dose/AUC$$

$$= 15.9 \text{ days} \times 6.75 \text{ megaBecquerels}/21.07 \text{ megaBecquerel-days/L} = 5.1 \text{ L}$$

$$A = 5.1 \text{ L} \times 42 \text{ g/L} = 214 \text{ g}$$

Amount in extravascular space = Total amount in body −
                                                  amount in intravascular space
$$= 214 - 105 = 109 \text{ g}$$

c. 13.5 g/day.

$$R_t = k_t \cdot A_{ss} = k_t \cdot V_{ss} \cdot C_{ss}$$

$$R_t = 0.063 \text{ day}^{-1} \times 5.1 \text{ L} \times 42 \text{ g/L}$$

9. a. Plot of S versus time is readily drawn from the data in Table 23–3.
   b. Table II–11 summarizes the data for the synthesis rate of S and the plasma concentration of S. The synthesis rate was calculated from the relationship

$$R_{syn} = \frac{dA_S}{dt} + k_s \cdot A_s$$

which for a small time interval, Δt, is approximated by

$$R_{syn} = \frac{\Delta A_s}{\Delta t} + k_s \cdot A_{s,av}$$

where R_{syn} is the average rate of synthesis over Δt;

$\dfrac{\Delta A_s}{\Delta t}$ is the average rate of change of A_s over Δt; and

$A_{s,av}$ is the average value of A_s over Δt. Its value is approximated by

$$A_{s,av} = [A_s(t_i) + A_s(t_i + 1)]/2$$

and it occurs at the midpoint time,

$$t_{mid} = [t_i + t_{i+1}]/2$$

where t_i and t_{i+1} are the ith and ith + 1 times.

Estimation of k_s. The first 50% fall of A_s is the same whether 100 mg or 200 mg of drug was injected. Hence during this time, inhibition of synthesis must be almost complete ($R_{syn} = 0$), then

$$\frac{dA_s}{dt} = -k_s \cdot As$$

Hence k_s is estimated from the slope of the initial straight line when A_s values are plotted against time on semilogarithmic paper.

Answer. $k_s = 0.170 \text{ hr}^{-1}$ ($t_{1/2} = 4.1 \text{ hr}$)

therefore, $R_{syn} = k_s \cdot A_s = 17\% \text{ hr}^{-1}$.

Table II-11.

Synthesis rate (percent of normal amount of S in body/hr)	17.0	1.45	1.35	2.2	2.8	4.2	6.0	9.5	12.1	14.9	16.2	16.9
Drug concentration at midpoint of time interval (mg/L)	0	7.05	6.4	5.8	5.0	3.7	2.6	1.95	1.2	0.7	0.38	0.21

c. $EC_{50} = 2 \text{ mg/L}$; $\gamma = 1.84$.

EC_{50} is concentration at which the synthesis is 50% of normal (8.5% of normal amount/hr)

The value of γ is obtained by substituting an effect-concentration data pair into the equation.

$$\frac{Effect}{E_{max}} = \frac{C^\gamma}{EC_{50}^\gamma + C^\gamma}$$

where Effect/E_{max} is one minus the synthesis rate as a fraction of the normal value, a measure of the degree of inhibition of synthesis. Using a concentration of 5 mg/L and an Effect/E_{max} of 0.844, the value of γ is 1.84.

d. Bolus = 33 mg; infusion rate = 1.65 mg/hr.

Desire 30% of normal values of As at steady state. This objective is achieved by decreasing the synthesis rate to 30% of the normal value, that is, to $0.3 \times 17.3\%$ $\text{hr}^{-1} = 5.2\% \text{ hr}^{-1}$. From plot in part b, 3.3 mg/L achieves this objective at steady state. Bolus dose (to produce 3.3 mg/L) = 3.3 mg/L × 10 L = 33 mg. Infusion rate (to sustain 3.3 mg/L) = $k \cdot V \cdot C_{ss}$ = 0.05 hr^{-1} × 33 mg = 1.65 mg/hr.

ANSWERS TO STUDY PROBLEMS (CHAP. 24)

1. *Dialysis*—Separation of large from small molecules by the preferential passive movement of small molecules through a semipermeable membrane.
Extracorporeal dialysis—Dialysis of substances outside the body. Substances are delivered in blood to the dialyzing system.
Hemodialysis—A form of extracorporeal dialysis in which blood and dialysate fluid each flow past opposite sides of a semipermeable membrane, permitting small molecules to be removed from the body.
Hemofiltration—Removal of substances in blood by filtration. Plasma water passes through the semipermeable membrane, as do substances not bound to plasma protein. Only when the molecule size of a solute is sufficiently large that it can no longer pass through the membrane does its filtration differ from that of plasma water.
Continuous ambulatory peritoneal dialysis—Continuous reinstillation, after a dwell time of 4 to 12 hr, of dialysate fluid into the peritoneal cavity. The peritoneal linings function as a semipermeable membrane, allowing small molecules to be removed from the body.
Dialysis clearance—Rate of removal of a substance in the dialysate relative to its concentration in the plasma entering the dialyzer under steady-state conditions. Blood dialysis clearance and unbound dialysis clearance are the parameters that relate the rate of removal to the drug concentration in blood and plasma water, respectively.
Dialyzer—A general term for the apparatus by which hemodialysis is carried out.
Dialyzer efficiency—Ratio of the rate of removal of substance to the rate of its presentation to the dialyzer under steady-state conditions.
Clinical dialyzability—A general term for the relative ability of dialysis to remove drug from the body. It is quantified by the ratio of the amount removed during the procedure relative to the amount initially in the body. The value of the ratio is the product of the fraction eliminated by dialysis and the fraction lost by all routes of elimination during the dialysis period.

2. a.

Table II-12.

	UNBOUND DIALYSIS CLEARANCE^a (L/hr)	DIALYSIS CLEARANCE^b (L/hr)	$\left(\frac{t_{1/2}}{t_{1/2,during}}\right)^c$	$t_{1/2}^{\,d}$ (hr)
S-Naproxen M.W. = 230 g/mole	6.3	0.019	1.03	14
Tobramycin M.W. = 468 g/mole	4.4	4.1	15	53
Verapamil M.W. = 455 g/mole	4.5	0.45	1.0	2.3

$^a Clu_D$ = dialysis clearance $\cdot \sqrt{\dfrac{113}{M.W.}}$

(150 mL/min or 9.0 L/hr)

$^b Cl_D = Clu_D \cdot fu$

$^c \left(\dfrac{t_{1/2}}{t_{1/2,during}}\right) = \dfrac{Cl + Cl_D}{Cl}$

$^d t_{1/2} = \dfrac{0.693 \cdot V}{Cl}$

b. Tobramycin is dialyzable. S-Naproxen is poorly dialyzable because of extensive plasma protein binding. Verapamil is poor because of a large V (extensive tissue binding).

DRUG	$k_D{}^a$	$f_D{}^b$	CLINICAL DIALYZABILITY $f_D(1 - e^{-k_D\tau})^c$
S-Naproxen	0.0517	0.0194	0.0036
Tobramycin	0.196	0.93	0.51
Verapamil	0.3	0.0043	0.003

$^a k_D = \dfrac{Cl + Cl_D}{V}$

^{b}Eq. 11.

^{c}Eq. 12.

3. a. 10.5 mL/min.

$$\int_0^6 C \cdot dt \simeq C_{av} \cdot 6 = 22 \text{ mg-hr/L}$$

$$Cl_D = \frac{\text{Amount recovered}}{\displaystyle\int_0^6 C \cdot dt} = \frac{14 \text{ mg}}{22 \text{ mg-hr/L}}$$

$$= 10.5 \text{ mL/min}$$

b. 3.5%.

$$Q_b = 0.305 \text{ L/min} = 18.3 \text{ L/hr}$$

$$\text{Efficiency} = \frac{V_D \cdot C_D}{Q_b \cdot \displaystyle\int_0^\tau C_{b,in} \cdot dt} = \frac{14 \text{ mg}}{18.3 \text{ L/hr} \times \dfrac{22 \text{ mg-hr/L}}{L}}$$

c. No. $C_{b,out}/C_{b,in} = 0.965$.

The ratio of $C_{b,out}$ and $C_{b,in}$ can be calculated from

$$\frac{C_{b,out}}{C_{b,in}} = 1 - \text{efficiency}$$

The concentrations of drug in blood entering and leaving the dialyzer are too close to obtain an accurate estimate of the difference. In addition, only minor differences in flow rates in and out, caused by loss of water into dialysate, can make concentration differences smaller or even negative.

d. 4%.

$$\frac{\text{Amount recovered}}{\text{Dose}} = \frac{14 \text{ mg}}{350 \text{ mg}} = 0.04$$

e. Yes. 10.5 mL/min measured versus 11.7 mL/min predicted.

$$Cl_D \simeq \frac{\text{Dialysis clearance}}{\text{of creatinine}} \cdot \sqrt{\frac{113}{252}} \times f_u$$

$$CL_D \approx 83 \text{ min} \times 0.67 \times 0.21$$

4. a. The manner of calculating dialysis clearance after i.p. administration is the principal cause of the difference in the values. The amount that entered the body during the first 4-hr dwell time after i.p. administration is unknown. It certainly is not equal to the dose, as was assumed by the authors.

   b. Clearance, too, is miscalculated, following i.p. administration. The *AUC* is less than that after i.v. administration because of the exchange of dialysate at 4 hr. After i.p. administration,

$$\frac{Dose}{AUC} = \frac{CL}{F}$$

It is evident that *F* is approximately equal to 0.6. This is the same factor by which the peritoneal dialysis clearance after i.p. administration was in error.

5. a. Yes, because 33% of initial amount is needed to cancel what is lost by dialysis.

$$\text{Nonrenal clearance} = (1 - fe(typical)) \cdot V \cdot 0.693/t_{1/2} (typical)$$

$$= 2.64 \text{ L/hr};$$

$$\frac{\text{Half-life}}{\text{off dialysis}} = \frac{t_{1/2} (typical)}{(1 - fe(typical))}$$

$$= 9.2 \text{ hr};$$

$$\begin{array}{c} \text{Fraction of amount} \\ \text{initially in body} \\ \text{eliminated by dialysis} \\ \text{(Eq. 12)} \end{array} = 0.36;$$

$$\begin{array}{c} \text{Fraction of amount} \\ \text{initially in body} \\ \text{required to cancel} \\ \text{the loss by dialysis} \\ \text{(Eq. 16)} \end{array} = 0.33.$$

   b. 150 mg. For a regimen of 240 mg every 6 hr, the average amount of theophylline in the body is 460 mg. The supplementary dose is 0.33 × 460 mg, or 150 mg.

   c. 240 mg initially and every 6 hr, with about 150 mg at the end of each dialysis treatment. Values should be adjusted to nearest dose strengths.

6. No. The clearance of the drug ($0.693 \, V/t_{1/2}$) is 0.16 L/hr, a value greater than that of dialysis clearance, <0.1 L/hr. With a usual half-life of 160 hr, one cannot expect the half-life on dialysis to shorten by much. Furthermore, the amount eliminated by dialysis in 24 hr would be minor.

7. a. 1.49 L/hr.

$$CL_D = \frac{\text{Amount in dialysate}}{AUC_{0-\tau}} = \frac{0.36 \text{ mg}}{0.242 \text{ mg-hr/L}}$$

   b. 21.7 L/hr.

$$V = \frac{V}{F} \cdot F = 350 \, L \times 0.8 = 280 \, L$$

$$CL_{total} = CL + CL_D = \frac{0.693 \cdot V}{t_{1/2}} + CL_D = \frac{0.693 \times 280 \, L}{9.6 \, hr} + 1.49 \, L/hr$$

c. 0.069.

$$f_D = \frac{CL_D}{CL + CL_D} = \frac{1.49 \, L/hr}{21.7 \, L/hr}$$

d. 0.022.

$$f_D \left(1 - e^{-\left[\frac{CL_D + CL}{V}\right] \cdot \tau}\right) = 0.069 \left(1 - e^{-21.7 \cdot 5/280}\right)$$

or

$$\frac{\text{Amount in dialysate}}{F \cdot \text{Dose}} = \frac{0.36 \, mg}{0.8 \times 20 \, mg}$$

8. a. See Fig. II–19.

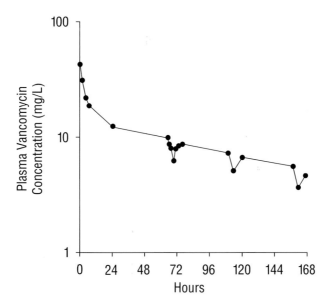

Fig. II–19.

b. Approximately 7 hrs. Estimate is limited by quality of data during the dialysis treatments. The best estimate is obtained during the dialysis treatment from 66 to 70 hr. Note that less than 1 half-life has elapsed.

c. Redistribution. A postdialysis rebound of concentration occurs because of redistribution of drug from tissues back into plasma. Because the plasma concentration returns to a value close to that expected had no drug been removed by dialysis, dialysis must not be very effective in removing vancomycin from the body.

d. No. The loss during each treatment appears to be quite small when compared to the amount in the body.

e. No. The removal of vancomycin by dialysis is not blood flow limited. Also, because the rate of return to plasma from tissues within the dialysis period is slow, increasing dialysis clearance would not materially increase drug removal from the whole body.

9. a. Elimination continuously slows from Group I to Group V. Under such changing conditions, the peak concentration and the peak time are expected to increase (see Fig. 4–8 in Chap. 4, Extravascular Dose).

   b. 4.7 L/hr.

$$CL_D = \frac{\text{Amount in dialysate}}{AUC(0 \text{ to } \tau)} = \frac{0.9 \times 30 \text{ mg}}{5.75 \text{ mg-hr/L}}$$

   c. 0.42.

$$\frac{t_{1/2,\text{during}}}{t_{1/2,\text{off}}} = \frac{CL}{CL_{HD} + CL}$$

$$\frac{2.05}{5.9} = \frac{CL}{4.7 + CL} \qquad CL = 2.48 \text{ L/hr}$$

$$f_D \cdot (1 - e^{-k_{Dt}}) = \frac{4.7}{4.7 + 2.48} (1 - e^{-0.693 \times 3/2.05})$$

   d. 3.50 L/hr.

$$CL_D = \frac{\text{Creatinine}}{\text{dialysis clearance}} \cdot \sqrt{\frac{113}{\text{M.W.}}} \times f_u$$

$$= 158 \text{ ml/min} \times 60 \text{ min/hr} \cdot \sqrt{\frac{113}{407}} \times 0.7$$

   e. 4.7 L/hr (measured) versus 3.5 L/hr (predicted). One explanation for the difference is that the clearance of creatinine begins to approach an upper limit imposed by blood (plasma) flow. Its value is therefore an underestimate of that expected when there is no flow limitation. The dialysis clearance of the drug is smaller than that of creatinine and therefore is not limited by blood flow to the same degree.

10. a. 4.02 L/hr.

$$\text{Amount in filtrate} = V_{\text{filtrate}} \cdot C_{\text{filtrate}} = Q_f \cdot \tau \cdot C_{\text{filtrate}}$$

$$= 86 \text{ mL/min} \times 60 \text{ min/hr} \times 3.5 \text{ hr} \times 0.47 \text{ mg/L} \times 1 \text{ L/1000 mL}$$

$$= 8.5 \text{ mg}$$

$$CL_{HF} = \frac{8.5 \text{ mg}}{2.11 \text{ mg-hr/L}}$$

   b. Extraction coefficient = 0.193.

$$\text{Efficiency} = \frac{CL_{HF} \text{ (blood)}}{Q_b}$$

$$CL_{HF} \text{ (blood)} = CL_{HF} \text{ (plasma)}$$

$$Q_b = 348 \text{ mL/min} \times 60 \text{ min/hr} \times 1 \text{ L/1000 mL}$$

$$= 20.9 \text{ L/hr}$$

$$\text{Efficiency} = \frac{CL_{HF}}{Q_b} = \frac{4.02}{20.9}$$

c. 0.183.

$$CL \text{ (absence)} = 0.298 \text{ L/min}$$
$$= 17.9 \text{ L/hr}$$

$$\frac{\text{Contribution of filtration}}{\text{to total elimination}} = \frac{CL_{HF}}{CL_{HF} + CL}$$

$$= \frac{4.02}{4.02 + 17.9}$$

d. Yes. By dosing at the end of a hemofiltration session, the amount lost in a treatment period would be small as the fraction remaining 20.5 hr after a dose is small (approximately 0.004). The drug is often given infrequently compared to the half-life (2.6 hr in this study) to end-stage renal disease patients.

$$\text{Fraction remaining} = e^{-kt} = e^{-(0.693/2.6) \times 20.5}$$

ANSWERS TO STUDY PROBLEMS (APPENDIX I-A)

1. 10.93 mg-hr/L. Using the trapezoidal rule, the AUC up to 12 hr is 8.21 mg-hr/L. The elimination rate constant, obtained from a semilogarithmic plot of the concentration-time data, is 0.136 hr^{-1}. Given that the last concentration (0.37 mg/L) is the zero-time concentration following an i.v. bolus dose, the area beyond this last observation $(C(0)/k)$ is 2.72 mg-hr/L.

2. 44.34 mg-hr/L. AUC to 24 hr = 44.17 mg-hr/L; extrapolated area beyond 24 hr = $C(24)/k = 0.04 \text{ mg/L}/0.23 \text{ hr}^{-1} = 0.17$ mg-hr/L, where $k = 0.693/t_{1/2}$, and $t1_{1/2} = 3$ hr, estimated from a semilogarithmic plot of the data.

3. Consider a set of n concentration-time values. Let $C(0)$, $C(t_1)$, $C(t_{n-1})$ and $C(t_n)$ be the concentrations at zero time, the first time, the $(n-1)$th time, and the nth time, respectively. Let Δt be the constant interval of time. Using the trapezoidal rule, the AUC is given by

$$\text{Total } AUC = AUC_1 + AUC_2 + \ldots AUC_{n-1} + AUC_n$$

or

$$\text{Total } AUC = \Delta t \left[\frac{C(0) + C(t_1)}{2} \right] + \Delta t \left[\frac{C(t_1) + C(t_2)}{2} \right] \cdots$$
$$+ \Delta t \left[\frac{C(t_{n-2}) + C(t_{n-1})}{2} \right] + \Delta t \left[\frac{C(t_{n-1}) + C(t_n)}{2} \right]$$

which on expansion and collection of terms reduces to

$$\text{Total } AUC = \Delta t \left[\frac{C(0)}{2} + C(t_1) + C(t_2) + \ldots C(t_{n-1}) + \frac{C(t_n)}{2} \right]$$

or

$$\text{Total } AUC = \Delta t \left[\frac{C(0) + C(t_n)}{2} + C(t_1) + C(t_2) + \ldots C(t_{n-1}) \right]$$

4. The completed Table A–5 should list the following values:

Table A–5.

TIME INTERVAL (hr)	AUC WITHIN TIME INTERVAL[a]		
	(CALCULATED AREA) $\frac{(64 - C(t))}{k}$	(TRAPEZOIDAL RULE)	(LOG TRAPEZOIDAL RULE)
0–2	108	109	108
0–4	185	192	185
0–8	277	320	277
0–12	323	432	323

[a]Note that up to an interval equal to the half-life, 4 hr, both numeric methods are reasonably accurate. By 3 half-lives the trapezoidal rule is 134% of the actual value.

ANSWERS TO STUDY PROBLEMS (APPENDIX I-B)

1. a. Half-life $= 6.5$ hr. Note scatter in semilogarithmic plot of rate of excretion against midpoint time of urine collection.
   b. $fe = 0.9$; $fe = Ae_\infty/\text{Dose} = 1797$ mg/2000 mg.
   c. Half-life $= 6.5$ hr. Note that the semilogarithmic plot of amount remaining to be excreted against time of urine collection is much smoother than the excretion rate plot.
2. a. Half-life $= 6$ hr. The value is obtained from the ln (excretion rate) versus time plot. An ARE plot cannot be drawn as Ae_∞ cannot be estimated.
   b. 11 mg. Using a half-life of 6.5 hr (problem 1), the elimination rate constant is 0.107 hr^{-1}. The value of e^{-kt} at 48 hr is then 0.006. As $ARE = Ae_\infty - Ae(t) = Ae_\infty \cdot e^{-kt}$ and Ae_∞ is about 1800 mg, then ARE is about $1800 \times 0.006 = 11$ mg. Note the approximation used in Problem 1, namely, that the amount excreted to 48 hr is Ae_∞, is reasonable. This follows, as 48 hr is approximately 7 half-lives.

ANSWERS TO STUDY PROBLEMS (APPENDIX I-C)

1. a. $ka = 1.4 \text{ hr}^{-1}$, $k = 0.35 \text{ hr}^{-1}$.
   b. Absorption began immediately because there was no lag time.

c. 1. Clearance = 5.9 L/hr.
    Assuming $F = 1$, Clearance = Dose/AUC = 100 mg/(17.05 mg-hr/L)
 2. V = Clearance/k = 17 L.
    If absorption is the rate-limiting step, then V = 5.9/1.4 = 4.2 L. This is an unlikely value.
2. Observations can be explained entirely by a competing reaction. With a competing reaction, the observed absorption rate constant $ka = ka' + kc$, and $F = ka'/ka$, where ka' is the true rate constant defining the absorption process and kc is the rate constant of the competing reaction. For both groups calculation indicates that $ka' = ka \cdot F = 0.35\ hr^{-1}$. Both the lower bioavailability and the apparent faster absorption of the drug in group A are due to more extensive degradation in the acidic gastric contents. Lesson: Be careful in interpreting the value of the absorption rate constant when a competing reaction is likely.
3. a. See Table C–5 below.

Table C–5. Estimation of Cumulative Absorption

TIME (hr)	PLASMA CONCENTRATION (mg/L)	AREA (mg-hr/L)	Aab/V (mg/L)	FRACTION OF BIOAVAILABLE DOSE ABSORBED
0.0	0.00	0.00	0.00	0.0
0.5	0.76	0.19	0.79	0.055
1	1.42	0.73	1.54	0.11
2	2.48	2.68	2.92	0.20
3	3.24	5.54	4.15	0.29
4	3.75	9.03	5.23	0.36
6	4.27	17.05	7.08	0.49
8	4.31	25.63	8.53	0.59
10	4.09	34.03	9.70	0.67
12	3.72	41.84	10.62	0.73
18	2.46	60.38	12.42	0.86
24	1.45	72.11	13.34	0.93
36	0.43	83.39	14.18	0.98
48	0.11	86.63	14.40	1.00

b. Disposition is described by a (linear) one-compartment model, with no change in disposition kinetics between treatments.
c. Approximately 100%.

$$F_{rel} = \frac{\left[\dfrac{AUC}{Dose}\right]_{CR}}{\left[\dfrac{AUC}{Dose}\right]_{soln}} = \frac{\left(\dfrac{86.63}{500}\right)}{\left(\dfrac{86.6}{500}\right)}$$

where CR = controlled release.
d. A semilogarithmic plot of fraction of bioavailable dose remaining to be absorbed *versus* time declines linearly, indicating that absorption, is a first-order process. The half-life of absorption is 6 hr.

$$\text{Fraction of bioavailable dose absorbed at time } t = \frac{\dfrac{Aab}{V}}{\left(\dfrac{k \cdot AUC(\infty)}{V}\right)} = \frac{C + k \cdot \int_0^t Cdt}{k \cdot AUC(\infty)}$$

The value of the denominator is 14.4 mg/L

Further, noting that if absorption is first order, then

$$\frac{Aab}{F \cdot \text{Dose}} = e^{-ka \cdot t}$$

A semilogarithmic plot of fraction of bioavailable dose remaining to be absorbed $[1 - Aab/F \cdot \text{Dose} = 1 - (C + k \cdot \int_0^t C \cdot dt)/(k \cdot AUC(\infty))]$ against time is a straight line with a slope of $-ka$. Such a plot (Fig. C–4) shows the decline is linear, with a half-life of 6 hr.

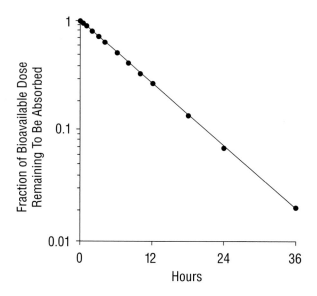

Fig. C–4.

4. a. Absorption kinetics are listed in Table C–6

Table C–6.

TIME (hr)	PLASMA CONCENTRATION (µg/L)	AUC (µg·hr/L)	$k \cdot AUC^a$ (µg/L)	$C + k \cdot AUC$ (µg/L)	FRACTION OF BIOAVAILABLE DRUG ABSORBED[b]	FRACTION OF DRUG ABSORBED[c]
0	0	0	0	0	0	0
0.5	0	0	0	0	0	0
2	0.49	0.37	0.13	0.62	0.05	0.025
4	0.99	1.85	0.67	1.70	0.13	0.065
6	1.83	4.67	1.68	3.5	0.28	0.14
8	1.84	8.34	3.00	4.8	0.38	0.19
10	1.93	12.1	4.36	5.9	0.47	0.24
14	1.52	19.0	6.84	8.4	0.67	0.34
18	1.43	24.9	8.96	10.4	0.83	0.42
24	1.63	31.2	11.2	12.9	1.02	0.51
26	0.65	33.5	12.1	12.7	1.01	0.50
28	0.29	34.5	12.4	12.7	1.01	0.50
30	0.10	34.8	12.5	12.6	1.00	0.50

[a] $k = 0.36$ hr^{-1} (0.693/1.9 hr)
[b] Fraction $= (C + k \cdot AUC)/k \cdot AUC(0-\infty)$; $AUC(0-\infty) = 34.83 + 0.1/0.36 = 35.1$ µg·hr/L, $k \cdot AUC(0-\infty) = 12.6$ µg/L.
[c] Fraction $= F \times (C + k \cdot AUC)/k \cdot AUC(0-\infty)$; where $F = 0.50$ (answer from Chap. 6, Problem 5c).

b. The absorption kinetics approximate, but do not exactly match, the expectation of constant-rate input over a period of 15 hr. A linear plot of the fraction bioavailable with time (not shown) indicates that after a delay of approximately 1 hr absorption does proceed at a nearly constant rate for 17 hr, during which time 83% of the bioavailable drug is absorbed. Between 17 and 24 hr, the remaining 17% is absorbed. As such, the device performs reasonably well. A semilogarithmic plot of the fraction absorbed with time shows an increasingly steeper slope, characteristic of a constant-rate process (Fig. C–5). Had absorption been a first-order process, the semilogarithmic decline would be linear.

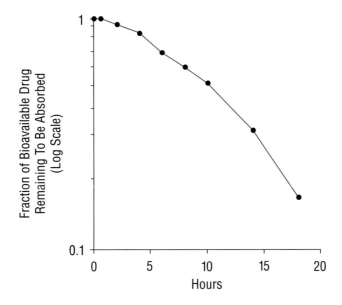

Fig. C–5.

ANSWERS TO STUDY PROBLEMS (APPENDIX I-D)

1.

$$MRT = \frac{\int_0^\infty C \cdot t \cdot dt}{\int_0^\infty C \cdot dt} \quad \text{(Eq. 8)}$$

$$C = C(0) \cdot e^{-kt}$$

$$MRT = \frac{C(0) \cdot \int_0^\infty e^{-kt} \cdot t \cdot dt}{C(0) \cdot \int_0^\infty e^{-kt} \cdot dt} = \frac{\int_0^\infty t \cdot e^{-kt} \cdot dt}{\int_0^\infty e^{-kt} \cdot dt}$$

$$= \frac{\left[\dfrac{-e^{-kt}}{k^2}(kt + 1)\right]_0^\infty}{\left[\dfrac{-e^{-kt}}{k}\right]_0^\infty} = \frac{1}{k}$$

2.

$$MRT = \frac{\int_0^{t_{inf}} (Dose - R_0 \cdot t)dt}{Dose}$$

Since $R_0 = Dose/t_{inf}$, then

$$MRT = \frac{Dose \int_0^{t_{inf}} \left(1 - \frac{t}{t_{inf}}\right) dt}{Dose}$$

$$= \left[t - \frac{t^2}{2t_{inf}}\right]_0^{t_{inf}} = \frac{2t_{inf}^2 - t_{inf}^2}{2 \cdot t_{inf}} = \frac{t_{inf}}{2}$$

3. a. 4 hr.

$$\text{Mean infusion time} = 2 \text{ hr} = (10 - 8) = \frac{t_{inf}}{2}$$

Therefore, $t_{inf} = 4$ hr.

  b. 2.77 hr.

Mean absorption time = 4 hr (12 − 8).

If absorption is first-order and obeys single compartment kinetics, mean absorption time = $1/ka$. Therefore, $ka = 0.25 \text{ hr}^{-1}$, and absorption half-life $(0.693/ka) = 2.77$ hr.

4.

$$C = I(e^{-kt} - e^{-ka \cdot t})$$

$$\text{where } I = \frac{F \cdot D \cdot ka}{V \cdot (ka - k)}$$

$$\text{Observed } MRT = \frac{\int_0^{\infty} C \cdot t \cdot dt}{\int_0^{\infty} C \cdot dt} = \frac{I}{I}\left[\frac{\int_0^{\infty} (e^{-kt} - e^{-ka \cdot t}) \cdot t \cdot dt}{\int_0^{\infty} (e^{-kt} - e^{-ka \cdot t}) \cdot dt}\right]$$

$$\text{Observed } MRT = \frac{\left[\frac{1}{k^2} - \frac{1}{ka^2}\right]}{\left[\frac{1}{k} - \frac{1}{ka}\right]} = \frac{\left[\frac{1}{k} + \frac{1}{ka}\right]\left[\frac{1}{k} - \frac{1}{ka}\right]}{\left[\frac{1}{k} - \frac{1}{ka}\right]} = \frac{1}{k} + \frac{1}{ka}$$

Neither Dose nor F is in the relationship.

5. a. $AUMC/AUC = 14.7$ hr; $MRT = 2.7$ hr. Table D–3 lists the calculated values of AUC and $AUMC$ following both the 24-hr constant-rate i.v. infusion and the administration of the rectal drug delivery device. The values were calculated using the trapezoidal rule (Appendix I–A). From this table, for the i.v. infusion $AUMC = 1041$ µg-hr²/L; $AUC = 70.6$ µg-hr/L.

$$MRT = \frac{AUMC}{AUC} - \frac{t_{inf}}{2} = 14.7 \text{ hr} - 24 \text{ hr}/2 = 2.7 \text{ hr.}$$

Table D–3.　Calculation of *AUC* and *AUMC* of Droperidol

TIME (hr)	24-hr i.v. INFUSION				RECTAL DELIVERY DEVICE			
	C ($\mu g \cdot L$)	AUC ($\mu g \cdot hr/L$)	$C \cdot t$ ($\mu g \cdot hr/L$)	$AUMC$ ($\mu g \cdot hr^2/L$)	C ($\mu g \cdot L$)	AUC ($\mu g \cdot hr/L$)	$C \cdot t$ ($\mu g \cdot hr/L$)	$AUMC$ ($\mu g \cdot hr^2/L$)
0	0	0	0	0	0	0	0	0
0.5	0.9	0.23	0.25	0.06	0	0	0	0
2	1.8	2.3	3.6	3.0	0.49	0.37	0.98	0.25
4	2.6	6.7	9.6	16.2	0.99	1.95	4.0	5.2
6	2.5	11.8	15.0	40.8	1.83	4.7	11.0	20.1
8	2.5	16.8	20.0	75.8	1.84	8.3	14.7	45.8
10	2.7	22.0	27.0	123	1.93	12.1	19.3	79.9
14	2.7	32.8	37.8	252	1.52	19.0	21.3	161
18	2.9	44.0	52.2	432	1.43	24.9	25.3	254
24	3.1	62.0	74.4	812	1.63	31.2	39.1	448
26	1.4	66.5	36.4	923	0.65	33.5	16.9	504
28	0.67	67.5	18.8	978	0.29	34.5	8.1	529
30	0.36	69.6	10.8	1008	0.1	34.8	3.0	540
∞	0	70.6[a]	0	1041[b]	0	35.1[c]	0	549[d]

[a]Extrapolated *AUC* beyond 30 hr = $C(30)/k$ = 0.36 $\mu g/L$/0.36 hr^{-1} = 1 $\mu g \cdot hr/L$

[b]Extrapolated *AUMC* beyond 30 hr = $\dfrac{C(30)}{k} \times \left[30 + \dfrac{1}{k}\right] = \dfrac{0.36 \ \mu g/L}{0.36 \ hr^{-1}}$ [30 hr + 2.8 hr] = 32.8 $\mu g \cdot hr^2/L$

[c]Extrapolated *AUC* beyond 30 hr = 0.1 $\mu g/L$/0.36 hr^{-1} = 0.28 $\mu g \cdot hr/L$.

[d]Extrapolated *AUMC* beyond 30 hr = $\dfrac{C(30)}{k}\left[30 + \dfrac{1}{k}\right] = \dfrac{0.1 \ \mu g/L}{0.36 \ hr^{-1}}$ [30 + 2.8] = 9.1 $\mu g \cdot hr^2/L$

b. Yes, reasonably well. Based on *MRT*, expected $t_{1/2}$ = 0.693 × *MRT* = 0.693 × 2.7 hr = 1.87 hr. That estimated from the decline of plasma concentration with time after stopping the infusion is 1.9 hr. The close agreement between the two values of $t_{1/2}$ suggests that the disposition kinetics of droperidol can be approximated by a one-compartment model. Had the disposition kinetics of the drug showed a marked polyexponential character, then the terminal half-life on stopping the infusion would be distinctly greater than 0.693 × *MRT*, which characterizes the body as a single compartment.

c. $(AUMC/AUC)_{\text{rectal device}}$ = 15.6 hr; mean input time = 12.9 hr. From Table D–3,

$$\frac{AUMC}{AUC} = \frac{549 \ \mu g \cdot hr^2/L}{35.1 \ \mu g \cdot hr/L}$$

$$\text{Mean input time} = \frac{AUMC}{AUC} - MRT = 15.6 \text{ hr} - 2.7 \text{ hr}$$

d. Mean absorption time = 3.9 hr. For a sequential process:

$$\text{Mean input time} = \text{mean release time} + \text{mean absorption time}$$

Hence

$$\text{Mean absorption time} = \text{mean input time} - \text{mean release time} = 12.9 \text{ hr} - 9 \text{ hr}$$

Note: In this calculation the *in vitro* input time is assumed to apply *in vivo*. In practice, it may not be so.

ANSWERS TO STUDY PROBLEMS (APPENDIX I-E)

1. $\dfrac{1}{1-r} - 1 = \dfrac{1-(1-r)}{(1-r)} = \dfrac{r}{1-r}$

2. From the answer to 1, and realizing that $F \cdot \text{Dose} \cdot ka/(ka - k)$ is common to both expressions,

$$\frac{1}{(1-r)} = 1 + \frac{r}{(1-r)}$$

Similarly,

$$\frac{1}{(1-s)} = 1 + \frac{s}{(1-s)}$$

Therefore,

$$\frac{1}{(1-r)} - \frac{1}{(1-s)} = \frac{r}{(1-r)} - \frac{s}{(1-s)}$$

ANSWERS TO STUDY PROBLEMS (APPENDIX I-F)

1. a. Table F–6 is Table F–4 completed.

Table F–6.

PERCENT OF DRUG IN BODY THAT IS . . .	NAFCILLIN	NAPROXEN	NITRAZEPAM
In plasma	12	27	2
Unbound	19	1	4
In extracellular fluid	34	67	6
Outside extracellular fluids	66	33	94
Bound to protein	11	27	2
Bound outside the extracellular fluids (in or on tissue cells, including blood cells)	54	32	91

^{a}For a 70-kg person.

b. Nitrazepam. See calculations in Table F–7.

Table F–7.

	$\dfrac{V_R{}^b}{fu_R}$	V (L)^a		
		BEFORE	AFTER^c	PERCENT INCREASE
Nafcillin	147	24.5	41.5	69
Naproxen	1226	11.2	14.9	33
Nitrazepam	958	133	259	94

^{a}70-kg person.
^{b}Estimated from

$V = 7.5 + 7.5 \cdot fu + \dfrac{V_R}{fu_R} \cdot fu.$

^{c}Value after fu is doubled.

2. Unbound volume of distribution (V/fu) is decreased from 2.5 to 1.5 L/kg, whereas unbound clearance shows essentially no change, 300 to 260 mL/h/kg. Tolbutamide is unquestionably of low extraction, since CL/Q_H is less than 0.02. The lack of change in unbound clearance indicates no effect of acute viral hepatitis on metabolic activity. The decrease in unbound volume is consistent with the change in fraction unbound for a drug with a small volume of distribution. The half-life shortens because the decrease in binding to plasma proteins decreases the unbound volume.

ANSWERS TO STUDY PROBLEM (APPENDIX I-G)

a. 40

$$\rho = \frac{H - 1 + (C_b/C)}{fu \cdot H} = \frac{0.45 - 1 + 2.35}{0.1 \times 0.45}$$

b. 1.81

$$C_b/C = 1 + H(fu \cdot \rho - 1) = 1 + 0.27 \ (0.1 \times 40 - 1)$$

The percent change in C_b/C is minor compared to that of the hematocrit. Note that had $fu \cdot \rho$ been equal to 1 (drug concentration in blood cells the same as that in plasma), there would have been no change in C_b/C when the hematocrit was altered. Furthermore, if $fu \cdot \rho$ is less than 1, then C_b/C increases with a decrease in H. Finally if $fu \cdot \rho$ is greater than 1, then C_b/C decreases with a decrease in H.

c. 6.31

$$C_b/C = 1 + H(fu \cdot \rho - 1) = 1 + 0.45 \ (0.32 \times 40 - 1)$$

The increased value of fu, resulting from the lowered plasma albumin concentration, greatly increases the ratio of C_b to C. Had ρ been a small value, the drug would have been largely confined to plasma and changes in fu would have had a minor effect on the ratio of C_b to C.

ANSWERS TO STUDY PROBLEMS (APPENDIX I-H)

1. a. $R_t = 1088$ mg/day, $V = 36$ L

$$R_t \ (\text{mg/day}) = \frac{(140 - \text{Age}) \times \text{weight (kg)}}{5.9}$$
$$= \frac{(140 - 33) \times 60}{5.9} = 1088 \text{ mg/day or } 45.3 \text{ mg/hr}$$

$$V \ (\text{L}) = 0.6 \times \text{Body Weight (kg)} = 0.6 \times 60 = 36 \text{ L}$$

b. $CL_{CR} = 16$ mL/min (0.98 L/hr)

$$CL_{CR}(d) = \frac{2R_t}{[C(t_1) + C(t_2)]} + \frac{2 \cdot V \cdot [C(t_1) - C(t_2)]}{\Delta t \cdot [C(t_1) + C(t_2)]}$$
$$C(t_1) = 26 \text{ mg/L}, \ C(t_2) = 42 \text{ mg/L}, \ \Delta t = 48 \text{ hr}$$

Therefore,

$$CL_{CR} \text{ (L/hr)} = \frac{2 \times 45.3 \text{ mg/hr}}{68 \text{ mg/L}} + \frac{2 \times 36\text{L} \times (-16 \text{ mg/L})}{48 \text{ hr} \times 68 \text{ mg/L}}$$
$$= 0.98 \text{ L/hr or } 16 \text{ mL/min}$$

c. The estimate is likely to be reasonable.

$$\text{Expected } C_{ss} = R_t/CL_{CR} = \frac{45.3 \text{ mg/hr}}{0.98 \text{ L/hr}} = 46 \text{ mg/L, or } 4.6 \text{ mg/dL}$$

$$\text{Expected } t_{1/2} = 0.693 \, V/CL_{CR} = \frac{0.693 \times 36\text{L}}{0.98 \text{ L/hr}} = 25 \text{ hr}$$

Hence, with a time interval (48 hr) of approximately 2 half-lives, one should be close to steady state. Furthermore, the second measurement of 4.2 mg/dL is close to the expected steady-state value.

2. a. $CL_{CR} = 0.45$ L/hr. During dialysis, the total clearance of creatinine $(CL_D + CL(d))$ is greater than that between dialyses $(CL(d))$. Accordingly, the serum creatinine concentration falls. Between treatment, the serum concentration rises back toward the predialysis concentration. This situation corresponds to an acute change in creatinine clearance, and hence Eq. 7 applies.

$$V \text{ (L)} = 0.6 \times \text{Body Weight (kg)} = 0.6 \times 67 = 40.2 \text{ L}$$

$$R_t \text{ (mg/day)} = \frac{(140 - \text{Age}) \times \text{Weight (kg)}}{5} = \frac{(140 - 55) \times 67}{5}$$
$$= 1139 \text{ mg/day or } 47 \text{ mg/hr}$$

$$CL_{CR} \text{ (L/hr)} = \frac{2 \times R_t}{(C(t_1) + (C(t_2))} + \frac{2 \times V \times [(C(t_1) - C(t_2)]}{\Delta t \times [C(t_1) + C(t_2)]}$$

Then, substituting $C(t_1) = 58$ mg/L, $C(t_2) = 86$ mg/L, $\Delta t = 72$ hr.

$$CL_{CR} \text{ (L/hr)} = \frac{2 \times 48 \text{ mg/hr}}{144 \text{ mg/L}} + \frac{2 \times 40.2 \text{ L} \times (-28 \text{ mg/L})}{72 \times 144 \text{ mg/L}}$$
$$= 0.45 \text{ L/hr or } 7.5 \text{ mL/min}$$

b. Yes. Concentration at end of dialysis period: Expected, 59 mg/L; observed, 58 mg/L. Before dialysis the serum creatinine concentration is anticipated to be a steady-state value,

$$C_{ss} = \frac{R_t}{CL_{CR}} = \frac{48 \text{ mg/hr}}{0.45 \text{ L/hr}} = 107 \text{ mg/L}$$

During dialysis:

$$CL = CL_{CR} + CL_D$$
$$= 0.44 \text{ L/hr} + 7.5 \text{ L/hr} = 7.94 \text{ L/hr}.$$

Hence, expected concentration at the end of a 3-hr dialysis period is

$$C = C_{ss}e^{-(CL/V)\times 3}$$
$$= 107 \text{ mg/L} \times e^{-(7.95 \text{ L/hr}/40.2 \text{ L})\times 3hr}$$
$$= 59 \text{ mg/L}$$

INDEX

Page numbers in *italics* indicate figures; numbers followed by t indicate tables.

absorption rate and, 94
determinants of, 86–87
Food
diurnal effects, 412
gastric emptying, 121, 130–132
variability in response, 209
Forced diuresis, 178
Formulation
absorption from solids, 128
drug metabolites, 370–371
variability in response, 208–209
Fraction excreted unchanged, 27
Fraction of dose remaining, 23
Fraction unbound, 146t
in plasma, 145–147
Fractional rate of removal, 23
Fractional turnover rate, 424–425
Furosemide
hysteresis, 362
infusion vs. single dose, 352–354, *353*
and phenobarbital interaction, 268
renal clearance, 172

Galanthamine, elimination kinetics, 26–28, *27*
Gallbladder, 168
drug disposition, 15
Gastric emptying, absorption from solids, 121, 130–132, 412
Gastrointestinal tract
absorption, 120–126, *121*
bioavailability, 123–126
gastric emptying, 121, 130–132, 412
intestinal, 121–123
of solids, 130–132
drug metabolism, 14–15, 157
Gender, and dosage, 240
Generic drugs, 46
Genetics, 220–229
drug interactions, 268
pharmacodynamics, 227–228, *228*
pharmacokinetic variations, 217
acetylation, 223–226, *225*
clinical implications, 226–227, 227t
oxidation, 222–223, *223*
phenotyping, 228
polymorphism, 220, 227, 227t
reading suggestions, 464
Genotype, 220
Gentamicin
absorption, 126
concentration monitoring, 302, 306
distribution kinetics, 327, 330–334
dosing interval and efficacy, 64
in hemodialysis patients, 450–451
modality of administration, 64, 65
therapeutic window, 59
Glomerular filtration, 170–172, *170*, *171*
Glucose
diffusion, 112–113
nonlinear renal clearance, 421
Glucuronidation, 168, 251, 385–386

Glycoproteins, protein and tissue binding, 398–403
Graded responses, 55, 343
drug interactions, 278–279, *278*
Granulocyte-macrophage colony-stimulating factor, 127, *127*
Griseofulvin
absorption, 49
dissolution, 132
solubility, cause of nonlinear bioavailability, 396
Growth hormone, 48
Guanethidine
chlorpromazine interaction, 269t

Halazepam metabolites, 380, 386
Half-life
absorption, 34
elimination, 19–20, 24, 26–27, 44
clearance and distribution, 178–181
urine data, 474–478
in multiple-dose regimens, 89–94, 101
See also Elimination.
Hematocrit
determinant of blood/plasma ratio, 509–511
Hemodialysis
concentration-dependent kinetics, 456
drug redistribution, 456
phenytoin, 458
postdialysis drug replacement, 449–452, 451t, *451*
Hemofiltration, 454–455
Hemoperfusion, 457
Henderson-Hasselbalch equation, 114
Heparin
nonlinear disposition, 422
Hepatic clearance, 161–169
biliary excretion and enterohepatic cycling, 168–169, *169*
binding in blood and, 163–165
enzyme activity, 165, *166*
first-pass, 167–168
individual variations, 215–217
memory aid, 165–167
Michaelis-Menten kinetics, 165–166, *166*, 406–411
perfusion, 162–163, *162*, 163t
perfusion rate-limited, 162–163
physiologic variables influencing, 161–168
protein binding, 163–165, *164*
well-stirred model, 165
Heterozygous, definition, 220
Homozygous, definition, 220
Human volunteers, response and concentration studies, 54–56
Hydrochlorothiazide bioavailability, 124
Hydrolysis, 157
Hypersensitivity, therapeutic window, 57
Hypertension, malignant, 252
Hysteresis, 358–361
curve interpretation, 362–363, *362*